MOSBY'S GUIDE TO
NURSING
DIAGNOSIS

MOSBY'S GUIDE TO
NURSING
DIAGNOSIS

Fifth Edition

Gail B. Ladwig, MSN, RN

Betty J. Ackley, MSN, EdS, RN

Mary Beth Flynn Makic, PhD, RN, CNS, CCNS, FAAN

ELSEVIER

ELSEVIER

3251 Riverport Lane
St. Louis, Missouri 63043

MOSBY'S GUIDE TO NURSING DIAGNOSIS, FIFTH EDITION   ISBN: 978-0-323-39020-0

NANDA International, Inc. Nursing Diagnoses: Definitions & Classifications 2015-2017, Tenth Edition. Edited by T. Heather Herdman and Shigemi Kamitsuru. 2014 NANDA International, Inc. Published 2014 by John Wiley & Sons, Ltd. Companion website: www.wiley.com/go/nursingdiagnoses. In order to make safe and effective judgments using NANDA-I diagnoses it is essential that nurses refer to the definitions and defining characteristics of the diagnoses listed in this work.

Notices

Knowledge and best practice in this field are constantly changing. As new research and experience broaden our understanding, changes in research methods, professional practices, or medical treatment may become necessary.

Practitioners and researchers must always rely on their own experience and knowledge in evaluating and using any information, methods, compounds, or experiments described herein. In using such information or methods they should be mindful of their own safety and the safety of others, including parties for whom they have a professional responsibility.

With respect to any drug or pharmaceutical products identified, readers are advised to check the most current information provided (i) on procedures featured or (ii) by the manufacturer of each product to be administered to verify the recommended dose or formula, the method and duration of administration, and contraindications. It is the responsibility of practitioners, relying on their own experience and knowledge of their patients, to make diagnoses, to determine dosages and the best treatment for each individual patient, and to take all appropriate safety precautions.

To the fullest extent of the law, neither the Publisher nor the authors, contributors, or editors assume any liability for any injury and/or damage to persons or property as a matter of products liability, negligence, or otherwise, or from any use or operation of any methods, products, instructions, or ideas contained in the material herein.

Library of Congress Cataloging-in-Publication Data
Names: Ladwig, Gail B., author. | Ackley, Betty J., author. | Makic, Mary Beth Flynn, author.
Title: Mosby's guide to nursing diagnosis / Gail B. Ladwig, Betty J. Ackley, Mary Beth Flynn Makic.
Other titles: Guide to nursing diagnosis
Description: Fifth edition. | St. Louis, Missouri : Elsevier, [2017] | Abridgment of: Nursing diagnosis handbook / [edited by] Betty J. Ackley, Gail B. Ladwig, Mary Beth Flynn Makic. Eleventh edition. St. Louis, Missouri : Elsevier, [2017]. | Includes bibliographical references and index.
Identifiers: LCCN 2016000374 | ISBN 9780323390200 (pbk.)
Subjects: | MESH: Nursing Diagnosis–methods | Patient Care Planning | Handbooks
Classification: LCC RT48.6 | NLM WY 49 | DDC 616.07/5–dc23 LC record available at http://lccn.loc.gov/2016000374

Senior Content Strategist: Sandra Clark
Associate Content Development Specialist: Jennifer Wade
Publishing Services Manager: Jeff Patterson
Book Production Specialist: Carol O'Connell
Design Direction: Ashley Miner

Printed in Canada

Last digit is the print number: 9 8 7 6 5 4 3

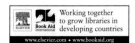

Working together to grow libraries in developing countries

www.elsevier.com • www.bookaid.org

In Memory of Betty J. Ackley

Dreams
Dreams come
Dreams go
Whispers, shouts, images
Dreams come
Dreams go
Follow, follow*

Betty believed in dreams. This textbook was our dream. We set out to write the best nursing diagnosis textbook ever. Our book is now in 1400 nursing programs. It has been high on Amazon's best seller list. I think her dream is realized. From a handout to students to an international publication. Thank you, dear friend Betty.

Betty passed away in December 2014, at her home,
with her husband (Dale) and daughter (Dawn) present.

Betty fought a gallant battle with pancreatic cancer for the last nine months.
She loved life, her family, and the profession of nursing.
She was an active member of NANDA-I for more than two decades.

The following is a quote from Dale Ackley, Betty's husband:

Betty saw a need and was able to help fill that need by working to complete this book and see it through to publication. She was very proud of each edition of the book. She always strived to make each edition as good as it could be. Betty was a loving daughter, grandmother, mother, and wife. She cared about people and was always helping everyone to be their very best. This book will continue to be her way of giving to the profession she loved. Nursing gave a lot to Betty, and she returned the love of nursing by writing the most helpful book she could write.

Dale Ackley

Also Dedicated to

Jerry Ladwig, my wonderful husband, who, after 51 years, is still supportive and helpful—he has been "my right-hand man" in every revision of this book. Also to my very special children, their spouses, and all of my grandchildren: Jerry, Kathy, Alexandra, Elizabeth, and Benjamin Ladwig; Christine, John, Sean, Ciara, and Bridget McMahon; Jennifer, Jim, Abby, Katelyn, Blake, and Connor Martin; Amy, Scott, Ford, and Vaughn Bertram—the greatest family anyone could ever hope for.

Gail B. Ladwig

My husband, Zlatko, and children, Alexander and Erik, whose unconditional love and support are ever present in my life. To my parents and sisters for always encouraging me to follow my passion. To Gail, for her incredible mentorship, guidance, and encouragement this past year. And finally to Betty, for believing in me and providing me with an opportunity to more fully contribute to this amazing textbook in support of nurses and the patients and families we serve.

Mary Beth Flynn Makic

---

*Gail Ladwig, 2015

ACKNOWLEDGMENTS

The authors would like to thank the following individuals for their contributions to *Nursing Diagnosis Handbook: An Evidence-Based Guide to Planning Care,* Eleventh Edition, by Betty J. Ackley, Gail B. Ladwig, and Mary Beth Flynn Makic, from which this book has been developed:

Betty J. Ackley, MSN, EdS, RN

Michelle Acorn, DNP, NP PHC/adult, BA, BScN/PHCNP, MN/ACNP, ENC(C), GNC(C), CAP, CGP

Keith A. Anderson, MSW, PhD

Amanda Andrews, MA, Ed, BSc, DN, RN, HEA Fellow

Jessica Bibbo, MA

Kathaleen C. Bloom, PhD, CNM

Lina Daou Boudiab, MSN, RN

Lisa Burkhart, PhD, RN, ANEF

Melodie Cannon, DNP, MSc/FNP, BHScN, RN(EC), NP-PHC, CEN, GNC(C)

Stacey M. Carroll, PhD, ANP-BC

Stephanie C. Christensen, PhD, CCC-SLP

June M. Como, EdD, RN, CNS

Maureen F. Cooney, DNP, FNP-BC

Ruth M. Curchoe, RN, BSN, MSN, CIC

Mary Alice DeWys, RN, BS, CIMI

Susan M. Dirkes, RN, MS, CCRN

Roberta Dobrzanski, MSN, RN

Julianne E. Doubet, BSN, RN, CEN, NREMT-P

Lorraine Duggan, MSN, ACNP-BC

Shelly Eisbach, PhD, RN, PMHNP-BC

Dawn Fairlie, ANP, FNP, GNP, DNS(c)

Arlene T. Farren, RN, PhD, AOCN, CTN-A

Debora Yvonne Fields, RN, BSN, MA, LICDC, CCMC

Noelle L. Fields, PhD, LCSW

Vanessa Flannery, MSN, PHCNS-BC, CNE

Shari D. Froelich, DNP, MSN, MSBA, ANP, BC, ACHPN, PMHNP, BC

Tracy P. George, DNP, APRN-BC, CNE

Susanne W. Gibbons, PhD, C-ANP/GNP

Barbara A. Given, PhD, RN, FAAN

Mila W. Grady, MSN, RN

Pauline McKinney Green, PhD, RN, CNE

Sherry A. Greenberg, PhD, RN, GNP-BC

Dianne Frances Hayward, RN, MSN, WHNP

Paula D. Hopper, MSN, RN, CNE

Wendie A. Howland, MN, RN-BC, CRRN, CCM, CNLCP, LNCC

Rebecca Johnson, PhD, RN, FAAN, FNAP

Nicole Jones, MSN, FNP-BC

Jane M. Kendall, RN, BS, CHT

Katharine Kolcaba, PhD, RN

Gail B. Ladwig, MSN, RN

Mary Beth Flynn Makic, PhD, RN, CNS, CCNS, FAAN

Mary P. Mancuso, MA, Counseling Psychology

Victoria K. Marshall, RN, BSN

Marina Martinez-Kratz, MS, RN, CNE

Ruth McCaffrey, DNP, ARNP, FNP-BC, GNP-BC, FAAN

Graham J. McDougall, Jr., PhD, RN, FAAN, FGSA

Laura Mcilvoy, PhD, RN, CCRN, CNRN

Marsha McKenzie, MA Ed, BSN, RN

Annie Muller, DNP, APN-BC

Katherina Nikzad-Terhune, PhD, LCSW

Barbara J. Olinzock, MSN, EdD, RN

Wolter Paans, MSc, PhD, RN

Margaret Elizabeth Padnos, RN, AB, BSN, MA

Chris Pasero, MS, RN-BC, FAAN

Kathleen L. Patusky, MA, PhD, RN, CNS

Sherry H. Pomeroy, PhD, RN

Ann Will Poteet, MS, RN, CNS

Lori M. Rhudy, PhD, RN, CNRN, ACNS-BC

Mary Jane Roth, RN, BSN, MA

Paula Riess Sherwood, RN, PhD, CNRN, FAAN

Debra Siela, PhD, RN, CCNS, ACNS-BC, CCRN-K, CNE, RRT

Kimberly Silvey, MSN, RN

A.B. St. Aubyn, BSc (Hons), RGN, RM, RHV, DPS:N (CHS), MSc, PGCert (Education), HEA Fellow

Andrea G. Steiner, MS, RD, LD, CNSC

Elaine E. Steinke, PhD, APRN, CNS-BC, FAHA, FAAN

Laura May Struble, PhD, GNP-BC

Denise Sullivan, MSN, ANP-BC

Dennis C. Tanner, PhD

Janelle M. Tipton, MSN, RN, AOCN

William J. Trees, DNP, FNP-BC, CNP, RN

Barbara Baele Vincensi, PhD, RN, FNP

Kerstin West-Wilson, RNC, IBCLC, BA Biology, BSN, MS Nutrition, Safe Kids NRP Car Seat Certified, BLS Instructor

Barbara J. Wheeler, RN, BN, MN, IBCLC

Suzanne White, MSN, RN, PHCNS-BC

Linda S. Williams, RN, MSN

David Wilson, MS, RNC

Ruth A. Wittmann-Price, PhD, RN, CNS, CNE, CHSE, ANEF, FAAN

Melody Zanotti, RN, LSW

Karen Zulkowski, DNS, RN

HOW TO USE *MOSBY'S GUIDE TO NURSING DIAGNOSIS*

ASSESS

Assess the client using the format provided by the clinical setting. Collect data including client's symptoms, clinical state, and known medical or psychiatric diagnoses.

DIAGNOSIS

Use Section I, Guide to Nursing Diagnoses, and locate the client's symptoms, clinical state, medical or psychiatric diagnoses, and anticipated or prescribed diagnostic studies or surgical interventions (listed in alphabetical order). Note suggestions for appropriate nursing diagnoses.

Then use Section II, Guide to Planning Care, to evaluate each suggested nursing diagnosis and "related to" etiology statement. Section II is a listing of care plans according to NANDA-I, arranged alphabetically by diagnostic concept, for each nursing diagnosis referred to in Section I. Determine the appropriateness of each nursing diagnosis by comparing the Defining Characteristics and/or Risk Factors to the client data collected.

DETERMINE OUTCOMES

Use Section II, Guide to Planning Care, to find appropriate outcomes for the client.

PLAN INTERVENTIONS

Use Section II, Guide to Planning Care, to find appropriate interventions for the client.

GIVE NURSING CARE

Administer nursing care following the plan of care based on the interventions.

EVALUATE NURSING CARE

Evaluate nursing care administered using the Client Outcomes. If the outcomes were not met, and the nursing interventions were not effective, reassess the client and determine if the appropriate nursing diagnoses were made.

DOCUMENT

Document all of the previous steps using the format provided in the clinical setting.

CONTENTS

SECTION I Guide to Nursing Diagnoses, 1

An alphabetized list of medical, surgical, and psychiatric diagnoses; diagnostic procedures, clinical states, symptoms, and problems, with suggested nursing diagnoses.

SECTION II Guide to Planning Care, 163

The definition, defining characteristics, risk factors, related factors, client outcomes, interventions, geriatric interventions, pediatric interventions, critical care interventions, home care interventions, culturally competent nursing interventions (when appropriate), and client/family teaching and discharge planning for each alphabetized nursing diagnosis.

MOSBY'S GUIDE TO
NURSING
DIAGNOSIS

Guide to Nursing Diagnosis

Section I is an alphabetical listing of client symptoms, client problems, medical diagnoses, psychosocial diagnoses, and clinical states. Each of these will have a list of possible nursing diagnoses. You may use this section to find suggestions for nursing diagnoses for your client.

- Assess the client using the format provided by the clinical setting.
- Locate the client's symptoms, problems, clinical state, diagnoses, surgeries, and diagnostic testing in the alphabetical listing contained in this section.
- Note suggestions given for appropriate nursing diagnoses.
- Evaluate the suggested nursing diagnoses to determine whether they are appropriate for the client and have information that was found in the assessment.
- Use Section II (which contains an alphabetized list of all NANDA-I approved nursing diagnoses) to validate this information and check the definition, related factors, and defining characteristics. Determine whether the nursing diagnosis you have selected is appropriate for the client.

A

ABDOMINAL DISTENTION

Constipation r/t decreased activity, decreased fluid intake, decreased fiber intake, pathological process

Dysfunctional **Gastrointestinal** motility r/t decreased perfusion of intestines, medication effect

Nausea r/t irritation of gastrointestinal tract

Imbalanced **Nutrition:** less than body requirements r/t nausea, vomiting

Acute **Pain** r/t retention of air, gastrointestinal secretions

Delayed **Surgical** recovery r/t retention of gas, secretions

ABDOMINAL HYSTERECTOMY

See Hysterectomy

ABDOMINAL PAIN

Dysfunctional **Gastrointestinal** motility r/t decreased perfusion, medication effect

Acute **Pain** r/t injury, pathological process

ABDOMINAL SURGERY

Constipation r/t decreased activity, decreased fluid intake, anesthesia, opioids

Dysfunctional **Gastrointestinal** motility r/t medication or anesthesia effect, trauma from surgery

Imbalanced **Nutrition:** less than body requirements r/t high metabolic needs, decreased ability to ingest or digest food

Acute **Pain** r/t surgical procedure

Ineffective peripheral **Tissue Perfusion** r/t immobility, abdominal surgery

Risk for delayed **Surgical** recovery r/t extensive surgical procedure

Risk for **Infection:** Risk factor: invasive procedure

Readiness for enhanced **Knowledge:** expresses an interest in learning

See Surgery, Perioperative Care; Surgery, Postoperative Care; Surgery, Preoperative Care

ABDOMINAL TRAUMA

Disturbed **Body Image** r/t scarring, change in body function, need for temporary colostomy

Ineffective **Breathing** pattern r/t abdominal distention, pain

Deficient **Fluid** volume r/t hemorrhage, active fluid volume loss

Dysfunctional **Gastrointestinal** motility r/t decreased perfusion

Acute **Pain** r/t abdominal trauma

Risk for **Bleeding:** Risk factors: trauma and possible contusion/rupture of abdominal organs

Risk for **Infection:** Risk factor: possible perforation of abdominal structures

ABLATION, RADIOFREQUENCY CATHETER

Fear r/t invasive procedure

Risk for decreased **Cardiac** tissue perfusion: Risk factor: catheterization of heart

ABORTION, INDUCED

Compromised family **Coping** r/t unresolved feelings about decision

Acute **Pain** r/t surgical intervention

Chronic low **Self-Esteem** r/t feelings of guilt

Chronic **Sorrow** r/t loss of potential child

Risk for **Bleeding:** Risk factor: trauma from abortion

Risk for delayed **Development:** Risk factor: unplanned or unwanted pregnancy

Risk for **Infection:** Risk factors: open uterine blood vessels, dilated cervix

Risk for **Post-Trauma** syndrome: Risk factor: psychological trauma of abortion

Risk for **Spiritual** distress: Risk factor: perceived moral implications of decision

Readiness for enhanced **Knowledge:** expresses an interest in learning

ABORTION, SPONTANEOUS

Disturbed **Body Image** r/t perceived inability to carry pregnancy, produce child

Disabled family **Coping** r/t unresolved feelings about loss

Ineffective **Coping** r/t personal vulnerability

Interrupted **Family** processes r/t unmet expectations for pregnancy and childbirth

Fear r/t implications for future pregnancies

Grieving r/t loss of fetus

Acute **Pain** r/t uterine contractions, surgical intervention

Situational low **Self-Esteem** r/t feelings about loss of fetus

Chronic **Sorrow** r/t loss of potential child

Risk for **Bleeding**: Risk factor: trauma from abortion

Risk for **Infection**: Risk factors: septic or incomplete abortion of products of conception, open uterine blood vessels, dilated cervix

Risk for **Post-Trauma** syndrome: Risk factor: psychological trauma of abortion

Risk for **Spiritual** distress: Risk factor: loss of fetus

Readiness for enhanced **Knowledge**: expresses an interest in learning

ABRUPTIO PLACENTAE <36 WEEKS

Anxiety r/t unknown outcome, change in birth plans

Death **Anxiety** r/t unknown outcome, hemorrhage, or pain

Interrupted **Family** processes r/t unmet expectations for pregnancy and childbirth

Fear r/t threat to well-being of self and fetus

Impaired **Gas** exchange: placental r/t decreased uteroplacental area

Acute **Pain** r/t irritable uterus, hypertonic uterus

Impaired **Tissue** integrity: maternal r/t possible uterine rupture

Risk for **Bleeding**: Risk factor: separation of placenta from uterus causing bleeding

Risk for disproportionate **Growth**: Risk factor: uteroplacental insufficiency

Risk for **Infection**: Risk factor: partial separation of placenta

Risk for disturbed **Maternal–Fetal** dyad: Risk factors: trauma of process, lack of energy of mother

Risk for **Shock**: Risk factor: separation of placenta from uterus

Readiness for enhanced **Knowledge**: expresses an interest in learning

ABSCESS FORMATION

Ineffective **Protection** r/t inadequate nutrition, abnormal blood profile, drug therapy, depressed immune function

Impaired **Tissue** integrity r/t altered circulation, nutritional deficit or excess

Readiness for enhanced **Knowledge**: expresses an interest in learning

ABUSE, CHILD

See Child Abuse

ABUSE, SPOUSE, PARENT, OR SIGNIFICANT OTHER

Anxiety r/t threat to self-concept, situational crisis of abuse

Caregiver Role Strain r/t chronic illness, self-care deficits, lack of respite care, extent of caregiving required

Impaired verbal **Communication** r/t psychological barriers of fear

Compromised family **Coping** r/t abusive patterns

Defensive **Coping** r/t low self-esteem

Dysfunctional **Family** processes r/t inadequate coping skills

Insomnia r/t psychological stress

Post-Trauma syndrome r/t history of abuse

Powerlessness r/t lifestyle of helplessness

Chronic low **Self-Esteem** r/t negative family interactions

Risk for impaired emancipated **Decision-Making**: Risk factor: inability to verbalize needs and wants

A Risk for self-directed **Violence:** Risk factor: history of abuse

ACCESSORY MUSCLE USE (TO BREATHE)

Ineffective **Breathing** pattern (See **Breathing** pattern, ineffective, Section III)

See Asthma; Bronchitis; COPD (Chronic Obstructive Pulmonary Disease); Respiratory Infections, Acute Childhood

ACCIDENT PRONE

Frail Elderly syndrome r/t history of falls

Acute **Confusion** r/t altered level of consciousness

Ineffective **Coping** r/t personal vulnerability, situational crises

Ineffective **Impulse** control (See **Impulse** control, ineffective, Section III)

Risk for **Injury:** Risk factor: history of accidents

ACHALASIA

Ineffective **Coping** r/t chronic disease

Acute **Pain** r/t stasis of food in esophagus

Impaired **Swallowing** r/t neuromuscular impairment

Risk for **Aspiration:** Risk factor: nocturnal regurgitation

ACID-BASE IMBALANCES

Risk for **Electrolyte** imbalance: Risk factors: renal dysfunction, diarrhea, treatment-related side effects (e.g., medications, drains)

ACIDOSIS, METABOLIC

Acute **Confusion** r/t acid-base imbalance, associated electrolyte imbalance

Impaired **Memory** r/t effect of metabolic acidosis on brain function

Imbalanced **Nutrition:** less than body requirements r/t inability to ingest, absorb nutrients

Risk for **Electrolyte** imbalance: Risk factor: effect of metabolic acidosis on renal function

Risk for **Injury:** Risk factors: disorientation, weakness, stupor

Risk for decreased **Cardiac** tissue perfusion: Risk factor: dysrhythmias from hyperkalemia

Risk for **Shock:** Risk factors: abnormal metabolic state, presence of acid state impairing function, decreased tissue perfusion

ACIDOSIS, RESPIRATORY

Activity intolerance r/t imbalance between oxygen supply and demand

Impaired **Gas** exchange r/t ventilation-perfusion imbalance

Impaired **Memory** r/t hypoxia

Risk for decreased **Cardiac** tissue perfusion: Risk factor: dysrhythmias associated with respiratory acidosis

ACNE

Disturbed **Body Image** r/t biophysical changes associated with skin disorder

Ineffective **Health** management r/t insufficient knowledge of therapeutic regimen

Impaired **Skin** integrity r/t hormonal changes (adolescence, menstrual cycle)

ACS (ACUTE CORONARY SYNDROME)

See MI (Myocardial Infarction)

ACQUIRED IMMUNODEFICIENCY SYNDROME

See AIDS (Acquired Immunodeficiency Syndrome)

ACROMEGALY

Activity intolerance (See **Activity** intolerance, Section III)

Ineffective **Airway** clearance r/t airway obstruction by enlarged tongue

Disturbed **Body Image** r/t changes in body function and appearance

Impaired physical **Mobility** r/t joint pain

Risk for decreased **Cardiac** tissue perfusion: Risk factor: increased atherosclerosis from abnormal health status

Risk for unstable blood **Glucose** level: Risk factor: abnormal physical health status

Sexual dysfunction r/t changes in hormonal secretions

Risk for **Overweight:** Risk factor: energy expenditure less than energy intake

ACTIVITY INTOLERANCE, POTENTIAL TO DEVELOP

Activity intolerance (See **Activity** intolerance, Section III)

ACUTE ABDOMINAL PAIN

Deficient **Fluid** volume r/t air and fluids trapped in bowel, inability to drink

Acute **Pain** r/t pathological process

Risk for dysfunctional **Gastrointestinal** motility: Risk factor: ineffective gastrointestinal tissue perfusion

See Abdominal Pain

ACUTE ALCOHOL INTOXICATION

Ineffective **Breathing** pattern r/t depression of the respiratory center from excessive alcohol intake

Acute **Confusion** r/t central nervous system depression

Dysfunctional **Family** processes r/t abuse of alcohol

Risk for **Aspiration:** Risk factor: depressed reflexes with acute vomiting

Risk for **Infection:** Risk factor: impaired immune system from malnutrition associated with chronic excessive alcohol intake

Risk for **Injury:** Risk factor: chemical (alcohol)

ACUTE BACK PAIN

Anxiety r/t situational crisis, back injury

Constipation r/t decreased activity, effect of pain medication

Ineffective **Coping** r/t situational crisis, back injury

Impaired physical **Mobility** r/t pain

Acute **Pain** r/t back injury

Readiness for enhanced **Knowledge:** expresses an interest in learning

ACUTE CONFUSION

See Confusion, Acute

ACUTE CORONARY SYNDROME

Decreased **Cardiac** output r/t cardiac disorder

Risk for decreased **Cardiac** tissue perfusion (See **Cardiac** tissue perfusion, risk for decreased, Section III)

ACUTE LYMPHOCYTIC LEUKEMIA (ALL)

See Cancer; Chemotherapy; Child with Chronic Condition; Leukemia

ACUTE RENAL FAILURE/ACUTE KIDNEY FAILURE

See Kidney Failure

ACUTE RESPIRATORY DISTRESS SYNDROME

See ARDS (Acute Respiratory Distress Syndrome)

ADAMS-STOKES SYNDROME

See Dysrhythmia

ADDICTION

See Alcoholism; Drug Abuse

ADDISON'S DISEASE

Activity intolerance r/t weakness, fatigue

Disturbed **Body Image** r/t increased skin pigmentation

Deficient **Fluid** volume r/t failure of regulatory mechanisms

Imbalanced **Nutrition:** less than body requirements r/t chronic illness

Risk for **Injury:** Risk factor: weakness

Readiness for enhanced **Knowledge:** expresses an interest in learning

ADENOIDECTOMY

Acute **Pain** r/t surgical incision

Ineffective **Airway** clearance r/t hesitation or reluctance to cough as a result of pain, fear

Nausea r/t anesthesia effects, drainage from surgery

Acute **Pain** r/t surgical incision

Risk for **Aspiration:** Risk factors: postoperative drainage, impaired swallowing

Risk for **Bleeding:** Risk factor: surgical incision

Risk for deficient **Fluid** volume: Risk factors: decreased intake as a result of painful swallowing, effects of anesthesia

Risk for imbalanced **Nutrition:** less than body requirements: Risk factor: reluctance to swallow

Readiness for enhanced **Knowledge:** expresses an interest in learning

ADHESIONS, LYSIS OF

See Abdominal Surgery

ADJUSTMENT DISORDER

Anxiety r/t inability to cope with psychosocial stressor

Labile **Emotional Control** r/t emotional disturbance

Risk-prone **Health** behavior r/t assault to self-esteem

Disturbed personal **Identity** r/t psychosocial stressor (specific to individual)

Situational low **Self-Esteem** r/t change in role function

Impaired **Social** interaction r/t absence of significant others or peers

ADJUSTMENT IMPAIRMENT

Risk-prone **Health** behavior (See **Health** behavior, risk-prone, Section III)

ADOLESCENT, PREGNANT

Anxiety r/t situational and maturational crisis, pregnancy

Disturbed **Body Image** r/t pregnancy superimposed on developing body

Decisional Conflict: keeping child versus giving up child versus abortion r/t lack of experience with decision-making, interference with decision-making, multiple or divergent sources of information, lack of support system

Disabled family **Coping** r/t highly ambivalent family relationships, chronically unresolved feelings of guilt, anger, despair

Ineffective **Coping** r/t situational and maturational crisis, personal vulnerability

Ineffective **Denial** r/t fear of consequences of pregnancy becoming known

Interrupted **Family** processes r/t unmet expectations for adolescent, situational crisis

Fear r/t labor and delivery

Deficient **Knowledge** r/t pregnancy, infant growth and development, parenting

Imbalanced **Nutrition:** less than body requirements r/t lack of knowledge of nutritional needs during pregnancy and as growing adolescent

Ineffective **Role** performance r/t pregnancy

Situational low **Self-Esteem** r/t feelings of shame and guilt about becoming or being pregnant

Impaired **Social** interaction r/t self-concept disturbance

Social isolation r/t absence of supportive significant others

Risk for impaired **Attachment:** Risk factor: anxiety associated with the parent role

Risk for delayed **Development:** Risk factor: unplanned or unwanted pregnancy

Risk for urge urinary **Incontinence:** Risk factor: pressure on bladder by growing uterus

Risk for disturbed **Maternal–Fetal** dyad: Risk factors: immaturity, substance use

Risk for impaired **Parenting:** Risk factors: adolescent parent, unplanned or unwanted pregnancy, single parent

Readiness for enhanced **Childbearing** process: reports appropriate prenatal lifestyle

Readiness for enhanced **Knowledge:** expresses an interest in learning

ADOPTION, GIVING CHILD UP FOR

Decisional Conflict r/t unclear personal values or beliefs, perceived threat to value system, support system deficit

Ineffective **Coping** r/t stress of loss of child

Interrupted **Family** processes r/t conflict within family regarding relinquishment of child

Grieving r/t loss of child, loss of role of parent

Insomnia r/t depression or trauma of relinquishment of child

Social isolation r/t making choice that goes against values of significant others

Chronic **Sorrow** r/t loss of relationship with child

Risk for **Spiritual** distress: Risk factor: perceived moral implications of decision

Readiness for enhanced **Spiritual** well-being: harmony with self regarding final decision

ADRENOCORTICAL INSUFFICIENCY

Deficient **Fluid** volume r/t insufficient ability to reabsorb water

Ineffective **Protection** r/t inability to tolerate stress

Delayed **Surgical** recovery r/t inability to respond to stress

Risk for **Shock:** Risk factors: deficient fluid volume, decreased cortisol to initiate stress response to insult to body

See Addison's Disease; Shock, Hypovolemic

ADVANCE DIRECTIVES

Death **Anxiety** r/t planning for end-of-life health decisions

Decisional Conflict r/t unclear personal values or beliefs, perceived threat to value system, support system deficit

Grieving r/t possible loss of self, significant other

Readiness for enhanced **Spiritual** well-being: harmonious interconnectedness with self, others, higher power, God

AFFECTIVE DISORDERS

See Depression (Major Depressive Disorder); Dysthymic Disorder; Manic Disorder, Bipolar I; SAD (Seasonal Affective Disorder)

AGE-RELATED MACULAR DEGENERATION

See Macular Degeneration

AGGRESSIVE BEHAVIOR

Fear r/t real or imagined threat to own well-being

Risk for other-directed **Violence** (See **Violence,** other-directed, risk for, Section III)

AGING

Death **Anxiety** r/t fear of unknown, loss of self, impact on significant others

Impaired **Dentition** r/t ineffective oral hygiene

Risk for **Frail Elderly** syndrome: Risk factors: >70 years, activity intolerance, impaired vision

Grieving r/t multiple losses, impending death

Ineffective **Health** management r/t powerlessness

Hearing Loss r/t exposure to loud noises, aging

Functional urinary **Incontinence** r/t impaired vision, impaired cognition, neuromuscular limitations, altered environmental factors

Impaired **Resilience** r/t aging, multiple losses

Sleep deprivation r/t aging-related sleep-stage shifts

Ineffective **Thermoregulation** r/t aging

Vision Loss r/t aging *(see care plan in Appendix)*

Risk for **Caregiver Role Strain:** Risk factor: inability to handle increasing needs of significant other

Risk for Impaired emancipated **Decision-Making:** Risk factor: inability to process information regarding health care decisions

Risk for **Injury:** Risk factors: vision loss, hearing loss, decreased balance, decreased sensation in feet

Risk for **Loneliness:** Risk factors: inadequate support system, role transition, health alterations, depression, fatigue

Readiness for enhanced community **Coping:** providing social support and other resources identified as needed for elderly client

Readiness for enhanced family **Coping:** ability to gratify needs, address adaptive tasks

Readiness for enhanced **Health** management: knowledge about medication, nutrition, exercise, coping strategies

Readiness for enhanced **Knowledge:** specify need to improve health

Readiness for enhanced **Nutrition:** need to improve health

Readiness for enhanced **Relationship:** demonstrates understanding of partner's insufficient function

Readiness for enhanced **Sleep:** need to improve sleep

Readiness for enhanced **Spiritual** well-being: one's experience of life's meaning, harmony with self, others, higher power, God, environment

Readiness for enhanced **Urinary** elimination: need to improve health

AGITATION

Acute **Confusion** r/t side effects of medication, hypoxia, decreased cerebral perfusion, alcohol abuse or withdrawal, substance abuse or withdrawal, sensory deprivation or overload

Sleep deprivation r/t sustained inadequate sleep hygiene, sundown syndrome

AGORAPHOBIA

Anxiety r/t real or perceived threat to physical integrity

Ineffective **Coping** r/t inadequate support systems

Fear r/t leaving home, going out in public places

Impaired **Social** interaction r/t disturbance in self-concept

Social isolation r/t altered thought process

AGRANULOCYTOSIS

Delayed **Surgical** recovery r/t abnormal blood profile

Risk for **Infection:** Risk factor: abnormal blood profile

Readiness for enhanced **Knowledge:** expresses an interest in learning

AIDS (ACQUIRED IMMUNODEFICIENCY SYNDROME)

Death **Anxiety** r/t fear of premature death

Disturbed **Body Image** r/t chronic contagious illness, cachexia

Caregiver Role Strain r/t unpredictable illness course, presence of situation stressors

Diarrhea r/t inflammatory bowel changes

Interrupted **Family** processes r/t distress about diagnosis of human immunodeficiency virus (HIV) infection

Fatigue r/t disease process, stress, decreased nutritional intake

Fear r/t powerlessness, threat to well-being

Grieving: family/parental r/t potential or impending death of loved one

Grieving: individual r/t loss of physical and psychosocial well-being

Hopelessness r/t deteriorating physical condition

Imbalanced **Nutrition:** less than body requirements r/t decreased ability to eat and absorb nutrients as a result of anorexia, nausea, diarrhea; oral candidiasis

Chronic **Pain** r/t tissue inflammation and destruction

Impaired **Resilience** r/t chronic illness

Situational low **Self-Esteem** r/t crisis of chronic contagious illness

Ineffective **Sexuality** pattern r/t possible transmission of disease

Social isolation r/t self-concept disturbance, therapeutic isolation

Chronic **Sorrow** r/t chronic illness

Spiritual distress r/t challenged beliefs or moral system

Risk for deficient **Fluid** volume: Risk factors: diarrhea, vomiting, fever, bleeding

Risk for **Infection:** Risk factor: inadequate immune system

Risk for **Loneliness:** Risk factor: social isolation

Risk for impaired **Oral Mucous Membrane:** Risk factor: immunological deficit

Risk for impaired **Skin** integrity: Risk factors: immunological deficit, diarrhea

Risk for **Spiritual** distress: Risk factor: physical illness

Readiness for enhanced **Knowledge:** expresses an interest in learning

See AIDS, Child; Cancer; Pneumonia

AIDS DEMENTIA

Chronic **Confusion** r/t viral invasion of nervous system

See Dementia

AIDS, CHILD

Impaired **Parenting** r/t congenital acquisition of infection secondary to intravenous (IV) drug use, multiple sexual partners, history of contaminated blood transfusion

See AIDS (Acquired Immunodeficiency Syndrome); Child with Chronic Condition; Hospitalized Child; Terminally Ill Child, Adolescent; Terminally Ill Child, Infant/Toddler; Terminally Ill Child, Preschool Child; Terminally Ill Child, School-Age Child/Preadolescent; Terminally Ill Child/Death of Child, Parent

AIRWAY OBSTRUCTION/ SECRETIONS

Ineffective **Airway** clearance (See **Airway** clearance, ineffective, Section III)

ALCOHOL WITHDRAWAL

Anxiety r/t situational crisis, withdrawal

Acute **Confusion** r/t effects of alcohol withdrawal

Ineffective **Coping** r/t personal vulnerability

Dysfunctional **Family** processes r/t abuse of alcohol

Insomnia r/t effect of alcohol withdrawal, anxiety

Imbalanced **Nutrition:** less than body requirements r/t poor dietary habits

Chronic low **Self-Esteem** r/t repeated unmet expectations

Risk for deficient **Fluid** volume: Risk factors: excessive diaphoresis, agitation, decreased fluid intake

Risk for other-directed **Violence:** Risk factor: substance withdrawal

Risk for self-directed **Violence:** Risk factor: substance withdrawal

Readiness for enhanced **Knowledge:** expresses an interest in learning

A

ALCOHOLISM

Anxiety r/t loss of control

Risk-prone **Health** behavior r/t lack of motivation to change behaviors, addiction

Acute **Confusion** r/t alcohol abuse

Chronic **Confusion** r/t neurological effects of chronic alcohol intake

Defensive **Coping** r/t denial of reality of addiction

Disabled family **Coping** r/t codependency issues due to alcoholism

Ineffective **Coping** r/t use of alcohol to cope with life events

Labile **Emotional Control** r/t substance abuse

Ineffective **Denial** r/t refusal to acknowledge addiction

Dysfunctional **Family** processes r/t alcohol abuse

Impaired **Home** maintenance r/t memory deficits, fatigue

Insomnia r/t irritability, nightmares, tremors

Impaired **Memory** r/t alcohol abuse

Self-Neglect r/t effects of alcohol abuse

Imbalanced **Nutrition:** less than body requirements r/t anorexia, inappropriate diet with increased carbohydrates

Powerlessness r/t alcohol addiction

Ineffective **Protection** r/t malnutrition, sleep deprivation

Chronic low **Self-Esteem** r/t failure at life events

Social isolation r/t unacceptable social behavior, values

Risk for **Injury:** Risk factor: alteration in sensory or perceptual function

Risk for **Loneliness:** Risk factor: unacceptable social behavior

Risk for other-directed **Violence:** Risk factors: reactions to substances used, impulsive behavior, disorientation, impaired judgment

Risk for self-directed **Violence:** Risk factors: reactions to substances used, impulsive behavior, disorientation, impaired judgment

ALCOHOLISM, DYSFUNCTIONAL FAMILY PROCESSES

Dysfunctional **Family** processes (See **Family** processes, dysfunctional, Section III)

ALKALOSIS

See Metabolic Alkalosis

ALL (ACUTE LYMPHOCYTIC LEUKEMIA)

See Cancer; Chemotherapy; Child with Chronic Condition; Leukemia

ALLERGIES

Latex Allergy response r/t hypersensitivity to natural rubber latex

Risk for **Allergy** response: Risk factors: chemical factors, dander, environmental substances, foods, insect stings, medications

Risk for **Latex Allergy** response: Risk factor: repeated exposure to products containing latex

Readiness for enhanced **Knowledge:** expresses an interest in learning

ALOPECIA

Disturbed **Body Image** r/t loss of hair, change in appearance

Readiness for enhanced **Knowledge:** expresses an interest in learning

ALTERED MENTAL STATUS

See Confusion, Acute; Confusion, Chronic; Memory Deficit

ALS (AMYOTROPHIC LATERAL SCLEROSIS)

See Amyotrophic Lateral Sclerosis (ALS)

ALZHEIMER'S DISEASE

Caregiver role strain r/t duration and extent of caregiving required

Chronic **Confusion** r/t loss of cognitive function

Compromised family **Coping** r/t interrupted family processes

Frail Elderly syndrome r/t alteration in cognitive functioning

Impaired **Home** maintenance r/t impaired cognitive function, inadequate support systems

Hopelessness r/t deteriorating condition

Insomnia r/t neurological impairment, daytime naps

Impaired **Memory** r/t neurological disturbance

Impaired physical **Mobility** r/t severe neurological dysfunction

Self-Neglect r/t loss of cognitive function

Powerlessness r/t deteriorating condition

Self-Care deficit: specify r/t loss of cognitive function, psychological impairment

Social isolation r/t fear of disclosure of memory loss

Wandering r/t cognitive impairment, frustration, physiological state

Risk for chronic functional **Constipation:** Risk factor: impaired cognitive functioning

Risk for **Injury:** Risk factor: confusion

Risk for **Loneliness:** Risk factor: potential social isolation

Risk for **Relocation** stress syndrome: Risk factors: impaired psychosocial health, decreased health status

Risk for other-directed **Violence:** Risk factors: frustration, fear, anger, loss of cognitive function

Readiness for enhanced **Knowledge:** Caregiver: expresses an interest in learning

See Dementia

AMD (AGE-RELATED MACULAR DEGENERATION)

See Macular Degeneration

AMENORRHEA

Imbalanced **Nutrition:** less than body requirements r/t inadequate food intake

See Sexuality, Adolescent

AMI (ACUTE MYOCARDIAL INFARCTION)

See MI (Myocardial Infarction)

AMNESIA

Acute **Confusion** r/t alcohol abuse, delirium, dementia, drug abuse

Dysfunctional **Family** processes r/t alcohol abuse, inadequate coping skills

Impaired **Memory** r/t excessive environmental disturbance, neurological disturbance

Post-Trauma syndrome r/t history of abuse, catastrophic illness, disaster, accident

AMNIOCENTESIS

Anxiety r/t threat to self and fetus, unknown future

Decisional Conflict r/t choice of treatment pending results of test

Risk for **Infection:** Risk factor: invasive procedure

AMNIONITIS

See Chorioamnionitis

AMNIOTIC MEMBRANE RUPTURE

See Premature Rupture of Membranes

AMPUTATION

Disturbed **Body Image** r/t negative effects of amputation, response from others

Grieving r/t loss of body part, future lifestyle changes

Impaired physical **Mobility** r/t musculoskeletal impairment, limited movement

Acute **Pain** r/t surgery, phantom limb sensation

A

Chronic **Pain** r/t surgery, phantom limb sensation

Ineffective peripheral **Tissue Perfusion** r/t impaired arterial circulation

Impaired **Skin** integrity r/t poor healing, prosthesis rubbing

Risk for **Bleeding:** Risk factor: vulnerable surgical site

Risk for Impaired **Tissue** integrity: Risk factor: mechanical factors impacting site

Readiness for enhanced **Knowledge:** expresses an interest in learning

AMYOTROPHIC LATERAL SCLEROSIS (ALS)

Death **Anxiety** r/t impending progressive loss of function leading to death

Ineffective **Breathing** pattern r/t compromised muscles of respiration

Impaired verbal **Communication** r/t weakness of muscles of speech, deficient knowledge of ways to compensate and alternative communication devices

Decisional Conflict: ventilator therapy r/t unclear personal values or beliefs, lack of relevant information

Impaired **Resilience** r/t perceived vulnerability

Chronic **Sorrow** r/t chronic illness

Impaired **Swallowing** r/t weakness of muscles involved in swallowing

Impaired spontaneous **Ventilation** r/t weakness of muscles of respiration

Risk for **Aspiration:** Risk factor: impaired swallowing

Risk for **Spiritual** distress: Risk factor: chronic debilitating condition

See Neurologic Disorders

ANAL FISTULA

See Hemorrhoidectomy

ANAPHYLACTIC SHOCK

Deficient **Fluid** volume r/t compromised regulatory mechanism

Ineffective **Airway** clearance r/t laryngeal edema, bronchospasm

Latex Allergy response r/t abnormal immune mechanism response

Impaired spontaneous **Ventilation** r/t acute airway obstruction from anaphylaxis process

ANAPHYLAXIS PREVENTION

Risk for **Allergy** response (See **Allergy** response, risk for, Section III)

ANASARCA

Excess **Fluid** volume r/t excessive fluid intake, cardiac/renal dysfunction, loss of plasma proteins

Risk for impaired **Skin** integrity: Risk factor: impaired circulation to skin from edema

ANEMIA

Anxiety r/t cause of disease

Impaired **Comfort** r/t feelings of always being cold from decreased hemoglobin and decreased metabolism

Fatigue r/t decreased oxygen supply to the body, increased cardiac workload

Impaired **Memory** r/t change in cognition from decreased oxygen supply to the body

Delayed **Surgical** recovery r/t decreased oxygen supply to body, increased cardiac workload

Risk for **Bleeding** (See **Bleeding**, risk for, Section III)

Risk for **Injury:** Risk factor: alteration in peripheral sensory perception

Readiness for enhanced **Knowledge:** expresses an interest in learning

ANEMIA, IN PREGNANCY

Anxiety r/t concerns about health of self and fetus

Fatigue r/t decreased oxygen supply to the body, increased cardiac workload

Risk for delayed **Development:** Risk factor: reduction in the oxygen-carrying capacity of blood

Risk for **Infection:** Risk factor: reduction in oxygen-carrying capacity of blood

Risk for disturbed **Maternal–Fetal** dyad: Risk factor: compromised oxygen transport

Readiness for enhanced **Knowledge:** expresses an interest in learning

ANEMIA, SICKLE CELL

See Anemia; Sickle Cell Anemia/Crisis

ANENCEPHALY

See Neural Tube Defects

ANEURYSM, ABDOMINAL SURGERY

Risk for deficient **Fluid** volume: Risk factor: hemorrhage r/t potential abnormal blood loss

Risk for **Infection:** Risk factor: invasive procedure

Risk for ineffective **Gastrointestinal** perfusion (See **Gastrointestinal** perfusion, ineffective, risk for, Section III)

Risk for ineffective **Renal** perfusion: Risk factor: prolonged ischemia of kidneys

See Abdominal Surgery

ANEURYSM, CEREBRAL

See Craniectomy/Craniotomy; Subarachnoid Hemorrhage

ANGER

Anxiety r/t situational crisis

Defensive **Coping** r/t inability to acknowledge responsibility for actions and results of actions

Labile **Emotional Control** r/t stressors

Fear r/t environmental stressor, hospitalization

Grieving r/t significant loss

Risk-prone **Health** behavior r/t assault to self-esteem, disability requiring change in lifestyle, inadequate support system

Powerlessness r/t health care environment

Risk for compromised **Human Dignity:** Risk factors: inadequate participation in decision-making, perceived dehumanizing treatment, perceived humiliation, exposure of the body, cultural incongruity

Risk for **Post-Trauma** syndrome: Risk factor: inadequate social support

Risk for other-directed **Violence:** Risk factors: history of violence, rage reaction

Risk for self-directed **Violence:** Risk factors: history of violence, history of abuse, rage reaction

ANGINA

Activity intolerance r/t acute pain, dysrhythmias

Anxiety r/t situational crisis

Decreased **Cardiac** output r/t myocardial ischemia, medication effect, dysrhythmia

Ineffective **Coping** r/t personal vulnerability to situational crisis of new diagnosis, deteriorating health

Ineffective **Denial** r/t deficient knowledge of need to seek help with symptoms

Grieving r/t pain, loss of health

Acute **Pain** r/t myocardial ischemia

Ineffective **Sexuality** pattern r/t disease process, medications, loss of libido

Readiness for enhanced **Knowledge:** expresses an interest in learning

ANGIOCARDIOGRAPHY (CARDIAC CATHETERIZATION)

See Cardiac Catheterization

ANGIOPLASTY, CORONARY

Fear r/t possible outcome of interventional procedure

Ineffective peripheral **Tissue Perfusion** r/t vasospasm, hematoma formation

Risk for **Bleeding:** Risk factors: possible damage to coronary artery, hematoma formation

A

Risk for decreased **Cardiac** tissue perfusion: Risk factors: ventricular ischemia, dysrhythmias

Readiness for enhanced **Knowledge:** expresses an interest in learning

ANOMALY, FETAL/NEWBORN (PARENT DEALING WITH)

Anxiety r/t threat to role functioning, situational crisis

Decisional Conflict: interventions for fetus or newborn r/t lack of relevant information, spiritual distress, threat to value system

Disabled family **Coping** r/t chronically unresolved feelings about loss of perfect baby

Ineffective **Coping** r/t personal vulnerability in situational crisis

Interrupted **Family** processes r/t unmet expectations for perfect baby, lack of adequate support systems

Fear r/t real or imagined threat to baby, implications for future pregnancies, powerlessness

Grieving r/t loss of ideal child

Hopelessness r/t long-term stress, deteriorating physical condition of child, lost spiritual belief

Deficient **Knowledge** r/t limited exposure to situation

Impaired **Parenting** r/t interruption of bonding process

Powerlessness r/t complication threatening fetus or newborn

Parental **Role** conflict r/t separation from newborn, intimidation with invasive or restrictive modalities, specialized care center policies

Situational low **Self-Esteem** r/t perceived inability to produce a perfect child

Social isolation r/t alterations in child's physical appearance, altered state of wellness

Chronic **Sorrow** r/t loss of ideal child, inadequate bereavement support

Spiritual distress r/t test of spiritual beliefs

Risk for impaired **Attachment:** Risk factor: ill infant unable to effectively initiate parental contact as result of altered behavioral organization

Risk for disorganized **Infant** behavior: Risk factor: congenital disorder

Risk for impaired **Parenting:** Risk factors: interruption of bonding process; unrealistic expectations for self, infant, or partner; perceived threat to own emotional survival; severe stress; lack of knowledge

Risk for **Spiritual** distress: Risk factor: lack of normal child to raise and carry on family name

ANORECTAL ABSCESS

Disturbed **Body Image** r/t odor and drainage from rectal area

Acute **Pain** r/t inflammation of perirectal area

Risk for **Constipation:** Risk factor: fear of painful elimination

Readiness for enhanced **Knowledge:** expresses an interest in learning

ANOREXIA

Deficient **Fluid** volume r/t inability to drink

Imbalanced **Nutrition:** less than body requirements r/t loss of appetite, nausea, vomiting, laxative abuse

Delayed **Surgical** recovery r/t inadequate nutritional intake

Risk for delayed **Surgical** recovery: Risk factor: inadequate nutritional intake

ANOREXIA NERVOSA

Activity intolerance r/t fatigue, weakness

Disturbed **Body Image** r/t misconception of actual body appearance

Constipation r/t lack of adequate food, fiber, and fluid intake

Defensive **Coping** r/t psychological impairment, eating disorder

Disabled family **Coping** r/t highly ambivalent family relationships

Ineffective **Denial** r/t fear of consequences of therapy, possible weight gain

Diarrhea r/t laxative abuse

Interrupted **Family** processes r/t situational crisis

Ineffective family **Health** management r/t family conflict, excessive demands on family associated with complexity of condition and treatment

Imbalanced **Nutrition:** less than body requirements r/t inadequate food intake, excessive exercise

Chronic low **Self-Esteem** r/t repeated unmet expectations

Ineffective **Sexuality** pattern r/t loss of libido from malnutrition

Risk for **Infection:** Risk factor: malnutrition resulting in depressed immune system

Risk for **Spiritual** distress: Risk factor: low self-esteem

See Maturational Issues, Adolescent

ANOSMIA (SMELL, LOSS OF ABILITY TO)

Imbalanced **Nutrition:** less than body requirements r/t loss of appetite associated with loss of smell

ANTEPARTUM PERIOD

See Pregnancy, Normal; Prenatal Care, Normal

ANTERIOR REPAIR, ANTERIOR COLPORRHAPHY

Urinary Retention r/t edema of urinary structures

Risk for urge urinary **Incontinence:** Risk factor: trauma to bladder

Readiness for enhanced **Knowledge:** expresses an interest in learning

See Vaginal Hysterectomy

ANTICOAGULANT THERAPY

Risk for **Bleeding:** Risk factor: altered clotting function from anticoagulant

Risk for deficient **Fluid** volume: hemorrhage: Risk factor: altered clotting mechanism

Readiness for enhanced **Knowledge:** expresses an interest in learning

ANTISOCIAL PERSONALITY DISORDER

Defensive **Coping** r/t excessive use of projection

Ineffective **Coping** r/t frequently violating the norms and rules of society

Labile **Emotional Control** r/t psychiatric disorder

Hopelessness r/t abandonment

Impaired **Social** interaction r/t sociocultural conflict, chemical dependence, inability to form relationships

Spiritual distress r/t separation from religious or cultural ties

Ineffective **Health** management r/t excessive demands on family

Risk for **Loneliness:** Risk factor: inability to interact appropriately with others

Risk for impaired **Parenting:** Risk factors: inability to function as parent or guardian, emotional instability

Risk for **Self-Mutilation:** Risk factors: self-hatred, depersonalization

Risk for other-directed **Violence:** Risk factors: history of violence, altered thought patterns

ANURIA

See Kidney Failure

ANXIETY

See Anxiety, Section III

ANXIETY DISORDER

Ineffective **Activity** planning r/t unrealistic perception of events

Anxiety r/t unmet security and safety needs

Death **Anxiety** r/t fears of unknown, powerlessness

A

Decisional **Conflict** r/t low self-esteem, fear of making a mistake

Defensive **Coping** r/t overwhelming feelings of dread

Disabled family **Coping** r/t ritualistic behavior, actions

Ineffective **Coping** r/t inability to express feelings appropriately

Ineffective **Denial** r/t overwhelming feelings of hopelessness, fear, threat to self

Insomnia r/t psychological impairment, emotional instability

Impaired **Mood** regulation r/t functional impairment, impaired social functioning, alteration in sleep pattern

Labile **Emotional Control** r/t emotional instability

Powerlessness r/t lifestyle of helplessness

Self-Care deficit r/t ritualistic behavior, activities

Sleep deprivation r/t prolonged psychological discomfort

Risk for **Spiritual** distress: Risk factor: psychological distress

Readiness for enhanced **Knowledge:** expresses an interest in learning

AORTIC ANEURYSM REPAIR (ABDOMINAL SURGERY)

See Abdominal Surgery; Aneurysm, Abdominal Surgery

AORTIC VALVULAR STENOSIS

See Congenital Heart Disease/Cardiac Anomalies

APHASIA

Anxiety r/t situational crisis of aphasia

Impaired verbal **Communication** r/t decrease in circulation to brain

Ineffective **Coping** r/t loss of speech

Ineffective **Health** maintenance r/t deficient knowledge regarding information on aphasia and alternative communication techniques

APLASTIC ANEMIA

Activity intolerance r/t imbalance between oxygen supply and demand

Fear r/t ability to live with serious disease

Risk for **Bleeding:** Risk factor: inadequate clotting factors

Risk for **Infection:** Risk factor: inadequate immune function

Readiness for enhanced **Knowledge:** expresses an interest in learning

APNEA IN INFANCY

See Premature Infant (Child); Premature Infant (Parent); SIDS (Sudden Infant Death Syndrome)

APNEUSTIC RESPIRATIONS

Ineffective **Breathing** pattern r/t perception or cognitive impairment, neurological impairment

APPENDECTOMY

Deficient **Fluid** volume r/t fluid restriction, hypermetabolic state, nausea, vomiting

Acute **Pain** r/t surgical incision

Delayed **Surgical** recovery r/t rupture of appendix

Risk for **Infection:** Risk factors: perforation or rupture of appendix, surgical incision, peritonitis

Readiness for enhanced **Knowledge:** expresses an interest in learning

See Hospitalized Child; Surgery, Postoperative Care

APPENDICITIS

Deficient **Fluid** volume r/t anorexia, nausea, vomiting

Acute **Pain** r/t inflammation

Risk for **Infection:** Risk factor: possible perforation of appendix

Readiness for enhanced **Knowledge:** expresses an interest in learning

APPREHENSION

Anxiety r/t threat to self-concept, threat to health status, situational crisis

Death **Anxiety** r/t apprehension over loss of self, consequences to significant others

ARDS (ACUTE RESPIRATORY DISTRESS SYNDROME)

Ineffective **Airway** clearance r/t excessive tracheobronchial secretions

Death **Anxiety** r/t seriousness of physical disease

Impaired **Gas** exchange r/t damage to alveolar capillary membrane, change in lung compliance

Impaired spontaneous **Ventilation** r/t damage to alveolar capillary membrane

See Ventilated Client, Mechanically

ARRHYTHMIA

See Dysrhythmia

ARTERIAL INSUFFICIENCY

Ineffective peripheral **Tissue Perfusion** r/t interruption of arterial flow

Delayed **Surgical** recovery r/t ineffective tissue perfusion

ARTHRITIS

Activity intolerance r/t chronic pain, fatigue, weakness

Disturbed **Body Image** r/t ineffective coping with joint abnormalities

Impaired physical **Mobility** r/t joint impairment

Chronic **Pain** r/t progression of joint deterioration

Self-Care deficit: specify r/t pain with movement, damage to joints

Readiness for enhanced **Knowledge:** expresses an interest in learning

See JRA (Juvenile Rheumatoid Arthritis)

ARTHROCENTESIS

Acute **Pain** r/t invasive procedure

ARTHROPLASTY (TOTAL HIP REPLACEMENT)

See Total Joint Replacement (Total Hip/Total Knee/Shoulder); Surgery, Perioperative; Surgery, Postoperative Care; Surgery, Preoperative Care

ARTHROSCOPY

Impaired physical **Mobility** r/t surgical trauma of knee

Readiness for enhanced **Knowledge:** expresses an interest in learning

ASCITES

Ineffective **Breathing** pattern r/t increased abdominal girth

Imbalanced **Nutrition:** less than body requirements r/t loss of appetite

Chronic **Pain** r/t altered body function

Readiness for enhanced **Knowledge:** expresses an interest in learning

See Cancer; Cirrhosis

ASPERGER'S SYNDROME

Ineffective **Relationship** r/t poor communication skills, lack of empathy

See Autism

ASPHYXIA, BIRTH

Ineffective **Breathing** pattern r/t depression of breathing reflex secondary to anoxia

Ineffective **Coping** r/t uncertainty of child outcome

Fear (parental) r/t concern over safety of infant

Impaired **Gas** exchange r/t poor placental perfusion, lack of initiation of breathing by newborn

Grieving r/t loss of perfect child, concern of loss of future abilities

Impaired spontaneous **Ventilation** r/t brain injury

Risk for impaired **Attachment:** Risk factors: ill infant who is unable to initiate parental contact, hospitalization in critical care environment

Risk for delayed **Development**: Risk factor: lack of oxygen to brain

Risk for disproportionate **Growth**: Risk factor: lack of oxygen to brain

Risk for disorganized **Infant** behavior: Risk factor: lack of oxygen to brain

Risk for **Injury**: Risk factor: lack of oxygen to brain

Risk for ineffective **Cerebral** tissue perfusion: Risk factor: poor placental perfusion or cord compression resulting in lack of oxygen to brain

ASPIRATION, DANGER OF

Risk for **Aspiration** (See **Aspiration**, risk for, Section III)

ASSAULT VICTIM

Post-Trauma syndrome r/t assault

Rape-Trauma syndrome r/t rape

Impaired **Resilience** r/t frightening experience, post-trauma stress response

Risk for **Post-Trauma** syndrome: Risk factors: perception of event, inadequate social support, unsupportive environment, diminished ego strength, duration of event

Risk for **Spiritual** distress: Risk factors: physical, psychological stress

ASSAULTIVE CLIENT

Risk for **Injury**: Risk factors: confused thought process, impaired judgment

Risk for other-directed **Violence**: Risk factors: paranoid ideation, anger

ASTHMA

Activity intolerance r/t fatigue, energy shift to meet muscle needs for breathing to overcome airway obstruction

Ineffective **Airway** clearance r/t tracheobronchial narrowing, excessive secretions

Anxiety r/t inability to breathe effectively, fear of suffocation

Disturbed **Body Image** r/t decreased participation in physical activities

Ineffective **Breathing** pattern r/t anxiety

Ineffective **Coping** r/t personal vulnerability to situational crisis

Ineffective **Health** management (See **Health** management, ineffective, Section III)

Impaired **Home** maintenance r/t deficient knowledge regarding control of environmental triggers

Sleep deprivation r/t ineffective breathing pattern, cough

Readiness for enhanced **Health** management (See **Health** management, readiness for enhanced, Section III)

Readiness for enhanced **Knowledge**: expresses an interest in learning

See Child with Chronic Condition; Hospitalized Child

ATAXIA

Anxiety r/t change in health status

Disturbed **Body Image** r/t staggering gait

Impaired physical **Mobility** r/t neuromuscular impairment

Risk for **Falls**: Risk factors: gait alteration, instability

ATELECTASIS

Ineffective **Breathing** pattern r/t loss of functional lung tissue, depression of respiratory function or hypoventilation because of pain

Impaired **Gas** exchange r/t decreased alveolar-capillary surface

Anxiety r/t alteration in respiratory pattern

ATHEROSCLEROSIS

See MI (Myocardial Infarction); CVA (Cerebrovascular Accident); Peripheral Vascular Disease (PVD)

ATHLETE'S FOOT

Impaired **Skin** integrity r/t effects of fungal agent

Readiness for enhanced **Knowledge:** expresses an interest in learning

See Itching; Pruritus

ATN (ACUTE TUBULAR NECROSIS)

See Kidney Failure

ATRIAL FIBRILLATION

See Dysrhythmia

ATRIAL SEPTAL DEFECT

See Congenital Heart Disease/Cardiac Anomalies

ATTENTION DEFICIT DISORDER

Risk-prone **Health** behavior r/t intense emotional state

Disabled family **Coping** r/t significant person with chronically unexpressed feelings of guilt, anxiety, hostility, and despair

Ineffective **Impulse** control r/t (See **Impulse** control, ineffective, Section III)

Chronic low **Self-Esteem** r/t difficulty in participating in expected activities, poor school performance

Social isolation r/t unacceptable social behavior

Risk for delayed **Development:** Risk factor: behavior disorders

Risk for **Falls:** Risk factor: rapid non-thinking behavior

Risk for **Loneliness:** Risk factor: social isolation

Risk for impaired **Parenting:** Risk factor: lack of knowledge of factors contributing to child's behavior

Risk for **Spiritual** distress: Risk factor: poor relationships

AUDITORY PROBLEMS

See Hearing Impairment

AUTISM

Impaired verbal **Communication** r/t speech and language delays

Compromised family **Coping** r/t parental guilt over etiology of disease, inability to accept or adapt to child's condition, inability to help child and other family members seek treatment

Disturbed personal **Identity** r/t inability to distinguish between self and environment, inability to identify own body as separate from those of other people, inability to integrate concept of self

Self-Neglect r/t impaired socialization

Impaired **Social** interaction r/t communication barriers, inability to relate to others, failure to develop peer relationships

Risk for delayed **Development:** Risk factor: autism

Risk for **Loneliness:** Risk factor: difficulty developing relationships with other people

Risk for **Self-Mutilation:** Risk factor: autistic state

Risk for other-directed **Violence:** Risk factors: frequent destructive rages toward others secondary to extreme response to changes in routine, fear of harmless things

Risk for self-directed **Violence:** Risk factors: frequent destructive rages toward self, secondary to extreme response to changes in routine, fear of harmless things

See Child with Chronic Condition

AUTONOMIC DYSREFLEXIA

Autonomic Dysreflexia r/t bladder distention, bowel distention, noxious stimuli

Risk for **Autonomic Dysreflexia:** Risk factors: bladder distention, bowel distention, noxious stimuli

AUTONOMIC HYPERREFLEXIA

See Autonomic Dysreflexia

B

B

BABY CARE

Readiness for enhanced **Childbearing** process: demonstrates appropriate feeding and baby care techniques, along with attachment to infant and providing a safe environment

Anxiety r/t situational crisis, back injury

Ineffective **Coping** r/t situational crisis, back injury

Impaired physical **Mobility** r/t pain

Acute **Pain** r/t back injury

Chronic **Pain** r/t back injury

Risk for **Constipation:** Risk factors: decreased activity, side effect of pain medication

Risk for **Disuse** syndrome: Risk factor: severe pain

Readiness for enhanced **Knowledge:** expresses an interest in learning

BACTEREMIA

Risk for **Infection:** Risk factor: compromised immune system

Risk for **Shock:** Risk factor: development of systemic inflammatory response from presence of bacteria in bloodstream

See Infection; Infection, Potential for

BARREL CHEST

See Aging (if appropriate); COPD (Chronic Obstructive Pulmonary Disease)

BATHING/HYGIENE PROBLEMS

Impaired **Mobility** r/t chronic physically limiting condition

Self-Neglect (See **Self-Neglect,** Section III)

Bathing **Self-Care** deficit (See **Self-Care** deficit, bathing, Section III)

BATTERED CHILD SYNDROME

Dysfunctional **Family** processes r/t inadequate coping skills

Sleep deprivation r/t prolonged psychological discomfort

Chronic **Sorrow** r/t situational crises

Risk for **Post-Trauma** syndrome: Risk factors: physical abuse, incest, rape, molestation

Risk for **Self-Mutilation:** Risk factors: feelings of rejection, dysfunctional family

Risk for **Suicide:** Risk factor: childhood abuse

See Child Abuse

BATTERED PERSON

See Abuse, Spouse, Parent, or Significant Other

BEDBUGS, INFESTATION

Impaired **Home** maintenance r/t deficient knowledge regarding prevention of bedbug infestation

Impaired **Skin** integrity r/t bites of bedbugs

See Itching; Pruritus

BED MOBILITY, IMPAIRED

Impaired bed **Mobility** (See **Mobility,** bed, impaired, Section III)

BED REST, PROLONGED

Deficient **Diversional** activity r/t prolonged bed rest

Impaired bed **Mobility** r/t neuromuscular impairment

Social isolation r/t prolonged bed rest

Risk for chronic functional **Constipation:** Risk factor: insufficient physical activity

Risk for **Disuse** syndrome: Risk factor: prolonged immobility

Risk for **Frail Elderly** syndrome: Risk factor: prolonged immobility

Risk for **Loneliness:** Risk factor: prolonged bed rest

Risk for **Overweight:** Risk factor: energy expenditure below energy intake

Risk for **Pressure** ulcer: Risk factor: prolonged immobility

BEDSORES

See Pressure Ulcer

BEDWETTING

Ineffective **Health** maintenance r/t unachieved developmental level, neuromuscular immaturity, diseases of the urinary system

BELL'S PALSY

Disturbed **Body Image** r/t loss of motor control on one side of face

Imbalanced **Nutrition:** less than body requirements r/t difficulty with chewing

Acute **Pain** r/t inflammation of facial nerve

Risk for **Injury** (eye): Risk factors: decreased tears, decreased blinking of eye

Readiness for enhanced **Knowledge:** expresses an interest in learning

BENIGN PROSTATIC HYPERTROPHY

See BPH (Benign Prostatic Hypertrophy); Prostatic Hypertrophy

BEREAVEMENT

Grieving r/t loss of significant person

Insomnia r/t grief

Risk for complicated **Grieving:** Risk factors: emotional instability, lack of social support

Risk for **Spiritual** distress: Risk factor: death of a loved one

BILIARY ATRESIA

Anxiety r/t surgical intervention, possible liver transplantation

Impaired **Comfort** r/t inflammation of skin, itching

Imbalanced **Nutrition:** less than body requirements r/t decreased absorption of fat and fat-soluble vitamins, poor feeding

Risk for **Bleeding:** Risk factors: vitamin K deficiency, altered clotting mechanisms

Risk for ineffective **Breathing** pattern: Risk factors: enlarged liver, development of ascites

Risk for impaired **Skin** integrity: Risk factor: pruritus

See Child with Chronic Condition; Cirrhosis (as complication); Hospitalized Child; Terminally Ill Child, Adolescent; Infant/Toddler; Preschool Child; School-Age Child/Preadolescent; Death of Child, Parent

BILIARY CALCULUS

See Cholelithiasis

BILIARY OBSTRUCTION

See Jaundice

BILIRUBIN ELEVATION IN NEONATE

Neonatal **Jaundice** (See **Jaundice,** Neonatal, Section III)

BIOPSY

Fear r/t outcome of biopsy

Readiness for enhanced **Knowledge:** expresses an interest in learning

BIOTERRORISM

Contamination r/t exposure to bioterrorism

Risk for **Infection:** Risk factor: exposure to harmful biological agent

Risk for **Post-Trauma** syndrome: Risk factor: perception of event of bioterrorism

BIPOLAR DISORDER I (MOST RECENT EPISODE, DEPRESSED OR MANIC)

Ineffective **Activity** planning r/t unrealistic perception of events

Fatigue r/t psychological demands

Risk-prone **Health** behavior r/t low state of optimism

Ineffective **Health** maintenance r/t lack of ability to make good judgments regarding ways to obtain help

Self-Care deficit: specify r/t depression, cognitive impairment

Chronic low **Self-Esteem** r/t repeated unmet expectations

Social isolation r/t ineffective coping

Risk for complicated **Grieving:** Risk factor: lack of previous resolution of former grieving response

Risk for **Loneliness:** Risk factors: stress, conflict

Risk for **Spiritual** distress: Risk factor: mental illness

Risk for **Suicide:** Risk factors: psychiatric disorder, poor support system

See Depression (Major Depressive Disorder); Manic Disorder, Bipolar I

BIRTH ASPHYXIA

See Asphyxia, Birth

BIRTH CONTROL

See Contraceptive Method

BLADDER CANCER

Urinary Retention r/t clots obstructing urethra

See Cancer; TURP (Transurethral Resection of the Prostate)

BLADDER DISTENTION

Urinary Retention r/t high urethral pressure caused by weak detrusor, inhibition of reflex arc, blockage, strong sphincter

BLADDER TRAINING

Disturbed **Body Image** r/t difficulty maintaining control of urinary elimination

Functional urinary **Incontinence** r/t altered environment; sensory, cognitive, mobility deficit

Stress urinary **Incontinence** r/t degenerative change in pelvic muscles and structural supports

Urge urinary **Incontinence** r/t decreased bladder capacity, increased urine concentration, overdistention of bladder

Readiness for enhanced **Knowledge:** expresses an interest in learning

BLADDER TRAINING, CHILD

See Toilet Training

BLEEDING TENDENCY

Risk for **Bleeding** (See **Bleeding**, risk for, Section III)

Risk for delayed **Surgical** recovery: Risk factor: bleeding tendency

BLEPHAROPLASTY

Disturbed **Body Image** r/t effects of surgery

Readiness for enhanced **Knowledge:** expresses an interest in learning

BLINDNESS

Interrupted **Family** processes r/t shift in health status of family member (change in visual acuity)

Impaired **Home** maintenance r/t decreased vision

Ineffective **Role** performance r/t alteration in health status (change in visual acuity)

Self-Care deficit: specify r/t inability to see to be able to perform activities of daily living

Vision Loss r/t impaired sensory reception, transmission, or integration (*see care plan in Appendix*)

Risk for delayed **Development:** Risk factor: vision impairment

Risk for **Injury:** Risk factor: sensory dysfunction

Readiness for enhanced **Knowledge:** expresses an interest in learning

See Vision Impairment

BLOOD DISORDER

Ineffective **Protection** r/t abnormal blood profile

Risk for **Bleeding:** Risk factor: abnormal blood profile

See ITP (Idiopathic Thrombocytopenic Purpura), Hemophilia, Lacerations, Shock, Hypovolemic

BLOOD PRESSURE ALTERATION

See Hypotension; HTN (Hypertension)

BLOOD SUGAR CONTROL

Risk for unstable blood **Glucose** level (See **Glucose** level, blood, unstable, risk for, Section III)

BLOOD TRANSFUSION

Anxiety r/t possibility of harm from transfusion

See Anemia

BODY DYSMORPHIC DISORDER

Anxiety r/t perceived defect of body

Disturbed **Body Image** r/t overinvolvement in physical appearance

Chronic low **Self-Esteem** r/t lack of self valuing because of perceived body defects

Social isolation r/t distancing self from others because of perceived self body defects

Risk for **Suicide:** Risk factor: perceived defects of body affecting self-valuing and hopes

BODY IMAGE CHANGE

Disturbed **Body Image** (See **Body Image,** disturbed, Section III)

BODY TEMPERATURE, ALTERED

Ineffective **Thermoregulation** (See **Thermoregulation,** ineffective, Section III)

BONE MARROW BIOPSY

Fear r/t unknown outcome of results of biopsy

Acute **Pain** r/t bone marrow aspiration

Readiness for enhanced **Knowledge:** expresses an interest in learning

See disease necessitating bone marrow biopsy (e.g., Leukemia)

BORDERLINE PERSONALITY DISORDER

Ineffective **Activity** planning r/t unrealistic perception of events

Anxiety r/t perceived threat to self-concept

Defensive **Coping** r/t difficulty with relationships, inability to accept blame for own behavior

Ineffective **Coping** r/t use of maladjusted defense mechanisms (e.g., projection, denial)

Powerlessness r/t lifestyle of helplessness

Social isolation r/t immature interests

Ineffective family **Health** management r/t manipulative behavior of client

Risk for **Caregiver Role Strain:** Risk factors: inability of care receiver to accept criticism, care receiver taking advantage of others to meet own needs or having unreasonable expectations

Risk for **Self-Mutilation:** Risk factors: ineffective coping, feelings of self-hatred

Risk for **Spiritual** distress: Risk factor: poor relationships associated with abnormal behaviors

Risk for self-directed **Violence:** Risk factors: feelings of need to punish self, manipulative behavior

BOREDOM

Deficient **Diversional** activity r/t environmental lack of diversional activity

Impaired **Mood** regulation r/t emotional instability

Social isolation r/t altered state of wellness

BOTULISM

Deficient **Fluid** volume r/t profuse diarrhea

Readiness for enhanced **Knowledge:** expresses an interest in learning

BOWEL INCONTINENCE

Bowel **Incontinence** r/t decreased awareness of need to defecate, loss of sphincter control, fecal impaction

Readiness for enhanced **Knowledge:** expresses an interest in learning

BOWEL OBSTRUCTION

Constipation r/t decreased motility, intestinal obstruction

Deficient **Fluid** volume r/t inadequate fluid volume intake, fluid loss in bowel

Imbalanced **Nutrition:** less than body requirements r/t nausea, vomiting

Acute **Pain** r/t pressure from distended abdomen

BOWEL RESECTION

See Abdominal Surgery

BOWEL SOUNDS, ABSENT OR DIMINISHED

Constipation r/t decreased or absent peristalsis

Deficient **Fluid** volume r/t inability to ingest fluids, loss of fluids in bowel

Delayed **Surgical** recovery r/t inability to obtain adequate nutritional status

Risk for dysfunctional **Gastrointestinal** motility (See **Gastrointestinal** motility, dysfunctional, risk for, Section III)

BOWEL SOUNDS, HYPERACTIVE

Diarrhea r/t increased gastrointestinal motility

BOWEL TRAINING

Bowel **Incontinence** r/t loss of control of rectal sphincter

Readiness for enhanced **Knowledge:** expresses an interest in learning

BOWEL TRAINING, CHILD

See Toilet Training

BPH (BENIGN PROSTATIC HYPERTROPHY)

Ineffective **Health** maintenance r/t deficient knowledge regarding self-care with prostatic hypertrophy

Insomnia r/t nocturia

Urinary Retention r/t obstruction of urethra

Risk for urge urinary **Incontinence:** Risk factors: detrusor muscle instability with impaired contractility, involuntary sphincter relaxation

Risk for **Infection:** Risk factors: urinary residual after voiding, bacterial invasion of bladder

Readiness for enhanced **Knowledge:** expresses an interest in learning

See Prostatic Hypertrophy

BRADYCARDIA

Decreased **Cardiac** output r/t slow heart rate supplying inadequate amount of blood for body function

Risk for ineffective **Cerebral** tissue perfusion: Risk factors: decreased cardiac output secondary to bradycardia, vagal response

Readiness for enhanced **Knowledge:** expresses an interest in learning

BRADYPNEA

Ineffective **Breathing** pattern r/t neuromuscular impairment, pain, musculoskeletal impairment, perception or cognitive impairment, anxiety, fatigue or decreased energy, effects of drugs

See Sleep Apnea (See **Airway** clearance, ineffective, Section III)

BRAIN INJURY

See Intracranial Pressure, Increased

BRAIN SURGERY

See Craniectomy/Craniotomy

BRAIN TUMOR

Acute **Confusion** r/t pressure from tumor

Fear r/t threat to well-being

Grieving r/t potential loss of physiosocial-psychosocial well-being

Decreased **Intracranial** adaptive capacity r/t presence of brain tumor

Acute **Pain** r/t pressure from tumor

Vision Loss r/t tumor growth compressing optic nerve and/or brain tissue

Risk for **Injury:** Risk factors: sensory-perceptual alterations, weakness

Risk for **Hyperthermia:** Risk factor: loss of thermoregulation with hypothalamic dysfunction

See Cancer; Chemotherapy; Child with Chronic Condition; Craniectomy/ Craniotomy; Hospitalized Child; Radiation Therapy; Terminally Ill Child, Adolescent; Terminally Ill Child, Infant/ Toddler; Terminally Ill Child, Preschool Child; Terminally Ill Child, School-Age Child/Preadolescent; Terminally Ill Child/ Death of Child, Parent

BRAXTON HICKS CONTRACTIONS

Activity intolerance r/t increased contractions with increased gestation

Anxiety r/t uncertainty about beginning labor

Fatigue r/t lack of sleep

Stress urinary **Incontinence** r/t increased pressure on bladder with contractions

Insomnia r/t contractions when lying down

Ineffective **Sexuality** pattern r/t fear of contractions associated with loss of infant

BREAST BIOPSY

Fear r/t potential for diagnosis of cancer

Risk for **Spiritual** distress: Risk factor: fear of diagnosis of cancer

Readiness for enhanced **Knowledge:** expresses an interest in learning

BREAST CANCER

Death **Anxiety** r/t diagnosis of cancer

Ineffective **Coping** r/t treatment, prognosis

Fear r/t diagnosis of cancer

Sexual dysfunction r/t loss of body part, partner's reaction to loss

Chronic **Sorrow** r/t diagnosis of cancer, loss of body integrity

Risk for **Spiritual** distress: Risk factor: fear of diagnosis of cancer

Readiness for enhanced **Knowledge:** expresses an interest in learning

See Cancer; Chemotherapy; Mastectomy; Radiation Therapy

BREAST EXAMINATION, SELF

See SBE (Self-Breast Examination)

BREAST LUMPS

Fear r/t potential for diagnosis of cancer

Readiness for enhanced **Knowledge:** expresses an interest in learning

BREAST PUMPING

Risk for **Infection:** Risk factors: possible contaminated breast pump, incomplete emptying of breast

Risk for impaired **Skin** integrity: Risk factor: high suction

Readiness for enhanced **Knowledge:** expresses an interest in learning

BREASTFEEDING, EFFECTIVE

Readiness for enhanced **Breastfeeding** (See **Breastfeeding,** readiness for enhanced, Section III)

BREASTFEEDING, INEFFECTIVE

Ineffective **Breastfeeding** (See **Breastfeeding,** ineffective, Section III)

See Infant Feeding Pattern, Ineffective; Painful Breasts, Engorgement; Painful Breasts, Sore Nipples

BREASTFEEDING, INTERRUPTED

Interrupted **Breastfeeding** (See **Breastfeeding,** interrupted, Section III)

BREAST MILK, INSUFFICIENT

Insufficient **Breast Milk** (See **Breast Milk,** insufficient, Section III)

BREATH SOUNDS, DECREASED OR ABSENT

See Atelectasis; Pneumothorax

BREATHING PATTERN ALTERATION

Ineffective **Breathing** pattern r/t neuromuscular impairment, pain, musculoskeletal impairment, perception or cognitive impairment, anxiety, decreased energy or fatigue

B

BREECH BIRTH

Fear: maternal r/t danger to infant, self

Impaired **Gas** exchange: fetal r/t compressed umbilical cord

Risk for **Aspiration:** fetal: Risk factor: birth of body before head

Risk for delayed **Development:** Risk factor: compressed umbilical cord

Risk for impaired **Tissue** integrity: fetal: Risk factor: difficult birth

Risk for impaired **Tissue** integrity: maternal: Risk factor: difficult birth

BRONCHITIS

Ineffective **Airway** clearance r/t excessive thickened mucus secretion

Readiness for enhanced **Health** management: wishes to stop smoking

Readiness for enhanced **Knowledge:** expresses an interest in learning

BRONCHOPULMONARY DYSPLASIA

Activity intolerance r/t imbalance between oxygen supply and demand

Excess **Fluid** volume r/t sodium and water retention

Imbalanced **Nutrition:** less than body requirements r/t poor feeding, increased caloric needs as a result of increased work of breathing

See Child with Chronic Condition; Hospitalized Child; Respiratory Conditions of the Neonate

BRONCHOSCOPY

Risk for **Aspiration:** Risk factor: temporary loss of gag reflex

Risk for **Injury:** Risk factors: complication of pneumothorax, laryngeal edema, hemorrhage (if biopsy done)

BRUITS, CAROTID

Risk for ineffective **Cerebral** tissue perfusion: Risk factor: interruption of carotid blood flow to brain

BRYANT'S TRACTION

See Traction and Casts

BUCK'S TRACTION

See Traction and Casts

BUERGER'S DISEASE

See Peripheral Vascular Disease (PVD)

BULIMIA

Disturbed **Body Image** r/t misperception about actual appearance, body weight

Compromised family **Coping** r/t chronically unresolved feelings of guilt, anger, hostility

Defensive **Coping** r/t eating disorder

Diarrhea r/t laxative abuse

Fear r/t food ingestion, weight gain

Imbalanced **Nutrition:** less than body requirements r/t induced vomiting, excessive exercise, laxative abuse

Powerlessness r/t urge to purge self after eating

Chronic low **Self-Esteem** r/t lack of positive feedback

See Maturational Issues, Adolescent

BUNION

Readiness for enhanced **Knowledge:** expresses an interest in learning

BUNIONECTOMY

Impaired physical **Mobility** r/t sore foot

Impaired **Walking** r/t pain associated with surgery

Risk for **Infection:** Risk factors: surgical incision, advanced age

Readiness for enhanced **Knowledge:** expresses an interest in learning

BURN RISK

Risk for **Thermal** injury (See **Thermal** injury, risk for, Section III)

BURNS

Anxiety r/t burn injury, treatments

Disturbed **Body Image** r/t altered physical appearance

Deficient **Diversional** activity r/t long-term hospitalization

Fear r/t pain from treatments, possible permanent disfigurement

Deficient **Fluid** volume r/t loss of protective skin

Grieving r/t loss of bodily function, loss of future hopes and plans

Hypothermia r/t impaired skin integrity

Impaired physical **Mobility** r/t pain, musculoskeletal impairment, contracture formation

Imbalanced **Nutrition:** less than body requirements r/t increased metabolic needs, anorexia, protein and fluid loss

Acute **Pain** r/t burn injury, treatments

Chronic **Pain** r/t burn injury, treatments

Ineffective peripheral **Tissue Perfusion** r/t circumferential burns, impaired arterial/venous circulation

Post-Trauma syndrome r/t life-threatening event

Impaired **Skin** integrity r/t injury of skin

Delayed **Surgical** recovery r/t ineffective tissue perfusion

Risk for ineffective **Airway** clearance: Risk factors: potential tracheobronchial obstruction, edema

Risk for deficient **Fluid** volume: Risk factors: loss from skin surface, fluid shift

Risk for **Infection:** Risk factors: loss of intact skin, trauma, invasive sites

Risk for **Peripheral Neurovascular** dysfunction: Risk factor: eschar formation with circumferential burn

Risk for **Post-Trauma** syndrome: Risk factors: perception, duration of event that caused burns

Readiness for enhanced **Knowledge:** expresses an interest in learning

See Hospitalized Child; Safety, Childhood

BURSITIS

Impaired physical **Mobility** r/t inflammation in joint

Acute **Pain** r/t inflammation in joint

BYPASS GRAFT

See Coronary Artery Bypass Grafting (CABG)

C

CABG (CORONARY ARTERY BYPASS GRAFTING)

See Coronary Artery Bypass Grafting (CABG)

CACHEXIA

Frail Elderly syndrome r/t fatigue, feeding self-care deficit

Imbalanced **Nutrition:** less than body requirements r/t inability to ingest food because of physiological factors

Risk for **Infection:** Risk factor: inadequate nutrition

CALCIUM ALTERATION

See Hypercalcemia; Hypocalcemia

CANCER

Activity intolerance r/t side effects of treatment, weakness from cancer

Death **Anxiety** r/t unresolved issues regarding dying

Disturbed **Body Image** r/t side effects of treatment, cachexia

Decisional Conflict r/t selection of treatment choices, continuation or discontinuation of treatment, "do not resuscitate" decision

Constipation r/t side effects of medication, altered nutrition, decreased activity

Compromised family **Coping** r/t prolonged disease or disability progression that exhausts supportive ability of significant others

Ineffective **Coping** r/t personal vulnerability in situational crisis, terminal illness

C

Ineffective **Denial** r/t complicated grieving process

Fear r/t serious threat to well-being

Grieving r/t potential loss of significant others, high risk for infertility

Ineffective **Health** maintenance r/t deficient knowledge regarding prescribed treatment

Hopelessness r/t loss of control, terminal illness

Insomnia r/t anxiety, pain

Impaired physical **Mobility** r/t weakness, neuromusculoskeletal impairment, pain

Imbalanced **Nutrition:** less than body requirements r/t loss of appetite, difficulty swallowing, side effects of chemotherapy, obstruction by tumor

Impaired **Oral Mucous Membrane** r/t chemotherapy, effects of radiation, oral pH changes, decreased oral secretions

Chronic **Pain** r/t metastatic cancer

Powerlessness r/t treatment, progression of disease

Ineffective **Protection** r/t cancer suppressing immune system

Ineffective **Role** performance r/t change in physical capacity, inability to resume prior role

Self-Care deficit: specify r/t pain, intolerance to activity, decreased strength

Impaired **Skin** integrity r/t immunological deficit, immobility

Social isolation r/t hospitalization, lifestyle changes

Chronic **Sorrow** r/t chronic illness of cancer

Spiritual distress r/t test of spiritual beliefs

Risk for **Bleeding:** Risk factor: bone marrow depression from chemotherapy

Risk for **Disuse** syndrome: Risk factors: immobility, fatigue

Risk for impaired **Home** maintenance: Risk factor: lack of familiarity with community resources

Risk for **Infection:** Risk factor: inadequate immune system

Risk for compromised **Resilience:** Risk factors: multiple stressors, pain, chronic illness

Risk for **Spiritual** distress: Risk factor: physical illness of cancer

Readiness for enhanced **Knowledge:** expresses an interest in learning

Readiness for enhanced **Spiritual** well-being: desire for harmony with self, others, higher power, God, when faced with serious illness

See Chemotherapy; Child with Chronic Condition; Hospitalized Child; Leukemia; Radiation Therapy; Terminally Ill Child, Adolescent; Terminally Ill Child, Infant/ Toddler; Terminally Ill Child, Preschool Child; Terminally Ill Child, School-Age Child/Preadolescent; Terminally Ill Child/ Death of Child, Parent

CANDIDIASIS, ORAL

Readiness for enhanced **Knowledge:** expresses an interest in learning

Impaired **Oral Mucous Membrane** r/t overgrowth of infectious agent, depressed immune function

Acute **Pain** r/t oral condition

CAPILLARY REFILL TIME, PROLONGED

Impaired **Gas** exchange r/t ventilation perfusion imbalance

Ineffective peripheral **Tissue Perfusion** r/t interruption of arterial flow

See Shock, Hypovolemic

CARBON MONOXIDE POISONING

See Smoke Inhalation

CARDIAC ARREST

Post-Trauma syndrome r/t experiencing serious life event

See Dysrhythmia, MI

CARDIAC CATHETERIZATION

Fear r/t invasive procedure, uncertainty of outcome of procedure

Risk for **Injury:** hematoma: Risk factor: invasive procedure

Risk for decreased **Cardiac** tissue perfusion: Risk factors: ventricular ischemia, dysrhythmia

Risk for **Peripheral Neurovascular** dysfunction: Risk factor: vascular obstruction

Risk for Impaired **Tissue** integrity: Risk factor: invasive procedure

Readiness for enhanced **Knowledge:** expresses an interest in learning postprocedure care, treatment, and prevention of coronary artery disease

CARDIAC DISORDERS

Decreased **Cardiac** output r/t cardiac disorder

Risk for decreased **Cardiac** tissue perfusion: Risk factor: cardiac disorder

See specific cardiac disorder

CARDIAC DISORDERS IN PREGNANCY

Activity intolerance r/t cardiac pathophysiology, increased demand for cardiac output because of pregnancy, weakness, fatigue

Death **Anxiety** r/t potential danger of condition

Compromised family **Coping** r/t prolonged hospitalization or maternal incapacitation that exhausts supportive capacity of significant others

Ineffective **Coping** r/t personal vulnerability

Interrupted **Family** processes r/t hospitalization, maternal incapacitation, changes in roles

Fatigue r/t physiological, psychological, and emotional demands

Fear r/t potential maternal effects, potential poor fetal or maternal outcome

Powerlessness r/t illness-related regimen

Ineffective **Role** performance r/t changes in lifestyle, expectations from disease process with superimposed pregnancy

Situational low **Self-Esteem** r/t situational crisis, pregnancy

Social isolation r/t limitations of activity, bed rest or hospitalization, separation from family and friends

Risk for decreased **Cardiac** tissue perfusion: Risk factor: strain on compromised heart from work of pregnancy, delivery

Risk for delayed **Development:** Risk factor: poor maternal oxygenation

Risk for deficient **Fluid** volume: Risk factor: sudden changes in circulation after delivery of placenta

Risk for excess **Fluid** volume: Risk factors: compromised regulatory mechanism with increased afterload, preload, circulating blood volume

Risk for impaired **Gas** exchange: Risk factor: pulmonary edema

Risk for disproportionate **Growth:** Risk factor: poor maternal oxygenation

Risk for disturbed **Maternal–Fetal** dyad: Risk factor: compromised oxygen transport

Risk for compromised **Resilience:** Risk factors: multiple stressors, fear

Risk for **Spiritual** distress: Risk factor: fear of diagnosis for self and infant

Readiness for enhanced **Knowledge:** expresses an interest in learning

CARDIAC DYSRHYTHMIA

See Dysrhythmia

CARDIAC OUTPUT, DECREASED

Decreased **Cardiac** output r/t cardiac dysfunction

Decreased **Cardiac** output (See **Cardiac** output, decreased, Section III)

Oliguria r/t cardiac dysfunction

Risk for decreased **Cardiac** output (See **Cardiac** output, risk for decreased, Section III)

C

CARDIAC TAMPONADE

Decreased **Cardiac** output r/t fluid in pericardial sac

See Pericarditis

CARDIOGENIC SHOCK

See Shock, Cardiogenic

CARDIOVASCULAR FUNCTION: RISK FOR IMPAIRED

Risk for Impaired **Cardiovascular** Function (See impaired **Cardiovascular** function, risk for, Section III)

CAREGIVER ROLE STRAIN

Caregiver Role Strain (See **Caregiver Role Strain,** Section III)

Risk for compromised **Resilience:** Risk factor: stress of prolonged caregiving

CARIOUS TEETH

See Cavities in Teeth

CAROTID ENDARTERECTOMY

Fear r/t surgery in vital area

Risk for ineffective **Airway** clearance: Risk factor: hematoma compressing trachea

Risk for **Bleeding:** Risk factors: possible hematoma formation, trauma to region

Risk for ineffective **Cerebral** tissue perfusion: Risk factors: hemorrhage, clot formation

Readiness for enhanced **Knowledge:** expresses an interest in learning

CARPAL TUNNEL SYNDROME

Impaired physical **Mobility** r/t neuromuscular impairment

Chronic **Pain** r/t unrelieved pressure on median nerve

Self-Care deficit: bathing, dressing, feeding r/t pain

CARPOPEDAL SPASM

See Hypocalcemia

CASTS

Deficient **Diversional** activity r/t physical limitations from cast

Impaired physical **Mobility** r/t limb immobilization

Self-Care deficit: bathing, dressing, feeding r/t presence of cast(s) on upper extremities

Self-Care deficit: toileting r/t presence of cast(s) on lower extremities

Impaired **Walking** r/t cast(s) on lower extremities, fracture of bones

Risk for **Peripheral Neurovascular** dysfunction: Risk factors: mechanical compression from cast, trauma from fracture

Risk for impaired **Skin** integrity: Risk factor: unrelieved pressure on skin from cast

Readiness for enhanced **Knowledge:** expresses an interest in learning

See Traction and Casts

CATARACT EXTRACTION

Anxiety r/t threat of permanent vision loss, surgical procedure

Vision Loss r/t edema from surgery (*see care plan in Appendix*)

Risk for **Injury:** Risk factors: increased intraocular pressure, accommodation to new visual field

Readiness for enhanced **Knowledge:** expresses an interest in learning

See Vision Impairment

CATARACTS

Vision Loss r/t impaired sensory input (*see care plan in Appendix*)

See Vision Impairment

CATATONIC SCHIZOPHRENIA

Impaired verbal **Communication** r/t cognitive impairment

Impaired **Memory** r/t cognitive impairment

Impaired physical **Mobility** r/t cognitive impairment, maintenance of rigid posture, inappropriate or bizarre postures

Imbalanced **Nutrition:** less than body requirements r/t decrease in outside stimulation, loss of perception of hunger, resistance to instructions to eat

Social isolation r/t inability to communicate, immobility

See Schizophrenia

CATHETERIZATION, URINARY

Risk for **Infection:** Risk factor: invasive procedure

Readiness for enhanced **Knowledge:** expresses an interest in learning

CAVITIES IN TEETH

Impaired **Dentition** r/t ineffective oral hygiene, barriers to self-care, economic barriers to professional care, nutritional deficits, dietary habits

CELIAC DISEASE

Diarrhea r/t malabsorption of food, immune effects of gluten on gastrointestinal system

Imbalanced **Nutrition:** less than body requirements r/t malabsorption due to immune effects of gluten

Readiness for enhanced **Knowledge:** expresses an interest in learning

CELLULITIS

Acute **Pain** r/t inflammatory changes in tissues from infection

Impaired **Tissue** integrity r/t inflammatory process damaging skin and underlying tissue

Ineffective peripheral **Tissue Perfusion** r/t edema of extremities

Risk for **Vascular Trauma:** Risk factor: infusion of antibiotics

Readiness for enhanced **Knowledge:** expresses an interest in learning

CELLULITIS, PERIORBITAL

Acute **Pain** r/t edema and inflammation of skin/tissues

Impaired **Skin** integrity r/t inflammation or infection of skin, tissues

Vision Loss r/t decreased visual field secondary to edema of eyelids (*see care plan in Appendix*)

Readiness for enhanced **Knowledge:** expresses an interest in learning

See Hospitalized Child

CENTRAL LINE INSERTION

Risk for **Infection:** Risk factor: invasive procedure

Risk for **Vascular Trauma** (See **Vascular Trauma,** risk for, Section III)

Readiness for enhanced **Knowledge:** expresses an interest in learning

CEREBRAL ANEURYSM

See Craniectomy/Craniotomy; Intracranial Pressure, Increased; Subarachnoid Hemorrhage

CEREBRAL PALSY

Impaired verbal **Communication** r/t impaired ability to articulate or speak words because of facial muscle involvement

Deficient **Diversional** activity r/t physical impairments, limitations on ability to participate in recreational activities

Impaired physical **Mobility** r/t spasticity, neuromuscular impairment or weakness

Imbalanced **Nutrition:** less than body requirements r/t spasticity, feeding or swallowing difficulties

Self-Care deficit: specify r/t neuromuscular impairments, sensory deficits

Impaired **Social** interaction r/t impaired communication skills, limited physical activity, perceived differences from peers

Chronic **Sorrow** r/t presence of chronic disability

C

Risk for **Falls:** Risk factor: impaired physical mobility

Risk for **Injury:** Risk factors: muscle weakness, inability to control spasticity

Risk for impaired **Parenting:** Risk factor: caring for child with overwhelming needs resulting from chronic change in health status

Risk for **Spiritual** distress: Risk factor: psychological stress associated with chronic illness

See Child with Chronic Condition

CEREBRAL PERFUSION

Risk for ineffective **Cerebral** tissue perfusion (See **Cerebral** tissue perfusion, ineffective, risk for, Section III)

CEREBROVASCULAR ACCIDENT (CVA)

See CVA (Cerebrovascular Accident)

CERVICITIS

Ineffective **Health** maintenance r/t deficient knowledge regarding care and prevention of condition

Ineffective **Sexuality** pattern r/t abstinence during acute stage

Risk for **Infection:** Risk factors: spread of infection, recurrence of infection

CESAREAN DELIVERY

Disturbed **Body Image** r/t surgery, unmet expectations for childbirth

Interrupted **Family** processes r/t unmet expectations for childbirth

Fear r/t perceived threat to own well-being, outcome of birth

Impaired physical **Mobility** r/t pain

Acute **Pain** r/t surgical incision

Ineffective **Role** performance r/t unmet expectations for childbirth

Situational low **Self-Esteem** r/t inability to deliver child vaginally

Risk for **Bleeding:** Risk factor: surgery

Risk for imbalanced **Fluid** volume: Risk factors: loss of blood, fluid shifts

Risk for **Infection:** Risk factor: surgical incision

Risk for **Urinary Retention:** Risk factor: regional anesthesia

Readiness for enhanced **Childbearing** process: a pattern of preparing for, maintaining, and strengthening care of newborn

Readiness for enhanced **Knowledge:** expresses an interest in learning

CHEMICAL DEPENDENCE

See Alcoholism; Drug Abuse; Cocaine Abuse; Substance Abuse

CHEMOTHERAPY

Death **Anxiety** r/t chemotherapy not accomplishing desired results

Disturbed **Body Image** r/t loss of weight, loss of hair

Fatigue r/t disease process, anemia, drug effects

Nausea r/t effects of chemotherapy

Imbalanced **Nutrition:** less than body requirements r/t side effects of chemotherapy

Impaired **Oral Mucous Membrane** r/t effects of chemotherapy

Ineffective **Protection** r/t suppressed immune system, decreased platelets

Risk for **Bleeding:** Risk factors: tumor eroding blood vessel, stress effects on gastrointestinal system

Risk for **Infection:** Risk factor: immunosuppression

Risk for **Vascular Trauma:** Risk factor: infusion of irritating medications

Readiness for enhanced **Knowledge:** expresses an interest in learning

See Cancer

CHEST PAIN

Fear r/t potential threat of death

Acute **Pain** r/t myocardial injury, ischemia

Risk for decreased **Cardiac** tissue perfusion: Risk factor: ventricular ischemia

See Angina; MI (Myocardial Infarction)

CHEST TUBES

Ineffective **Breathing** pattern r/t asymmetrical lung expansion secondary to pain

Impaired **Gas** exchange r/t decreased functional lung tissue

Acute **Pain** r/t presence of chest tubes, injury

Risk for **Injury:** Risk factor: presence of invasive chest tube

CHEYNE-STOKES RESPIRATION

Ineffective **Breathing** pattern r/t critical illness

See Heart Failure

CHF (CONGESTIVE HEART FAILURE)

See Heart Failure

CHICKENPOX

See Communicable Diseases, Childhood

CHILD ABUSE

Interrupted **Family** processes r/t inadequate coping skills

Fear r/t threat of punishment for perceived wrongdoing

Insomnia r/t hypervigilance, fear

Imbalanced **Nutrition:** less than body requirements r/t inadequate caretaking

Acute **Pain** r/t physical injuries

Impaired **Parenting** r/t psychological impairment, physical or emotional abuse of parent, substance abuse, unrealistic expectations of child

Post-Trauma syndrome r/t physical abuse, incest, rape, molestation

Chronic low **Self-Esteem** r/t lack of positive feedback, excessive negative feedback

Impaired **Skin** integrity r/t altered nutritional state, physical abuse

Social isolation: family imposed r/t fear of disclosure of family dysfunction and abuse

Risk for delayed **Development:** Risk factors: shaken baby syndrome, abuse

Risk for disproportionate **Growth:** Risk factor: abuse

Risk for **Poisoning:** Risk factors: inadequate safeguards, lack of proper safety precautions, accessibility of illicit substances because of impaired home maintenance

Risk for **Suffocation:** Risk factors: unattended child, unsafe environment

Risk for **Trauma:** Risk factors: inadequate precautions, cognitive or emotional difficulties

CHILDBEARING PROBLEMS

Ineffective **Childbearing** process (See **Childbearing** process, ineffective, Section III)

Risk for ineffective **Childbearing** process: See **Childbearing** process, risk for ineffective, Section III)

CHILD NEGLECT

See Child Abuse; Failure to Thrive, Nonorganic

CHILD WITH CHRONIC CONDITION

Activity intolerance r/t fatigue associated with chronic illness

Compromised family **Coping** r/t prolonged overconcern for child; distortion of reality regarding child's health problem, including extreme denial about its existence or severity

Disabled family **Coping** r/t prolonged disease or disability progression that exhausts supportive capacity of significant others

Ineffective **Coping:** child r/t situational or maturational crises

Decisional Conflict r/t treatment options, conflicting values

Deficient **Diversional** activity r/t immobility, monotonous environment, frequent or

C

lengthy treatments, reluctance to participate, self-imposed social isolation

Interrupted **Family** processes r/t intermittent situational crisis of illness, disease, hospitalization

Ineffective **Health** maintenance r/t exhausting family resources (finances, physical energy, support systems)

Impaired **Home** maintenance r/t overtaxed family members (e.g., exhausted, anxious)

Hopelessness: child r/t prolonged activity restriction, long-term stress, lack of involvement in or passively allowing care as a result of parental overprotection

Insomnia: child or parent r/t time-intensive treatments, exacerbation of condition, 24-hour care needs

Deficient **Knowledge** r/t knowledge or skill acquisition regarding health practices, acceptance of limitations, promotion of maximal potential of child, self-actualization of rest of family

Imbalanced **Nutrition:** less than body requirements r/t anorexia, fatigue from physical exertion

Risk for **Overweight** r/t effects of steroid medications on appetite

Chronic **Pain** r/t physical, biological, chemical, or psychological factors

Powerlessness: child r/t health care environment, illness-related regimen, lifestyle of learned helplessness

Parental **Role** conflict r/t separation from child as a result of chronic illness, home care of child with special needs, interruptions of family life resulting from home care regimen

Chronic low **Self-Esteem** r/t actual or perceived differences; peer acceptance; decreased ability to participate in physical, school, and social activities

Ineffective **Sexuality** pattern: parental r/t disrupted relationship with sexual partner

Impaired **Social** interaction r/t developmental lag or delay, perceived differences

Social isolation: family r/t actual or perceived social stigmatization, complex care requirements

Chronic **Sorrow** r/t developmental stages and missed opportunities or milestones that bring comparisons with social or personal norms, unending caregiving as reminder of loss

Risk for delayed **Development:** Risk factor: chronic illness

Risk for disproportionate **Growth:** Risk factor: chronic illness

Risk for **Infection:** Risk factor: debilitating physical condition

Risk for impaired **Parenting:** Risk factors: impaired or disrupted bonding, caring for child with perceived overwhelming care needs

Readiness for enhanced family **Coping:** impact of crisis on family values, priorities, goals, or relationships; changes in family choices to optimize wellness

CHILDBIRTH

Readiness for enhanced **Childbearing** process (See **Childbearing** process, readiness for enhanced, Section III)

See Labor, Normal; Postpartum, Normal Care

CHILLS

Hyperthermia r/t infectious process

CHLAMYDIA INFECTION

See STD (Sexually Transmitted Disease)

CHLOASMA

Disturbed **Body Image** r/t change in skin color

CHOKING OR COUGHING WITH EATING

Impaired **Swallowing** r/t neuromuscular impairment

Risk for **Aspiration:** Risk factors: depressed cough and gag reflexes

CHOLECYSTECTOMY

Imbalanced **Nutrition:** less than body requirements r/t high metabolic needs, decreased ability to digest fatty foods

Acute **Pain** r/t trauma from surgery

Risk for deficient **Fluid** volume: Risk factors: restricted intake, nausea, vomiting

Readiness for enhanced **Knowledge:** expresses an interest in learning

See Abdominal Surgery

CHOLELITHIASIS

Nausea r/t obstruction of bile

Imbalanced **Nutrition:** less than body requirements r/t anorexia, nausea, vomiting

Acute **Pain** r/t obstruction of bile flow, inflammation in gallbladder

Readiness for enhanced **Knowledge:** expresses an interest in learning

CHORIOAMNIONITIS

Anxiety r/t threat to self and infant

Grieving r/t guilt about potential loss of ideal pregnancy and birth

Hyperthermia r/t infectious process

Situational low **Self-Esteem** r/t guilt about threat to infant's health

Risk for **Infection:** Risk factors: infection transmission from mother to fetus, infection in fetal environment

CHRONIC CONFUSION

See Confusion, Chronic

CHRONIC FUNCTIONAL CONSTIPATION

(See **Constipation,** chronic functional, section III)

(See **Constipation,** chronic functional, risk for, section III)

CHRONIC LYMPHOCYTIC LEUKEMIA

See Cancer; Chemotherapy; Leukemia

CHRONIC OBSTRUCTIVE PULMONARY DISEASE (COPD)

See COPD (Chronic Obstructive Pulmonary Disease)

C

CHRONIC PAIN

See Pain, Chronic

CHRONIC RENAL FAILURE (CHRONIC KIDNEY DISEASE)

See Renal Failure

CHVOSTEK'S SIGN

See Hypocalcemia

CIRCUMCISION

Acute **Pain** r/t surgical intervention

Risk for **Bleeding:** Risk factor: surgical trauma

Risk for **Infection:** Risk factor: surgical wound

Readiness for enhanced **Knowledge:** parent: expresses an interest in learning

CIRRHOSIS

Chronic **Confusion** r/t chronic organic disorder with increased ammonia levels, substance abuse

Defensive **Coping** r/t inability to accept responsibility to stop substance abuse

Fatigue r/t malnutrition

Ineffective **Health** maintenance r/t deficient knowledge regarding correlation between lifestyle habits and disease process

Nausea r/t irritation to gastrointestinal system

Imbalanced **Nutrition:** less than body requirements r/t loss of appetite, nausea, vomiting

Chronic **Pain** r/t liver enlargement

Chronic low **Self-Esteem** r/t chronic illness

Chronic **Sorrow** r/t presence of chronic illness

Risk for **Bleeding:** Risk factors: impaired blood coagulation, bleeding from portal hypertension

Risk for **Injury:** Risk factors: substance intoxication, potential delirium tremens

Risk for impaired **Oral Mucous Membrane:** Risk factors: altered nutrition, inadequate oral care

Risk for impaired **Skin** integrity: Risk factors: altered nutritional state, altered metabolic state

CLEFT LIP/CLEFT PALATE

Ineffective **Airway** clearance r/t common feeding and breathing passage, postoperative laryngeal, incisional edema

Ineffective **Breastfeeding** r/t infant anomaly

Impaired verbal **Communication** r/t inadequate palate function, possible hearing loss from infected eustachian tubes

Fear: parental r/t special care needs, surgery

Grieving r/t loss of perfect child

Ineffective infant **Feeding** pattern r/t cleft lip, cleft palate

Impaired physical **Mobility** r/t imposed restricted activity, use of elbow restraints

Impaired **Oral Mucous Membrane** r/t surgical correction

Acute **Pain** r/t surgical correction, elbow restraints

Impaired **Skin** integrity r/t incomplete joining of lip, palate ridges

Chronic **Sorrow** r/t birth of child with congenital defect

Risk for **Aspiration:** Risk factor: common feeding and breathing passage

Risk for disturbed **Body Image:** Risk factors: disfigurement, speech impediment

Risk for delayed **Development:** Risk factor: inadequate nutrition resulting from difficulty feeding

Risk for deficient **Fluid** volume: Risk factor: inability to take liquids in usual manner

Risk for disproportionate **Growth:** Risk factor: inability to feed with normal techniques

Risk for **Infection:** Risk factors: invasive procedure, disruption of eustachian tube development, aspiration

Readiness for enhanced **Knowledge:** parent: expresses an interest in learning

CLOTTING DISORDER

Fear r/t threat to well-being

Risk for **Bleeding:** Risk factor: impaired clotting

Readiness for enhanced **Knowledge:** expresses an interest in learning

See Anticoagulant Therapy; DIC (Disseminated Intravascular Coagulation); Hemophilia

COCAINE ABUSE

Ineffective **Breathing** pattern r/t drug effect on respiratory center

Chronic **Confusion** r/t excessive stimulation of nervous system by cocaine

Ineffective **Coping** r/t inability to deal with life stresses

Risk for decreased **Cardiac** tissue perfusion r/t increase in sympathetic response in the body damaging the heart

See Drug Abuse; Substance Abuse

COCAINE BABY

See Crack Baby; Infant of Substance-Abusing Mother

CODEPENDENCY

Caregiver Role Strain r/t codependency

Impaired verbal **Communication** r/t psychological barriers

Ineffective **Coping** r/t inadequate support systems

Decisional Conflict r/t support system deficit

Ineffective **Denial** r/t unmet self-needs

Powerlessness r/t lifestyle of helplessness

COLD, VIRAL

Readiness for enhanced **Comfort** (See **Comfort**, readiness for enhanced, Section III)

Readiness for enhanced **Knowledge:** expresses an interest in learning

COLECTOMY

Constipation r/t decreased activity, decreased fluid intake

Imbalanced **Nutrition:** less than body requirements r/t high metabolic needs, decreased ability to ingest or digest food

Acute **Pain** r/t recent surgery

Risk for **Infection:** Risk factor: invasive procedure

Readiness for enhanced **Knowledge:** expresses an interest in learning

See Abdominal Surgery

COLITIS

Diarrhea r/t inflammation in colon

Deficient **Fluid** volume r/t frequent stools

Acute **Pain** r/t inflammation in colon

Readiness for enhanced **Knowledge:** expresses an interest in learning

See Crohn's Disease; Inflammatory Bowel Disease (Child and Adult)

COLLAGEN DISEASE

See specific disease (e.g., lupus erythematosus; JRA [juvenile rheumatoid arthritis]); Congenital Heart Disease/ Cardiac Anomalies

COLOSTOMY

Disturbed **Body Image** r/t presence of stoma, daily care of fecal material

Ineffective **Sexuality** pattern r/t altered body image, self-concept

Social isolation r/t anxiety about appearance of stoma and possible leakage of stool

Risk for **Constipation:** Risk factor: inappropriate diet

Risk for **Diarrhea:** Risk factor: inappropriate diet

Risk for impaired **Skin** integrity: Risk factor: irritation from bowel contents

Readiness for enhanced **Knowledge:** expresses an interest in learning

COLPORRHAPHY, ANTERIOR

See Vaginal Hysterectomy

COMA

Death Anxiety: significant others r/t unknown outcome of coma state

Interrupted **Family** processes r/t illness or disability of family member

Functional urinary **Incontinence** r/t presence of comatose state

Self-Care deficit: r/t neuromuscular impairment

Ineffective family **Health** management r/t complexity of therapeutic regimen

Risk for **Aspiration:** Risk factors: impaired swallowing, loss of cough or gag reflex

Risk for **Disuse** syndrome: Risk factor: altered level of consciousness impairing mobility

Risk for **Hypothermia:** Risk factors: inactivity, possible pharmaceutical agents, possible hypothalamic injury

Risk for **Injury:** Risk factor: potential seizure activity

Risk for corneal **Injury:** Risk factor: suppressed corneal reflex

Risk for urinary tract **Injury:** Risk factor: long-term use of urinary catheter

Risk for impaired **Oral Mucous Membrane:** Risk factors: dry mouth, inability to do own mouth care

Risk for **Pressure** ulcer: Risk factor: prolonged immobility

Risk for impaired **Skin** integrity: Risk factor: immobility

Risk for **Spiritual** distress: significant others: Risk factors: loss of ability to relate to loved one, unknown outcome of coma

Risk for impaired **Tissue** integrity: Risk factor: impaired physical mobility

See Head Injury, Subarachnoid Hemorrhage, Increased Intracranial Pressure

C

COMFORT, LOSS OF

Impaired **Comfort** (See **Comfort,** impaired, Section III)

Readiness for enhanced **Comfort** (See **Comfort,** readiness for enhanced, Section III)

COMMUNICABLE DISEASES, CHILDHOOD (E.G., MEASLES, MUMPS, RUBELLA, CHICKENPOX, SCABIES, LICE, IMPETIGO)

Impaired **Comfort** r/t pruritus, inflammation or infection of skin, subdermal organisms

Deficient **Diversional** activity r/t imposed isolation from peers, disruption in usual play activities, fatigue, activity intolerance

Ineffective **Health** maintenance r/t nonadherence to appropriate immunization schedules, lack of prevention of transmission of infection

Acute **Pain** r/t impaired skin integrity, edema

Risk for **Infection:** transmission to others: Risk factor: contagious organisms

See Meningitis/Encephalitis; Respiratory Infections, Acute Childhood; Reye's Syndrome

COMMUNICATION

Readiness for enhanced **Communication** (See **Communication**, readiness for enhanced, Section III)

COMMUNICATION PROBLEMS

Impaired verbal **Communication** (See **Communication**, verbal, impaired, Section III)

COMMUNITY COPING

Ineffective community **Coping** (See **Coping,** community, ineffective, Section III)

Readiness for enhanced community **Coping:** community sense of power to manage stressors, social supports available, resources available for problem solving

COMMUNITY HEALTH PROBLEMS

Deficient community **Health** (See **Health,** deficient, community, Section III)

COMPARTMENT SYNDROME

Fear r/t possible loss of limb, damage to limb

Acute **Pain** r/t pressure in compromised body part

Ineffective peripheral **Tissue Perfusion** r/t increased pressure within compartment

COMPULSION

See OCD (Obsessive-Compulsive Disorder)

CONDUCTION DISORDERS (CARDIAC)

See Dysrhythmia

CONFUSION, ACUTE

Acute **Confusion** r/t older than 70 years of age with hospitalization, alcohol abuse, delirium, dementia, drug abuse

Frail Elderly syndrome r/t impaired memory

CONFUSION, CHRONIC

Chronic **Confusion** r/t dementia, Korsakoff's psychosis, multi-infarct dementia, cerebrovascular accident, head injury

Frail Elderly syndrome r/t impaired memory

Impaired **Memory** r/t fluid and electrolyte imbalance, neurological disturbances, excessive environmental disturbances, anemia, acute or chronic hypoxia, decreased cardiac output

Impaired **Mood** regulation r/t emotional instability

See Alzheimer's Disease; Dementia

CONFUSION, POSSIBLE

Risk for acute **Confusion:** Risk factor (See **Confusion,** acute, risk for, Section III)

CONGENITAL HEART DISEASE/ CARDIAC ANOMALIES

Activity intolerance r/t fatigue, generalized weakness, lack of adequate oxygenation

Ineffective **Breathing** pattern r/t pulmonary vascular disease

Decreased **Cardiac** output r/t cardiac dysfunction

Excess **Fluid** volume r/t cardiac dysfunction, side effects of medication

Impaired **Gas** exchange r/t cardiac dysfunction, pulmonary congestion

Imbalanced **Nutrition:** less than body requirements r/t fatigue, generalized weakness, inability of infant to suck and feed, increased caloric requirements

Risk for delayed **Development:** Risk factor: inadequate oxygen and nutrients to tissues

Risk for deficient **Fluid** volume: Risk factor: side effects of diuretics

Risk for disproportionate **Growth:** Risk factor: inadequate oxygen and nutrients to tissues

Risk for disorganized **Infant** behavior: Risk factor: invasive procedures

Risk for **Poisoning:** Risk factor: potential toxicity of cardiac medications

Risk for ineffective **Thermoregulation:** Risk factor: neonatal age

See Child with Chronic Condition; Hospitalized Child

CONGESTIVE HEART FAILURE (CHF)/HEART FAILURE (HF)

See CHF (Congestive Heart Failure)

CONJUNCTIVITIS

Acute **Pain** r/t inflammatory process

Vision Loss r/t change in visual acuity resulting from inflammation

CONSCIOUSNESS, ALTERED LEVEL OF

Acute **Confusion** r/t alcohol abuse, delirium, dementia, drug abuse, head injury

Chronic **Confusion** r/t multi-infarct dementia, Korsakoff's psychosis, head injury, cerebrovascular accident, neurological deficit, **Frail Elderly** syndrome

Functional urinary **Incontinence** r/t neurological dysfunction

Decreased **Intracranial** adaptive capacity r/t brain injury

Impaired **Memory** r/t neurological disturbances

Self-Care deficit: specify r/t neuromuscular impairment

Risk for **Aspiration:** Risk factors: impaired swallowing, loss of cough or gag reflex

Risk for **Disuse** syndrome: Risk factor: impaired mobility resulting from altered level of consciousness

Risk for **Falls:** Risk factor: diminished mental status

Risk for impaired **Oral Mucous Membrane:** Risk factors: dry mouth, interrupted oral care

Risk for ineffective **Cerebral** tissue perfusion: Risk factors: increased intracranial pressure, altered cerebral perfusion

Risk for impaired **Skin** integrity: Risk factor: immobility

See Coma, Head Injury, Subarachnoid Hemorrhage, Increased Intracranial Pressure

CONSTIPATION

Constipation (See **Constipation,** Section II)

CONSTIPATION, CHRONIC FUNCTIONAL

Constipation (See **Constipation,** chronic functional, Section III)

CONSTIPATION, PERCEIVED

Perceived **Constipation** (See perceived **Constipation,** Section III)

CONSTIPATION, RISK FOR

Risk for **Constipation** (See **Constipation,** risk for, Section III)

Risk for chronic functional **Constipation** (See **Constipation**, chronic functional, risk for, Section III)

C CONTAMINATION

Contamination (See **Contamination**, Section III)

Risk for **Contamination** (See **Contamination**, risk for, Section III)

CONTINENT ILEOSTOMY (KOCK POUCH)

Ineffective **Coping** r/t stress of disease, exacerbations caused by stress

Imbalanced **Nutrition:** less than body requirements r/t malabsorption from disease process

Risk for **Injury:** Risk factors: failure of valve, stomal cyanosis, intestinal obstruction

Readiness for enhanced **Knowledge:** expresses an interest in learning

See Abdominal Surgery, Crohn's Disease

CONTRACEPTIVE METHOD

Decisional Conflict: method of contraception r/t unclear personal values or beliefs, lack of experience or interference with decision-making, lack of relevant information, support system deficit

Ineffective **Sexuality** pattern r/t fear of pregnancy

Readiness for enhanced **Health** management: requesting information about available and appropriate birth control methods

CONVULSIONS

Anxiety r/t concern over controlling convulsions

Impaired **Memory** r/t neurological disturbance

Risk for **Aspiration:** Risk factor: impaired swallowing

Risk for delayed **Development:** Risk factor: seizures

Risk for **Injury:** Risk factor: seizure activity

Readiness for enhanced **Knowledge:** expresses an interest in learning

See Seizure Disorders, Adult; Seizure Disorders, Childhood

COPD (CHRONIC OBSTRUCTIVE PULMONARY DISEASE)

Activity intolerance r/t imbalance between oxygen supply and demand

Ineffective **Airway** clearance r/t bronchoconstriction, increased mucus, ineffective cough, infection

Anxiety r/t breathlessness, change in health status

Death **Anxiety** r/t seriousness of medical condition, difficulty being able to "catch breath," feeling of suffocation

Interrupted **Family** processes r/t role changes

Impaired **Gas** exchange r/t ventilation-perfusion inequality

Ineffective **Health** management (See **Health** management, ineffective, Section III)

Imbalanced **Nutrition:** less than body requirements r/t decreased intake because of dyspnea, unpleasant taste in mouth left by medications, increased need for calories from work of breathing

Powerlessness r/t progressive nature of disease

Self-Care deficit: r/t fatigue from the increased work of breathing

Chronic low **Self-Esteem** r/t chronic illness

Sleep deprivation r/t breathing difficulties when lying down

Impaired **Social** interaction r/t social isolation because of oxygen use, activity intolerance

Chronic **Sorrow** r/t presence of chronic illness

Risk for **Infection:** Risk factor: stasis of respiratory secretions

Readiness for enhanced **Health** management (See **Health** management, readiness for enhanced, Section III)

COPING

Readiness for enhanced **Coping**
(See **Coping**, readiness for enhanced,
Section III)

COPING PROBLEMS

Compromised family **Coping** (see **Coping**,
compromised family, Section III)

Defensive **Coping** (See **Coping**, defensive,
Section III)

Disabled family **Coping** (See **Coping**,
disabled family, Section III)

Ineffective **Coping** (See **Coping**, ineffective,
Section III)

Ineffective community **Coping** (see **Coping**,
ineffective community, Section III)

CORNEAL INJURY

Risk for corneal **Injury** (See corneal **Injury**,
risk for, Section III)

CORNEAL REFLEX, ABSENT

Risk for **Injury**: Risk factors: accidental
corneal abrasion, drying of cornea

CORNEAL TRANSPLANT

Risk for **Infection**: Risk factors: invasive
procedure, surgery

Readiness for enhanced **Health**
management: describes need to rest and
avoid strenuous activities during healing
phase

CORONARY ARTERY BYPASS GRAFTING (CABG)

Decreased **Cardiac** output r/t dysrhythmia,
depressed cardiac function, change in
preload, contractility or afterload

Fear r/t outcome of surgical
procedure

Deficient **Fluid** volume r/t intraoperative
blood loss, use of diuretics in surgery

Acute **Pain** r/t traumatic surgery

Risk for **Perioperative Positioning** injury:
Risk factors: hypothermia, extended supine
position

Risk for impaired **Tissue** integrity: Risk
factor: surgical procedure

Readiness for enhanced **Knowledge**:
expresses an interest in learning

C

COSTOVERTEBRAL ANGLE TENDERNESS

See Kidney Stone; Pyelonephritis

COUGH, INEFFECTIVE

Ineffective **Airway** clearance r/t decreased
energy, fatigue, normal aging changes

*See Bronchitis; COPD (Chronic
Obstructive Pulmonary Disease);
Pulmonary Edema*

CRACK ABUSE

*See Cocaine Abuse; Drug Abuse;
Substance Abuse*

CRACK BABY

Disorganized **Infant** behavior r/t
prematurity, drug withdrawal, lack of
attachment

Risk for impaired **Attachment**: Risk factors:
parent's inability to meet infant's needs,
substance abuse

Risk for disturbed **Maternal–Fetal** dyad:
Risk factor: substance abuse

See Infant of Substance-Abusing Mother

CRACKLES IN LUNGS, COARSE

Ineffective **Airway** clearance r/t excessive
secretions in airways, ineffective cough

*See Heart Failure; Pneumonia;
Pulmonary Edema*

CRACKLES IN LUNGS, FINE

Ineffective **Breathing** pattern r/t fatigue,
surgery, decreased energy

*See Bronchitis or Pneumonia (if from
pulmonary infection); CHF (Congestive
Heart Failure) (if cardiac in origin);
Infection*

CRANIECTOMY/CRANIOTOMY

Frail Elderly syndrome r/t alteration in
cognition

C

Fear r/t threat to well-being

Decreased **Intracranial** adaptive capacity r/t brain injury, intracranial hypertension

Impaired **Memory** r/t neurological surgery

Acute **Pain** r/t recent brain surgery, increased intracranial pressure

Risk for ineffective **Cerebral** tissue perfusion: Risk factors: cerebral edema, increased intracranial pressure

Risk for **Injury:** Risk factor: potential confusion

See Coma (if relevant)

CREPITATION, SUBCUTANEOUS

See Pneumothorax

CRISIS

Anxiety r/t threat to or change in environment, health status, interaction patterns, situation, self-concept, or role functioning; threat of death of self or significant other

Death **Anxiety** r/t feelings of hopelessness associated with crisis

Compromised family **Coping** r/t situational or developmental crisis

Ineffective **Coping** r/t situational or maturational crisis

Fear r/t crisis situation

Grieving r/t potential significant loss

Impaired individual **Resilience** r/t onset of crisis

Situational low **Self-Esteem** r/t perception of inability to handle crisis

Stress overload (See **Stress** overload, Section III)

Risk for **Spiritual** distress: Risk factors: physical or psychological stress, natural disasters, situational losses, maturational losses

CROHN'S DISEASE

Anxiety r/t change in health status

Ineffective **Coping** r/t repeated episodes of diarrhea

Diarrhea r/t inflammatory process

Ineffective **Health** maintenance r/t deficient knowledge regarding management of disease

Imbalanced **Nutrition:** less than body requirements r/t diarrhea, altered ability to digest and absorb food

Acute **Pain** r/t increased peristalsis

Powerlessness r/t chronic disease

Risk for deficient **Fluid** volume: Risk factor: abnormal fluid loss with diarrhea

CROUP

See Respiratory Infections, Acute Childhood

CRYOSURGERY FOR RETINAL DETACHMENT

See Retinal Detachment

CUSHING'S SYNDROME

Activity intolerance r/t fatigue, weakness

Disturbed **Body Image** r/t change in appearance from disease process

Excess **Fluid** volume r/t failure of regulatory mechanisms

Sexual dysfunction r/t loss of libido

Impaired **Skin** integrity r/t thin vulnerable skin from effects of increased cortisol

Risk for **Infection:** Risk factor: suppression of immune system caused by increased cortisol levels

Risk for **Injury:** Risk factors: decreased muscle strength, brittle bones

Readiness for enhanced **Knowledge:** expresses an interest in learning

CUTS (WOUNDS)

See Lacerations

CVA (CEREBROVASCULAR ACCIDENT)

Anxiety r/t situational crisis, change in physical or emotional condition

Disturbed **Body Image** r/t chronic illness, paralysis

Caregiver Role Strain r/t cognitive problems of care receiver, need for significant home care

Impaired verbal **Communication** r/t pressure damage, decreased circulation to brain in speech center informational sources

Chronic **Confusion** r/t neurological changes

Constipation r/t decreased activity

Ineffective **Coping** r/t disability

Interrupted **Family** processes r/t illness, disability of family member

Frail Elderly syndrome r/t alteration in cognitive functioning

Grieving r/t loss of health

Impaired **Home** maintenance r/t neurological disease affecting ability to perform activities of daily living

Functional urinary **Incontinence** r/t neurological dysfunction

Reflex urinary **Incontinence** r/t loss of feeling to void

Impaired **Memory** r/t neurological disturbances

Impaired physical **Mobility** r/t loss of balance and coordination

Unilateral Neglect r/t disturbed perception from neurological damage

Self-Care deficit: specify r/t decreased strength and endurance, paralysis

Impaired **Social** interaction r/t limited physical mobility, limited ability to communicate

Impaired **Swallowing** r/t neuromuscular dysfunction

Impaired **Transfer Ability** r/t limited physical mobility

Vision Loss r/t pressure damage to visual centers in the brain (*see care plan in Appendix*)

Impaired **Walking** r/t loss of balance and coordination

Risk for **Aspiration:** Risk factors: impaired swallowing, loss of gag reflex

Risk for chronic functional **Constipation:** Risk factor: immobility

Risk for **Disuse** syndrome: Risk factor: paralysis

Risk for **Falls:** Risk factors: paralysis, decreased balance

Risk for **Injury:** Risk factors: vision loss, decreased tissue perfusion with loss of sensation

Risk for ineffective **Cerebral** tissue perfusion: Risk factor: clot, emboli, or hemorrhage from cerebral vessel

Risk for impaired **Skin** integrity: Risk factor: immobility

Readiness for enhanced **Knowledge:** expresses an interest in learning

CYANOSIS, CENTRAL WITH CYANOSIS OF ORAL MUCOUS MEMBRANES

Impaired **Gas** exchange r/t alveolar-capillary membrane changes

CYANOSIS, PERIPHERAL WITH CYANOSIS OF NAIL BEDS

Ineffective peripheral **Tissue Perfusion** r/t interruption of arterial flow, severe vasoconstriction, cold temperatures

CYSTIC FIBROSIS

Activity intolerance r/t imbalance between oxygen supply and demand

Ineffective **Airway** clearance r/t increased production of thick mucus

Anxiety r/t dyspnea, oxygen deprivation

Disturbed **Body Image** r/t changes in physical appearance, treatment of chronic lung disease (clubbing, barrel chest, home oxygen therapy)

Impaired **Gas** exchange r/t ventilation-perfusion imbalance

Impaired **Home** maintenance r/t extensive daily treatment, medications necessary for health

Imbalanced **Nutrition:** less than body requirements r/t anorexia; decreased absorption of nutrients, fat; increased work of breathing

Chronic **Sorrow** r/t presence of chronic disease

Risk for **Caregiver Role Strain**: Risk factors: illness severity of care receiver, unpredictable course of illness

Risk for deficient **Fluid** volume: Risk factors: decreased fluid intake, increased work of breathing

Risk for **Infection**: Risk factors: thick, tenacious mucus; harboring of bacterial organisms; immunocompromised state

Risk for **Spiritual** distress: Risk factor: presence of chronic disease

See Child with Chronic Condition; Hospitalized Child; Terminally Ill Child, Adolescent; Terminally Ill Child, Infant/ Toddler; Terminally Ill Child, Preschool Child; Terminally Ill Child, School-Age Child/Preadolescent; Terminally Ill Child/ Death of Child, Parent

CYSTITIS

Acute **Pain**: dysuria r/t inflammatory process in bladder and urethra

Impaired **Urinary** elimination: frequency r/t urinary tract infection

Urge urinary **Incontinence**: Risk factor: infection in bladder

Readiness for enhanced **Knowledge**: expresses an interest in learning

CYSTOCELE

Stress urinary **Incontinence** r/t prolapsed bladder

Readiness for enhanced **Knowledge**: expresses an interest in learning

CYSTOSCOPY

Urinary Retention r/t edema in urethra obstructing flow of urine

Risk for **Infection**: Risk factor: invasive procedure

Readiness for enhanced **Knowledge**: expresses an interest in learning

D

DEAFNESS

Impaired verbal **Communication** r/t impaired hearing

Hearing Loss r/t alteration in sensory reception, transmission, integration

Risk for delayed **Development**: Risk factor: impaired hearing

Risk for **Injury**: Risk factor: alteration in sensory perception

DEATH

Risk for **Sudden Infant Death** syndrome (SIDS) (See **Sudden Infant Death** syndrome, risk for, Section III)

DEATH, ONCOMING

Death **Anxiety** r/t unresolved issues surrounding dying

Compromised family **Coping** r/t client's inability to provide support to family

Ineffective **Coping** r/t personal vulnerability

Fear r/t threat of death

Grieving r/t loss of significant other

Powerlessness r/t effects of illness, oncoming death

Social isolation r/t altered state of wellness

Spiritual distress r/t intense suffering

Readiness for enhanced **Spiritual** well-being: desire of client and family to be in harmony with each other and higher power, God

See Terminally Ill Child, Adolescent; Terminally Ill Child, Infant/Toddler; Terminally Ill Child, Preschool Child; Terminally Ill Child, School-Age Child/ Preadolescent; Terminally Ill Child/Death of Child, Parent

DECISIONS, DIFFICULTY MAKING

Decisional Conflict r/t support system deficit, perceived threat to value system, multiple or divergent sources of information, lack of relevant information, unclear personal values or beliefs

Readiness for enhanced **Decision-Making** (See **Decision-Making,** readiness for enhanced, Section III)

DECUBITUS ULCER

See Pressure Ulcer

DEEP VEIN THROMBOSIS (DVT)

See DVT (Deep Vein Thrombosis)

DEFENSIVE BEHAVIOR

Defensive **Coping** r/t nonacceptance of blame, denial of problems or weakness

Ineffective **Denial** r/t inability to face situation realistically

DEHISCENCE, ABDOMINAL

Fear r/t threat of death, severe dysfunction

Acute **Pain** r/t stretching of abdominal wall

Impaired **Skin** integrity r/t altered circulation, malnutrition, opening in incision

Delayed **Surgical** recovery r/t altered circulation, malnutrition, opening in incision

Impaired **Tissue** integrity r/t exposure of abdominal contents to external environment

Risk for deficient **Fluid** volume: Risk factor: altered circulation associated with opening of wound and exposure of abdominal contents

Risk for **Infection:** Risk factors: loss of skin integrity, open surgical wound

DEHYDRATION

Deficient **Fluid** volume r/t active fluid volume loss

Impaired **Oral Mucous Membrane** r/t decreased salivation, fluid deficit

Risk for chronic functional **Constipation:** Risk factor: decreased fluid volume

Risk for imbalanced body **Temperature:** Risk factor: hyperthermia due to sensible water loss

See Burns; Heat Stroke; Vomiting; Diarrhea

DELIRIUM

Acute **Confusion** r/t effects of medication, response to hospitalization, alcohol abuse, substance abuse, sensory deprivation or overload, infection, polypharmacy

Impaired **Memory** r/t delirium

Sleep deprivation r/t sustained inadequate sleep hygiene

Risk for **Injury:** Risk factor: altered level of consciousness

DELIRIUM TREMENS (DT)

See Alcohol Withdrawal

DELIVERY

See Labor, Normal

DELUSIONS

Impaired verbal **Communication** r/t psychological impairment, delusional thinking

Acute **Confusion** r/t alcohol abuse, delirium, dementia, drug abuse

Ineffective **Coping** r/t distortion and insecurity of life events

Fear r/t content of intrusive thoughts

Risk for other-directed **Violence:** Risk factor: delusional thinking

Risk for self-directed **Violence:** Risk factor: delusional thinking

DEMENTIA

Chronic **Confusion** r/t neurological dysfunction

Interrupted **Family** processes r/t disability of family member

Frail Elderly syndrome r/t alteration in cognitive functioning

Impaired **Home** maintenance r/t inadequate support system, neurological dysfunction

Imbalanced **Nutrition:** less than body requirements r/t neurological impairment

Functional urinary **Incontinence** r/t neurological dysfunction

Insomnia r/t neurological impairment, naps during the day

Impaired physical **Mobility** r/t alteration in cognitive function

Self-Neglect r/t cognitive impairment

Self-Care deficit: specify r/t psychological or neuromuscular impairment

Chronic **Sorrow:** Significant other r/t chronic long-standing disability, loss of mental function

Impaired **Swallowing** r/t neuromuscular changes associated with long-standing dementia

Risk for **Caregiver Role Strain:** Risk factors: number of caregiving tasks, duration of caregiving required

Risk for Chronic Functional **Constipation:** Risk factor: decreased fluid intake

Risk for **Falls:** Risk factor: diminished mental status

Risk for **Frail Elderly** syndrome: risk factors: cognitive impairment

Risk for **Injury:** Risk factors: confusion, decreased muscle coordination

Risk for impaired **Skin** integrity: Risk factors: altered nutritional status, immobility

DENIAL OF HEALTH STATUS

Ineffective **Denial** r/t lack of perception about the health status effects of illness

Ineffective **Health** management r/t denial of seriousness of health situation

DENTAL CARIES

Impaired **Dentition** r/t ineffective oral hygiene, barriers to self-care, economic barriers to professional care, nutritional deficits, dietary habits

Ineffective **Health** maintenance r/t lack of knowledge regarding prevention of dental disease

DEPRESSION (MAJOR DEPRESSIVE DISORDER)

Death **Anxiety** r/t feelings of lack of self-worth

Constipation r/t inactivity, decreased fluid intake

Fatigue r/t psychological demands

Ineffective **Health** maintenance r/t lack of ability to make good judgments regarding ways to obtain help

Hopelessness r/t feeling of abandonment, long-term stress

Impaired **Mood** Regulation r/t emotional instability

Insomnia r/t inactivity

Self-Neglect r/t depression, cognitive impairment

Powerlessness r/t pattern of helplessness

Chronic low **Self-Esteem** r/t repeated unmet expectations

Sexual dysfunction r/t loss of sexual desire

Social isolation r/t ineffective coping

Chronic **Sorrow** r/t unresolved grief

Risk for complicated **Grieving:** Risk factor: lack of previous resolution of former grieving response

Risk for **Suicide:** Risk factors: grieving, hopelessness

DERMATITIS

Anxiety r/t situational crisis imposed by illness

Impaired **Comfort** r/t itching

Impaired **Skin** integrity r/t side effect of medication, allergic reaction

Readiness for enhanced **Knowledge:** expresses an interest in learning

See Itching

DESPONDENCY

Hopelessness r/t long-term stress

See Depression (Major Depressive Disorder)

DESTRUCTIVE BEHAVIOR TOWARD OTHERS

Risk-prone **Health** behavior r/t intense emotional state

Ineffective **Coping** r/t situational crises, maturational crises, disturbance in pattern of appraisal of threat

Risk for other-directed **Violence** (See **Violence**, other-directed, risk for, Section III)

DEVELOPMENTAL CONCERNS

Risk for delayed **Development** (See **Development**, delayed, risk for, Section III)

See Growth and Development Lag

DIABETES IN PREGNANCY

See Gestational Diabetes (Diabetes in Pregnancy)

DIABETES INSIPIDUS

Deficient **Fluid** volume r/t inability to conserve fluid

Ineffective **Health** maintenance r/t deficient knowledge regarding care of disease, importance of medications

DIABETES MELLITUS

Ineffective **Health** maintenance r/t complexity of therapeutic regimen

Ineffective **Health** management (See **Health** management, ineffective, Section III)

Imbalanced **Nutrition:** less than body requirements r/t inability to use glucose (type 1 [insulin-dependent] diabetes)

Risk for **Overweight** r/t excessive intake of nutrients (type 2 diabetes)

Ineffective peripheral **Tissue** perfusion r/t impaired arterial circulation

Powerlessness r/t perceived lack of personal control

Sexual dysfunction r/t neuropathy associated with disease

Vision Loss r/t ineffective tissue perfusion of retina

Risk for unstable blood **Glucose** level (See **Glucose** level, blood, unstable, risk for, Section III)

Risk for **Infection:** Risk factors: hyperglycemia, impaired healing, circulatory changes

Risk for **Injury:** Risk factors: hypoglycemia or hyperglycemia from failure to consume adequate calories, failure to take insulin

Risk for dysfunctional **Gastrointestinal** motility: Risk factor: complication of diabetes

Risk for impaired **Skin** integrity: Risk factor: loss of pain perception in extremities

Risk for delayed **Surgical** recovery: Risk factor: impaired healing due to circulatory changes

Readiness for enhanced **Health** management (See **Health** management, readiness for enhanced, Section III)

Readiness for enhanced **Knowledge:** expresses an interest in learning

See Hyperglycemia; Hypoglycemia

DIABETES MELLITUS, JUVENILE (IDDM TYPE 1)

Risk-prone **Health** behavior r/t inadequate comprehension, inadequate social support, low self-efficacy, impaired adjustment attributable to adolescent maturational crises

Disturbed **Body Image** r/t imposed deviations from biophysical and psychosocial norm, perceived differences from peers

Impaired **Comfort** r/t insulin injections, peripheral blood glucose testing

Ineffective **Health** maintenance r/t (See **Health** maintenance, ineffective, Section III)

Imbalanced **Nutrition:** less than body requirements r/t inability of body to adequately metabolize and use glucose and nutrients, increased caloric needs of child to promote growth and physical activity participation with peers

Readiness for enhanced **Knowledge:** expresses an interest in learning

See Diabetes Mellitus; Child with Chronic Condition; Hospitalized Child

D

DIABETIC COMA

Acute **Confusion** r/t hyperglycemia, presence of excessive metabolic acids

Deficient **Fluid** volume r/t hyperglycemia resulting in polyuria

Ineffective **Health** management r/t lack of understanding of preventive measures, adequate blood sugar control

Risk for unstable blood **Glucose** level (See **Glucose** level, blood, unstable, risk for, Section III)

Risk for **Infection:** Risk factors: hyperglycemia, changes in vascular system

See Diabetes Mellitus

DIABETIC KETOACIDOSIS

See Ketoacidosis, Diabetic

DIABETIC RETINOPATHY

Grieving r/t loss of vision

Ineffective **Health** maintenance r/t deficient knowledge regarding preserving vision with treatment if possible, use of low-vision aids

Vision Loss r/t change in sensory reception

See Vision Impairment; Blindness

DIALYSIS

See Hemodialysis; Peritoneal Dialysis

DIAPHRAGMATIC HERNIA

See Hiatal Hernia

DIARRHEA

Diarrhea r/t infection, change in diet, gastrointestinal disorders, stress, medication effect, impaction

Deficient **Fluid** volume r/t excessive loss of fluids in liquid stools

Risk for **Electrolyte** imbalance: Risk factor: effect of loss of electrolytes from frequent stools

DIC (DISSEMINATED INTRAVASCULAR COAGULATION)

Fear r/t threat to well-being

Deficient **Fluid** volume: hemorrhage r/t depletion of clotting factors

Risk for **Bleeding:** Risk factors: microclotting within vascular system, depleted clotting factors

Risk for ineffective **Gastrointestinal** perfusion (See **Gastrointestinal** perfusion, ineffective, risk for, Section III)

DIGITALIS TOXICITY

Decreased **Cardiac** output r/t drug toxicity affecting cardiac rhythm, rate

Ineffective **Health** management r/t deficient knowledge regarding action, appropriate method of administration of digitalis

DIGNITY, LOSS OF

Risk for compromised **Human Dignity** (See **Human Dignity,** compromised, risk for, Section III)

DILATION AND CURETTAGE (D&C)

Acute **Pain** r/t uterine contractions

Risk for **Bleeding:** Risk factor: surgical procedure

Risk for **Infection:** Risk factor: surgical procedure

Risk for ineffective **Sexuality** pattern: Risk factors: painful coitus, fear associated with surgery on genital area

Readiness for enhanced **Knowledge:** expresses an interest in learning

DIRTY BODY (FOR PROLONGED PERIOD)

Self-Neglect r/t mental illness, substance abuse, cognitive impairment

DISCHARGE PLANNING

Impaired **Home Maintenance** r/t family member's disease or injury interfering with home maintenance

Deficient **Knowledge** r/t lack of exposure to information for home care

Relocation stress syndrome: Risk factors: insufficient predeparture counseling, insufficient support system, unpredictability of experience

Readiness for enhanced **Knowledge:** expresses an interest in learning

DISCOMFORTS OF PREGNANCY

Disturbed **Body Image** r/t pregnancy-induced body changes

Impaired **Comfort** r/t enlarged abdomen, swollen feet

Fatigue r/t hormonal, metabolic, body changes

Stress urinary **Incontinence** r/t enlarged uterus, fetal movement

Insomnia r/t psychological stress, fetal movement, muscular cramping, urinary frequency, shortness of breath

Nausea r/t hormone effect

Acute **Pain:** headache r/t hormonal changes of pregnancy

Acute **Pain:** leg cramps r/t nerve compression, calcium/phosphorus/potassium imbalance

Risk for **Constipation:** Risk factors: decreased intestinal motility, inadequate fiber in diet

Risk for **Injury:** Risk factors: faintness and/or syncope caused by vasomotor lability or postural hypotension, venous stasis in lower extremities

DISLOCATION OF JOINT

Acute **Pain** r/t dislocation of a joint

Self-Care deficit: r/t inability to use a joint

Risk for **Injury:** Risk factor: unstable joint

DISSECTING ANEURYSM

Fear r/t threat to well-being

See Abdominal Surgery; Aneurysm, Abdominal Surgery

DISSEMINATED INTRAVASCULAR COAGULATION (DIC)

See DIC (Disseminated Intravascular Coagulation)

DISSOCIATIVE IDENTITY DISORDER (NOT OTHERWISE SPECIFIED)

Anxiety r/t psychosocial stress

Ineffective **Coping** r/t personal vulnerability in crisis of accurate self-perception

Disturbed personal **Identity** r/t inability to distinguish self caused by multiple personality disorders, depersonalization, disturbance in memory

Impaired **Memory** r/t altered state of consciousness

See Multiple Personality Disorder (Dissociative Identity Disorder)

DISTRESS

Anxiety r/t situational crises, maturational crises

Death **Anxiety** r/t denial of one's own mortality or impending death

DISUSE SYNDROME, POTENTIAL TO DEVELOP

Risk for **Disuse** syndrome: Risk factors: paralysis, mechanical immobilization, prescribed immobilization, severe pain, altered level of consciousness

DIVERSIONAL ACTIVITY, LACK OF

Deficient **Diversional** activity r/t environmental lack of diversional activity as in frequent hospitalizations, lengthy treatments

DIVERTICULITIS

Constipation r/t dietary deficiency of fiber and roughage

Diarrhea r/t increased intestinal motility caused by inflammation

Deficient **Knowledge** r/t diet needed to control disease, medication regimen

Imbalanced **Nutrition:** less than body requirements r/t loss of appetite

Acute **Pain** r/t inflammation of bowel

Risk for deficient **Fluid Volume:** Risk factor: diarrhea

DIZZINESS

Decreased **Cardiac** output r/t alteration in heart rate and rhythm, altered stroke volume

Deficient **Knowledge** r/t actions to take to prevent or modify dizziness and prevent falls

D

Impaired physical **Mobility** r/t dizziness

Risk for **Falls:** Risk factor: difficulty maintaining balance

Risk for ineffective **Cerebral** tissue perfusion: Risk factor: interruption of cerebral arterial blood flow

DOMESTIC VIOLENCE

Impaired verbal **Communication** r/t psychological barriers of fear

Compromised family **Coping** r/t abusive patterns

Defensive **Coping** r/t low self-esteem

Dysfunctional **Family** processes r/t inadequate coping skills

Fear r/t threat to self-concept, situational crisis of abuse

Insomnia r/t psychological stress

Post-Trauma syndrome r/t history of abuse

Powerlessness r/t lifestyle of helplessness

Situational low **Self-Esteem** r/t negative family interactions

Risk for compromised **Resilience:** Risk factor: effects of abuse

Risk for other-directed **Violence:** Risk factor: history of abuse

DOWN SYNDROME

See Child with Chronic Condition; Intellectual Disability

DRESS SELF (INABILITY TO)

Dressing **Self-Care** deficit r/t intolerance to activity, decreased strength and endurance, pain, discomfort, perceptual or cognitive impairment, neuromuscular impairment, musculoskeletal impairment, depression, severe anxiety

DRIBBLING OF URINE

Overflow urinary **Incontinence** r/t degenerative changes in pelvic muscles and urinary structures

Stress urinary **Incontinence** r/t degenerative changes in pelvic muscles and urinary structures

DROOLING

Impaired **Swallowing** r/t neuromuscular impairment, mechanical obstruction

Risk for **Aspiration:** Risk factor: impaired swallowing

DROPOUT FROM SCHOOL

Impaired individual **Resilience** (See **Resilience,** individual, impaired, Section III)

Anxiety r/t conflict about life goals

Ineffective **Coping** r/t inadequate resources

DRUG ABUSE

Anxiety r/t threat to self-concept, lack of control of drug use

Risk-prone **Health** behavior r/t addiction

Ineffective **Coping** r/t situational crisis

Ineffective **Denial** r/t use of drugs affecting quality of own life and that of significant others

Insomnia r/t effects of drugs

Imbalanced **Nutrition:** less than body requirements r/t poor eating habits

Powerlessness r/t feeling unable to change patterns of drug abuse

Impaired individual **Resilience** (See **Resilience,** individual, impaired, Section III)

Sexual dysfunction r/t actions and side effects of drug abuse

Sleep deprivation r/t prolonged psychological discomfort

Impaired **Social** interaction r/t disturbed thought processes from drug abuse

Spiritual distress r/t separation from religious, cultural ties

Risk for **Injury:** Risk factors: hallucinations, drug effects

Risk for other-directed **Violence:** Risk factor: poor impulse control

See Cocaine Abuse; Substance Abuse

DRUG WITHDRAWAL

Anxiety r/t physiological withdrawal

Acute **Confusion** r/t effects of substance withdrawal

Ineffective **Coping** r/t situational crisis, withdrawal

Insomnia r/t effects of medication/ substance withdrawal

Imbalanced **Nutrition:** less than body requirements r/t poor eating habits

Risk for other-directed **Violence:** Risk factors: poor impulse control, hallucinations

Risk for self-directed **Violence:** Risk factors: poor impulse control, hallucinations

See Drug Abuse

DRY EYE

Risk for dry **Eye:** Risk factors: (See dry **Eye,** risk for, Section III)

Risk for Corneal **Injury:** Risk factor: suppressed corneal reflex

Readiness for enhanced **Knowledge:** expresses an interest in learning

See Conjunctivitis; Keratoconjunctivitis Sicca

DT (DELIRIUM TREMENS)

See Alcohol Withdrawal

DVT (DEEP VEIN THROMBOSIS)

Constipation r/t inactivity, bed rest

Impaired physical **Mobility** r/t pain in extremity

Acute **Pain** r/t vascular inflammation, edema

Ineffective peripheral **Tissue** perfusion r/t deficient knowledge of aggravating factors

Delayed **Surgical** recovery r/t impaired physical mobility

Readiness for enhanced **Knowledge:** expresses an interest in learning

Risk for imbalanced body **Temperature:** Risk factor: inactivity

See Anticoagulant Therapy

DYING CLIENT

See Terminally Ill Adult; Terminally Ill Adolescent; Terminally Ill Child, Infant/ Toddler; Terminally Ill Child, Preschool Child; Terminally Ill Child, School-Age Child/Preadolescent; Terminally Ill Child/ Death of Child, Parent

DYSFUNCTIONAL EATING PATTERN

Imbalanced **Nutrition:** less than body requirements r/t psychological factors

Risk for **Overweight:** Risk factor: psychological factors

See Anorexia Nervosa; Bulimia; Maturational Issues, Adolescent; Obesity

DYSFUNCTIONAL FAMILY UNIT

See Family Problems

DYSFUNCTIONAL VENTILATORY WEANING

Dysfunctional **Ventilatory** weaning response r/t physical, psychological, situational factors

DYSMENORRHEA

Nausea r/t prostaglandin effect

Acute **Pain** r/t cramping from hormonal effects

Readiness for enhanced **Knowledge:** expresses an interest in learning

DYSPAREUNIA

Sexual **Dysfunction** r/t lack of lubrication during intercourse, alteration in reproductive organ function

DYSPEPSIA

Anxiety r/t pressures of personal role

Acute **Pain** r/t gastrointestinal disease, consumption of irritating foods

Readiness for enhanced **Knowledge:** expresses an interest in learning

D

DYSPHAGIA

Impaired **Swallowing** r/t neuromuscular impairment

Risk for **Aspiration:** Risk factor: loss of gag or cough reflex

DYSPHASIA

Impaired verbal **Communication** r/t decrease in circulation to brain

Impaired social **Interaction** r/t difficulty in communicating

DYSPNEA

Activity intolerance r/t imbalance between oxygen supply and demand

Ineffective **Breathing** pattern r/t compromised cardiac or pulmonary function, decreased lung expansion, neurological impairment affecting respiratory center, extreme anxiety

Fear r/t threat to state of well-being, potential death

Impaired **Gas** exchange r/t alveolar-capillary damage

Insomnia r/t difficulty breathing, positioning required for effective breathing

Sleep deprivation r/t ineffective breathing pattern

DYSRHYTHMIA

Activity intolerance r/t decreased cardiac output

Decreased **Cardiac** output r/t alteration in heart rate, rhythm

Fear r/t threat of death, change in health status

Risk for ineffective **Cerebral** tissue perfusion: Risk factor: decreased blood supply to the brain from dysrhythmia

Readiness for enhanced **Knowledge:** expresses an interest in learning

DYSTHYMIC DISORDER

Ineffective **Coping** r/t impaired social interaction

Ineffective **Health** maintenance r/t inability to make good judgments regarding ways to obtain help

Insomnia r/t anxious thoughts

Chronic low **Self-Esteem** r/t repeated unmet expectations

Ineffective **Sexuality** pattern r/t loss of sexual desire

Social isolation r/t ineffective coping

See Depression (Major Depressive Disorder)

DYSTOCIA

Anxiety r/t difficult labor, deficient knowledge regarding normal labor pattern

Ineffective **Coping** r/t situational crisis

Fatigue r/t prolonged labor

Grieving r/t loss of ideal labor experience

Acute **Pain** r/t difficult labor, medical interventions

Powerlessness r/t perceived inability to control outcome of labor

Risk for **Bleeding:** Risk factor: hemorrhage secondary to uterine atony

Risk for ineffective **Cerebral** tissue perfusion (fetal): Risk factor: difficult labor and birth

Risk for delayed **Development** (infant): Risk factor: difficult labor and birth

Risk for disproportionate **Growth:** Risk factor: difficult labor and birth

Risk for **Infection:** Risk factor: prolonged rupture of membranes

Risk for impaired **Tissue** integrity (maternal and fetal): Risk factor: difficult labor

DYSURIA

Impaired **Urinary** elimination r/t infection/inflammation of the urinary tract

Risk for urge urinary **Incontinence:** Risk factor: detrusor hyperreflexia from infection in the urinary tract

Acute **Pain** r/t infection/inflammation of the urinary tract

E

ECMO (EXTRACORPOREAL MEMBRANE OXYGENATOR)

Death **Anxiety** r/t emergency condition, hemorrhage

Decreased **Cardiac** output r/t altered contractility of the heart

Impaired **Gas** exchange (See **Gas** exchange, impaired, Section III)

See Respiratory Conditions of the Neonate

E. COLI INFECTION

Fear r/t serious illness, unknown outcome

Deficient **Knowledge** r/t how to prevent disease; care of self with serious illness

See Gastroenteritis; Gastroenteritis, Child; Hospitalized Child

EAR SURGERY

Acute **Pain** r/t edema in ears from surgery

Hearing Loss r/t invasive surgery of ears, dressings

Risk for delayed **Development**: Risk factor: hearing impairment

Risk for **Falls**: Risk factor: dizziness from excessive stimuli to vestibular apparatus

Readiness for enhanced **Knowledge**: expresses an interest in learning

See Hospitalized Child

EARACHE

Acute **Pain** r/t trauma, edema, infection

Hearing Loss r/t altered sensory reception, transmission

EBOLA VIRUS DISEASE

Fear r/t serious threat to well-being

Ineffective **Health** maintenance r/t knowledge deficit regarding transmission, symptoms, and treatment

Social isolation r/t fear of incurable disease

Deficient **Fluid** volume r/t active fluid loss, vomiting, diarrhea, and failure of regulatory mechanisms

Risk for **Infection**: Risk factor: lack of knowledge concerning transmission of disease

ECLAMPSIA

Interrupted **Family** processes r/t unmet expectations for pregnancy and childbirth

Fear r/t threat of well-being to self and fetus

Risk for **Aspiration**: Risk factor: seizure activity

Risk for ineffective **Cerebral** tissue perfusion: fetal: Risk factor: uteroplacental insufficiency

Risk for delayed **Development**: Risk factor: uteroplacental insufficiency

Risk for excess **Fluid** volume: Risk factor: decreased urine output as a result of renal dysfunction

Risk for disproportionate **Growth**: Risk factor: uteroplacental insufficiency

ECT (ELECTROCONVULSIVE THERAPY)

Decisional Conflict r/t lack of relevant information

Fear r/t real or imagined threat to well-being

Impaired **Memory** r/t effects of treatment

See Depression (Major Depressive Disorder)

ECTOPIC PREGNANCY

Death **Anxiety** r/t emergency condition, hemorrhage

Disturbed **Body Image** r/t negative feelings about body and reproductive functioning

Fear r/t threat to self, surgery, implications for future pregnancy

Acute **Pain** r/t stretching or rupture of implantation site

Ineffective **Role** performance r/t loss of pregnancy

Situational low **Self-Esteem** r/t loss of pregnancy, inability to carry pregnancy to term

Chronic **Sorrow** r/t loss of pregnancy, potential loss of fertility

Risk for **Bleeding:** Risk factors: possible rupture of implantation site, surgical trauma

Risk for ineffective **Coping:** Risk factor: loss of pregnancy

Risk for interrupted **Family** processes: Risk factor: situational crisis

Risk for **Infection:** Risk factors: traumatized tissue, surgical procedure

Risk for **Spiritual** distress: Risk factor: grief process

ECZEMA

Disturbed **Body Image** r/t change in appearance from inflamed skin

Impaired **Comfort:** pruritus r/t inflammation of skin

Impaired **Skin** integrity r/t side effect of medication, allergic reaction

Readiness for enhanced **Knowledge:** expresses an interest in learning

ED (ERECTILE DYSFUNCTION)

See Erectile Dysfunction (ED); Impotence

EDEMA

Excess **Fluid** volume r/t excessive fluid intake, cardiac dysfunction, renal dysfunction, loss of plasma proteins

Ineffective **Health** maintenance r/t deficient knowledge regarding treatment of edema

Risk for impaired **Skin** integrity: Risk factors: impaired circulation, fragility of skin

See Heart Failure; Kidney Failure

ELDER ABUSE

See Abuse, Spouse, Parent, or Significant Other

ELDERLY

See Aging; Frail Elderly Syndrome

ELECTROCONVULSIVE THERAPY

See ECT (Electroconvulsive Therapy)

ELECTROLYTE IMBALANCE

Risk for **Electrolyte** imbalance (See **Electrolyte** imbalance, risk for, Section III)

EMANCIPATED DECISION-MAKING, IMPAIRED

Risk for impaired emancipated **Decision-Making:** Risk factor: inability or unwillingness to verbalize needs and wants

Readiness for enhanced emancipated **Decision-Making**

EMACIATED PERSON

Frail Elderly syndrome r/t living alone, malnutrition, alteration in cognitive functioning

Imbalanced **Nutrition:** less than body requirements r/t inability to ingest food, digest food, absorb nutrients because of biological, psychological, economic factors

EMBOLECTOMY

Fear r/t threat of great bodily harm from embolus

Ineffective peripheral **Tissue Perfusion** r/t presence of embolus

Risk for **Bleeding:** Risk factors: postoperative complication, surgical area

See Surgery, Postoperative Care

EMBOLI

See Pulmonary Embolism

EMBOLISM IN LEG OR ARM

Ineffective peripheral **Tissue Perfusion** r/t arterial obstruction from clot

See Deep Vein Thrombosis

EMESIS

Nausea (See **Nausea**, Section III)

See Vomiting

EMOTIONAL PROBLEMS

See Coping Problems

EMPATHY

Readiness for enhanced community **Coping:** social supports, being available for problem solving

Readiness for enhanced family **Coping:** basic needs met, desire to move to higher level of health

Readiness for enhanced **Spiritual Well-Being:** desire to establish interconnectedness through spirituality

EMPHYSEMA

See COPD (Chronic Obstructive Pulmonary Disease)

EMPTINESS

Social isolation r/t inability to engage in satisfying personal relationships

Chronic **Sorrow** r/t unresolved grief

Spiritual distress r/t separation from religious or cultural ties

ENCEPHALITIS

See Meningitis/Encephalitis

ENDOCARDIAL CUSHION DEFECT

See Congenital Heart Disease/Cardiac Anomalies

ENDOCARDITIS

Activity intolerance r/t reduced cardiac reserve, prescribed bed rest

Decreased **Cardiac** output r/t inflammation of lining of heart and change in structure of valve leaflets, increased myocardial workload

Risk for imbalanced **Nutrition:** less than body requirements: Risk factors: fever, hypermetabolic state associated with fever

Risk for ineffective **Cerebral** tissue perfusion: Risk factor: possible presence of emboli in cerebral circulation

Risk for ineffective peripheral **Tissue** perfusion: Risk factor: possible presence of emboli in peripheral circulation

Readiness for enhanced **Knowledge:** expresses an interest in learning

ENDOMETRIOSIS

Grieving r/t possible infertility

Nausea r/t prostaglandin effect

Acute **Pain** r/t onset of menses with distention of endometrial tissue

Sexual dysfunction r/t painful intercourse

Readiness for enhanced **Knowledge:** expresses an interest in learning

ENDOMETRITIS

Anxiety r/t fear of unknown

Ineffective **Thermoregulation** r/t infectious process

Acute **Pain** r/t infectious process in reproductive tract

Readiness for enhanced **Knowledge:** expresses an interest in learning

ENURESIS

Ineffective **Health** maintenance r/t unachieved developmental task, neuromuscular immaturity, diseases of urinary system

See Toilet Training

ENVIRONMENTAL INTERPRETATION PROBLEMS

(See chronic **Confusion**)

EPIDIDYMITIS

Anxiety r/t situational crisis, pain, threat to future fertility

Acute **Pain** r/t inflammation in scrotal sac

Ineffective **Sexuality** pattern r/t edema of epididymis and testes

Readiness for enhanced **Knowledge:** expresses an interest in learning

EPIGLOTTITIS

See Respiratory Infections, Acute Childhood (Croup, Epiglottis, Pertussis, Pneumonia, Respiratory Syncytial Virus)

EPILEPSY

Anxiety r/t threat to role functioning

Ineffective **Health** management r/t deficient knowledge regarding seizure control

Impaired **Memory** r/t seizure activity

Risk for **Aspiration:** Risk factors: impaired swallowing, excessive secretions

Risk for delayed **Development:** Risk factor: seizure disorder

Risk for **Injury:** Risk factor: environmental factors during seizure

Readiness for enhanced **Knowledge:** expresses an interest in learning

See Seizure Disorders, Adult; Seizure Disorders, Childhood

EPISIOTOMY

Anxiety r/t fear of pain

Disturbed **Body Image** r/t fear of resuming sexual relations

Impaired physical **Mobility** r/t pain, swelling, tissue trauma

Acute **Pain** r/t tissue trauma

Sexual dysfunction r/t altered body structure, tissue trauma

Impaired **Skin** integrity r/t perineal incision

Risk for **Infection:** Risk factor: tissue trauma

EPISTAXIS

Fear r/t large amount of blood loss

Risk for deficient **Fluid** volume: Risk factor: excessive blood loss

EPSTEIN-BARR VIRUS

See Mononucleosis

ERECTILE DYSFUNCTION (ED)

Situational low **Self-Esteem** r/t physiological crisis, inability to practice usual sexual activity

Sexual dysfunction r/t altered body function

Readiness for enhanced **Knowledge:** information regarding treatment for erectile dysfunction

See Impotence

ESOPHAGEAL VARICES

Fear r/t threat of death from hematemesis

Risk for **Bleeding:** Risk factors: portal hypertension, distended variceal vessels that can easily rupture

See Cirrhosis

ESOPHAGITIS

Acute **Pain** r/t inflammation of esophagus

Readiness for enhanced **Knowledge:** expresses an interest in learning

ETOH WITHDRAWAL

See Alcohol Withdrawal

EVISCERATION

See Dehiscence, Abdominal

EXHAUSTION

Impaired individual **Resilience** (See **Resilience,** individual, impaired, Section III)

Disturbed **Sleep** pattern (See **Sleep** pattern, disturbed, Section III)

EXPOSURE TO HOT OR COLD ENVIRONMENT

Hyperthermia r/t exposure to hot environment, abnormal reaction to anesthetics

Hypothermia r/t exposure to cold environment

Risk for imbalanced **Body** temperature: Risk factors: extremes of environmental temperature, inappropriate clothing for environmental temperature

EXTERNAL FIXATION

Disturbed **Body Image** r/t trauma, change to affected part

Risk for **Infection:** Risk factor: presence of pins inserted into bone

See Fracture

EXTRACORPOREAL MEMBRANE OXYGENATOR (ECMO)

See ECMO (Extracorporeal Membrane Oxygenator)

EYE DISCOMFORT

Risk for dry **Eye** (See **Eye,** dry, risk for, Section III)

Risk for corneal **Injury:** Risk factors: exposure of the eyeball, blinking less than five times per minute

EYE SURGERY

Anxiety r/t possible loss of vision

Self-Care deficit: specify r/t impaired vision

Vision Loss r/t surgical procedure, eye pathology

Risk for **Injury:** Risk factor: impaired vision

Readiness for enhanced **Knowledge:** expresses an interest in learning

See Hospitalized Child; Vision Impairment

F

FAILURE TO THRIVE, CHILD

Disorganized **Infant** behavior (See **Infant** behavior, disorganized, Section III)

Insomnia r/t inconsistency of caretaker; lack of quiet, consistent environment

Imbalanced **Nutrition:** less than body requirements r/t inadequate type or amounts of food for infant or child, inappropriate feeding techniques

Impaired **Parenting** r/t lack of parenting skills, inadequate role modeling

Chronic low **Self-Esteem:** parental r/t feelings of inadequacy, support system deficiencies, inadequate role model

Social isolation r/t limited support systems, self-imposed situation

Risk for impaired **Attachment:** Risk factor: inability of parents to meet infant's needs

Risk for delayed **Development** (See **Development,** delayed, risk for, Section III)

Risk for disproportionate **Growth** (See **Growth,** disproportionate, risk for, Section III)

FALLS, RISK FOR

Risk for **Falls** (See **Falls,** risk for, Section III)

FAMILY PROBLEMS

Compromised family **Coping** (See **Coping,** family, compromised, Section III)

Disabled family **Coping** (See **Coping,** family, disabled, Section III)

Interrupted **Family Processes** r/t situation transition and/or crises, developmental transition and/or crises

Ineffective family **Health** management (See, family **Health** management, ineffective, Section III)

Readiness for enhanced family **Coping:** needs sufficiently gratified, adaptive tasks effectively addressed to enable goals of self-actualization to surface

FAMILY PROCESS

Dysfunctional **Family** processes (See **Family** processes, dysfunctional, Section III)

Interrupted **Family** processes (See **Family** processes, interrupted, Section III)

Readiness for enhanced **Family** processes (See **Family** processes, readiness for enhanced, Section III)

Readiness for enhanced **Relationship** (See **Relationship,** readiness for enhanced, Section III)

FATIGUE

Fatigue (See **Fatigue,** Section III)

FEAR

Death **Anxiety** r/t fear of death

Fear r/t identifiable physical or psychological threat to person

F

FEBRILE SEIZURES

*See Seizure Disorders, Childhood
(Epilepsy, Febrile Seizures, Infantile
Spasms)*

FECAL IMPACTION

See Impaction of Stool

(See **Constipation,** Section III)

(See **Constipation,** chronic functional,
Section III)

FECAL INCONTINENCE

Bowel **Incontinence** r/t neurological
impairment, gastrointestinal disorders,
anorectal trauma, weakened perineal
muscles

FEEDING PROBLEMS, NEWBORN

Ineffective **Breastfeeding** (See
Breastfeeding, ineffective, Section III)

Insufficient **Breastfeeding** (See
Breastfeeding, insufficient, Section III)

Disorganized **Infant** behavior r/t
prematurity, immature neurological system

Ineffective infant **Feeding** pattern r/t
prematurity, neurological impairment or
delay, oral hypersensitivity, prolonged
nothing-by-mouth status

Impaired **Swallowing** r/t prematurity

Risk for delayed **Development:** Risk factor:
inadequate nutrition

Risk for deficient **Fluid** volume: Risk factor:
inability to take in adequate amount of
fluids

Risk for disproportionate **Growth:** Risk
factor: feeding problems

FEMORAL POPLITEAL BYPASS

Anxiety r/t threat to or change in health
status

Acute **Pain** r/t surgical trauma, edema in
surgical area

Ineffective peripheral **Tissue Perfusion** r/t
impaired arterial circulation

Risk for **Bleeding:** Risk factor: surgery on
arteries

Risk for **Infection:** Risk factor: invasive
procedure

FETAL ALCOHOL SYNDROME

*See Infant of Substance-Abusing
Mother*

FETAL DISTRESS/ NONREASSURING FETAL HEART RATE PATTERN

Fear r/t threat to fetus

Ineffective peripheral **Tissue Perfusion:** fetal
r/t interruption of umbilical cord blood
flow

FEVER

Ineffective **Thermoregulation** r/t infectious
process

Risk for Imbalanced body **Temperature:**
Risk factors: acute brain injury,
pharmaceutical agent

FIBROCYSTIC BREAST DISEASE

See Breast Lumps

FILTHY HOME ENVIRONMENT

Impaired **Home** maintenance
(See **Home** maintenance, impaired,
Section III)

Self-Neglect r/t mental illness, substance
abuse, cognitive impairment

FINANCIAL CRISIS IN THE HOME ENVIRONMENT

Impaired **Home** maintenance r/t insufficient
finances

FISTULECTOMY

See Hemorrhoidectomy

FLAIL CHEST

Ineffective **Breathing** pattern r/t chest
trauma

Fear r/t difficulty breathing

Impaired **Gas** exchange r/t loss of effective
lung function

Impaired spontaneous **Ventilation** r/t
paradoxical respirations

FLASHBACKS

Post-Trauma syndrome r/t catastrophic event

FLAT AFFECT

Hopelessness r/t prolonged activity restriction creating isolation, failing or deteriorating physiological condition, long-term stress, abandonment, lost belief in transcendent values or higher power or God

Risk for Loneliness: Risk factors: social isolation, lack of interest in surroundings

See Depression (Major Depressive Disorder); Dysthymic Disorder

FLESH-EATING BACTERIA (NECROTIZING FASCIITIS)

See Necrotizing Fasciitis (Flesh-Eating Bacteria)

FLUID BALANCE

Readiness for enhanced **Fluid** balance (See **Fluid** balance, readiness for enhanced, Section III)

FLUID VOLUME DEFICIT

Deficient **Fluid** volume r/t active fluid loss, vomiting, diarrhea, failure of regulatory mechanisms

Risk for Shock: Risk factors: hypovolemia, sepsis, systemic inflammatory response syndrome (SIRS)

FLUID VOLUME EXCESS

Excess **Fluid** volume r/t compromised regulatory mechanism, excess sodium intake

FLUID VOLUME IMBALANCE, RISK FOR

Risk for imbalanced **Fluid** volume: Risk factor: major invasive surgeries

FOOD ALLERGIES

Diarrhea r/t immune effects of offending food on gastrointestinal system

Risk for **Allergy** response: Risk factor: specific foods

Readiness for enhanced **Knowledge:** expresses an interest in learning

See Anaphylactic Shock if relevant

FOODBORNE ILLNESS

Diarrhea r/t infectious material in gastrointestinal tract

Deficient **Fluid** volume r/t active fluid loss from vomiting and diarrhea

Deficient **Knowledge** r/t care of self with serious illness, prevention of further incidences of foodborne illness

Nausea r/t contamination irritating stomach

Risk for dysfunctional **Gastrointestinal** motility: Risk factor: contaminated food

See Gastroenteritis; Gastroenteritis, Child; Hospitalized Child; E. coli Infection

FOOD INTOLERANCE

Risk for dysfunctional **Gastrointestinal** motility: Risk factor: food intolerance

FOREIGN BODY ASPIRATION

Ineffective **Airway** clearance r/t obstruction of airway

Ineffective **Health** maintenance r/t parental deficient knowledge regarding high-risk items

Risk for **Suffocation:** Risk factor: inhalation of small objects

See Safety, Childhood

FORMULA FEEDING OF INFANT

Grieving: maternal r/t loss of desired breastfeeding experience

Risk for **Constipation:** infant: Risk factor: iron-fortified formula

Risk for **Infection:** infant: Risk factors: lack of passive maternal immunity, supine feeding position, contamination of formula

Readiness for enhanced **Knowledge:** expresses an interest in learning

G

FRACTURE

Deficient **Diversional** activity r/t immobility

Impaired physical **Mobility** r/t limb immobilization

Acute **Pain** r/t muscle spasm, edema, trauma

Post-Trauma syndrome r/t catastrophic event

Impaired **Walking** r/t limb immobility

Risk for ineffective peripheral **Tissue Perfusion:** Risk factors: immobility, presence of cast

Risk for **Peripheral Neurovascular** dysfunction: Risk factors: mechanical compression, treatment of fracture

Risk for impaired **Skin** integrity: Risk factors: immobility, presence of cast

Readiness for enhanced **Knowledge:** expresses an interest in learning

FRACTURED HIP

See Hip Fracture

FRAIL ELDERLY SYNDROME

Activity intolerance r/t sensory changes

Risk for **Frail Elderly** syndrome (see **Frail Elderly** syndrome, risk for, Section III)

Risk for **Injury:** Risk factors: impaired vision, impaired gait

Risk for **Powerlessness:** Risk factor: inability to maintain independence

FREQUENCY OF URINATION

Stress urinary **Incontinence** r/t degenerative change in pelvic muscles and structural support

Urge urinary **Incontinence** r/t decreased bladder capacity, irritation of bladder stretch receptors causing spasm, alcohol, caffeine, increased fluids, increased urine concentration, overdistended bladder

Impaired **Urinary** elimination r/t urinary tract infection

Urinary retention r/t high urethral pressure caused by weak detrusor, inhibition of reflex arc, strong sphincter, blockage

FRIENDSHIP

Readiness for enhanced **Relationship:** expresses desire to enhance communication between partners

FROSTBITE

Acute **Pain** r/t decreased circulation from prolonged exposure to cold

Ineffective peripheral **Tissue Perfusion** r/t damage to extremities from prolonged exposure to cold

Impaired **Tissue** integrity r/t freezing of skin and tissues

See Hypothermia

FROTHY SPUTUM

See CHF (Congestive Heart Failure); Pulmonary Edema; Seizure Disorders, Adult; Seizure Disorders, Childhood (Epilepsy, Febrile Seizures, Infantile Spasms)

FUSION, LUMBAR

Anxiety r/t fear of surgical procedure, possible recurring problems

Impaired physical **Mobility** r/t limitations from surgical procedure, presence of brace

Acute **Pain** r/t discomfort at bone donor site, surgical operation

Risk for **Injury:** Risk factor: improper body mechanics

Risk for **Perioperative Positioning** injury: Risk factor: immobilization during surgery

Readiness for enhanced **Knowledge:** expresses an interest in learning

G

GAG REFLEX, DEPRESSED OR ABSENT

Impaired **Swallowing** r/t neuromuscular impairment

Risk for **Aspiration:** Risk factors: depressed cough or gag reflex

GALLOP RHYTHM

Decreased **Cardiac** output r/t decreased contractility of heart

GALLSTONES

See Cholelithiasis

GANG MEMBER

Impaired individual **Resilience**
(See **Resilience,** individual, impaired, Section III)

GANGRENE

Fear r/t possible loss of extremity

Ineffective peripheral **Tissue** perfusion r/t obstruction of arterial flow

See Diabetes Mellitus; Peripheral Vascular Disease

GAS EXCHANGE, IMPAIRED

Impaired **Gas** exchange r/t ventilation-perfusion imbalance

GASTRIC ULCER

See GI Bleed (Gastrointestinal Bleeding); Ulcer, Peptic (Duodenal or Gastric)

GASTRITIS

Imbalanced **Nutrition:** less than body requirements r/t vomiting, inadequate intestinal absorption of nutrients, restricted dietary regimen

Acute **Pain** r/t inflammation of gastric mucosa

Risk for deficient **Fluid** volume:
Risk factors: excessive loss from gastrointestinal tract from vomiting, decreased intake

GASTROENTERITIS

Diarrhea r/t infectious process involving intestinal tract

Deficient **Fluid** volume r/t excessive loss from gastrointestinal tract from diarrhea, vomiting

Nausea r/t irritation to gastrointestinal system

Imbalanced **Nutrition:** less than body requirements r/t vomiting, inadequate intestinal absorption of nutrients, restricted dietary intake

Acute **Pain** r/t increased peristalsis causing cramping

Risk for **Electrolyte** imbalance: Risk factor: loss of gastrointestinal fluids high in electrolytes

Readiness for enhanced **Knowledge:** expresses an interest in learning

See Gastroenteritis, Child

GASTROENTERITIS, CHILD

Impaired **Skin** integrity: diaper rash r/t acidic excretions on perineal tissues

Readiness for enhanced **Knowledge:** expresses an interest in learning

Acute **Pain** r/t increased peristalsis causing cramping

See Gastroenteritis; Hospitalized Child

GASTROESOPHAGEAL REFLUX (GERD)

Ineffective **Airway** clearance r/t reflux of gastric contents into esophagus and tracheal or bronchial tree

Ineffective **Health** maintenance r/t deficient knowledge regarding anti-reflux regimen (e.g., positioning, change in diet)

Acute **Pain** r/t irritation of esophagus from gastric acids

Risk for **Aspiration:** Risk factor: entry of gastric contents in tracheal or bronchial tree

GASTROESOPHAGEAL REFLUX, CHILD

Ineffective **Airway** clearance r/t reflux of gastric contents into esophagus and tracheal or bronchial tree

Anxiety: parental r/t possible need for surgical intervention

Deficient **Fluid** volume r/t persistent vomiting

G

Imbalanced **Nutrition:** less than body requirements r/t poor feeding, vomiting

Risk for **Aspiration:** Risk factor: entry of gastric contents in tracheal or bronchial tree

Risk for impaired **Parenting:** Risk factors: disruption in bonding as a result of irritable or inconsolable infant, lack of sleep for parents

Readiness for enhanced **Knowledge:** expresses an interest in learning

See Child with Chronic Condition; Hospitalized Child

GASTROINTESTINAL BLEEDING (GI BLEED)

See GI Bleed (Gastrointestinal Bleeding)

GASTROINTESTINAL HEMORRHAGE

See GI Bleed (Gastrointestinal Bleeding)

GASTROINTESTINAL SURGERY

Risk for **Injury:** Risk factor: inadvertent insertion of nasogastric tube through gastric incision line

Risk for ineffective **Gastrointestinal** perfusion (See **Gastrointestinal** perfusion, ineffective, risk for, Section III)

See Abdominal Surgery

GASTROSCHISIS/OMPHALOCELE

Ineffective **Airway** clearance r/t complications of anesthetic effects

Impaired **Gas** exchange r/t effects of anesthesia, subsequent atelectasis

Grieving r/t threatened loss of infant, loss of perfect birth or infant because of serious medical condition

Risk for deficient **Fluid** volume: Risk factors: inability to feed because of condition, subsequent electrolyte imbalance

Risk for **Infection:** Risk factor: disrupted skin integrity with exposure of abdominal contents

Risk for **Injury:** Risk factors: disrupted skin integrity, ineffective protection

GASTROSTOMY

Risk for impaired **Skin** integrity: Risk factor: presence of gastric contents on skin

See Tube Feeding

GENITAL HERPES

See Herpes Simplex II

GENITAL WARTS

See STD (Sexually Transmitted Disease)

GERD

See Gastroesophageal Reflux (GERD)

GESTATIONAL DIABETES (DIABETES IN PREGNANCY)

Anxiety r/t threat to self and/or fetus

Impaired **Nutrition:** less than body requirements r/t decreased insulin production and glucose uptake in cells

Risk for **Overweight:** fetal: r/t excessive glucose uptake

Impaired **Nutrition:** more than body requirements: fetal r/t excessive glucose uptake

Risk for delayed **Development:** fetal: Risk factor: endocrine disorder of mother

Risk for unstable blood **Glucose:** Risk factor: excessive intake of carbohydrates

Risk for disproportionate **Growth:** fetal: Risk factor: endocrine disorder of mother

Risk for disturbed **Maternal–Fetal** dyad: Risk factor: impaired glucose metabolism

Risk for impaired **Tissue** integrity: fetal: Risk factors: large infant, congenital defects, birth injury

Risk for impaired **Tissue** integrity: maternal: Risk factor: delivery of large infant

Readiness for enhanced **Knowledge:** expresses an interest in learning

See Diabetes Mellitus

GI BLEED (GASTROINTESTINAL BLEEDING)

Fatigue r/t loss of circulating blood volume, decreased ability to transport oxygen

Fear r/t threat to well-being, potential death

Deficient **Fluid** volume r/t gastrointestinal bleeding, hemorrhage

Imbalanced **Nutrition:** less than body requirements r/t nausea, vomiting

Acute **Pain** r/t irritated mucosa from acid secretion

Risk for ineffective **Coping:** Risk factors: personal vulnerability in crisis, bleeding, hospitalization

Readiness for enhanced **Knowledge:** expresses an interest in learning

GINGIVITIS

Impaired **Oral Mucous Membrane** r/t ineffective oral hygiene

GLAUCOMA

Deficient **Knowledge** r/t treatment and self-care for disease

Vision Loss r/t untreated increased intraocular pressure *(see care plan in Appendix)*

See Vision Impairment

GLOMERULONEPHRITIS

Excess **Fluid** volume r/t renal impairment

Imbalanced **Nutrition:** less than body requirements r/t anorexia, restrictive diet

Acute **Pain** r/t edema of kidney

Readiness for enhanced **Knowledge:** expresses an interest in learning

GLUTEN ALLERGY

See Celiac Disease

GONORRHEA

Acute **Pain** r/t inflammation of reproductive organs

Risk for **Infection:** Risk factor: spread of organism throughout reproductive organs

Readiness for enhanced **Knowledge:** expresses an interest in learning

See STD (Sexually Transmitted Disease)

GOUT

Impaired physical **Mobility** r/t musculoskeletal impairment

Chronic **Pain** r/t inflammation of affected joint

Readiness for enhanced **Knowledge:** expresses an interest in learning

GRANDIOSITY

Defensive **Coping** r/t inaccurate perception of self and abilities

GRAND MAL SEIZURE

See Seizure Disorders, Adult; Seizure Disorders, Childhood (Epilepsy, Febrile Seizures, Infantile Spasms)

GRANDPARENTS RAISING GRANDCHILDREN

Anxiety r/t change in role status

Decisional Conflict r/t support system deficit

Parental **Role** conflict r/t change in parental role

Compromised family **Coping** r/t family role changes

Interrupted **Family** processes r/t family role shifts

Ineffective **Role** performance r/t role transition, aging

Ineffective family **Health** management r/t excessive demands on individual or family

Risk for impaired **Parenting:** Risk factor: role strain

Risk for **Powerlessness:** Risk factors: role strain, situational crisis, aging

Risk for **Spiritual** distress: Risk factor: life change

Readiness for enhanced **Parenting:** physical and emotional needs of children are met

G

GRAVES' DISEASE

See Hyperthyroidism

GRIEVING

Grieving r/t anticipated or actual significant loss, change in life status, style, or function

GRIEVING, COMPLICATED

Complicated **Grieving** r/t expected or sudden death of a significant other with whom there was a volatile relationship, emotional instability, lack of social support

Risk for complicated **Grieving:** Risk factors: death of a significant other with whom there was a volatile relationship, emotional instability, lack of social support

GROOM SELF (INABILITY TO)

Bathing **Self-Care** deficit (See **Self-Care** deficit, bathing, Section III)

Dressing **Self-Care** deficit (See **Self-Care** deficit, dressing, Section III)

GROWTH AND DEVELOPMENT LAG

Risk for disproportionate **Growth** (See **Growth,** disproportionate, risk for, Section III)

GUILLAIN-BARRÉ SYNDROME

Impaired **Spontaneous Ventilation** r/t weak respiratory muscles

Risk for **Aspiration** r/t ineffective cough, depressed gag reflex

See Neurologic Disorders

GUILT

Grieving r/t potential loss of significant person, animal, prized material possession, change in life role

Impaired individual **Resilience** (See **Resilience,** individual, impaired, Section III)

Situational low **Self-Esteem** r/t unmet expectations of self

Risk for complicated **Grieving:** Risk factors: actual loss of significant person, animal, prized material possession, change in life role

Risk for **Post-Trauma** syndrome: Risk factor: exaggerated sense of responsibility for traumatic event

Readiness for enhanced **Spiritual** well-being: desire to be in harmony with self, others, higher power or God

H1N1

See Influenza

HAIR LOSS

Disturbed **Body Image** r/t psychological reaction to loss of hair

Imbalanced **Nutrition:** less than body requirements r/t inability to ingest food because of biological, psychological, economic factors

HALITOSIS

Impaired **Dentition** r/t ineffective oral hygiene

Impaired **Oral Mucous Membrane** r/t ineffective oral hygiene

HALLUCINATIONS

Anxiety r/t threat to self-concept

Acute **Confusion** r/t alcohol abuse, delirium, dementia, mental illness, drug abuse

Ineffective **Coping** r/t distortion and insecurity of life events

Risk for **Self-Mutilation:** Risk factor: command hallucinations

Risk for other-directed **Violence:** Risk factors: catatonic excitement, manic excitement, rage or panic reactions, response to violent internal stimuli

Risk for self-directed **Violence:** Risk factors: catatonic excitement, manic excitement, rage or panic reactions, response to violent internal stimuli

HEAD INJURY

Ineffective **Breathing** pattern r/t pressure damage to breathing center in brainstem

Acute **Confusion** r/t increased intracranial pressure

Decreased **Intracranial** adaptive capacity r/t increased intracranial pressure

Risk for ineffective **Cerebral** tissue perfusion: Risk factors: effects of increased intracranial pressure, trauma to brain

Vision Loss r/t pressure damage to sensory centers in brain (*see care plan in Appendix*)

See Neurologic Disorders

HEADACHE

Acute **Pain** r/t lack of knowledge of pain control techniques or methods to prevent headaches

Ineffective **Health** management r/t lack of knowledge, identification, elimination of aggravating factors

HEALTH BEHAVIOR, RISK-PRONE

Risk-prone **Health** behavior: Risk factors (See **Health** behavior, risk-prone, Section III)

HEALTH MAINTENANCE PROBLEMS

Ineffective **Health** maintenance (See **Health** maintenance, ineffective, Section III)

Ineffective **Health** management (See **Health** management, ineffective, Section III)

HEALTH-SEEKING PERSON

Readiness for enhanced **Health** management (See **Health** management, readiness for enhanced, Section III)

HEARING IMPAIRMENT

Impaired verbal **Communication** r/t inability to hear own voice

Hearing Loss (See **Hearing Loss**, Section III)

Social isolation r/t difficulty with communication

HEART ATTACK

See MI (Myocardial Infarction)

HEARTBURN

Nausea r/t gastrointestinal irritation

Acute **Pain:** heartburn r/t inflammation of stomach and esophagus

Risk for imbalanced **Nutrition:** less than body requirements: Risk factor: pain after eating

Readiness for enhanced **Knowledge:** expresses an interest in learning

See Gastroesophageal Reflux (GERD)

HEART FAILURE

Activity intolerance r/t weakness, fatigue

Decreased **Cardiac** output r/t impaired cardiac function, increased preload, decreased contractility, increased afterload

Constipation r/t activity intolerance

Fatigue r/t disease process with decreased cardiac output

Fear r/t threat to one's own well-being

Excess **Fluid** volume r/t impaired excretion of sodium and water

Impaired **Gas** exchange r/t excessive fluid in interstitial space of lungs

Powerlessness r/t illness-related regimen

Risk for **Shock** (cardiogenic): Risk factors: decreased contractility of heart, increased afterload

Readiness for enhanced **Health** management (See **Health** management, readiness for enhanced, Section III)

See Child with Chronic Condition; Congenital Heart Disease/Cardiac Anomalies; Hospitalized Child

HEART SURGERY

See Coronary Artery Bypass Grafting (CABG)

H

HEAT STROKE

Deficient **Fluid** volume r/t profuse diaphoresis from high environmental temperature

Hyperthermia r/t vigorous activity, high environmental temperature, inappropriate clothing

HEMATEMESIS

See GI Bleed (Gastrointestinal Bleeding)

HEMATURIA

See Kidney Stone; UTI (Urinary Tract Infection)

HEMIANOPIA

Anxiety r/t change in vision

Unilateral Neglect r/t effects of disturbed perceptual abilities

Visual Loss r/t impaired sensory reception, transmission, integration

Risk for **Injury:** Risk factor: disturbed sensory perception

HEMIPLEGIA

Anxiety r/t change in health status

Disturbed **Body Image** r/t functional loss of one side of body

Impaired physical **Mobility** r/t loss of neurological control of involved extremities

Self-Care deficit: specify: r/t neuromuscular impairment

Impaired **Sitting** r/t partial paralysis

Impaired **Standing** r/t partial paralysis

Impaired **Transfer** ability r/t partial paralysis

Unilateral Neglect r/t effects of disturbed perceptual abilities

Impaired **Walking** r/t loss of neurological control of involved extremities

Risk for **Falls:** Risk factor: impaired mobility

Risk for impaired **Skin** integrity: Risk factors: alteration in sensation, immobility; pressure over bony prominence

See CVA (Cerebrovascular Accident)

HEMODIALYSIS

Ineffective **Coping** r/t situational crisis

Interrupted **Family** processes r/t changes in role responsibilities as a result of therapy regimen

Excess **Fluid** volume r/t renal disease with minimal urine output

Powerlessness r/t treatment regimen

Risk for **Caregiver Role Strain:** Risk factor: complexity of care receiver treatment

Risk for **Electrolyte** imbalance: Risk factor: effect of metabolic state on kidney function

Risk for deficient **Fluid** volume: Risk factor: excessive removal of fluid during dialysis

Risk for **Infection:** Risk factors: exposure to blood products, risk for developing hepatitis B or C, impaired immune system

Risk for **Injury:** Risk factors: clotting of blood access, abnormal surface for blood flow

Risk for impaired **Tissue** integrity: Risk factor: mechanical factor associated with fistula formation

Readiness for enhanced **Knowledge:** expresses an interest in learning

See Renal Failure; Renal Failure, Child with Chronic Condition

HEMODYNAMIC MONITORING

Risk for **Infection:** Risk factor: invasive procedure

Risk for **Injury:** Risk factors: inadvertent wedging of catheter, dislodgment of catheter, disconnection of catheter

Risk for impaired **Tissue** integrity: Risk factor: invasive procedure

See Shock; Cardiogenic, Hypovolemic, Septic, Systemic Inflammatory Response Syndrome (SIRS)

HEMOLYTIC UREMIC SYNDROME

Fatigue r/t decreased red blood cells

Fear r/t serious condition with unknown outcome

H

Deficient **Fluid** volume r/t vomiting, diarrhea

Nausea r/t effects of uremia

Risk for **Injury:** Risk factors: decreased platelet count, seizure activity

Risk for impaired **Skin** integrity: Risk factor: diarrhea

See Hospitalized Child; Renal Failure, Acute/Chronic, Child

HEMOPHILIA

Fear r/t high risk for AIDS infection from contaminated blood products

Impaired physical **Mobility** r/t pain from acute bleeds, imposed activity restrictions, joint pain

Acute **Pain** r/t bleeding into body tissues

Risk for **Bleeding:** Risk factors: deficient clotting factors, child's developmental level, age-appropriate play, inappropriate use of toys or sports equipment

Readiness for enhanced **Knowledge:** expresses an interest in learning

See Child with Chronic Condition; Hospitalized Child; Maturational Issues, Adolescent

HEMOPTYSIS

Fear r/t serious threat to well-being

Risk for ineffective **Airway** clearance: Risk factor: obstruction of airway with blood and mucus

Risk for deficient **Fluid** volume: Risk factor: excessive loss of blood

HEMORRHAGE

Fear r/t threat to well-being

Deficient **Fluid** volume r/t massive blood loss

See Hypovolemic Shock

HEMORRHOIDECTOMY

Anxiety r/t embarrassment, need for privacy

Constipation r/t fear of pain with defecation

Acute **Pain** r/t surgical procedure

Urinary Retention r/t pain, anesthetic effect

Risk for **Bleeding:** Risk factors: inadequate clotting, trauma from surgery

Readiness for enhanced **Knowledge:** expresses an interest in learning

HEMORRHOIDS

Impaired **Comfort** r/t itching in rectal area

Constipation r/t painful defecation, poor bowel habits

Impaired **Sitting** r/t pain and pressure

Readiness for enhanced **Knowledge:** expresses an interest in learning

HEMOTHORAX

Deficient **Fluid** volume r/t blood in pleural space

See Pneumothorax

HEPATITIS

Activity intolerance r/t weakness or fatigue caused by infection

Deficient **Diversional** activity r/t isolation

Fatigue r/t infectious process, altered body chemistry

Imbalanced **Nutrition:** less than body requirements r/t anorexia, impaired use of proteins and carbohydrates

Acute **Pain** r/t edema of liver, bile irritating skin

Social isolation r/t treatment-imposed isolation

Risk for deficient **Fluid** volume: Risk factor: excessive loss of fluids from vomiting and diarrhea

Readiness for enhanced **Knowledge:** expresses an interest in learning

HERNIA

See Hiatal Hernia; Inguinal Hernia Repair

HERNIATED DISK

See Low Back Pain

H

HERNIORRHAPHY

See Inguinal Hernia Repair

HERPES IN PREGNANCY

Fear r/t threat to fetus, impending surgery

Situational low **Self-Esteem** r/t threat to fetus as a result of disease process

Risk for **Infection** (infant): Risk factors: transplacental transfer during primary herpes, exposure to active herpes during birth process

See Herpes Simplex II

HERPES SIMPLEX I

Impaired **Oral Mucous Membrane** r/t inflammatory changes in mouth

HERPES SIMPLEX II

Ineffective **Health** maintenance r/t deficient knowledge regarding treatment, prevention, spread of disease

Acute **Pain** r/t active herpes lesion

Situational low **Self-Esteem** r/t expressions of shame or guilt

Sexual dysfunction r/t disease process

Impaired **Tissue** integrity r/t active herpes lesion

Impaired **Urinary** elimination r/t pain with urination

HERPES ZOSTER

See Shingles

HHNS (HYPEROSMOLAR HYPERGLYCEMIC NONKETOTIC SYNDROME)

See Hyperosmolar Hyperglycemic Nonketotic Syndrome (HHNS)

HIATAL HERNIA

Ineffective **Health** maintenance r/t deficient knowledge regarding care of disease

Nausea r/t effects of gastric contents in esophagus

Imbalanced **Nutrition:** less than body requirements r/t pain after eating

Acute **Pain** r/t gastroesophageal reflux

HIP FRACTURE

Acute **Confusion** r/t sensory overload, sensory deprivation, medication side effects, advanced age, pain

Constipation r/t immobility, opioids, anesthesia

Fear r/t outcome of treatment, future mobility, present helplessness

Impaired physical **Mobility** r/t surgical incision, temporary absence of weight bearing, pain when walking

Acute **Pain** r/t injury, surgical procedure, movement

Powerlessness r/t health care environment

Self-Care deficit: specify r/t musculoskeletal impairment

Impaired **Transfer** ability r/t immobilization of hip

Impaired **Walking** r/t temporary absence of weight bearing

Risk for **Bleeding:** Risk factors: postoperative complication, surgical blood loss

Risk for **Infection:** Risk factor: invasive procedure

Risk for **Injury:** Risk factors: activities such as greater than 90-degree flexion of hips that can result in dislodged prosthesis, unsteadiness when ambulating

Risk for **Perioperative Positioning** injury: Risk factors: immobilization, muscle weakness, emaciation

Risk for **Peripheral Neurovascular** dysfunction: Risk factors: trauma, vascular obstruction, fracture

Risk for impaired **Skin** integrity: Risk factor: immobility

HIP REPLACEMENT

See Total Joint Replacement (Total Hip/ Total Knee/Shoulder)

HIRSCHSPRUNG'S DISEASE

Constipation: bowel obstruction r/t inhibited peristalsis as a result of congenital absence of parasympathetic ganglion cells in distal colon

Grieving r/t loss of perfect child, birth of child with congenital defect even though child expected to be normal within 2 years

Imbalanced **Nutrition:** less than body requirements r/t anorexia, pain from distended colon

Acute **Pain** r/t distended colon, incisional postoperative pain

Impaired **Skin** integrity r/t stoma, potential skin care problems associated with stoma

Readiness for enhanced **Knowledge:** expresses an interest in learning

See Hospitalized Child

HIRSUTISM

Disturbed **Body Image** r/t excessive hair

HITTING BEHAVIOR

Acute **Confusion** r/t dementia, alcohol abuse, drug abuse, delirium

Risk for other-directed **Violence** (See **Violence,** other-directed, risk for, Section III)

HIV (HUMAN IMMUNODEFICIENCY VIRUS)

Fear r/t possible death

Ineffective **Protection** r/t depressed immune system

See AIDS (Acquired Immunodeficiency Syndrome)

HODGKIN'S DISEASE

See Anemia; Cancer; Chemotherapy

HOMELESSNESS

Impaired **Home** maintenance r/t impaired cognitive or emotional functioning, inadequate support system, insufficient finances

HOME MAINTENANCE PROBLEMS

Impaired **Home** maintenance (See **Home** maintenance, impaired, Section III)

Self-Neglect r/t mental illness, substance abuse, cognitive impairment

Powerlessness r/t interpersonal interactions

Risk for **Trauma:** Risk factor: being in high-crime neighborhood

HOPE

Readiness for enhanced **Hope** (See **Hope,** readiness for enhanced, Section III)

HOPELESSNESS

Hopelessness (See **Hopelessness,** Section III)

HOSPITALIZED CHILD

Activity intolerance r/t fatigue associated with acute illness

Anxiety: separation (child) r/t familiar surroundings and separation from family and friends

Compromised family **Coping** r/t possible prolonged hospitalization that exhausts supportive capacity of significant people

Ineffective **Coping:** parent r/t possible guilt regarding hospitalization of child, parental inadequacies

Deficient **Diversional** activity r/t immobility, monotonous environment, frequent or lengthy treatments, reluctance to participate, therapeutic isolation, separation from peers

Interrupted **Family** processes r/t situational crisis of illness, disease, hospitalization

Fear r/t deficient knowledge or maturational level with fear of unknown, mutilation, painful procedures, surgery

Hopelessness: child r/t prolonged activity restriction, uncertain prognosis

Insomnia: child or parent r/t 24-hour care needs of hospitalization

H

Acute **Pain** r/t treatments, diagnostic or therapeutic procedures, disease process

Powerlessness: child r/t health care environment, illness-related regimen

Risk for impaired **Attachment:** Risk factor: separation

Risk for delayed **Development:** regression: Risk factors: disruption of normal routine, unfamiliar environment or caregivers, developmental vulnerability of young children

Risk for **Injury:** Risk factors: unfamiliar environment, developmental age, lack of parental knowledge regarding safety (e.g., side rails, IV site/pole)

Risk for imbalanced **Nutrition:** less than body requirements: Risk factors: anorexia, absence of familiar foods, cultural preferences

Readiness for enhanced family **Coping:** impact of crisis on family values, priorities, goals, relationships in family

See Child with Chronic Condition

HOSTILE BEHAVIOR

Risk for other-directed **Violence:** Risk factor: antisocial personality disorder

HTN (HYPERTENSION)

Ineffective **Health** management (See **Health** management, ineffective, Section III)

Readiness for enhanced **Health** management (See **Health** management, readiness for enhanced, Section III)

Risk for **Overweight:** Risk factor: lack of knowledge of relationship between diet and disease process

HUMAN IMMUNODEFICIENCY VIRUS (HIV)

See AIDS (Acquired Immunodeficiency Syndrome); HIV (Human Immunodeficiency Virus)

HUMILIATING EXPERIENCE

Risk for compromised **Human Dignity** (See **Human Dignity,** compromised, risk for, Section III)

HUNTINGTON'S DISEASE

Decisional Conflict r/t whether to have children

See Neurologic Disorders

HYDROCELE

Acute **Pain** r/t severely enlarged hydrocele

Ineffective **Sexuality** pattern r/t recent surgery on area of scrotum

HYDROCEPHALUS

Decisional Conflict r/t unclear or conflicting values regarding selection of treatment modality

Interrupted **Family** processes r/t situational crisis

Imbalanced **Nutrition:** less than body requirements r/t inadequate intake as a result of anorexia, nausea, vomiting, feeding difficulties

Risk for delayed **Development:** Risk factor: sequelae of increased intracranial pressure

Risk for disproportionate **Growth:** Risk factor: sequelae of increased intracranial pressure

Risk for **Infection:** Risk factor: sequelae of invasive procedure (shunt placement)

Risk for ineffective **Cerebral** tissue perfusion: Risk factors: interrupted flow, hypervolemia of cerebral ventricles

Risk for **Falls:** Risk factors: acute illness, alteration in cognitive functioning

See Normal Pressure Hydrocephalus (NPH); Child with Chronic Condition; Hospitalized Child; Mental Retardation (if appropriate); Premature Infant (Child); Premature Infant (Parent)

HYGIENE, INABILITY TO PROVIDE OWN

Frail Elderly syndrome r/t living alone

Self-Neglect (See **Self-Neglect,** Section III)

Bathing **Self-Care** deficit (See **Self-Care** deficit, bathing, Section III)

HYPERACTIVE SYNDROME

Decisional Conflict r/t multiple or divergent sources of information regarding education, nutrition, medication regimens; willingness to change own food habits; limited resources

Parental Role conflict: when siblings present r/t increased attention toward hyperactive child

Compromised family **Coping** r/t unsuccessful strategies to control excessive activity, behaviors, frustration, anger

Ineffective **Impulse** control r/t disorder of development, environment that might cause frustration or irritation

Ineffective **Role** performance: parent r/t stressors associated with dealing with hyperactive child, perceived or projected blame for causes of child's behavior, unmet needs for support or care, lack of energy to provide for those needs

Chronic low **Self-Esteem** r/t inability to achieve socially acceptable behaviors; frustration; frequent reprimands, punishment, or scolding for uncontrolled activity and behaviors; mood fluctuations and restlessness; inability to succeed academically; lack of peer support

Impaired **Social** interaction r/t impulsive and overactive behaviors, concomitant emotional difficulties, distractibility and excitability

Risk for delayed **Development**: Risk factor: behavior disorders

Risk for impaired **Parenting**: Risk factor: disruptive or uncontrollable behaviors of child

Risk for other-directed **Violence**: parent or child: Risk factors: frustration with disruptive behavior, anger, unsuccessful relationships

HYPERBILIRUBINEMIA (INFANT)

Anxiety: parent r/t threat to infant, unknown future

Parental **Role** conflict r/t interruption of family life because of care regimen

Neonatal **Jaundice** r/t abnormal breakdown of red blood cells following birth

Imbalanced **Nutrition:** less than body requirements (infant) r/t disinterest in feeding because of jaundice-related lethargy

Risk for disproportionate **Growth**: infant: Risk factor: disinterest in feeding because of jaundice-related lethargy

Risk for imbalanced body **Temperature:** infant: Risk factor: phototherapy

Risk for **Injury**: infant: Risk factors: kernicterus, phototherapy lights

HYPERCALCEMIA

Decreased **Cardiac** output r/t bradydysrhythmia

Impaired physical **Mobility** r/t decreased muscle tone

Imbalanced **Nutrition:** less than body requirements r/t gastrointestinal manifestations of hypercalcemia (nausea, anorexia, ileus)

Risk for **Disuse** syndrome: Risk factor: comatose state impairing mobility

HYPERCAPNIA

Fear r/t difficulty breathing

Impaired **Gas** exchange r/t ventilation-perfusion imbalance, retention of carbon dioxide

See ARDS; COPD; Sleep Apnea

HYPEREMESIS GRAVIDARUM

Anxiety r/t threat to self and infant, hospitalization

Deficient **Fluid** volume r/t excessive vomiting

Impaired **Home** maintenance r/t chronic nausea, inability to function

Nausea r/t hormonal changes of pregnancy

Imbalanced **Nutrition:** less than body requirements r/t excessive vomiting

Powerlessness r/t health care regimen

Social isolation r/t hospitalization

Risk for **Electrolyte** imbalance: Risk factor: vomiting

H

H

HYPERGLYCEMIA

Ineffective **Health** management r/t complexity of therapeutic regimen, decisional conflicts, economic difficulties, unsupportive family, insufficient cues to action, deficient knowledge, mistrust, lack of acknowledgment of seriousness of condition

Risk for unstable blood **Glucose** level (See **Glucose** level, blood, unstable, risk for, Section III)

See Diabetes Mellitus

HYPERKALEMIA

Risk for **Activity** intolerance: Risk factor: muscle weakness

Risk for decreased **Cardiac** tissue perfusion: Risk factor: abnormal electrolyte level affecting heart rate and rhythm

Risk for excess **Fluid** volume: Risk factor: untreated renal failure

HYPERNATREMIA

Risk for deficient **Fluid** volume: Risk factors: abnormal water loss, inadequate water intake

HYPEROSMOLAR HYPERGLYCEMIC NONKETOTIC SYNDROME (HHNS)

Acute **Confusion** r/t dehydration, electrolyte imbalance

Deficient **Fluid** volume r/t polyuria, hyperglycemia, inadequate fluid intake

Risk for **Electrolyte** imbalance: Risk factor: effect of metabolic state on kidney function

Risk for **Injury**: seizures: Risk factors: hyperosmolar state, electrolyte imbalance

See Diabetes Mellitus; Diabetes Mellitus, Juvenile (IDDM Type 1)

HYPERPHOSPHATEMIA

Deficient **Knowledge** r/t dietary changes needed to control phosphate levels

See Renal Failure

HYPERSENSITIVITY TO SLIGHT CRITICISM

Defensive **Coping** r/t situational crisis, psychological impairment, substance abuse

HYPERTENSION (HTN)

See HTN (Hypertension)

Risk for decreased **Cardiac** output: Risk factors: decreased contractility and altered conductivity associated with myocardial damage

Risk for impaired **Cardiovascular** function: Risk factors: obesity, inadequate physical activity and failure to alter diet

HYPERTHERMIA

Hyperthermia (See **Hyperthermia**, Section III)

HYPERTHYROIDISM

Anxiety r/t increased stimulation, loss of control

Diarrhea r/t increased gastric motility

Insomnia r/t anxiety, excessive sympathetic discharge

Imbalanced **Nutrition:** less than body requirements r/t increased metabolic rate, increased gastrointestinal activity

Risk for **Injury:** eye damage: Risk factor: protruding eyes without sufficient lubrication

Readiness for enhanced **Knowledge:** expresses an interest in learning

HYPERVENTILATION

Ineffective **Breathing** pattern r/t anxiety, acid-base imbalance

See Anxiety Disorder; Dyspnea; Heart Failure

HYPOCALCEMIA

Activity intolerance r/t neuromuscular irritability

Ineffective **Breathing** pattern r/t laryngospasm

Imbalanced **Nutrition:** less than body requirements r/t effects of vitamin D deficiency, renal failure, malabsorption, laxative use

HYPOGLYCEMIA

Acute **Confusion** r/t insufficient blood glucose to brain

Ineffective **Health** management r/t deficient knowledge regarding disease process, self-care

Imbalanced **Nutrition:** less than body requirements r/t imbalance of glucose and insulin level

Risk for unstable blood **Glucose** level (See **Glucose** level, blood, unstable, risk for, Section III)

See Diabetes Mellitus; Diabetes Mellitus, Juvenile (IDDM Type 1)

HYPOKALEMIA

Activity intolerance r/t muscle weakness

Risk for decreased **Cardiac** tissue perfusion: Risk factor: possible dysrhythmia from electrolyte imbalance

HYPOMAGNESEMIA

Imbalanced **Nutrition:** less than body requirements r/t deficient knowledge of nutrition, alcoholism

See Alcoholism

HYPOMANIA

Insomnia r/t psychological stimulus

See Manic Disorder, Bipolar I

HYPONATREMIA

Acute **Confusion** r/t electrolyte imbalance

Excess **Fluid** volume r/t excessive intake of hypotonic fluids

Risk for **Injury:** Risk factors: seizures, new onset of confusion

HYPOPLASTIC LEFT LUNG

See Congenital Heart Disease/Cardiac Anomalies

HYPOTENSION

Decreased **Cardiac** output r/t decreased preload, decreased contractility

Risk for deficient **Fluid** volume: Risk factor: excessive fluid loss

Risk for ineffective **Cerebral** tissue perfusion: Risk factors: hypovolemia, decreased contractility, decreased afterload

Risk for ineffective **Gastrointestinal** perfusion (See **Gastrointestinal** perfusion, ineffective, risk for, Section III)

Risk for ineffective **Renal** perfusion: Risk factor: prolonged ischemia of kidneys

Risk for **Shock** (See **Shock,** risk for, Section III)

See Dehydration; Heart Failure; MI

HYPOTHERMIA

Hypothermia (See **Hypothermia,** Section III)

Risk for **Hypothermia** (see **Hypothermia,** risk for, Section III)

HYPOTHYROIDISM

Activity intolerance r/t muscular stiffness, shortness of breath on exertion

Constipation r/t decreased gastric motility

Impaired **Gas** exchange r/t respiratory depression

Impaired **Skin** integrity r/t edema, dry or scaly skin

Risk for **Overweight:** Risk factor: decreased metabolic process

HYPOVOLEMIC SHOCK

See Shock, Hypovolemic

HYPOXIA

Acute **Confusion** r/t decreased oxygen supply to brain

Fear r/t breathlessness

Impaired **Gas** exchange r/t altered oxygen supply, inability to transport oxygen

Risk for **Shock** (See **Shock,** risk for, Section III)

H

HYSTERECTOMY

Constipation r/t opioids, anesthesia, bowel manipulation during surgery

Ineffective **Coping** r/t situational crisis of surgery

Grieving r/t change in body image, loss of reproductive status

Acute **Pain** r/t surgical injury

Sexual dysfunction r/t disturbance in self-concept

Urinary retention r/t edema in area, anesthesia, opioids, pain

Risk for **Bleeding:** Risk factor: surgical procedure

Risk for **Constipation:** Risk factors: opioids, anesthesia, bowel manipulation during surgery

Risk for ineffective peripheral **Tissue** perfusion: Risk factor: deficient knowledge of aggravating factors

Readiness for enhanced **Knowledge:** Expresses an interest in learning

See Surgery, Perioperative; Surgery, Preoperative; Surgery, Postoperative

I

IBS (IRRITABLE BOWEL SYNDROME)

Constipation r/t low-residue diet, stress

Diarrhea r/t increased motility of intestines associated with disease process, stress

Ineffective **Health** management r/t deficient knowledge, powerlessness

Chronic **Pain** r/t spasms, increased motility of bowel

Risk for **Electrolyte** imbalance: Risk factor: diarrhea

Readiness for enhanced **Health** management: expresses desire to manage illness and prevent onset of symptoms

ICD (IMPLANTABLE CARDIOVERTER/DEFIBRILLATOR)

Anxiety r/t possible dysrhythmia, threat of death

Decreased **Cardiac** output r/t possible dysrhythmia

Readiness for enhanced **Knowledge:** expresses an interest in learning

IDDM (INSULIN-DEPENDENT DIABETES)

See Diabetes Mellitus

IDENTITY DISTURBANCE/ PROBLEMS

Disturbed personal **Identity** r/t situational crisis, psychological impairment, chronic illness, pain

Risk for disturbed personal **Identity** (See **Identity,** personal, risk for disturbed, Section III)

IDIOPATHIC THROMBOCYTOPENIC PURPURA (ITP)

See ITP (Idiopathic Thrombocytopenic Purpura)

ILEAL CONDUIT

Disturbed **Body Image** r/t presence of stoma

Ineffective **Health** management r/t new skills required to care for appliance and self

Ineffective **Sexuality** pattern r/t altered body function and structure

Social isolation r/t alteration in physical appearance, fear of accidental spill of urine

Risk for **Latex Allergy** response: Risk factor: repeated exposures to latex associated with treatment and management of disease

Risk for impaired **Skin** integrity: Risk factor: difficulty obtaining tight seal of appliance

Readiness for enhanced **Knowledge:** expresses an interest in learning

ILEOSTOMY

Disturbed **Body Image** r/t presence of stoma

Diarrhea r/t dietary changes, alteration in intestinal motility

Deficient **Knowledge** r/t limited practice of stoma care, dietary modifications

Ineffective **Sexuality** pattern r/t altered body function and structure

Social isolation r/t alteration in physical appearance, fear of accidental spill of ostomy contents

Risk for impaired **Skin** integrity: Risk factors: difficulty obtaining tight seal of appliance, caustic drainage

Readiness for enhanced **Knowledge:** expresses an interest in learning

ILEUS

Deficient **Fluid** volume r/t loss of fluids from vomiting, fluids trapped in bowel

Dysfunctional **Gastrointestinal** motility r/t effects of surgery, decreased perfusion of intestines, medication effect, immobility

Nausea r/t gastrointestinal irritation

Acute **Pain** r/t pressure, abdominal distention

Readiness for enhanced **Knowledge:** expresses an interest in learning

IMMOBILITY

Ineffective **Breathing** pattern r/t inability to deep breathe in supine position

Acute **Confusion:** elderly r/t sensory deprivation from immobility

Constipation r/t immobility

Risk for **Frail Elderly** syndrome: Risk factors: low physical activity, bed rest

Impaired physical **Mobility** r/t medically imposed bed rest

Ineffective peripheral **Tissue Perfusion** r/t interruption of venous flow

Powerlessness r/t forced immobility from health care environment

Impaired **Walking** r/t limited physical mobility, deconditioning of body

Risk for **Disuse** syndrome: Risk factor: immobilization

Risk for impaired **Skin** integrity: Risk factors: pressure over bony prominences, shearing forces when moved, pressure from devices

Risk for Impaired **Tissue** Integrity: Risk factors: mechanical factors from pressure over bony prominences, shearing forces when moved, pressure from devices

Risk for **Overweight:** Risk factor: energy expenditure less than energy intake

Readiness for enhanced **Knowledge:** expresses an interest in learning

IMMUNIZATION

See Readiness for enhanced **Health** management, Section III

IMMUNOSUPPRESSION

Risk for **Infection:** Risk factors: immunosuppression, exposure to disease outbreak

Impaired **Social** interaction r/t therapeutic isolation

IMPACTION OF STOOL

Constipation r/t decreased fluid intake, less than adequate amounts of fiber and bulk-forming foods in diet, medication effect, or immobility

IMPERFORATE ANUS

Anxiety r/t ability to care for newborn

Deficient **Knowledge** r/t home care for newborn

Impaired **Skin** integrity r/t pruritus

IMPAIRED SITTING

Impaired physical **Mobility** r/t musculoskeletal, cognitive, or neuromuscular disorder

IMPAIRED STANDING

Activity intolerance r/t insufficient physiological or psychological energy

Powerlessness r/t loss of function

IMPETIGO

Impaired **Skin** integrity r/t infectious disease

Readiness for enhanced **Knowledge:** expresses an interest in learning

See Communicable Diseases, Childhood

IMPLANTABLE CARDIOVERTER/ DEFIBRILLATOR (ICD)

See ICD (Implantable Cardioverter/ Defibrillator)

IMPOTENCE

Situational low **Self-Esteem** r/t physiological crisis, inability to practice usual sexual activity

Sexual dysfunction r/t altered body function

Readiness for enhanced **Knowledge:** treatment information for erectile dysfunction

See Erectile Dysfunction (ED)

IMPULSIVENESS

Ineffective **Impulse** control r/t (See **Impulse** control, ineffective, Section III)

INACTIVITY

Activity intolerance r/t imbalance between oxygen supply and demand, sedentary lifestyle, weakness, immobility

Hopelessness r/t deteriorating physiological condition, long-term stress, social isolation

Impaired physical **Mobility** r/t intolerance to activity, decreased strength and endurance, depression, severe anxiety, musculoskeletal impairment, perceptual or cognitive impairment, neuromuscular impairment, pain, discomfort

Risk for **Constipation:** Risk factor: insufficient physical activity

INCOMPETENT CERVIX

See Premature Dilation of the Cervix (Incompetent Cervix)

INCONTINENCE OF STOOL

Disturbed **Body Image** r/t inability to control elimination of stool

Bowel **Incontinence** r/t decreased awareness of need to defecate, loss of sphincter control

Toileting **Self-Care** deficit r/t cognitive impairment, neuromuscular impairment, perceptual impairment, weakness

Situational low **Self-Esteem** r/t inability to control elimination of stool

Risk for impaired **Skin** integrity: Risk factor: presence of stool

INCONTINENCE OF URINE

Functional urinary **Incontinence** r/t altered environment; sensory, cognitive, or mobility deficits

Overflow urinary **Incontinence** r/t relaxation of pelvic muscles and changes in urinary structures

Reflex urinary **Incontinence** r/t neurological impairment

Stress urinary **Incontinence** (See **Incontinence,** urinary, stress, Section III)

Urge urinary **Incontinence** (See **Incontinence,** urinary, urge, Section III)

Toileting **Self-Care** deficit r/t cognitive impairment

Situational low **Self-Esteem** r/t inability to control passage of urine

Risk for impaired **Skin** integrity: Risk factor: presence of urine on perineal skin

INDIGESTION

Nausea r/t gastrointestinal irritation

Imbalanced **Nutrition:** less than body requirements r/t discomfort when eating

INDUCTION OF LABOR

Anxiety r/t medical interventions, powerlessness

Decisional Conflict r/t perceived threat to idealized birth

Ineffective **Coping** r/t situational crisis of medical intervention in birthing process

Acute **Pain** r/t contractions

Situational low **Self-Esteem** r/t inability to carry out normal labor

Risk for **Injury:** maternal and fetal: Risk factors: hypertonic uterus, potential prematurity of newborn

Readiness for enhanced **Family** processes: family support during induction of labor

INFANT APNEA

See Premature Infant (Child); Respiratory Conditions of the Neonate; SIDS (Sudden Infant Death Syndrome)

INFANT BEHAVIOR

Disorganized **Infant** behavior r/t pain, oral/motor problems, feeding intolerance, environmental overstimulation, lack of containment or boundaries, prematurity, invasive or painful procedures

Risk for disorganized **Infant** behavior: Risk factors: pain, oral/motor problems, environmental overstimulation, lack of containment or boundaries

Readiness for enhanced organized **Infant** behavior: stable physiologic measures, use of some self-regulatory measures

INFANT CARE

Readiness for enhanced **Childbearing** process: a pattern of preparing for, maintaining, and strengthening care of newborn infant

INFANT FEEDING PATTERN, INEFFECTIVE

Ineffective infant **Feeding** pattern r/t prematurity, neurological impairment or delay, oral hypersensitivity, prolonged nothing-by-mouth order

INFANT OF DIABETIC MOTHER

Decreased **Cardiac** output r/t cardiomegaly

Deficient **Fluid** volume r/t increased urinary excretion and osmotic diuresis

Imbalanced **Nutrition:** less than body requirements r/t hypotonia, lethargy, poor

sucking, postnatal metabolic changes from hyperglycemia to hypoglycemia and hyperinsulinism

Risk for delayed **Development:** Risk factor: prolonged and severe postnatal hypoglycemia

Risk for impaired **Gas** exchange: Risk factors: increased incidence of cardiomegaly, prematurity

Risk for unstable blood **Glucose** level: Risk factor: metabolic change from hyperglycemia to hypoglycemia and hyperinsulinism

Risk for disproportionate **Growth:** Risk factor: prolonged and severe postnatal hypoglycemia

Risk for disturbed **Maternal–Fetal** dyad: Risk factor: impaired glucose metabolism

See Premature Infant (Child); Respiratory Conditions of the Neonate

INFANT OF SUBSTANCE-ABUSING MOTHER (FETAL ALCOHOL SYNDROME, CRACK BABY, OTHER DRUG WITHDRAWAL INFANTS)

Ineffective **Airway** clearance r/t pooling of secretions from the lack of adequate cough reflex, effects of viral or bacterial lower airway infection as a result of altered protective state

Interrupted **Breastfeeding** r/t use of drugs or alcohol by mother

Diarrhea r/t effects of withdrawal, increased peristalsis from hyperirritability

Ineffective infant **Feeding** pattern r/t uncoordinated or ineffective sucking reflex

Disorganized **Infant** behavior r/t exposure and or withdrawal from toxic substances (alcohol and drugs)

Ineffective **Childbearing** process r/t inconsistent prenatal health visits, suboptimal maternal nutrition, substance abuse

Insomnia r/t hyperirritability or hypersensitivity to environmental stimuli

Imbalanced **Nutrition:** less than body requirements r/t feeding problems; uncoordinated or ineffective suck and swallow; effects of diarrhea, vomiting, or colic associated with maternal substance abuse

Impaired **Parenting** r/t impaired or absent attachment behaviors, inadequate support systems

Risk for delayed **Development:** Risk factor: substance abuse

Risk for disproportionate **Growth:** Risk factor: substance abuse

Risk for **Infection:** skin, meningeal, respiratory: Risk factor: stress effects of withdrawal

See Cerebral Palsy; Child with Chronic Condition; Crack Baby; Failure to Thrive, Nonorganic; Hospitalized Child; Hyperactive Syndrome; Premature Infant (Child); SIDS (Sudden Infant Death Syndrome)

INFANTILE POLYARTERITIS

See Kawasaki Disease

INFECTION

Hyperthermia r/t increased metabolic rate

Ineffective **Protection** r/t inadequate nutrition, abnormal blood profiles, drug therapies, treatments

Impaired **Social** interaction r/t therapeutic isolation

Risk for **Vascular Trauma:** Risk factor: infusion of antibiotics

INFECTION, POTENTIAL FOR

Risk for **Infection** (See **Infection,** risk for, Section III)

INFERTILITY

Ineffective **Health** management r/t deficient knowledge about infertility

Powerlessness r/t infertility

Chronic **Sorrow** r/t inability to conceive a child

Spiritual distress r/t inability to conceive a child

INFLAMMATORY BOWEL DISEASE (CHILD AND ADULT)

Ineffective **Coping** r/t repeated episodes of diarrhea

Diarrhea r/t effects of inflammatory changes of the bowel

Deficient **Fluid** volume r/t frequent and loose stools

Imbalanced **Nutrition:** less than body requirements r/t anorexia, decreased absorption of nutrients from gastrointestinal tract

Acute **Pain** r/t abdominal cramping and anal irritation

Impaired **Skin** integrity r/t frequent stools, development of anal fissures

Social isolation r/t diarrhea

See Child with Chronic Condition; Crohn's Disease; Hospitalized Child; Maturational Issues, Adolescent

INFLUENZA

Deficient **Fluid** volume r/t inadequate fluid intake

Ineffective **Health** management r/t lack of knowledge regarding preventive immunizations

Ineffective **Thermoregulation** r/t infectious process

Acute **Pain** r/t inflammatory changes in joints

Readiness for enhanced **Knowledge:** information to prevent or treat influenza

INGUINAL HERNIA REPAIR

Impaired physical **Mobility** r/t pain at surgical site and fear of causing hernia to rupture

Acute **Pain** r/t surgical procedure

Urinary retention r/t possible edema at surgical site

Risk for **Infection:** Risk factor: surgical procedure

INJURY

Risk for **Falls:** Risk factors: orthostatic hypotension, impaired physical mobility, diminished mental status

Risk for **Injury:** Risk factor: environmental conditions interacting with client's adaptive and defensive resources

Risk for corneal **Injury:** Risk factors: blinking less than five times per minute, mechanical ventilation, pharmaceutical agent, prolonged hospitalization

Risk for **Thermal** injury: Risk factors: cognitive impairment, inadequate supervision, developmental level

Risk for urinary tract **Injury:** Risk factor: inflammation and/or infection from long-term use of urinary catheter

INSANITY

See Mental Illness, Psychosis

INSOMNIA

(See **Insomnia,** Section III)

INSULIN SHOCK

See Hypoglycemia

INTELLECTUAL DISABILITY

Impaired verbal **Communication** r/t developmental delay

Interrupted **Family** processes r/t crisis of diagnosis and situational transition

Grieving r/t loss of perfect child, birth of child with congenital defect or subsequent head injury

Deficient community **Health** r/t lack of programs to address developmental deficiencies

Impaired **Home** maintenance r/t insufficient support systems

Self-Neglect r/t learning disability

Self-Care deficit: bathing, dressing, feeding, toileting r/t perceptual or cognitive impairment

Self-Mutilation r/t inability to express tension verbally

Social isolation r/t delay in accomplishing developmental tasks

Spiritual distress r/t chronic condition of child with special needs

Stress overload r/t intense, repeated stressor (chronic condition)

Impaired **Swallowing** r/t neuromuscular impairment

Risk for ineffective **Activity** planning r/t inability to process information

Risk for delayed **Development:** Risk factor: cognitive or perceptual impairment

Risk for disproportionate **Growth:** Risk factor: mental retardation

Risk for impaired **Religiosity:** Risk factor: social isolation

Risk for **Self-Mutilation:** Risk factors: separation anxiety, depersonalization

Readiness for enhanced family **Coping:** adaptation and acceptance of child's condition and needs

See Child with Chronic Condition; Safety, Childhood

INTERMITTENT CLAUDICATION

Deficient **Knowledge** r/t lack of knowledge of cause and treatment of peripheral vascular diseases

Acute **Pain** r/t decreased circulation to extremities with activity

Ineffective peripheral **Tissue Perfusion** r/t interruption of arterial flow

Risk for **Injury:** Risk factor: tissue hypoxia

Readiness for enhanced **Knowledge:** prevention of pain and impaired circulation

See Peripheral Vascular Disease (PVD)

INTERNAL CARDIOVERTER/ DEFIBRILLATOR (ICD)

See ICD (Implantable Cardioverter/ Defibrillator)

INTERNAL FIXATION

Impaired **Walking** r/t repair of fracture

Risk for **Infection:** Risk factors: traumatized tissue, broken skin

See Fracture

INTERSTITIAL CYSTITIS

Acute **Pain** r/t inflammatory process

Impaired **Urinary** elimination r/t inflammation of bladder

Risk for **Infection:** Risk factor: suppressed inflammatory response

Readiness for enhanced **Knowledge:** expresses an interest in learning

INTERVERTEBRAL DISK EXCISION

See Laminectomy

INTESTINAL OBSTRUCTION

See Ileus; Bowel Obstruction

INTESTINAL PERFORATION

See Peritonitis

INTOXICATION

Anxiety r/t loss of control of actions

Acute **Confusion** r/t alcohol abuse

Ineffective **Coping** r/t use of mind-altering substances as a means of coping

Impaired **Memory** r/t effects of alcohol on mind

Risk for **Aspiration:** Risk factors: diminished mental status, vomiting

Risk for **Falls:** Risk factor: diminished mental status

Risk for other-directed **Violence:** Risk factor: inability to control thoughts and actions

INTRAAORTIC BALLOON COUNTERPULSATION

Anxiety r/t device providing cardiovascular assistance

Decreased **Cardiac** output r/t heart dysfunction needing counterpulsation

Compromised family **Coping** r/t seriousness of significant other's medical condition

Impaired physical **Mobility** r/t restriction of movement because of mechanical device

Risk for **Peripheral Neurovascular** dysfunction: Risk factors: vascular obstruction of balloon catheter, thrombus formation, emboli, edema

Risk for **Infection:** Risk factor: invasive procedure

Risk for impaired **Tissue** integrity: Risk factor: invasive procedure

INTRACRANIAL PRESSURE, INCREASED

Ineffective **Breathing** pattern r/t pressure damage to breathing center in brainstem

Acute **Confusion** r/t increased intracranial pressure

Decreased **Intracranial** adaptive capacity r/t sustained increase in intracranial pressure

Impaired **Memory** r/t neurological disturbance

Vision Loss r/t pressure damage to sensory centers in brain

Risk for ineffective **Cerebral** tissue perfusion: Risk factors: body position, cerebral vessel circulation deficits

See Head Injury; Subarachnoid Hemorrhage

INTRAUTERINE GROWTH RETARDATION

Anxiety: maternal r/t threat to fetus

Ineffective **Coping:** maternal r/t situational crisis, threat to fetus

Impaired **Gas** exchange r/t insufficient placental perfusion

Imbalanced **Nutrition:** less than body requirements r/t insufficient placenta

Situational low **Self-Esteem:** maternal r/t guilt about threat to fetus

Spiritual distress r/t unknown outcome of fetus

Risk for **Powerlessness:** Risk factor: unknown outcome of fetus

INTRAVENOUS THERAPY

Risk for **Vascular Trauma:** Risk factor: infusion of irritating chemicals

INTUBATION, ENDOTRACHEAL OR NASOGASTRIC

Disturbed **Body Image** r/t altered appearance with mechanical devices

Impaired verbal **Communication** r/t endotracheal tube

Imbalanced **Nutrition:** less than body requirements r/t inability to ingest food because of the presence of tubes

Impaired **Oral Mucous Membrane** r/t presence of tubes

Acute **Pain** r/t presence of tube

IODINE REACTION WITH DIAGNOSTIC TESTING

Risk for adverse reaction to iodinated **Contrast Media** (See reaction to iodinated **Contrast Media**, risk for adverse, Section III)

IRREGULAR PULSE

See Dysrhythmia

IRRITABLE BOWEL SYNDROME (IBS)

See IBS (Irritable Bowel Syndrome)

ISOLATION

Impaired individual **Resilience** (See **Resilience,** individual, impaired, Section III)

Social isolation (See **Social** isolation, Section III)

ITCHING

Impaired **Comfort** r/t inflammation of skin causing itching

Risk for impaired **Skin** integrity: Risk factor: scratching, dry skin

ITP (IDIOPATHIC THROMBOCYTOPENIC PURPURA)

Deficient **Diversional** activity r/t activity restrictions, safety precautions

Ineffective **Protection** r/t decreased platelet count

Risk for **Bleeding:** Risk factors: decreased platelet count, developmental level, age-appropriate play

See Hospitalized Child

J

JAUNDICE

Imbalanced **Nutrition,** less than body requirements r/t decreased appetite with liver disorder

Risk for **Bleeding:** Risk factor: impaired liver function

Risk for impaired **Liver** function: Risk factors: possible viral infection, medication effect

Risk for impaired **Skin** integrity: Risk factors: pruritus, itching

See Cirrhosis; Hepatitis

JAUNDICE, NEONATAL

Neonatal **Jaundice** (See **Jaundice,** neonatal, Section III)

Risk for ineffective **Gastrointestinal** perfusion: Risk factor: liver dysfunction

Readiness for enhanced **Health** management (parents): expresses desire to manage treatment: assessment of jaundice when infant is discharged from the hospital, when to call the physician, and possible preventive measures such as frequent breastfeeding

See Hyperbilirubinemia

JAW PAIN AND HEART ATTACKS

See Angina; Chest Pain; MI (Myocardial Infarction)

JAW SURGERY

Deficient **Knowledge** r/t emergency care for wired jaws (e.g., cutting bands and wires), oral care

Imbalanced **Nutrition:** less than body requirements r/t jaws wired closed, difficulty eating

Acute **Pain** r/t surgical procedure

Impaired **Swallowing** r/t edema from surgery

Risk for **Aspiration:** Risk factor: wired jaws

JITTERY

Anxiety r/t unconscious conflict about essential values and goals, threat to or change in health status

Death **Anxiety** r/t unresolved issues relating to end of life

Risk for **Post-Trauma** syndrome: Risk factors: occupation, survivor's role in event, inadequate social support

JOCK ITCH

Ineffective **Health** management r/t prevention and treatment of disorder

Impaired **Skin** integrity r/t moisture and irritating or tight-fitting clothing

See Itching

JOINT DISLOCATION

See Dislocation of Joint

JOINT PAIN

See Arthritis; Bursitis; JRA (Juvenile Rheumatoid Arthritis); Osteoarthritis; Rheumatoid Arthritis

JOINT REPLACEMENT

Risk for **Peripheral Neurovascular** dysfunction: Risk factor: orthopedic surgery

Risk for impaired **Tissue** integrity: Risk factor: invasive procedure

See Total Joint Replacement (Total Hip/ Total Knee/Shoulder)

JRA (JUVENILE RHEUMATOID ARTHRITIS)

Impaired **Comfort** r/t altered health status

Fatigue r/t chronic inflammatory disease

Impaired physical **Mobility** r/t pain, restricted joint movement

Acute **Pain** r/t swollen or inflamed joints, restricted movement, physical therapy

Self-Care deficit: feeding, bathing, dressing, toileting r/t restricted joint movement, pain

Risk for compromised **Human Dignity:** Risk factors: perceived intrusion by clinicians, invasion of privacy

Risk for **Injury:** Risk factors: impaired physical mobility, splints, adaptive devices, increased bleeding potential from antiinflammatory medications

Risk for compromised **Resilience:** Risk factor: chronic condition

Risk for situational low **Self-Esteem:** Risk factor: disturbed body image

Risk for impaired **Skin** integrity: Risk factors: splints, adaptive devices

See Child with Chronic Condition; Hospitalized Child

K

KAPOSI'S SARCOMA

Risk for complicated **Grieving:** Risk factor: loss of social support

Risk for impaired **Religiosity:** Risk factors: illness/hospitalization, ineffective coping

Risk for impaired **Resilience:** Risk factor: serious illness

See AIDS (Acquired Immunodeficiency Syndrome)

KAWASAKI DISEASE

Anxiety: parental r/t progression of disease, complications of arthritis, and cardiac involvement

Impaired **Comfort** r/t altered health status

Hyperthermia r/t inflammatory disease process

Imbalanced **Nutrition:** less than body requirements r/t impaired oral mucous membranes

Impaired **Oral Mucous Membrane** r/t inflamed mouth and pharynx; swollen lips that become dry, cracked, fissured

Acute **Pain** r/t enlarged lymph nodes; erythematous skin rash that progresses to desquamation, peeling, denuding of skin

Impaired **Skin** integrity r/t inflammatory skin changes

Risk for imbalanced **Fluid** volume: Risk factor: hypovolemia

Risk for decreased **Cardiac** tissue perfusion: Risk factor: cardiac involvement

See Hospitalized Child

KELOIDS

Disturbed **Body Image** r/t presence of scar tissue at site of a healed skin injury

Readiness for enhanced **Health** management: desire to have information to manage condition

KERATOCONJUNCTIVITIS SICCA (DRY EYE SYNDROME)

Risk for dry **Eye:** Risk factors: aging, staring at a computer screen for long intervals

Risk for **Infection:** Risk factor: dry eyes that are more vulnerable to infection

Risk for corneal **Injury:** Risk factors: dry eye, exposure of the eyeball

Vision Loss r/t dry eye resulting in film or obstruction of vision *(see care plan in Appendix)*

See Conjunctivitis

KERATOPLASTY

See Corneal Transplant

KETOACIDOSIS, ALCOHOLIC

See Alcohol Withdrawal; Alcoholism

KETOACIDOSIS, DIABETIC

Deficient **Fluid** volume r/t excess excretion of urine, nausea, vomiting, increased respiration

Impaired **Memory** r/t fluid and electrolyte imbalance

Imbalanced **Nutrition:** less than body requirements r/t body's inability to use nutrients

Risk for unstable blood **Glucose** level: Risk factor: deficient knowledge of diabetes management (e.g., action plan)

Risk for **Powerlessness:** Risk factor: illness-related regimen

Risk for impaired **Resilience:** Risk factor: complications of disease

See Diabetes Mellitus

KEYHOLE HEART SURGERY

K

See MIDCAB (Minimally Invasive Direct Coronary Artery Bypass)

KIDNEY DISEASE SCREENING

Risk for ineffective **Renal** perfusion: Risk factors: hypovolemia, hypertension, alteration in metabolism

Readiness for enhanced **Health** management: seeks information for screening

KIDNEY FAILURE

Activity intolerance r/t effects of anemia, heart failure

Death **Anxiety** r/t unknown outcome of disease

Decreased **Cardiac** output r/t effects of heart failure, elevated potassium levels interfering with conduction system

Impaired **Comfort** r/t pruritus

Ineffective **Coping** r/t depression resulting from chronic disease

Fatigue r/t effects of chronic uremia and anemia

Excess **Fluid** volume r/t decreased urine output, sodium retention, inappropriate fluid intake

Ineffective **Health** management r/t complexity of health care regimen, inadequate number of cues to action, perceived barriers, powerlessness

Imbalanced **Nutrition:** less than body requirements r/t anorexia, nausea, vomiting, altered taste sensation, dietary restrictions

Impaired **Oral Mucous Membrane** r/t irritation from nitrogenous waste products

Chronic **Sorrow** r/t chronic illness

Spiritual distress r/t dealing with chronic illness

Impaired **Urinary** elimination r/t effects of disease, need for dialysis

Risk for **Electrolyte** imbalance: Risk factor: renal dysfunction

Risk for **Infection:** Risk factor: altered immune functioning

Risk for **Injury:** Risk factors: bone changes, neuropathy, muscle weakness

Risk for impaired **Oral Mucous Membrane:** Risk factors: dehydration, effects of uremia

Risk for **Powerlessness:** Risk factor: chronic illness

Risk for **Sepsis:** Risk factor: infection

KIDNEY FAILURE ACUTE/ CHRONIC, CHILD

Disturbed **Body Image** r/t growth retardation, bone changes, visibility of dialysis access devices (shunt, fistula), edema

Deficient **Diversional Activity** r/t immobility during dialysis

See Child with Chronic Condition; Hospitalized Child

KIDNEY FAILURE, NONOLIGURIC

Anxiety r/t change in health status

Risk for deficient **Fluid** volume: Risk factor: loss of large volumes of urine

See Kidney Failure

KIDNEY STONE

Acute **Pain** r/t obstruction from kidney calculi

Impaired **Urinary** elimination: urgency and frequency r/t anatomical obstruction, irritation caused by stone

Risk for **Infection:** Risk factor: obstruction of urinary tract with stasis of urine

Readiness for enhanced **Knowledge:** expresses an interest in learning about prevention of stones

KIDNEY TRANSPLANTATION, DONOR

Impaired emancipated **Decision-Making** r/t harvesting of kidney from traumatized donor

Moral Distress r/t conflict among decision makers, end-of-life decisions, time constraints for decision-making

Spiritual distress r/t grieving from loss of significant person

Readiness for enhanced **Communication:** expressing thoughts and feelings about situation

Readiness for enhanced family **Coping:** decision to allow organ donation

Readiness for enhanced emancipated **Decision-Making:** expresses desire to enhance understanding and meaning of choices

Readiness for enhanced **Resilience:** decision to donate organs

Readiness for enhanced **Spirituality:** inner peace resulting from allowance of organ donation

See Nephrectomy

KIDNEY TRANSPLANTATION, RECIPIENT

Anxiety r/t possible rejection, procedure

Ineffective **Health** maintenance r/t long-term home treatment after transplantation, diet, signs of rejection, use of medications

Deficient **Knowledge** r/t specific nutritional needs, possible paralytic ileus, fluid or sodium restrictions

Impaired **Urinary** elimination r/t possible impaired renal function

Risk for **Bleeding:** Risk factor: surgical procedure

Risk for **Infection:** Risk factor: use of immunosuppressive therapy to control rejection

Risk for ineffective **Renal** perfusion: Risk factor: transplanted kidney

Risk for **Shock:** Risk factor: possible hypovolemia

Risk for **Spiritual** distress: Risk factor: obtaining transplanted kidney from someone's traumatic loss

Readiness for enhanced **Spiritual** well-being: acceptance of situation

KIDNEY TRANSPLANT

Ineffective **Protection** r/t immunosuppressive therapy

Risk for ineffective **Renal** perfusion: Risk factor: complications from transplant procedure

Readiness for enhanced **Decision-making:** expresses desire to enhance understanding of choices

Readiness for enhanced **Family** processes: adapting to life without dialysis

Readiness for enhanced **Health** management: desire to manage the treatment and prevention of complications after transplantation

Readiness for enhanced **Spiritual** well-being: heightened coping, living without dialysis

See Kidney Failure, Kidney Transplantation, Donor; Kidney Transplantation, Recipient; Nephrectomy; Perioperative Care; Surgery, Postoperative Care; Surgery, Preoperative Care

KIDNEY TUMOR

See Wilms' Tumor

KISSING DISEASE

See Mononucleosis

KNEE REPLACEMENT

See Total Joint Replacement (Total Hip/ Total Knee/Shoulder)

KNOWLEDGE

Readiness for enhanced **Knowledge** (See **Knowledge,** readiness for enhanced, Section III)

KNOWLEDGE, DEFICIENT

Ineffective **Health** maintenance r/t lack of or significant alteration in communication skills (written, verbal, and/or gestural)

Deficient **Knowledge** (See **Knowledge,** deficient, Section III)

Readiness for enhanced **Knowledge** (See **Knowledge,** readiness for enhanced, Section III)

KOCK POUCH

See Continent Ileostomy (Kock Pouch)

KORSAKOFF'S SYNDROME

Acute **Confusion** r/t alcohol abuse

Dysfunctional **Family** processes r/t alcoholism as possible cause of syndrome

Impaired **Memory** r/t neurological changes associated with excessive alcohol intake

Self-Neglect r/t cognitive impairment from chronic alcohol abuse

Risk for **Falls:** Risk factor: cognitive impairment from chronic alcohol abuse

Risk for **Injury:** Risk factors: sensory dysfunction, lack of coordination when ambulating from chronic alcohol abuse

Risk for impaired **Liver** function: Risk factor: substance abuse (alcohol)

Risk for imbalanced **Nutrition:** less than body requirements: Risk factor: lack of adequate balanced intake from chronic alcohol abuse

L

LABOR, INDUCTION OF

See Induction of Labor

LABOR, NORMAL

Anxiety r/t fear of the unknown, situational crisis

Impaired **Comfort** r/t labor

Fatigue r/t childbirth

Deficient **Knowledge** r/t lack of preparation for labor

Labor **Pain** r/t uterine contractions, stretching of cervix and birth canal

Impaired **Tissue** integrity r/t passage of infant through birth canal, episiotomy

Risk for ineffective **Childbearing** process (See **Childbearing** process, Section III)

Risk for **Falls:** Risk factors: excessive loss or shift in intravascular fluid volume, orthostatic hypotension

Risk for deficient **Fluid** volume: Risk factor: excessive loss of blood

Risk for **Infection:** Risk factors: multiple vaginal examinations, tissue trauma, prolonged rupture of membranes

Risk for **Injury:** fetal: Risk factor: hypoxia

Risk for **Post-Trauma** syndrome: Risk factors: trauma or violence associated with labor pains, medical or surgical interventions, history of sexual abuse

Readiness for enhanced **Childbearing** process: responds appropriately, is proactive, bonds with infant, uses support systems

Readiness for enhanced family **Coping:** significant other provides support during labor

Readiness for enhanced **Health** management: prenatal care and childbirth education birth process

Readiness for enhanced **Power:** expresses readiness to enhance participation in choices regarding treatment during labor

LABOR PAIN

Labor **Pain** r/t uterine contractions, stretching of cervix and birth canal

LABYRINTHITIS

Ineffective **Health** management r/t delay in seeking treatment for respiratory and ear infections

Risk for **Injury** r/t dizziness

Readiness for enhanced **Health** management: management of episodes

See Ménière's Disease

LACERATIONS

Readiness for enhanced **Health** management: appropriate care of injury

Risk for **Infection:** Risk factor: broken skin

Risk for **Trauma:** Risk factor: children playing with dangerous objects

LACTATION

See Breastfeeding, Ineffective; Breastfeeding, Interrupted; Breastfeeding, Readiness for Enhanced

LACTIC ACIDOSIS

Decreased **Cardiac** output r/t altered heart rate/rhythm, preload, and contractility

Risk for **Electrolyte** imbalance: Risk factor: impaired regulatory mechanism

Risk for decreased **Cardiac** tissue perfusion: Risk factor: hypoxia

See Ketoacidosis, Diabetes Mellitus

LACTOSE INTOLERANCE

Readiness for enhanced **Knowledge:** interest in identifying lactose intolerance, treatment, and substitutes for milk products

See Abdominal Distention; Diarrhea

LAMINECTOMY

Anxiety r/t change in health status, surgical procedure

Impaired **Comfort** r/t surgical procedure

Deficient **Knowledge** r/t appropriate postoperative and postdischarge activities

Impaired physical **Mobility** r/t neuromuscular impairment

Acute **Pain** r/t localized inflammation and edema

Urinary retention r/t competing sensory impulses, effects of opioids or anesthesia

Risk for **Bleeding:** Risk factor: surgery

Risk for **Infection:** Risk factors: invasive procedure, surgery

Risk for **Perioperative Positioning** injury: Risk factor: prone position

See Surgery, Perioperative; Surgery, Postoperative; Surgery, Preoperative

LANGUAGE IMPAIRMENT

See Speech Disorders

LAPAROSCOPIC LASER CHOLECYSTECTOMY

See Cholecystectomy; Laser Surgery

LAPAROSCOPY

Urge urinary **Incontinence** r/t pressure on the bladder from gas

Acute **Pain:** shoulder r/t gas irritating the diaphragm

Risk for ineffective **Gastrointestinal** perfusion: Risk factor: complications from procedure

LAPAROTOMY

See Abdominal Surgery

LARGE BOWEL RESECTION

See Abdominal Surgery

LARYNGECTOMY

Ineffective **Airway** clearance r/t surgical removal of glottis, decreased humidification

Death **Anxiety** r/t unknown results of surgery

Disturbed **Body Image** r/t change in body structure and function

Impaired **Comfort** r/t surgery

Impaired verbal **Communication** r/t removal of larynx

Interrupted **Family** processes r/t surgery, serious condition of family member, difficulty communicating

Grieving r/t loss of voice, fear of death

Ineffective **Health** management r/t deficient knowledge regarding self-care with laryngectomy

Imbalanced **Nutrition:** less than body requirements r/t absence of oral feeding, difficulty swallowing, increased need for fluids

Impaired **Oral Mucous Membrane** r/t absence of oral feeding

Chronic **Sorrow** r/t change in body image

Impaired **Swallowing** r/t edema, laryngectomy tube

Risk for **Electrolyte** imbalance: Risk factor: fluid imbalance

Risk for complicated **Grieving:** Risk factors: loss, major life event

Risk for compromised **Human Dignity:** Risk factor: inability to communicate

Risk for **Infection:** Risk factors: invasive procedure, surgery

Risk for **Powerlessness:** Risk factors: chronic illness, change in communication

Risk for impaired **Resilience:** Risk factor: change in health status

Risk for situational low **Self-Esteem:** Risk factor: disturbed body image

LASER SURGERY

Impaired **Comfort** r/t surgery

Constipation r/t laser intervention in vulval and perianal areas

Deficient **Knowledge** r/t preoperative and postoperative care associated with laser procedure

Acute **Pain** r/t heat from laser

Risk for **Bleeding:** Risk factor: surgery

Risk for **Infection:** Risk factor: delayed heating reaction of tissue exposed to laser

Risk for **Injury:** Risk factor: accidental exposure to laser beam

LASIK EYE SURGERY (LASER-ASSISTED IN SITU KERATOMILEUSIS)

Impaired **Comfort** r/t surgery

Decisional Conflict r/t decision to have surgery

Risk for **Infection**: Risk factors: invasive procedure, surgery

Readiness for enhanced **Health** management: surgical procedure preoperative and postoperative teaching and expectations

LATEX ALLERGY

Latex Allergy response (See **Latex Allergy** response, Section III)

Risk for **Latex Allergy** response (See **Latex Allergy** response, risk for, Section III)

Readiness for enhanced **Knowledge**: prevention and treatment of exposure to latex products

LAXATIVE ABUSE

Perceived **Constipation** r/t health belief, faulty appraisal, impaired thought processes

LEAD POISONING

Contamination r/t flaking, peeling paint in presence of young children

Impaired **Home** maintenance r/t presence of lead paint

Risk for delayed **Development**: Risk factor: lead poisoning

LEFT HEART CATHETERIZATION

See Cardiac Catheterization

LEGIONNAIRES' DISEASE

Contamination r/t contaminated water in air-conditioning systems

See Pneumonia

LENS IMPLANT

See Cataract Extraction; Vision Impairment

LETHARGY/LISTLESSNESS

Frail Elderly syndrome r/t alteration in cognitive function

Fatigue r/t decreased metabolic energy production

Insomnia r/t internal or external stressors

Risk for ineffective **Cerebral** tissue perfusion: Risk factor: carbon dioxide retention and/or lack of oxygen supply to brain

LEUKEMIA

Ineffective **Protection** r/t abnormal blood profile

Fatigue r/t abnormal blood profile and/or side effects of chemotherapy treatment

Risk for imbalanced **Fluid** volume: Risk factors: nausea, vomiting, bleeding, side effects of treatment

Risk for **Infection**: Risk factor: ineffective immune system

Risk for impaired **Resilience**: Risk factor: serious illness

See Cancer; Chemotherapy

LEUKOPENIA

Ineffective **Protection** r/t leukopenia

Risk for **Infection**: Risk factor: low white blood cell count

LEVEL OF CONSCIOUSNESS, DECREASED

See Confusion, Acute; Confusion, Chronic

LICE

Impaired **Comfort** r/t inflammation, pruritus

Readiness for enhanced **Health** management: preventing and treating infestation

Impaired **Home** maintenance r/t close unsanitary, overcrowded conditions

Self-Neglect r/t lifestyle

See Communicable Diseases, Childhood

LIFESTYLE, SEDENTARY

Sedentary lifestyle (See **Sedentary** lifestyle, Section III)

Risk for ineffective peripheral **Tissue Perfusion**: Risk factor: lack of movement

LIGHTHEADEDNESS

See Dizziness; Vertigo

LIMB REATTACHMENT PROCEDURES

Anxiety r/t unknown outcome of reattachment procedure, use and appearance of limb

Disturbed **Body Image** r/t unpredictability of function and appearance of reattached body part

Grieving r/t unknown outcome of reattachment procedure

Spiritual distress r/t anxiety about condition

Stress overload r/t multiple coexisting stressors, physical demands

Risk for **Bleeding:** Risk factor: severed vessels

Risk for **Perioperative Positioning** injury: Risk factor: immobilization

Risk for **Peripheral Neurovascular** dysfunction: Risk factors: trauma, orthopedic and neurovascular surgery, compression of nerves and blood vessels

Risk for **Powerlessness:** Risk factor: unknown outcome of procedure

Risk for impaired **Religiosity:** Risk factors: suffering, hospitalization

See Surgery, Postoperative Care

LIPOSUCTION

Disturbed **Body Image** r/t dissatisfaction with unwanted fat deposits in body

Risk for impaired **Resilience:** Risk factor: body image disturbance

Readiness for enhanced **Decision-Making:** expresses desire to make decision regarding liposuction

Readiness for enhanced **Self-Concept:** satisfaction with new body image

See Surgery, Perioperative Care; Surgery, Postoperative Care; Surgery, Preoperative Care

LITHOTRIPSY

Readiness for enhanced **Health** management: expresses desire for information related to procedure and aftercare and prevention of stones

See Kidney Stone

LIVER BIOPSY

Anxiety r/t procedure and results

Risk for deficient **Fluid** volume: Risk factor: hemorrhage from biopsy site

Risk for **Infection:** Risk factor: invasive procedure

Risk for **Powerlessness:** Risk factor: inability to control outcome of procedure

LIVER CANCER

Risk for **Bleeding:** Risk factor: liver dysfunction

Risk for **Falls:** Risk factor: confusion associated with liver dysfunction

Risk for ineffective **Gastrointestinal** perfusion: Risk factor: liver dysfunction

Risk for impaired **Liver** function: Risk factor: disease process

Risk for impaired **Resilience:** Risk factor: serious illness

See Cancer; Chemotherapy; Radiation Therapy

LIVER DISEASE

See Cirrhosis; Hepatitis

LIVER FUNCTION

Risk for impaired **Liver** function (See **Liver** function, impaired, risk for, Section III)

LIVER TRANSPLANT

Impaired **Comfort** r/t surgical pain

Decisional Conflict r/t acceptance of donor liver

Ineffective **Protection** r/t immunosuppressive therapy

Risk for impaired **Liver** function: Risk factors: possible rejection, infection

L

Readiness for enhanced **Family** processes: change in physical needs of family member

Readiness for enhanced **Health** management: desire to manage the treatment and prevention of complications after transplantation

Readiness for enhanced **Spiritual** well-being: heightened coping

See Surgery, Perioperative Care; Surgery, Postoperative Care; Surgery, Preoperative Care

LIVING WILL

Moral Distress r/t end-of-life decisions

Readiness for enhanced **Decision-Making**: expresses desire to enhance understanding of choices for decision making

Readiness for enhanced **Relationship**: shares information with others

Readiness for enhanced **Religiosity**: request to meet with religious leaders or facilitators

Readiness for enhanced **Resilience**: uses effective communication

Readiness for enhanced **Spiritual** well-being: acceptance of and preparation for end of life

See Advance Directives

LOBECTOMY

See Thoracotomy

LONELINESS

Spiritual distress r/t loneliness, social alienation

Risk for **Loneliness** (See **Loneliness**, risk for, Section III)

Risk for impaired **Religiosity**: Risk factor: lack of social interaction

Readiness for enhanced **Hope**: expresses desire to enhance interconnectedness with others

Readiness for enhanced **Relationship**: expresses satisfaction with complementary relationship between partners

LOOSE STOOLS (BOWEL MOVEMENTS)

Diarrhea r/t increased gastric motility

Risk for dysfunctional **Gastrointestinal** motility (See **Gastrointestinal** motility, dysfunctional, risk for, Section III)

See Diarrhea

LOSS OF BLADDER CONTROL

See Incontinence of Urine

LOSS OF BOWEL CONTROL

See Incontinence of Stool

LOU GEHRIG'S DISEASE

See Amyotrophic Lateral Sclerosis (ALS)

LOW BACK PAIN

Impaired **Comfort** r/t back pain

Ineffective **Health** maintenance r/t deficient knowledge regarding self-care with back pain

Impaired physical **Mobility** r/t back pain

Chronic **Pain** r/t degenerative processes, musculotendinous strain, injury, inflammation, congenital deformities

Urinary Retention r/t possible spinal cord compression

Risk for **Powerlessness**: Risk factor: living with chronic pain

Readiness for enhanced **Health** management: expresses desire for information to manage pain

LOW BLOOD PRESSURE

See Hypotension

LOW BLOOD SUGAR

See Hypoglycemia

LOWER GI BLEEDING

See GI Bleed (Gastrointestinal Bleeding)

LUMBAR PUNCTURE

Anxiety r/t invasive procedure and unknown results

Deficient **Knowledge** r/t information about procedure

Acute **Pain** r/t possible loss of cerebrospinal fluid

Risk for ineffective **Cerebral** tissue perfusion: Risk factor: treatment-related side effects

Risk for **Infection**: Risk factor: invasive procedure

LUMPECTOMY

Decisional Conflict r/t treatment choices

Readiness for enhanced **Knowledge**: preoperative and postoperative care

Readiness for enhanced **Spiritual** well-being: hope of benign diagnosis

See Cancer

LUNG CANCER

See Cancer; Chemotherapy; Radiation Therapy; Thoracotomy

LUNG SURGERY

See Thoracotomy

LUPUS ERYTHEMATOSUS

Disturbed **Body Image** r/t change in skin, rash, lesions, ulcers, mottled erythema

Fatigue r/t increased metabolic requirements

Ineffective **Health** maintenance r/t deficient knowledge regarding medication, diet, activity

Acute **Pain** r/t inflammatory process

Powerlessness r/t unpredictability of course of disease

Impaired **Religiosity** r/t ineffective coping with disease

Chronic **Sorrow** r/t presence of chronic illness

Spiritual distress r/t chronicity of disease, unknown etiology

Risk for decreased **Cardiac** tissue perfusion: Risk factor: altered circulation

Risk for impaired **Resilience**: Risk factor: chronic disease

Risk for impaired **Skin** integrity: Risk factors: chronic inflammation, edema, altered circulation

LYME DISEASE

Impaired **Comfort** r/t inflammation

Fatigue r/t increased energy requirements

Deficient **Knowledge** r/t lack of information concerning disease, prevention, treatment

Acute **Pain** r/t inflammation of joints, urticaria, rash

Risk for decreased **Cardiac** output: Risk factor: dysrhythmia

Risk for **Powerlessness**: Risk factor: possible chronic condition

LYMPHEDEMA

Disturbed **Body Image** r/t change in appearance of body part with edema

Excess **Fluid** volume r/t compromised regulatory system; inflammation, obstruction, or removal of lymph glands

Deficient **Knowledge** r/t management of condition

Risk for **Infection**: Risk factor: abnormal lymphatic system allowing stasis of fluids with decreased resistance to infection

Risk for situational low **Self-Esteem**: Risk factor: disturbed body image

LYMPHOMA

See Cancer

M

MACULAR DEGENERATION

Ineffective **Coping** r/t visual loss

Compromised family **Coping** r/t deteriorating vision of family member

Risk-prone **Health** behavior r/t deteriorating vision while trying to maintain usual lifestyle

Hopelessness r/t deteriorating vision

Sedentary lifestyle r/t visual loss

Self-Neglect r/t change in vision

Social isolation r/t inability to drive because of visual changes

Vision Loss r/t impaired visual function

Risk for **Falls:** Risk factor: visual difficulties

Risk for **Injury:** Risk factor: inability to distinguish traffic lights and safety signs

Risk for **Powerlessness:** Risk factor: deteriorating vision

Risk for impaired **Religiosity:** Risk factor: possible lack of transportation to church

Risk for impaired **Resilience:** Risk factor: changing vision

Readiness for enhanced **Health** management: appropriate choices of daily activities for meeting the goals of a treatment program

MAGNETIC RESONANCE IMAGING (MRI)

See MRI (Magnetic Resonance Imaging)

MAJOR DEPRESSIVE DISORDER

See Depression (Major Depressive Disorder)

MALABSORPTION SYNDROME

Diarrhea r/t lactose intolerance, gluten sensitivity, resection of small bowel

Dysfunctional **Gastrointestinal** motility r/t disease state

Deficient **Knowledge** r/t lack of information about diet and nutrition

Imbalanced **Nutrition:** less than body requirements r/t inability of body to absorb nutrients because of physiological factors

Risk for **Electrolyte** imbalance: Risk factors: hypovolemia, hyponatremia, hypokalemia

Risk for imbalanced **Fluid** volume: Risk factors: diarrhea, hypovolemia

Risk for disproportionate **Growth:** Risk factor: malnutrition from malabsorption

See Abdominal Distention

MALADAPTIVE BEHAVIOR

See Crisis; Post-Trauma Syndrome; Suicide Attempt

MALAISE

See Fatigue

MALARIA

Contamination r/t geographic area

Risk for **Contamination:** Risk factors: increased environmental exposure (not wearing protective clothing, not using insecticide or repellant on skin and in room in areas where infected mosquitoes are present); inadequate defense mechanisms (inappropriate use of prophylactic regimen)

Risk for impaired **Liver** function: Risk factor: complications of disease

Readiness for enhanced community **Coping:** uses resources available for problem solving

Readiness for enhanced **Health** management: expresses desire to enhance immunization status/vaccination status

Readiness for enhanced **Resilience:** immunization status

See Anemia

MALE INFERTILITY

See Erectile Dysfunction (ED); Infertility

MALIGNANCY

See Cancer

MALIGNANT HYPERTENSION (ARTERIOLAR NEPHROSCLEROSIS)

Decreased **Cardiac** output r/t altered afterload, altered contractility

Fatigue r/t disease state, increased blood pressure

Excess **Fluid** volume r/t decreased kidney function

Risk for ineffective **Cerebral** tissue perfusion: Risk factor: elevated blood pressure damaging cerebral vessels

Risk for acute **Confusion:** Risk factor: increased blood urea nitrogen or creatinine levels

Risk for imbalanced **Fluid** volume: Risk factors: hypertension, altered kidney function

Risk for ineffective **Renal** perfusion: Risk factor: elevated blood pressure damaging the kidney

Readiness for enhanced **Health** management: expresses desire to manage the illness, high blood pressure

MALIGNANT HYPERTHERMIA

Hyperthermia r/t anesthesia reaction associated with inherited condition

Risk for ineffective **Renal** perfusion: Risk factors: hyperthermia, muscle destruction (rhabdomyolysis)

Readiness for enhanced **Health** management: knowledge of risk factors

MALNUTRITION

Insufficient **Breast Milk** r/t (See **Breast Milk,** insufficient, Section III)

Frail Elderly syndrome r/t undetected malnutrition

Deficient **Knowledge** r/t misinformation about normal nutrition, social isolation, lack of food preparation facilities

Imbalanced **Nutrition:** less than body requirements r/t inability to ingest food, digest food, or absorb nutrients because of biological, psychological, or economic factors; institutionalization (i.e., lack of menu choices)

Ineffective **Protection** r/t inadequate nutrition

Ineffective **Health** management r/t inadequate nutrition

Self-Neglect r/t inadequate nutrition

Risk for disproportionate **Growth:** Risk factor: malnutrition

Risk for **Powerlessness:** Risk factor: possible inability to provide adequate nutrition

MAMMOGRAPHY

Readiness for enhanced **Health** management: follows guidelines for screening

Readiness for enhanced **Resilience:** responsibility for self-care

MANIC DISORDER, BIPOLAR I

Anxiety r/t change in role function

Ineffective **Coping** r/t situational crisis

Ineffective **Denial** r/t fear of inability to control behavior

Interrupted **Family** processes r/t family member's illness

Risk-prone **Health** behavior r/t low self-efficacy

Ineffective **Health** management r/t unpredictability of client, excessive demands on family, chronic illness, social support deficit

Impaired **Home** maintenance r/t altered psychological state, inability to concentrate

Disturbed personal **Identity** r/t manic state

Insomnia r/t constant anxious thoughts

Imbalanced **Nutrition:** less than body requirements r/t lack of time and motivation to eat, constant movement

Impaired individual **Resilience** r/t psychological disorder

Ineffective **Role** performance r/t impaired social interactions

Self-Neglect r/t manic state

Sleep deprivation r/t hyperagitated state

Risk for ineffective **Activity** planning r/t inability to process information

Risk for **Caregiver Role Strain:** Risk factor: unpredictability of condition

Risk for imbalanced **Fluid** volume: Risk factor: hypovolemia

Risk for **Powerlessness:** Risk factor: inability to control changes in mood

Risk for **Spiritual** distress: Risk factor: depression

M

Risk for **Suicide:** Risk factor: bipolar disorder

Risk for self-directed **Violence:** Risk factors: hallucinations, delusions

Risk for other-directed **Violence:** Risk factor: pathologic intoxication

Readiness for enhanced **Hope:** expresses desire to enhance problem-solving goals

MANIPULATIVE BEHAVIOR

Defensive **Coping** r/t superior attitude toward others

Ineffective **Coping** r/t inappropriate use of defense mechanisms

Self-Mutilation r/t use of manipulation to obtain nurturing relationship with others

Self-Neglect r/t maintaining control

Impaired **Social** interaction r/t self-concept disturbance

Risk for **Loneliness:** Risk factor: inability to interact appropriately with others

Risk for situational low **Self-Esteem:** Risk factor: history of learned helplessness

Risk for **Self-Mutilation:** Risk factor: inability to cope with increased psychological or physiological tension in healthy manner

MARFAN SYNDROME

Decreased **Cardiac** output r/t dilation of the aortic root, dissection or rupture of the aorta

Risk for decreased **Cardiac** tissue perfusion: Risk factor: heart-related complications from Marfan syndrome

Readiness for enhanced **Health** management: describes reduction of risk factors

See Mitral Valve Prolapse; Scoliosis

MASTECTOMY

Disturbed **Body Image** r/t loss of sexually significant body part

Impaired **Comfort** r/t altered body image; difficult diagnosis

Death **Anxiety** r/t threat of mortality associated with breast cancer

Fatigue r/t increased metabolic requirements

Fear r/t change in body image, prognosis

Deficient **Knowledge** r/t self-care activities

Nausea r/t chemotherapy

Acute **Pain** r/t surgical procedure

Sexual dysfunction r/t change in body image, fear of loss of femininity

Chronic **Sorrow** r/t disturbed body image, unknown long-term health status

Spiritual distress r/t change in body image

Risk for **Infection:** Risk factors: surgical procedure, broken skin

Risk for impaired physical **Mobility:** Risk factors: nerve or muscle damage, pain

Risk for **Post-Trauma** syndrome: Risk factors: loss of body part, surgical wounds

Risk for **Powerlessness:** Risk factor: fear of unknown outcome of procedure

Risk for impaired **Resilience:** Risk factor: altered body image

See Cancer; Modified Radical Mastectomy; Surgery, Perioperative; Surgery, Postoperative; Surgery, Preoperative

MASTITIS

Anxiety r/t threat to self, concern over safety of milk for infant

Ineffective **Breastfeeding** r/t breast pain, conflicting advice from health care providers

Deficient **Knowledge** r/t antibiotic regimen, comfort measures

Acute **Pain** r/t infectious disease process, swelling of breast tissue

Ineffective **Role** performance r/t change in capacity to function in expected role

MATERNAL INFECTION

Ineffective **Protection** r/t invasive procedures, traumatized tissue

See Postpartum, Normal Care

MATURATIONAL ISSUES, ADOLESCENT

Ineffective **Coping** r/t maturational crises

Risk-prone **Health** behavior r/t inadequate comprehension, negative attitude toward health care

Interrupted **Family** processes r/t developmental crises of adolescence resulting from challenge of parental authority and values, situational crises from change in parental marital status

Deficient **Knowledge:** potential for enhanced health maintenance r/t information misinterpretation, lack of education regarding age-related factors

Impaired **Social** interaction r/t ineffective, unsuccessful, or dysfunctional interaction with peers

Social isolation r/t perceived alteration in physical appearance, social values not accepted by dominant peer group

Risk for Ineffective **Activity** planning: Risk factor: unrealistic perception of personal competencies

Risk for disturbed personal **Identity:** Risk factor: maturational issues

Risk for **Injury:** Risk factor: thrill-seeking behaviors

Risk for chronic low **Self-Esteem:** Risk factor: lack of sense of belonging in peer group

Risk for situational low **Self-Esteem:** Risk factor: developmental changes

Readiness for enhanced **Communication:** expressing willingness to communicate with parental figures

Readiness for enhanced **Relationship:** expresses desire to enhance communication with parental figures

See Sexuality, Adolescent; Substance Abuse (if relevant)

MAZE III PROCEDURE

See Dysrhythmia; Open Heart Surgery

MD (MUSCULAR DYSTROPHY)

See Muscular Dystrophy (MD)

MEASLES (RUBEOLA)

See Communicable Diseases, Childhood

MECONIUM ASPIRATION

See Respiratory Conditions of the Neonate

MECONIUM DELAYED

Risk for neonatal **Jaundice:** Risk factor: delayed meconium

MELANOMA

Disturbed **Body Image** r/t altered pigmentation, surgical incision

Fear r/t threat to well-being

Ineffective **Health** maintenance r/t deficient knowledge regarding self-care and treatment of melanoma

Acute **Pain** r/t surgical incision

Chronic **Sorrow** r/t disturbed body image, unknown long-term health status

Readiness for enhanced **Health** management: describes reduction of risk factors; protection from sunlight's ultraviolet rays

See Cancer

MELENA

Fear r/t presence of blood in feces

Risk for imbalanced **Fluid** volume: Risk factor: hemorrhage

See GI Bleed (Gastrointestinal Bleeding)

MEMORY DEFICIT

Impaired **Memory** (See **Memory,** impaired, Section III)

MÉNIÈRE'S DISEASE

Risk for **Injury:** Risk factor: symptoms of disease

Readiness for enhanced **Health** management: expresses desire to manage illness

See Dizziness; Nausea; Vertigo

M

M

MENINGITIS/ENCEPHALITIS

Ineffective **Airway** clearance r/t seizure activity

Impaired **Comfort** r/t altered health status

Excess **Fluid** volume r/t increased intracranial pressure, syndrome of inappropriate secretion of antidiuretic hormone

Decreased **Intracranial** adaptive capacity r/t sustained increase in intracranial pressure

Impaired **Mobility** r/t neuromuscular or central nervous system insult

Acute **Pain** r/t biological injury

Risk for **Aspiration:** Risk factor: seizure activity

Risk for acute **Confusion:** Risk factor: infection of brain

Risk for **Falls:** Risk factors: neuromuscular dysfunction, confusion

Risk for **Injury:** Risk factor: seizure activity

Risk for impaired **Resilience:** Risk factor: illness

Risk for **Shock:** Risk factor: infection

Risk for ineffective **Cerebral** tissue perfusion: Risk factors: cerebral tissue edema and inflammation of meninges, increased intracranial pressure, infection

See Hospitalized Child

MENINGOCELE

See Neural Tube Defects

MENOPAUSE

Impaired **Comfort** r/t symptoms associated with menopause

Insomnia r/t hormonal shifts

Impaired **Memory** r/t change in hormonal levels

Sexual dysfunction r/t menopausal changes

Ineffective **Sexuality** pattern r/t altered body structure, lack of lubrication, lack of knowledge of artificial lubrication

Ineffective **Thermoregulation** r/t changes in hormonal levels

Risk for urge urinary **Incontinence:** Risk factor: changes in hormonal levels affecting bladder function

Risk for **Overweight:** Risk factor: change in metabolic rate caused by fluctuating hormone levels

Risk for **Powerlessness:** Risk factor: changes associated with menopause

Risk for impaired **Resilience:** Risk factor: menopause

Risk for situational low **Self-Esteem:** Risk factors: developmental changes, menopause

Readiness for enhanced **Health** management: verbalized desire to manage menopause

Readiness for enhanced **Self-Care:** expresses satisfaction with body image

Readiness for enhanced **Spiritual** well-being: desire for harmony of mind, body, and spirit

MENORRHAGIA

Fear r/t loss of large amounts of blood

Risk for deficient **Fluid** volume: Risk factor: excessive loss of menstrual blood

MENTAL ILLNESS

Defensive **Coping** r/t psychological impairment, substance abuse

Ineffective **Coping** r/t situational crisis, coping with mental illness

Compromised family **Coping** r/t lack of available support from client

Disabled family **Coping** r/t chronically unexpressed feelings of guilt, anxiety, hostility, or despair

Ineffective **Denial** r/t refusal to acknowledge abuse problem, fear of the social stigma of disease

Risk-prone **Health** behavior r/t low self-efficacy

Disturbed personal **Identity** r/t psychoses

Ineffective **Relationship** r/t effects of mental illness in partner relationship

Chronic **Sorrow** r/t presence of mental illness

Stress overload r/t multiple coexisting stressors

Ineffective family **Health** management r/t chronicity of condition, unpredictability of client, unknown prognosis

Risk for **Loneliness:** Risk factor: social isolation

Risk for **Powerlessness:** Risk factor: lifestyle of helplessness

Risk for impaired **Resilience:** Risk factor: chronic illness

Risk for chronic low **Self-Esteem:** Risk factor: presence of mental illness/repeated negative reinforcement

METABOLIC ACIDOSIS

See Ketoacidosis, Alcoholic; Ketoacidosis, Diabetic; Risk for Shock; Risk for Sepsis

METABOLIC ALKALOSIS

Deficient **Fluid** volume r/t fluid volume loss, vomiting, gastric suctioning, failure of regulatory mechanisms

METASTASIS

See Cancer

METHICILLIN-RESISTANT *STAPHYLOCOCCUS AUREUS* (MRSA)

See MRSA (Methicillin-Resistant Staphylococcus aureus)

MI (MYOCARDIAL INFARCTION)

Activity intolerance r/t imbalance between oxygen supply and demand

Anxiety r/t threat of death, possible change in role status

Death **Anxiety** r/t seriousness of medical condition

Constipation r/t decreased peristalsis from decreased physical activity, medication effect, change in diet

Ineffective family **Coping** r/t spouse or significant other's fear of partner loss

Ineffective **Denial** r/t fear, deficient knowledge about heart disease

Interrupted **Family** processes r/t crisis, role change

Fear r/t threat to well-being

Ineffective **Health** maintenance r/t deficient knowledge regarding self-care and treatment

Acute **Pain** r/t myocardial tissue damage from inadequate blood supply

Situational low **Self-Esteem** r/t crisis of MI

Ineffective **Sexuality** pattern r/t fear of chest pain, possibility of heart damage

Risk for **Powerlessness:** Risk factor: acute illness

Risk for **Shock:** Risk factors: hypotension, myocardial dysfunction, hypoxia

Risk for **Spiritual** distress: Risk factor: physical illness

Risk for decreased **Cardiac** output: Risk factors: alteration in heart rate, rhythm, and contractility

Risk for decreased **Cardiac** tissue perfusion: Risk factors: coronary artery spasm, hypertension, hypotension, hypoxia

Readiness for enhanced **Knowledge:** expresses an interest in learning about condition

See Angioplasty (Coronary); Coronary Artery Bypass Grafting (CABG)

MIDCAB (MINIMALLY INVASIVE DIRECT CORONARY ARTERY BYPASS)

Risk for **Bleeding:** Risk factor: surgery

Readiness for enhanced **Health** management: preoperative and postoperative care associated with surgery

Risk for **Infection:** Risk factor: surgical procedure

See Angioplasty, Coronary; Coronary Artery Bypass Grafting (CABG)

MIDLIFE CRISIS

Ineffective **Coping** r/t inability to deal with changes associated with aging

M

Powerlessness r/t lack of control over life situation

Spiritual distress r/t questioning beliefs or value system

Risk for disturbed personal **Identity**

Risk for chronic low **Self-Esteem**: Risk factor: ineffective coping with loss

Readiness for enhanced **Relationship**: meets goals for lifestyle change

Readiness for enhanced **Spiritual** well-being: desire to find purpose and meaning to life

MIGRAINE HEADACHE

Ineffective **Health** maintenance r/t deficient knowledge regarding prevention and treatment of headaches

Readiness for enhanced **Health** management: expresses desire to manage illness

Acute **Pain**: headache r/t vasodilation of cerebral and extracerebral vessels

Risk for impaired **Resilience**: Risk factors: chronic illness, disabling pain

MILK INTOLERANCE

See Lactose Intolerance

MINIMALLY INVASIVE DIRECT CORONARY BYPASS (MIDCAB)

See MIDCAB (Minimally Invasive Direct Coronary Artery Bypass)

MISCARRIAGE

See Pregnancy Loss

MITRAL STENOSIS

Activity intolerance r/t imbalance between oxygen supply and demand

Anxiety r/t possible worsening of symptoms, activity intolerance, fatigue

Decreased **Cardiac** output r/t incompetent heart valves, abnormal forward or backward blood flow, flow into a dilated chamber, flow through an abnormal passage between chambers

Fatigue r/t reduced cardiac output

Ineffective **Health** maintenance r/t deficient knowledge regarding self-care with disorder

Risk for decreased **Cardiac** tissue perfusion: Risk factor: incompetent heart valve

Risk for **Infection**: Risk factors: invasive procedure, risk for endocarditis

MITRAL VALVE PROLAPSE

Anxiety r/t symptoms of condition: palpitations, chest pain

Fatigue r/t abnormal catecholamine regulation, decreased intravascular volume

Fear r/t lack of knowledge about mitral valve prolapse, feelings of having heart attack

Ineffective **Health** maintenance r/t deficient knowledge regarding methods to relieve pain and treat dysrhythmia and shortness of breath, need for prophylactic antibiotics before invasive procedures

Acute **Pain** r/t mitral valve regurgitation

Risk for ineffective **Cerebral** tissue perfusion: Risk factor: postural hypotension

Risk for **Infection**: Risk factor: invasive procedures

Risk for **Powerlessness**: Risk factor: unpredictability of onset of symptoms

Readiness for enhanced **Knowledge**: expresses interest in learning about condition

MOBILITY, IMPAIRED BED

Impaired bed **Mobility** (See **Mobility,** bed, impaired, Section III)

MOBILITY, IMPAIRED PHYSICAL

Impaired physical **Mobility** (See **Mobility,** physical, impaired, Section III)

Risk for **Falls**: Risk factor: impaired physical mobility

MOBILITY, IMPAIRED WHEELCHAIR

Impaired wheelchair **Mobility** (See **Mobility,** wheelchair, impaired, Section III)

MODIFIED RADICAL MASTECTOMY

Impaired emancipated **Decision-Making**

Readiness for enhanced **Communication:** willingness to enhance communication

See Mastectomy

MONONUCLEOSIS

Activity intolerance r/t generalized weakness

Impaired **Comfort** r/t sore throat, muscle aches

Fatigue r/t disease state, stress

Ineffective **Health** maintenance r/t deficient knowledge concerning transmission and treatment of disease

Acute **Pain** r/t enlargement of lymph nodes, oropharyngeal edema

Impaired **Swallowing** r/t enlargement of lymph nodes, oropharyngeal edema

Risk for **Injury:** Risk factor: possible rupture of spleen

Risk for **Loneliness:** Risk factor: social isolation

MOOD DISORDERS

Caregiver Role Strain r/t overwhelming needs of care receiver, unpredictability of mood alterations

Labile **Emotional Control** r/t (See Labile **Emotional Control,** Section III)

Risk-prone **Health** behavior r/t hopelessness, altered locus of control

Impaired **Mood** regulation r/t (See **Mood** regulation, impaired, Section III)

Self-Neglect r/t inability to care for self

Social isolation r/t alterations in mental status

Risk for situational low **Self-Esteem:** Risk factor: unpredictable changes in mood

Readiness for enhanced **Communication:** expresses feelings

See specific disorder: Depression (Major Depressive Disorder); Dysthymic Disorder; Hypomania; Manic Disorder, Bipolar I

MOON FACE

Disturbed **Body Image** r/t change in appearance from disease and medication(s)

Risk for situational low **Self-Esteem:** Risk factor: change in body image

See Cushing's Syndrome

MORAL/ETHICAL DILEMMAS

Impaired emancipated **Decision-Making** r/t questioning personal values and belief, which alter decision

Moral Distress r/t conflicting information guiding moral or ethical decision-making

Risk for **Powerlessness:** Risk factor: lack of knowledge to make a decision

Risk for **Spiritual** distress: Risk factor: moral or ethical crisis

Readiness for enhanced emancipated **Decision-Making:** expresses desire to enhance congruency of decisions with personal values and goals

Readiness for enhanced **Religiosity:** requests assistance in expanding religious options

Readiness for enhanced **Resilience:** vulnerable state

Readiness for enhanced **Spiritual** well-being: request for interaction with others regarding difficult decisions

MORNING SICKNESS

See Hyperemesis Gravidarum; Pregnancy, Normal

MOTION SICKNESS

See Labyrinthitis

MOTTLING OF PERIPHERAL SKIN

Ineffective peripheral **Tissue Perfusion** r/t interruption of arterial flow, decreased circulating blood volume

M

Risk for **Shock:** Risk factor: inadequate circulation to perfuse body

MOURNING

See Grieving

MOUTH LESIONS

See Mucous Membrane, Impaired Oral

MRI (MAGNETIC RESONANCE IMAGING)

Anxiety r/t fear of being in closed spaces

Readiness for enhanced **Health** management: describes reduction of risk factors associated with exam

Deficient **Knowledge** r/t unfamiliarity with information resources, exam information

Readiness for enhanced **Knowledge:** expresses interest in learning about exam

MRSA (METHICILLIN-RESISTANT *STAPHYLOCOCCUS AUREUS*)

Impaired **Skin** integrity r/t infection

Delayed **Surgical** recovery r/t infection

Ineffective **Thermoregulation** r/t severe infection stimulating immune system

Impaired **Tissue** integrity r/t wound, infection

Risk for **Loneliness:** Risk factor: physical isolation

Risk for impaired **Resilience:** Risk factor: illness

Risk for **Shock:** Risk factor: sepsis

MUCOCUTANEOUS LYMPH NODE SYNDROME

See Kawasaki Disease

MUCOUS MEMBRANE, IMPAIRED ORAL

Impaired **Oral Mucous Membrane** (See **Oral Mucous Membrane**, impaired, Section III)

MULTI-INFARCT DEMENTIA

See Dementia

MULTIPLE GESTATIONS

Anxiety r/t uncertain outcome of pregnancy

Death **Anxiety** r/t maternal complications associated with multiple gestations

Insufficient **Breast Milk** r/t multiple births

Ineffective **Childbearing** process r/t unavailable support system

Fatigue r/t physiological demands of a multifetal pregnancy and/or care of more than one infant

Impaired **Home** maintenance r/t fatigue

Stress urinary **Incontinence** r/t increased pelvic pressure

Insomnia r/t impairment of normal sleep pattern; parental responsibilities

Deficient **Knowledge** r/t caring for more than one infant

Neonatal **Jaundice** r/t feeding pattern not well established

Deficient **Knowledge** r/t caring for more than one infant

Imbalanced **Nutrition:** less than body requirements r/t physiological demands of a multifetal pregnancy

Stress overload r/t multiple coexisting stressors, family demands

Impaired **Walking** r/t increased uterine size

Risk for ineffective **Breastfeeding:** Risk factors: lack of support, physical demands of feeding more than one infant

Risk for delayed **Development:** fetus: Risk factor: multiple gestations

Risk for disproportionate **Growth:** fetus: Risk factor: multiple gestations

Risk for neonatal **Jaundice:** Risk factors: abnormal weight loss, prematurity, feeding pattern not well-established

Readiness for enhanced **Childbearing** process: demonstrates appropriate care for infants and mother

Readiness for enhanced **Family** processes: family adapting to change with more than one infant

MULTIPLE PERSONALITY DISORDER (DISSOCIATIVE IDENTITY DISORDER)

Anxiety r/t loss of control of behavior and feelings

Disturbed **Body Image** r/t psychosocial changes

Defensive **Coping** r/t unresolved past traumatic events, severe anxiety

Ineffective **Coping** r/t history of abuse

Hopelessness r/t long-term stress

Disturbed personal **Identity** r/t severe child abuse

Chronic low **Self-Esteem** r/t rejection, failure

Risk for **Self-Mutilation:** Risk factor: need to act out to relieve stress

Readiness for enhanced **Communication:** willingness to discuss problems associated with condition

See Dissociative Identity Disorder (Not Otherwise Specified)

MULTIPLE SCLEROSIS (MS)

Ineffective **Activity** planning r/t unrealistic perception of personal competence

Ineffective **Airway** clearance r/t decreased energy or fatigue

Impaired physical **Mobility** r/t neuromuscular impairment

Self-Neglect r/t functional impairment

Powerlessness r/t progressive nature of disease

Self-Care deficit: specify r/t neuromuscular impairment

Sexual dysfunction r/t biopsychosocial alteration of sexuality

Chronic **Sorrow** r/t loss of physical ability

Spiritual distress r/t perceived hopelessness of diagnosis

Urinary Retention r/t inhibition of the reflex arc

Risk for **Disuse** syndrome: Risk factor: physical immobility

Risk for **Injury:** Risk factors: altered mobility, sensory dysfunction

Risk for imbalanced **Nutrition:** less than body requirements: Risk factors: impaired swallowing, depression

Risk for **Powerlessness:** Risk factor: chronic illness

Risk for impaired **Religiosity:** Risk factor: illness

Risk for **Thermal Injury:** Risk factor: neuromuscular impairment

Readiness for enhanced **Health** management: expresses a desire to manage condition

Readiness for enhanced **Self-Care:** expresses desire to enhance knowledge of strategies and responsibility for self-care

Readiness for enhanced **Spiritual** well-being: struggling with chronic debilitating condition

See Neurologic Disorders

MUMPS

See Communicable Diseases, Childhood

MURMURS

Decreased **Cardiac** output r/t altered preload/afterload

Risk for decreased **Cardiac** tissue perfusion: Risk factor: incompetent valve

Risk for **Fatigue:** Risk factor: decreased cardiac output

MUSCULAR ATROPHY/WEAKNESS

Risk for **Disuse** syndrome: Risk factor: impaired physical mobility

Risk for **Falls:** Risk factor: impaired physical mobility

MUSCULAR DYSTROPHY (MD)

Activity intolerance r/t fatigue, muscle weakness

Ineffective **Activity** planning r/t unrealistic perception of personal competence

Ineffective **Airway** clearance r/t muscle weakness and decreased ability to cough

M

Constipation r/t immobility

Fatigue r/t increased energy requirements to perform activities of daily living

Impaired physical **Mobility** r/t muscle weakness and development of contractures

Imbalanced **Nutrition:** less than body requirements r/t impaired swallowing or chewing

Self-Care deficit: feeding, bathing, dressing, toileting r/t muscle weakness and fatigue

Self-Neglect r/t functional impairment

Impaired **Transfer** ability r/t muscle weakness

Impaired **Walking** r/t muscle weakness

Risk for **Aspiration:** Risk factor: impaired swallowing

Risk for decreased **Cardiac** tissue perfusion: Risk factor: hypoxia associated with cardiomyopathy

Risk for **Disuse** syndrome: Risk factor: complications of immobility

Risk for **Falls:** Risk factor: muscle weakness

Risk for **Infection:** Risk factor: pooling of pulmonary secretions as a result of immobility and muscle weakness

Risk for **Injury:** Risk factors: muscle weakness, unsteady gait

Risk for **Overweight:** Risk factor: inactivity

Risk for **Powerlessness:** Risk factor: chronic condition

Risk for impaired **Religiosity:** Risk factor: illness

Risk for impaired **Resilience:** Risk factor: chronic illness

Risk for situational low **Self-Esteem:** Risk factor: presence of chronic condition

Readiness for enhanced **Self-Concept:** acceptance of strength and abilities

Risk for impaired **Skin** integrity: Risk factors: immobility, braces or adaptive devices

See Child with Chronic Condition; Hospitalized Child

MVC (MOTOR VEHICLE CRASH)

See Fracture; Head Injury; Injury; Pneumothorax

MYASTHENIA GRAVIS

Ineffective **Airway** clearance r/t decreased ability to cough and swallow

Interrupted **Family** processes r/t crisis of dealing with diagnosis

Fatigue r/t paresthesia, aching muscles, weakness of muscles

Impaired physical **Mobility** r/t defective transmission of nerve impulses at the neuromuscular junction

Imbalanced **Nutrition:** less than body requirements r/t difficulty eating and swallowing

Impaired **Swallowing** r/t neuromuscular impairment

Risk for **Caregiver Role Strain:** Risk factors: severity of illness of client, overwhelming needs of client

Risk for impaired **Religiosity:** Risk factor: illness

Risk for impaired **Resilience:** Risk factor: new diagnosis of chronic, serious illness

Readiness for enhanced **Spiritual** well-being: heightened coping with serious illness

See Neurologic Disorders

MYCOPLASMA PNEUMONIA

See Pneumonia

MYELOCELE

See Neural Tube Defects

MYELOMENINGOCELE

See Neural Tube Defects

MYOCARDIAL INFARCTION (MI)

See MI (Myocardial Infarction)

MYOCARDITIS

Activity intolerance r/t reduced cardiac reserve and prescribed bed rest

Decreased **Cardiac** output r/t altered preload/afterload

Deficient **Knowledge** r/t treatment of disease

Risk for decreased **Cardiac** tissue perfusion: Risk factors: hypoxia, hypovolemia, cardiac tamponade

Readiness for enhanced **Knowledge:** treatment of disease

See Heart Failure, if appropriate

MYRINGOTOMY

Fear r/t hospitalization, surgical procedure

Ineffective **Health** maintenance r/t deficient knowledge regarding care after surgery

Acute **Pain** r/t surgical procedure

Risk for **Infection:** Risk factor: invasive procedure

See Ear Surgery

MYXEDEMA

See Hypothyroidism

N

NARCISSISTIC PERSONALITY DISORDER

Defensive **Coping** r/t grandiose sense of self

Impaired emancipated **Decision-Making** r/t lack of realistic problem-solving skills

Interrupted **Family** processes r/t taking advantage of others to achieve own goals

Risk-prone **Health** behavior r/t low self-efficacy

Disturbed personal **Identity** r/t psychological impairment

Ineffective **Relationship** r/t lack of mutual support/respect between partners

Impaired individual **Resilience** r/t psychological disorders

Impaired **Social** interaction r/t self-concept disturbance

Risk for **Loneliness:** Risk factors: emotional deprivation, social isolation

NARCOLEPSY

Anxiety r/t fear of lack of control over falling asleep

Disturbed **Sleep** pattern r/t uncontrollable desire to sleep

Risk for **Trauma:** Risk factor: falling asleep during potentially dangerous activity

Readiness for enhanced **Sleep:** expresses willingness to enhance sleep

NARCOTIC USE

See Opiate Use (preferred terminology)

NASOGASTRIC SUCTION

Impaired **Oral Mucous Membrane** r/t presence of nasogastric tube

Risk for **Electrolyte** imbalance: Risk factor: loss of gastrointestinal fluids that contain electrolytes

Risk for imbalanced **Fluid** volume: Risk factor: loss of gastrointestinal fluids without adequate replacement

Risk for dysfunctional **Gastrointestinal** motility: Risk factor: decreased intestinal motility

NAUSEA

Nausea (See **Nausea,** Section III)

NEAR-DROWNING

Ineffective **Airway** clearance r/t aspiration of fluid

Aspiration r/t aspiration of fluid into lungs

Fear: parental r/t possible death of child, possible permanent and debilitating sequelae

Impaired **Gas** exchange r/t laryngospasm, holding breath, aspiration, inflammation

Grieving r/t potential death of child, unknown sequelae, guilt about accident

Ineffective **Health** maintenance r/t parental deficient knowledge regarding safety measures appropriate for age

Hypothermia r/t central nervous system injury, prolonged submersion in cold water

N

Risk for delayed **Development:** Risk factors: hypoxemia, cerebral anoxia

Risk for disproportionate **Growth:** Risk factor: exposure to violence

Risk for complicated **Grieving:** Risk factors: potential death of child, unknown sequelae, guilt about accident

Risk for **Infection:** Risk factors: aspiration, invasive monitoring

Risk for ineffective **Cerebral** tissue perfusion: Risk factor: hypoxia

Readiness for enhanced **Spiritual** well-being: struggle with survival of life-threatening situation

See Child with Chronic Condition; Hospitalized Child; Safety, Childhood; Terminally Ill Child/Death of Child, Parent

NEARSIGHTEDNESS

Readiness for enhanced **Health** management: need for correction of myopia

NEARSIGHTEDNESS; CORNEAL SURGERY

See LASIK Eye Surgery (Laser-Assisted in Situ Keratomileusis)

NECK VEIN DISTENTION

Decreased **Cardiac** output r/t decreased contractility of heart resulting in increased preload

Excess **Fluid** volume r/t excess fluid intake, compromised regulatory mechanisms

See Congestive Heart Failure; Heart Failure

NECROSIS, KIDNEY TUBULAR; NECROSIS, ACUTE TUBULAR

See Kidney Failure

NECROTIZING ENTEROCOLITIS

Ineffective **Breathing** pattern r/t abdominal distention, hypoxia

Diarrhea r/t infection

Deficient **Fluid** volume r/t vomiting, gastrointestinal bleeding

Neonatal **Jaundice** r/t feeding pattern not well established

Imbalanced **Nutrition:** less than body requirements r/t decreased ability to absorb nutrients, decreased perfusion to gastrointestinal tract

Risk for dysfunctional **Gastrointestinal** motility: Risk factor: infection

Risk for ineffective **Gastrointestinal** perfusion: Risk factors: shunting of blood away from mesenteric circulation and toward vital organs as a result of perinatal stress, hypoxia

Risk for **Infection:** Risk factors: bacterial invasion of gastrointestinal tract, invasive procedures

See Hospitalized Child; Premature Infant (Child)

NEGATIVE FEELINGS ABOUT SELF

Chronic low **Self-Esteem** r/t long-standing negative self-evaluation

Self-Neglect r/t negative feelings

Readiness for enhanced **Self-Concept:** expresses willingness to enhance self-concept

NEGLECT, UNILATERAL

Unilateral Neglect (See **Unilateral Neglect**, Section III)

NEGLECTFUL CARE OF FAMILY MEMBER

Caregiver Role Strain r/t overwhelming care demands of family member, lack of social or financial support

Disabled family **Coping** r/t highly ambivalent family relationships, lack of respite care

Interrupted **Family** processes r/t situational transition or crisis

Deficient **Knowledge** r/t care needs

Impaired individual **Resilience** r/t vulnerability from neglect

Risk for compromised **Human Dignity:** Risk factor: inadequate participation in decision-making

NEONATAL JAUNDICE

Neonatal **Jaundice** (See neonatal **Jaundice**, Section III)

NEONATE

Readiness for enhanced **Childbearing** process: appropriate care of newborn

See Newborn, Normal; Newborn, Postmature; Newborn, Small for Gestational Age (SGA)

NEOPLASM

Fear r/t possible malignancy

See Cancer

NEPHRECTOMY

Anxiety r/t surgical recovery, prognosis

Ineffective **Breathing** pattern r/t location of surgical incision

Constipation r/t lack of return of peristalsis

Acute **Pain** r/t incisional discomfort

Spiritual distress r/t chronic illness

Risk for **Bleeding:** Risk factor: surgery

Risk for imbalanced **Fluid** volume: Risk factors: vascular losses, decreased intake

Risk for **Infection:** Risk factors: invasive procedure, lack of deep breathing because of location of surgical incision

Risk for ineffective **Renal** perfusion: Risk factor: kidney disease

NEPHROSTOMY, PERCUTANEOUS

Acute **Pain** r/t invasive procedure

Impaired **Urinary** elimination r/t nephrostomy tube

Risk for **Infection:** Risk factor: invasive procedure

NEPHROTIC SYNDROME

Activity intolerance r/t generalized edema

Disturbed **Body Image** r/t edematous appearance and side effects of steroid therapy

Excess **Fluid** volume r/t edema resulting from oncotic fluid shift caused by serum protein loss and kidney retention of salt and water

Imbalanced **Nutrition:** less than body requirements r/t anorexia, protein loss

Imbalanced **Nutrition:** more than body requirements r/t increased appetite attributable to steroid therapy

Social isolation r/t edematous appearance

Risk for **Infection:** Risk factor: altered immune mechanisms caused by disease and effects of steroids

Risk for ineffective **Renal** perfusion: Risk factor: kidney disease

Risk for impaired **Skin** integrity: Risk factor: edema

See Child with Chronic Condition; Hospitalized Child

N

NEURAL TUBE DEFECTS (MENINGOCELE, MYELOMENINGOCELE, SPINA BIFIDA, ANENCEPHALY)

Chronic functional **Constipation** r/t immobility or less than adequate mobility

Grieving r/t loss of perfect child, birth of child with congenital defect

Reflex urinary **Incontinence** r/t neurogenic impairment

Total urinary **Incontinence** r/t neurogenic impairment

Urge urinary **Incontinence** r/t neurogenic impairment

Impaired **Mobility** r/t neuromuscular impairment

Chronic low **Self-Esteem** r/t perceived differences, decreased ability to participate in physical and social activities at school

Impaired **Skin** integrity r/t incontinence

Risk for delayed **Development:** Risk factor: inadequate nutrition

Risk for disproportionate **Growth:** Risk factor: congenital disorder

Risk for **Latex Allergy** response: Risk factor: multiple exposures to latex products

Risk for imbalanced **Nutrition:** more than body requirements: Risk factor: diminished, limited, or impaired physical activity

Risk for **Powerlessness:** Risk factor: debilitating disease

Risk for impaired **Skin** integrity: lower extremities: Risk factor: decreased sensory perception

Readiness for enhanced family **Coping:** effective adaptive response by family members

Readiness for enhanced **Family** processes: family supports each other

See Child with Chronic Condition; Premature Infant (Child)

NEURALGIA

See Trigeminal Neuralgia

NEURITIS (PERIPHERAL NEUROPATHY)

Activity intolerance r/t pain with movement

Ineffective **Health** maintenance r/t deficient knowledge regarding self-care with neuritis

Acute **Pain** r/t stimulation of affected nerve endings, inflammation of sensory nerves

See Neuropathy, Peripheral

NEUROGENIC BLADDER

Reflex urinary **Incontinence** r/t neurological impairment

Urinary Retention r/t interruption in the lateral spinal tracts

Risk for **Latex Allergy** response: Risk factor: repeated exposures to latex associated with possible repeated catheterizations

NEUROLOGIC DISORDERS

Ineffective **Airway** clearance r/t perceptual or cognitive impairment, decreased energy, fatigue

Acute **Confusion** r/t dementia, alcohol abuse, drug abuse, delirium

Ineffective **Coping** r/t disability requiring change in lifestyle

Interrupted **Family** processes r/t situational crisis, illness, or disability of family member

Grieving r/t loss of usual body functioning

Impaired **Home** maintenance r/t client's or family member's disease

Risk for corneal **Injury:** Risk factor: lack of spontaneous blink reflex

Impaired **Memory** r/t neurological disturbance

Impaired physical **Mobility** r/t neuromuscular impairment

Imbalanced **Nutrition:** less than body requirements r/t impaired swallowing, depression, difficulty feeding self

Powerlessness r/t progressive nature of disease

Self-Care deficit: specify r/t neuromuscular dysfunction

Sexual dysfunction r/t biopsychosocial alteration of sexuality

Social isolation r/t altered state of wellness

Impaired **Swallowing** r/t neuromuscular dysfunction

Risk for **Disuse** syndrome: Risk factors: physical immobility, neuromuscular dysfunction

Risk for **Injury:** Risk factors: altered mobility, sensory dysfunction, cognitive impairment

Risk for ineffective **Cerebral** tissue perfusion: Risk factor: cerebral disease/ injury

Risk for impaired **Religiosity:** Risk factor: life transition

Risk for impaired **Skin** integrity: Risk factors: altered sensation, altered mental status, paralysis

See specific condition: Alcohol Withdrawal; Amyotrophic Lateral Sclerosis (ALS); CVA (Cerebrovascular Accident); Delirium; Dementia; Guillain-Barré Syndrome; Head Injury; Huntington's Disease; Spinal Cord Injury; Myasthenia Gravis; Muscular Dystrophy; Parkinson's Disease

NEUROPATHY, PERIPHERAL

Chronic **Pain** r/t damage to nerves in the peripheral nervous system as a result of medication side effects, vitamin deficiency, or diabetes

Ineffective **Thermoregulation** r/t decreased ability to regulate body temperature

Risk for **Injury:** Risk factors: lack of muscle control, decreased sensation

Risk for impaired **Skin** integrity: Risk factor: poor perfusion

Risk for **Thermal** Injury r/t nerve damage

See Peripheral Vascular Disease (PVD)

NEUROSURGERY

See Craniectomy/Craniotomy

NEWBORN, NORMAL

Breastfeeding r/t normal oral structure and gestational age greater than 34 weeks

Ineffective **Thermoregulation** r/t immaturity of neuroendocrine system

Risk for **Sudden Infant Death** syndrome: Risk factors: lack of knowledge regarding infant sleeping in prone or side-lying position, prenatal or postnatal infant smoke exposure, infant overheating or overwrapping, loose articles in the sleep environment

Risk for **Infection:** Risk factors: open umbilical stump, immature immune system

Risk for **Injury:** Risk factors: immaturity, need for caretaking

Readiness for enhanced **Childbearing** process: appropriate care of newborn

Readiness for enhanced organized **Infant** behavior: demonstrates adaptive response to pain

Readiness for enhanced **Parenting:** providing emotional and physical needs of infant

NEWBORN, POSTMATURE

Hypothermia r/t depleted stores of subcutaneous fat

Impaired **Skin** integrity r/t cracked and peeling skin as a result of decreased vernix

Risk for ineffective **Airway** clearance: Risk factor: meconium aspiration

Risk for unstable blood **Glucose** level: Risk factor: depleted glycogen stores

NEWBORN, SMALL FOR GESTATIONAL AGE (SGA)

Neonatal **Jaundice** r/t neonate age and difficulty feeding

Imbalanced **Nutrition:** less than body requirements r/t history of placental insufficiency

Ineffective **Thermoregulation** r/t decreased brown fat, subcutaneous fat

Risk for delayed **Development:** Risk factor: history of placental insufficiency

Risk for disproportionate **Growth:** Risk factor: history of placental insufficiency

Risk for **Injury:** Risk factors: hypoglycemia, perinatal asphyxia, meconium aspiration

Risk for **Sudden Infant Death** syndrome: Risk factor: low birth weight

NICOTINE ADDICTION

Risk-prone **Health** behavior r/t smoking

Ineffective **Health** maintenance r/t lack of ability to make a judgment about smoking cessation

Risk for impaired **Skin** integrity: Risk factor: poor tissue perfusion associated with nicotine

Powerlessness r/t perceived lack of control over ability to give up nicotine

N

Readiness for enhanced emancipated **Decision-Making:** expresses desire to enhance understanding and meaning of choices

Readiness for enhanced **Health** management: expresses desire to learn measures to stop smoking

NIDDM (NON-INSULIN-DEPENDENT DIABETES MELLITUS)

Readiness for enhanced **Health** management: expresses desire for information on exercise and diet to manage diabetes

See Diabetes Mellitus

NIGHTMARES

Post-Trauma syndrome r/t disaster, war, epidemic, rape, assault, torture, catastrophic illness, or accident

NIPPLE SORENESS

Impaired **Comfort** r/t physical condition

See Painful Breasts; Sore Nipples, Breastfeeding

NOCTURIA

Urge urinary **Incontinence** r/t decreased bladder capacity, irritation of bladder stretch receptors causing spasm, alcohol, caffeine, increased fluids, increased urine concentration, overdistention of bladder

Impaired **Urinary** elimination r/t sensory motor impairment, urinary tract infection

Risk for **Powerlessness:** Risk factor: inability to control nighttime voiding

NOCTURNAL MYOCLONUS

See Restless Leg Syndrome; Stress

NOCTURNAL PAROXYSMAL DYSPNEA

See PND (Paroxysmal Nocturnal Dyspnea)

NONCOMPLIANCE

Ineffective **Health** management (See **Health** management, ineffective, Section III)

NON–INSULIN-DEPENDENT DIABETES MELLITUS (NIDDM)

See Diabetes Mellitus

NORMAL PRESSURE HYDROCEPHALUS (NPH)

Impaired verbal **Communication** r/t obstruction of flow of cerebrospinal fluid affecting speech

Acute **Confusion** r/t increased intracranial pressure caused by obstruction to flow of cerebrospinal fluid

Impaired **Memory** r/t neurological disturbance

Risk for ineffective **Cerebral** tissue perfusion: Risk factor: fluid pressing on the brain

Risk for **Falls:** Risk factor: unsteady gait as a result of obstruction of cerebrospinal fluid

NOROVIRUS

See Viral Gastroenteritis

NSTEMI (NON-ST-ELEVATION MYOCARDIAL INFARCTION)

See MI (Myocardial Infarction)

NURSING

See Breastfeeding, Effective; Breastfeeding, Ineffective; Breastfeeding, Interrupted

NUTRITION

Readiness for enhanced **Nutrition** (See **Nutrition**, readiness for enhanced, Section III)

NUTRITION, IMBALANCED

Imbalanced **Nutrition:** less than body requirements (See **Nutrition:** less than body requirements, imbalanced, Section III)

Obesity (See **Obesity**, Section III)

Overweight (See **Overweight**, Section III)

Risk for **Overweight** (See **Overweight**, risk for, Section III)

O

OBESITY

Disturbed **Body Image** r/t eating disorder, excess weight

Risk-prone **Health** behavior: r/t negative attitude toward health care

Obesity (See **Obesity,** Section III)

Chronic low **Self-Esteem** r/t ineffective coping, overeating

Risk for ineffective peripheral **Tissue Perfusion:** Risk factor: sedentary lifestyle

Readiness for enhanced **Nutrition:** expresses willingness to enhance nutrition

OBS (ORGANIC BRAIN SYNDROME)

See Organic Mental Disorders; Dementia

OBSESSIVE-COMPULSIVE DISORDER (OCD)

See OCD (Obsessive-Compulsive Disorder)

OBSTRUCTION, BOWEL

See Bowel Obstruction

OBSTRUCTIVE SLEEP APNEA

Insomnia r/t blocked airway

Obesity r/t excessive intake related to metabolic need

See PND (Paroxysmal Nocturnal Dyspnea)

OCD (OBSESSIVE-COMPULSIVE DISORDER)

Ineffective **Activity** planning r/t unrealistic perception of events

Anxiety r/t threat to self-concept, unmet needs

Impaired emancipated **Decision-Making** r/t inability to make a decision for fear of reprisal

Disabled family **Coping** r/t family process being disrupted by client's ritualistic activities

Ineffective **Coping** r/t expression of feelings in an unacceptable way, ritualistic behavior

Risk-prone **Health** behavior r/t inadequate comprehension associated with repetitive thoughts

Powerlessness r/t unrelenting repetitive thoughts to perform irrational activities

Impaired individual **Resilience** r/t psychological disorder

Risk for situational low **Self-Esteem:** Risk factor: inability to control repetitive thoughts and actions

ODD (OPPOSITIONAL DEFIANT DISORDER)

Anxiety r/t feelings of anger and hostility toward authority figures

Ineffective **Coping** r/t lack of self-control or perceived lack of self-control

Disabled **Family** coping r/t feelings of anger, hostility; defiant behavior toward authority figures

Risk-prone **Health** behavior r/t multiple stressors associated with condition

Ineffective **Impulse** control r/t anger/compunction to engage in disruptive behaviors

Chronic or situational low **Self-Esteem** r/t poor self-control and disruptive behaviors

Impaired **Social** interaction r/t being touchy or easily annoyed, blaming others for own mistakes, constant trouble in school

Social isolation r/t unaccepted social behavior

Ineffective family **Health** management r/t difficulty in limit setting and managing oppositional behaviors

Risk for ineffective **Activity** planning: Risk factors: unrealistic perception of events, hedonism, insufficient social support

Risk for impaired **Parenting:** Risk factors: children's difficult behaviors and inability to set limits

Risk for **Powerlessness:** Risk factor: inability to deal with difficult behaviors

O

Risk for **Spiritual** distress: Risk factor: anxiety and stress in dealing with difficult behaviors

Risk for other-directed **Violence:** Risk factors: history of violence, threats of violence against others, history of antisocial behavior, history of indirect violence

OLDER ADULT

See Aging

OLIGURIA

Deficient **Fluid** volume r/t active fluid loss, failure of regulatory mechanism, inadequate intake

See Cardiac Output, Decreased; Kidney Failure; Shock, Hypovolemic

OMPHALOCELE

See Gastroschisis/Omphalocele

OOPHORECTOMY

Risk for ineffective **Sexuality** pattern: Risk factor: altered body function

See Surgery, Perioperative; Surgery, Postoperative; Surgery, Preoperative

OPCAB (OFF-PUMP CORONARY ARTERY BYPASS)

See Angioplasty, Coronary; Coronary Artery Bypass Grafting (CABG)

OPEN HEART SURGERY

Risk for decreased **Cardiac** tissue perfusion: Risk factor: cardiac surgery

See Coronary Artery Bypass Grafting (CABG); Dysrhythmia

OPEN REDUCTION OF FRACTURE WITH INTERNAL FIXATION (FEMUR)

Anxiety r/t outcome of corrective procedure

Impaired physical **Mobility** r/t postoperative position, abduction of leg, avoidance of acute flexion

Powerlessness r/t loss of control, unanticipated change in lifestyle

Risk for **Infection:** Risk factor: surgical procedure

Risk for **Perioperative Positioning** injury: Risk factor: immobilization

Risk for **Peripheral Neurovascular** dysfunction: Risk factors: mechanical compression, orthopedic surgery, immobilization

See Surgery, Postoperative Care

OPIATE USE

Chronic **Pain** syndrome r/t prolonged use of opiates

Risk for **Constipation:** Risk factor: effects of opiates on peristalsis

See Drug Abuse; Drug Withdrawal

OPPORTUNISTIC INFECTION

Delayed **Surgical** recovery r/t abnormal blood profiles, impaired healing

Risk for **Infection:** Risk factor: abnormal blood profiles

See AIDS (Acquired Immunodeficiency Syndrome); HIV (Human Immunodeficiency Virus)

OPPOSITIONAL DEFIANT DISORDER (ODD)

See ODD (Oppositional Defiant Disorder)

ORAL MUCOUS MEMBRANE, IMPAIRED

Impaired **Oral Mucous Membrane** (See **Oral Mucous Membrane,** impaired, Section III)

ORAL THRUSH

See Candidiasis, Oral

ORCHITIS

Readiness for enhanced **Health** management: follows recommendations for mumps vaccination

See Epididymitis

ORGANIC MENTAL DISORDERS

Frail Elderly syndrome r/t alteration in cognitive function

Impaired **Social** interaction r/t disturbed thought processes

Risk for disturbed personal **Identity**: Risk factor: delusions/fluctuating perceptions of stimuli

Risk for **Infection**: Risk factor: surgical procedure

See Dementia

ORTHOPEDIC TRACTION

Ineffective **Role** performance r/t limited physical mobility

Impaired **Social** interaction r/t limited physical mobility

Impaired **Transfer** ability r/t limited physical mobility

Risk for impaired **Religiosity**: Risk factor: immobility

See Traction and Casts

ORTHOPNEA

Ineffective **Breathing** pattern r/t inability to breathe with head of bed flat

Decreased **Cardiac** output r/t inability of heart to meet demands of body

ORTHOSTATIC HYPOTENSION

See Dizziness

OSTEOARTHRITIS

Acute **Pain** r/t movement

Impaired **Walking** r/t inflammation and damage to joints

See Arthritis

OSTEOMYELITIS

Deficient **Diversional** activity r/t prolonged immobilization, hospitalization

Fear: parental r/t concern regarding possible growth plate damage caused by infection, concern that infection may become chronic

Ineffective **Health** maintenance r/t continued immobility at home, possible extensive casts, continued antibiotics

Impaired physical **Mobility** r/t imposed immobility as a result of infected area

Acute **Pain** r/t inflammation in affected extremity

Ineffective **Thermoregulation** r/t infectious process

Risk for **Constipation**: Risk factor: immobility

Risk for **Infection**: Risk factor: inadequate primary and secondary defenses

Risk for impaired **Skin** integrity: Risk factor: irritation from splint or cast

See Hospitalized Child

OSTEOPOROSIS

Deficient **Knowledge** r/t diet, exercise, need to abstain from alcohol and nicotine

Impaired physical **Mobility** r/t pain, skeletal changes

Imbalanced **Nutrition**: less than body requirements r/t inadequate intake of calcium and vitamin D

Acute **Pain** r/t fracture, muscle spasms

Risk for **Injury**: fracture: Risk factors: lack of activity, risk of falling resulting from environmental hazards, neuromuscular disorders, diminished senses, cardiovascular responses to drugs

Risk for **Powerlessness**: Risk factor: debilitating disease

Readiness for enhanced **Health** management: expresses desire to manage the treatment of illness and prevent complications

OSTOMY

See Child with Chronic Condition; Colostomy; Ileal Conduit; Ileostomy

OTITIS MEDIA

Acute **Pain** r/t inflammation, infectious process

Risk for delayed **Development**: speech and language: Risk factor: frequent otitis media

O

Risk for **Infection:** Risk factors: eustachian tube obstruction, traumatic eardrum perforation, infectious disease process

Readiness for enhanced **Knowledge:** information on treatment and prevention of disease

OVARIAN CARCINOMA

Death **Anxiety** r/t unknown outcome, possible poor prognosis

Fear r/t unknown outcome, possible poor prognosis

Ineffective **Health Maintenance** r/t deficient knowledge regarding self-care, treatment of condition

Readiness for enhanced **Family Processes:** family functioning meets needs of client

Readiness for enhanced **Resilience:** participates in support groups

See Chemotherapy; Hysterectomy; Radiation Therapy

P

PACEMAKER

Anxiety r/t change in health status, presence of pacemaker

Death **Anxiety** r/t worry over possible malfunction of pacemaker

Deficient **Knowledge** r/t self-care program, when to seek medical attention

Acute **Pain** r/t surgical procedure

Risk for **Bleeding:** Risk factor: surgery

Risk for decreased **Cardiac** tissue perfusion: Risk factor: pacemaker malfunction

Risk for **Infection:** Risk factors: invasive procedure, presence of foreign body (catheter and generator)

Risk for **Powerlessness:** Risk factor: presence of electronic device to stimulate heart

Readiness for enhanced **Health** management: appropriate health care management of pacemaker

PAGET'S DISEASE

Disturbed **Body Image** r/t possible enlarged head, bowed tibias, kyphosis

Deficient **Knowledge** r/t appropriate diet high in protein and calcium, mild exercise

Chronic **Sorrow** r/t chronic condition with altered body image

Risk for **Trauma:** fracture: Risk factor: excessive bone destruction

PAIN, ACUTE

Acute **Pain** (See **Pain,** acute, Section III)

PAIN, CHRONIC

Chronic **Pain** (See **Pain,** chronic, Section III)

PAINFUL BREASTS, ENGORGEMENT

Acute **Pain** r/t distention of breast tissue

Ineffective **Role** performance r/t change in physical capacity to assume role of breastfeeding mother

Impaired **Tissue** integrity r/t excessive fluid in breast tissues

Risk for ineffective **Breastfeeding:** Risk factors: pain, infant's inability to latch on to engorged breast

Risk for **Infection:** Risk factor: milk stasis

PAINFUL BREASTS, SORE NIPPLES

Insufficient **Breast Milk** r/t long breastfeeding time/pain response

Ineffective **Breastfeeding** r/t pain

Acute **Pain** r/t cracked nipples

Ineffective **Role** performance r/t change in physical capacity to assume role of breastfeeding mother

Impaired **Skin** integrity r/t mechanical factors involved in suckling, breastfeeding management

Risk for **Infection:** Risk factor: break in skin

PALLOR OF EXTREMITIES

Ineffective peripheral **Tissue Perfusion** r/t interruption of vascular flow

See Shock; Peripheral Vascular Disease (PVD)

PALPITATIONS (HEART PALPITATIONS)

See Dysrhythmia

PANCREATIC CANCER

Death **Anxiety** r/t possible poor prognosis of disease process

Ineffective family **Coping** r/t poor prognosis

Fear r/t poor prognosis of the disease

Grieving r/t shortened life span

Deficient **Knowledge** r/t disease-induced diabetes, home management

Spiritual distress r/t poor prognosis

Risk for impaired **Liver** function: Risk factor: complications from underlying disease

See Cancer; Chemotherapy; Radiation Therapy; Surgery, Perioperative; Surgery, Postoperative; Surgery, Preoperative

PANCREATITIS

Ineffective **Breathing** pattern r/t splinting from severe pain, disease process, and inflammation

Ineffective **Denial** r/t ineffective coping, alcohol use

Diarrhea r/t decrease in pancreatic secretions resulting in steatorrhea

Deficient **Fluid** volume r/t vomiting, decreased fluid intake, fever, diaphoresis, fluid shifts

Ineffective **Health** maintenance r/t deficient knowledge concerning diet, alcohol use, medication

Nausea r/t irritation of gastrointestinal system

Imbalanced **Nutrition:** less than body requirements r/t inadequate dietary intake, increased nutritional needs as a result of acute illness, increased metabolic needs caused by increased body temperature, disease process

Acute **Pain** r/t irritation and edema of the inflamed pancreas

Chronic **Sorrow** r/t chronic illness

Readiness for enhanced **Comfort:** expresses desire to enhance comfort

PANIC DISORDER (PANIC ATTACKS)

Ineffective **Activity** planning r/t unrealistic perception of events

Anxiety r/t situational crisis

Ineffective **Coping** r/t personal vulnerability

Risk-prone **Health** behavior r/t low self-efficacy

Disturbed personal **Identity** r/t situational crisis

Post-Trauma syndrome r/t previous catastrophic event

Social isolation r/t fear of lack of control

Risk for **Loneliness:** Risk factor: inability to socially interact because of fear of losing control

Risk for **Post-Trauma** syndrome: Risk factors: perception of the event, diminished ego strength

Risk for **Powerlessness:** Risk factor: ineffective coping skills

Readiness for enhanced **Coping:** seeks problem-oriented and emotion-oriented strategies to manage condition

See Anxiety; Anxiety Disorder

PARALYSIS

Disturbed **Body Image** r/t biophysical changes, loss of movement, immobility

Impaired **Comfort** r/t prolonged immobility

Constipation r/t effects of spinal cord disruption, inadequate fiber in diet

Ineffective **Health** maintenance r/t deficient knowledge regarding self-care with paralysis

P

Impaired **Home** maintenance r/t physical disability

Reflex urinary **Incontinence** r/t neurological impairment

Impaired physical **Mobility** r/t neuromuscular impairment

Impaired wheelchair **Mobility** r/t neuromuscular impairment

Self-Neglect r/t functional impairment

Powerlessness r/t illness-related regimen

Self-Care deficit: specify r/t neuromuscular impairment

Sexual dysfunction r/t loss of sensation, biopsychosocial alteration

Chronic **Sorrow** r/t loss of physical mobility

Impaired **Transfer** ability r/t paralysis

Risk for **Autonomic Dysreflexia:** Risk factor: cause of paralysis

Risk for **Disuse** syndrome: Risk factor: paralysis

Risk for **Falls:** Risk factor: paralysis

Risk for **Injury:** Risk factors: altered mobility, sensory dysfunction

Risk for **Latex Allergy** response: Risk factor: possible repeated urinary catheterizations

Risk for **Post-Trauma** syndrome: Risk factor: event causing paralysis

Risk for impaired **Religiosity:** Risk factors: immobility, possible lack of transportation

Risk for impaired **Resilience:** Risk factor: chronic disability

Risk for situational low **Self-Esteem:** Risk factor: change in body image and function

Risk for impaired **Skin** integrity: Risk factors: altered circulation, altered sensation, immobility

Readiness for enhanced **Self-Care:** expresses desire to enhance knowledge and responsibility for strategies for self-care

See Child with Chronic Condition; Hemiplegia; Hospitalized Child; Neural Tube Defects; Spinal Cord Injury

PARALYTIC ILEUS

Constipation r/t decreased gastrointestinal motility

Deficient **Fluid** volume r/t loss of fluids from vomiting, retention of fluid in bowel

Dysfunctional **Gastrointestinal** motility r/t recent abdominal surgery, electrolyte imbalance

Nausea r/t gastrointestinal irritation

Acute **Pain** r/t pressure, abdominal distention, presence of nasogastric tube

See Bowel Obstruction

PARANOID PERSONALITY DISORDER

Ineffective **Activity** planning r/t unrealistic perception of events

Anxiety r/t uncontrollable intrusive, suspicious thoughts

Risk-prone **Health** behavior r/t intense emotional state

Disturbed personal **Identity** r/t difficulty with reality testing

Impaired individual **Resilience** r/t psychological disorder

Chronic low **Self-Esteem** r/t inability to trust others

Social isolation r/t inappropriate social skills

Risk for **Loneliness:** Risk factor: social isolation

Risk for other-directed **Violence:** Risk factor: being suspicious of others and their actions

PARAPLEGIA

See Spinal Cord Injury

PARATHYROIDECTOMY

Anxiety r/t surgery

Risk for ineffective **Airway** clearance: Risk factors: edema or hematoma formation, airway obstruction

Risk for **Bleeding:** Risk factor: surgery

Risk for impaired verbal **Communication:** Risk factors: possible laryngeal damage, edema

Risk for **Infection:** Risk factor: surgical procedure

See Hypocalcemia

PARENT ATTACHMENT

Risk for impaired **Attachment** (See **Attachment,** impaired, risk for, Section III)

Readiness for enhanced **Childbearing** process: demonstrates appropriate care of newborn

See Parental Role Conflict

PARENTAL ROLE CONFLICT

Parental **Role** conflict (See **Role** conflict, parental, Section III)

Ineffective **Relationship** r/t unrealistic expectations

Chronic **Sorrow** r/t difficult parent–child relationship

Risk for **Spiritual** distress: Risk factor: altered relationships

Readiness for enhanced **Parenting:** willingness to enhance parenting

PARENTING

Readiness for enhanced **Parenting** (See **Parenting,** readiness for enhanced, Section III)

PARENTING, IMPAIRED

Impaired **Parenting** (See **Parenting,** impaired, Section III)

Chronic **Sorrow** r/t difficult parent–child relationship

Risk for **Spiritual** distress: Risk factor: altered relationships

PARENTING, RISK FOR IMPAIRED

Risk for impaired **Parenting** (See **Parenting,** impaired, risk for, Section III)

See Parenting, Impaired

PARESTHESIA

Risk for **Injury:** Risk factors: inability to feel temperature changes, pain

Risk for impaired **Skin** integrity: Risk factor: impaired sensation

Risk for **Thermal** injury: Risk factor: neuromuscular impairment

PARKINSON'S DISEASE

Impaired verbal **Communication** r/t decreased speech volume, slowness of speech, impaired facial muscles

Constipation r/t weakness of muscles, lack of exercise, inadequate fluid intake, decreased autonomic nervous system activity

Frail Elderly syndrome r/t chronic illness

Imbalanced **Nutrition:** less than body requirements r/t tremor, slowness in eating, difficulty in chewing and swallowing

Chronic **Sorrow** r/t loss of physical capacity

Risk for **Injury:** Risk factors: tremors, slow reactions, altered gait

See Neurologic Disorders

PAROXYSMAL NOCTURNAL DYSPNEA (PND)

See PND (Paroxysmal Nocturnal Dyspnea)

PATENT DUCTUS ARTERIOSUS (PDA)

See Congenital Heart Disease/Cardiac Anomalies

PATIENT-CONTROLLED ANALGESIA (PCA)

See PCA (Patient-Controlled Analgesia)

PATIENT EDUCATION

Deficient **Knowledge** r/t lack of exposure to information misinterpretation, unfamiliarity with information resources to manage illness

Readiness for enhanced emancipated **Decision-Making:** expresses desire to enhance understanding of choices for decision-making

P

Readiness for enhanced **Knowledge** (specify): interest in learning

Readiness for enhanced **Health** management: expresses desire for information to manage the illness

PCA (PATIENT-CONTROLLED ANALGESIA)

Deficient **Knowledge** r/t self-care of pain control

Nausea r/t side effects of medication

Risk for **Injury:** Risk factor: possible complications associated with PCA

Risk for **Vascular Trauma:** Risk factors: insertion site, length of insertion time

Readiness for enhanced **Knowledge:** appropriate management of PCA

PECTUS EXCAVATUM

See Marfan Syndrome

PEDICULOSIS

See Lice

PEG (PERCUTANEOUS ENDOSCOPIC GASTROSTOMY)

See Tube Feeding

PELVIC INFLAMMATORY DISEASE (PID)

See PID (Pelvic Inflammatory Disease)

PENILE PROSTHESIS

Ineffective **Sexuality** pattern r/t use of penile prosthesis

Risk for **Infection:** Risk factor: invasive surgical procedure

Risk for situational low **Self-Esteem:** Risk factor: ineffective sexuality pattern

Readiness for enhanced **Health** management: seeks information regarding care and use of prosthesis

See Erectile Dysfunction (ED); Impotence

PEPTIC ULCER

See Ulcer, Peptic (Duodenal or Gastric)

PERCUTANEOUS TRANSLUMINAL CORONARY ANGIOPLASTY (PTCA)

See Angioplasty, Coronary

PERICARDIAL FRICTION RUB

Decreased **Cardiac** output

Acute Pain r/t inflammation, effusion

Risk for decreased **Cardiac** tissue perfusion: Risk factors: inflammation in pericardial sac, fluid accumulation compressing heart

PERICARDITIS

Activity intolerance r/t reduced cardiac reserve, prescribed bed rest

Decreased **Cardiac** output r/t impaired cardiac function from inflammation of pericardial sac

Risk for decreased **Cardiac** tissue perfusion: Risk factor: inflammation in pericardial sac

Deficient **Knowledge** r/t unfamiliarity with information sources

Risk for imbalanced **Nutrition:** less than body requirements: Risk factors: fever, hypermetabolic state associated with fever

Acute **Pain** r/t biological injury, inflammation

PERIODONTAL DISEASE

Risk for impaired **Oral Mucous Membranes** (See **Oral Mucous Membranes,** impaired, risk for, Section III)

PERIOPERATIVE HYPOTHERMIA

Risk for **Perioperative Hypothermia** (See **Perioperative Hypothermia,** risk for, Section III)

PERIOPERATIVE POSITIONING

Risk for **Perioperative Positioning** injury (See **Perioperative Positioning** injury, risk for, Section III)

PERIPHERAL NEUROPATHY

See Neuropathy, Peripheral

PERIPHERAL NEUROVASCULAR DYSFUNCTION

Risk for **Peripheral Neurovascular** dysfunction (See **Peripheral Neurovascular** dysfunction, risk for, Section III)

See Neuropathy, Peripheral; Peripheral Vascular Disease (PVD)

PERIPHERAL VASCULAR DISEASE (PVD)

Ineffective **Health** maintenance r/t deficient knowledge regarding self-care and treatment of disease

Chronic **Pain:** intermittent claudication r/t ischemia

Ineffective peripheral **Tissue Perfusion** r/t disease process

Risk for **Falls:** Risk factor: altered mobility

Risk for **Injury:** Risk factors: tissue hypoxia, altered mobility, altered sensation

Risk for **Peripheral Neurovascular** dysfunction: Risk factor: possible vascular obstruction

Risk for impaired **Tissue** integrity: Risk factor: altered circulation or sensation

Readiness for enhanced **Health** management: self-care and treatment of disease

See Neuropathy, Peripheral; Peripheral Neurovascular Dysfunction

PERITONEAL DIALYSIS

Ineffective **Breathing** pattern r/t pressure from dialysate

Impaired **Comfort** r/t instillation of dialysate, temperature of dialysate

Impaired **Home** maintenance r/t complex home treatment of client

Deficient **Knowledge** r/t treatment procedure, self-care with peritoneal dialysis

Chronic **Sorrow** r/t chronic disability

Risk for ineffective **Coping:** Risk factor: disability requiring change in lifestyle

Risk for unstable blood **Glucose** level: Risk factors: increased concentrations of glucose in dialysate, ineffective medication management

Risk for imbalanced **Fluid** volume: Risk factor: medical procedure

Risk for **Infection:** peritoneal: Risk factors: invasive procedure, presence of catheter, dialysate

Risk for **Powerlessness:** Risk factors: chronic condition, care involved

See Child with Chronic Condition; Hemodialysis; Hospitalized Child; Kidney Failure; Kidney Failure, Acute/Chronic, Child

PERITONITIS

Ineffective **Breathing** pattern r/t pain, increased abdominal pressure

Constipation r/t decreased oral intake, decrease of peristalsis

Deficient **Fluid** volume r/t retention of fluid in bowel with loss of circulating blood volume

Nausea r/t gastrointestinal irritation

Imbalanced **Nutrition:** less than body requirements r/t nausea, vomiting

Acute **Pain** r/t inflammation and infection of gastrointestinal system

Risk for dysfunctional **Gastrointestinal** motility: Risk factor: gastrointestinal disease

PERNICIOUS ANEMIA

Diarrhea r/t malabsorption of nutrients

Fatigue r/t imbalanced nutrition: less than body requirements

Impaired **Memory** r/t lack of adequate red blood cells

Nausea r/t altered oral mucous membrane, sore tongue, bleeding gums

Imbalanced **Nutrition:** less than body requirements r/t lack of appetite associated with nausea and altered oral mucous membrane

Impaired **Oral Mucous Membrane** r/t vitamin deficiency; inability to absorb vitamin B_{12} associated with lack of intrinsic factor

P

Risk for **Falls:** Risk factors: dizziness, lightheadedness

Risk for **Peripheral Neurovascular** dysfunction: Risk factor: anemia

PERSISTENT FETAL CIRCULATION

See Congenital Heart Disease/Cardiac Anomalies

PERSONAL IDENTITY PROBLEMS

Disturbed personal **Identity** (See **Identity,** personal, disturbed, Section III)

Risk for disturbed personal **Identity** (See disturbed personal **Identity,** risk for, Section III)

PERSONALITY DISORDER

Ineffective **Activity** planning r/t unrealistic perception of events

Impaired individual **Resilience** r/t psychological disorder

See specific disorder: Antisocial Personality Disorder; Borderline Personality Disorder; OCD (Obsessive-Compulsive Disorder); Paranoid Personality Disorder

PERTUSSIS (WHOOPING COUGH)

Risk for impaired emancipated **Decision-Making** r/t whether to administer usual childhood vaccinations

See Respiratory Infections, Acute Childhood

PESTICIDE CONTAMINATION

Contamination r/t use of environmental contaminants, pesticides

Risk for **Allergy** response r/t repeated exposure to pesticides

Risk for disproportionate **Growth:** Risk factor: environmental contamination

PETECHIAE

See Anticoagulant Therapy; Clotting Disorder; DIC (Disseminated Intravascular Coagulation); Hemophilia

PETIT MAL SEIZURE

Readiness for enhanced **Health** management: wears medical alert bracelet; limits hazardous activities such as driving, swimming, working at heights, operating equipment

See Epilepsy

PHARYNGITIS

See Sore Throat

PHENYLKETONURIA (PKU)

See PKU (Phenylketonuria)

PHEOCHROMOCYTOMA

Anxiety r/t symptoms from increased catecholamines—headache, palpitations, sweating, nervousness, nausea, vomiting, syncope

Ineffective **Health** maintenance r/t deficient knowledge regarding treatment and self-care

Insomnia r/t high levels of catecholamines

Nausea r/t increased catecholamines

Risk for decreased **Cardiac** tissue perfusion: Risk factor: hypertension

See Surgery, Perioperative; Surgery, Postoperative; Surgery, Preoperative

PHLEBITIS

See Thrombophlebitis

PHOBIA (SPECIFIC)

Fear r/t presence or anticipation of specific object or situation

Powerlessness r/t anxiety about encountering unknown or known entity

Impaired individual **Resilience** r/t psychological disorder

Readiness for enhanced **Power:** expresses readiness to enhance identification of choices that can be made for change

See Anxiety; Anxiety Disorder; Panic Disorder (Panic Attacks)

PHOTOSENSITIVITY

Ineffective **Health** maintenance r/t deficient knowledge regarding medications inducing photosensitivity

Risk for dry **Eye:** Risk factors: pharmaceutical agents, sunlight exposure

Risk for impaired **Skin** integrity: Risk factor: exposure to sun

PHYSICAL ABUSE

See Abuse, Child; Abuse, Spouse, Parent, or Significant Other

PICA

Anxiety r/t stress

Imbalanced **Nutrition:** less than body requirements r/t eating nonnutritive substances

Impaired **Parenting** r/t lack of supervision, food deprivation

Risk for **Constipation:** Risk factor: presence of undigestible materials in gastrointestinal tract

Risk for dysfunctional **Gastrointestinal** motility: Risk factor: abnormal eating behavior

Risk for **Infection:** Risk factor: ingestion of infectious agents via contaminated substances

Risk for **Poisoning:** Risk factor: ingestion of substances containing lead

See Anemia

PID (PELVIC INFLAMMATORY DISEASE)

Ineffective **Health** maintenance r/t deficient knowledge regarding self-care, treatment of disease

Acute **Pain** r/t biological injury, inflammation, edema, congestion of pelvic tissues

Ineffective **Sexuality** pattern r/t medically imposed abstinence from sexual activities until acute infection subsides, change in reproductive potential

Risk for **Infection:** Risk factors: insufficient knowledge to avoid exposure to pathogens; proper hygiene, nutrition, other health habits

See Maturational Issues, Adolescent; STD (Sexually Transmitted Disease)

PIH (PREGNANCY-INDUCED HYPERTENSION/PREECLAMPSIA)

Anxiety r/t fear of the unknown, threat to self and infant, change in role functioning

Death **Anxiety** r/t threat of preeclampsia

Deficient **Diversional** activity r/t bed rest

Interrupted **Family** processes r/t situational crisis

Impaired **Home** maintenance r/t bed rest

Deficient **Knowledge** r/t lack of experience with situation

Impaired physical **Mobility** r/t medically prescribed limitations

Impaired **Parenting** r/t prescribed bed rest

Powerlessness r/t complication threatening pregnancy, medically prescribed limitations

Ineffective **Role** performance r/t change in physical capacity to assume role of pregnant woman or resume other roles

Situational low **Self-Esteem** r/t loss of idealized pregnancy

Impaired **Social** interaction r/t imposed bed rest

Risk for imbalanced **Fluid** volume: Risk factors: hypertension, altered kidney function

Risk for **Injury:** fetal: Risk factors: decreased uteroplacental perfusion, seizures

Risk for **Injury:** maternal: Risk factors: vasospasm, high blood pressure

Readiness for enhanced **Knowledge:** exhibits desire for information on managing condition

PILOERECTION

Hypothermia r/t exposure to cold environment

P

PIMPLES

See Acne

PINK EYE

See Conjunctivitis

PINWORMS

Impaired **Comfort** r/t itching

Impaired **Home** maintenance r/t inadequate cleaning of bed linen and toilet seats

Insomnia r/t discomfort

Readiness for enhanced **Health** management: proper handwashing; short, clean fingernails; avoiding hand, mouth, nose contact with unwashed hands; appropriate cleaning of bed linen and toilet seats

PITUITARY TUMOR, BENIGN

See Cushing's Disease

PKU (PHENYLKETONURIA)

Risk for delayed **Development**: Risk factors: not following strict dietary program; eating foods extremely low in phenylalanine; avoiding eggs, milk, any foods containing aspartame (e.g., NutraSweet)

Readiness for enhanced **Health** management: testing for PKU and following prescribed dietary regimen

PLACENTA ABRUPTIO

Death **Anxiety** r/t threat of mortality associated with bleeding

Fear r/t threat to self and fetus

Ineffective **Health** maintenance r/t deficient knowledge regarding treatment and control of hypertension associated with placenta abruptio

Acute **Pain:** abdominal/back r/t premature separation of placenta before delivery

Risk for **Bleeding**: Risk factor: placenta abruptio

Risk for deficient **Fluid** volume: Risk factor: maternal blood loss

Risk for **Powerlessness:** Risk factors: complications of pregnancy, unknown outcome

Risk for **Shock:** Risk factor: hypovolemia

Risk for **Spiritual** distress: Risk factor: fear from unknown outcome of pregnancy

PLACENTA PREVIA

Death **Anxiety** r/t threat of mortality associated with bleeding

Disturbed **Body Image** r/t negative feelings about body and reproductive ability, feelings of helplessness

Ineffective **Coping** r/t threat to self and fetus

Deficient **Diversional** activity r/t long-term hospitalization

Interrupted **Family** processes r/t maternal bed rest, hospitalization

Fear r/t threat to self and fetus, unknown future

Impaired **Home** maintenance r/t maternal bed rest, hospitalization

Impaired physical **Mobility** r/t medical protocol, maternal bed rest

Ineffective **Role** performance r/t maternal bed rest, hospitalization

Situational low **Self-Esteem** r/t situational crisis

Spiritual distress r/t inability to participate in usual religious rituals, situational crisis

Risk for **Bleeding**: Risk factor: placenta previa

Risk for **Constipation**: Risk factors: bed rest, pregnancy

Risk for deficient **Fluid** volume: Risk factor: maternal blood loss

Risk for imbalanced **Fluid** volume: Risk factor: maternal blood loss

Risk for **Injury**: fetal and maternal: Risk factors: threat to uteroplacental perfusion, hemorrhage

Risk for disturbed **Maternal–Fetal** dyad: Risk factor: complication of pregnancy

Risk for impaired **Parenting:** Risk factors: maternal bed rest, hospitalization

Risk for ineffective peripheral **Tissue Perfusion:** placental: Risk factors: dilation of cervix, loss of placental implantation site

Risk for **Powerlessness:** Risk factors: complications of pregnancy, unknown outcome

Risk for **Shock:** Risk factor: hypovolemia

PLANTAR FASCIITIS

Impaired **Comfort** r/t inflamed structures of feet

Impaired physical **Mobility** r/t discomfort

Acute **Pain** r/t inflammation

Chronic **Pain** r/t inflammation

PLEURAL EFFUSION

Ineffective **Breathing** pattern r/t pain

Excess **Fluid** volume r/t compromised regulatory mechanisms; heart, liver, or kidney failure

Acute **Pain** r/t inflammation, fluid accumulation

PLEURAL FRICTION RUB

Ineffective **Breathing** pattern r/t pain

Acute **Pain** r/t inflammation, fluid accumulation

PLEURAL TAP

See Pleural Effusion

PLEURISY

Ineffective **Breathing** pattern r/t pain

Impaired **Gas** exchange r/t ventilation perfusion imbalance

Acute **Pain** r/t pressure on pleural nerve endings associated with fluid accumulation or inflammation

Impaired **Walking** r/t activity intolerance, inability to "catch breath"

Risk for ineffective **Airway** clearance: Risk factors: increased secretions, ineffective cough because of pain

Risk for **Infection:** Risk factor: exposure to pathogens

PMS (PREMENSTRUAL TENSION SYNDROME)

Fatigue r/t hormonal changes

Excess **Fluid** volume r/t alterations of hormonal levels inducing fluid retention

Deficient **Knowledge** r/t methods to deal with and prevent syndrome

Acute **Pain** r/t hormonal stimulation of gastrointestinal structures

Risk for **Powerlessness:** Risk factor: lack of knowledge and ability to deal with symptoms

Risk for impaired **Resilience:** Risk factor: PMS symptoms

Readiness for enhanced **Communication:** willingness to express thoughts and feelings about PMS

Readiness for enhanced **Health** management: desire for information to manage and prevent symptoms

PND (PAROXYSMAL NOCTURNAL DYSPNEA)

Anxiety r/t inability to breathe during sleep

Ineffective **Breathing** pattern r/t increase in carbon dioxide levels, decrease in oxygen levels

Insomnia r/t suffocating feeling from fluid in lungs on awakening from sleep

Sleep deprivation r/t inability to breathe during sleep

Risk for decreased **Cardiac** tissue perfusion: Risk factor: hypoxia

Risk for **Powerlessness:** Risk factor: inability to control nocturnal dyspnea

Readiness for enhanced **Sleep:** expresses willingness to learn measures to enhance sleep

PNEUMONECTOMY

See Thoracotomy

P

PNEUMONIA

Activity intolerance r/t imbalance between oxygen supply and demand

Ineffective **Airway** clearance r/t inflammation and presence of secretions

Impaired **Gas** exchange r/t decreased functional lung tissue

Ineffective **Health** management r/t deficient knowledge regarding self-care and treatment of disease

Imbalanced **Nutrition:** less than body requirements r/t loss of appetite

Impaired **Oral Mucous Membrane** r/t dry mouth from mouth breathing, decreased fluid intake

Ineffective **Thermoregulation** r/t infectious process

Risk for acute **Confusion:** Risk factors: underlying illness, hypoxia

Risk for deficient **Fluid** volume: Risk factor: inadequate intake of fluids

Risk for **Vascular Trauma:** Risk factor: irritation from intravenous antibiotics

See Respiratory Infections, Acute Childhood

PNEUMOTHORAX

Fear r/t threat to own well-being, difficulty breathing

Impaired **Gas** exchange r/t ventilation-perfusion imbalance, decreased functional lung tissue

Acute **Pain** r/t recent injury, coughing, deep breathing

Risk for **Injury:** Risk factor: possible complications associated with closed chest drainage system

See Chest Tubes

POISONING, RISK FOR

Risk for **Poisoning** (See **Poisoning,** risk for, Section III)

POLIOMYELITIS

See Paralysis

POLYDIPSIA

Readiness for enhanced **Fluid** balance: excessive thirst gone when diabetes is controlled

See Diabetes Mellitus

POLYPHAGIA

Readiness for enhanced **Nutrition:** knowledge of appropriate diet for diabetes

See Diabetes Mellitus

POLYURIA

Readiness for enhanced **Urinary** elimination: willingness to learn measures to enhance urinary elimination

See Diabetes Mellitus

POSTOPERATIVE CARE

See Surgery, Postoperative

POSTPARTUM DEPRESSION

Anxiety r/t new responsibilities of parenting

Disturbed **Body Image** r/t normal postpartum recovery

Ineffective **Childbearing** process r/t depression/lack of support system

Ineffective **Coping** r/t hormonal changes

Fatigue r/t childbirth, postpartum state, crying child

Risk-prone **Health** behavior r/t lack of support systems

Impaired **Home** maintenance r/t fatigue, care of newborn

Hopelessness r/t stress, exhaustion

Deficient **Knowledge** r/t lifestyle changes

Impaired **Parenting** r/t hormone-induced depression

Ineffective **Role** performance r/t new responsibilities of parenting

Sexual dysfunction r/t fear of another pregnancy, postpartum pain, lochia flow

Sleep deprivation r/t environmental stimulation of newborn

Impaired **Social** interaction r/t change in role functioning

Risk for disturbed personal **Identity** r/t role change/depression/inability to cope

Risk for situational low **Self-Esteem:** Risk factor: decreased power over feelings of sadness

Risk for **Spiritual** distress: Risk factors: altered relationships, social isolation

Readiness for enhanced **Hope:** expresses desire to enhance hope and interconnectedness with others

See Depression (Major Depressive Disorder)

POSTPARTUM HEMORRHAGE

Activity intolerance r/t anemia from loss of blood

Death **Anxiety** r/t threat of mortality associated with bleeding

Disturbed **Body Image** r/t loss of ideal childbirth

Insufficient **Breast Milk** r/t fluid volume depletion

Interrupted **Breastfeeding** r/t separation from infant for medical treatment

Decreased **Cardiac** output r/t hypovolemia

Fear r/t threat to self, unknown future

Deficient **Fluid** volume r/t uterine atony, loss of blood

Impaired **Home** maintenance r/t lack of stamina

Deficient **Knowledge** r/t lack of exposure to situation

Acute **Pain** r/t nursing and medical interventions to control bleeding

Ineffective peripheral **Tissue Perfusion** r/t hypovolemia

Risk for **Bleeding:** Risk factor: postpartum complications

Risk for impaired **Childbearing:** Risk factor: postpartum complication

Risk for imbalanced **Fluid** volume: Risk factor: maternal blood loss

Risk for **Infection:** Risk factors: loss of blood, depressed immunity

Risk for impaired **Parenting:** Risk factor: weakened maternal condition

Risk for **Powerlessness:** Risk factor: acute illness

Risk for **Shock:** Risk factor: hypovolemia

POSTPARTUM, NORMAL CARE

Anxiety r/t change in role functioning, parenting

Effective **Breastfeeding** r/t basic breastfeeding knowledge, support of partner and health care provider

Fatigue r/t childbirth, new responsibilities of parenting, body changes

Acute **Pain** r/t episiotomy, lacerations, bruising, breast engorgement, headache, sore nipples, epidural or intravenous site, hemorrhoids

Sexual dysfunction r/t recent childbirth

Impaired **Tissue** integrity r/t episiotomy, lacerations

Sleep deprivation r/t care of infant

Impaired **Urinary** elimination r/t effects of anesthesia, tissue trauma

Risk for **Constipation:** Risk factors: hormonal effects on smooth muscles, fear of straining with defecation, effects of anesthesia

Risk for **Infection:** Risk factors: tissue trauma, blood loss

Readiness for enhanced family **Coping:** adaptation to new family member

Readiness for enhanced **Hope:** desire to increase hope

Readiness for enhanced **Parenting:** expresses willingness to enhance parenting skills

POST-TRAUMA SYNDROME

Post-Trauma syndrome (See **Post-Trauma** syndrome, Section III)

POST-TRAUMA SYNDROME, RISK FOR

Risk for **Post-Trauma** syndrome (See **Post-Trauma** syndrome, risk for, Section III)

P

POST-TRAUMATIC STRESS DISORDER (PTSD)

See PTSD (Post-Traumatic Stress Disorder)

POTASSIUM, INCREASE/DECREASE

See Hyperkalemia; Hypokalemia

POWER/POWERLESSNESS

Powerlessness (See **Powerlessness,** Section III)

Risk for **Powerlessness** (See **Powerlessness,** risk for, Section III)

Readiness for enhanced **Power** (See **Power,** readiness for enhanced, Section III)

PREECLAMPSIA

See PIH (Pregnancy-Induced Hypertension/Preeclampsia)

PREGNANCY, CARDIAC DISORDERS

See Cardiac Disorders in Pregnancy

PREGNANCY-INDUCED HYPERTENSION/PREECLAMPSIA (PIH)

See PIH (Pregnancy-Induced Hypertension/Preeclampsia)

PREGNANCY LOSS

Anxiety r/t threat to role functioning, health status, situational crisis

Compromised family **Coping** r/t lack of support by significant other because of personal suffering

Ineffective **Coping** r/t situational crisis

Grieving r/t loss of pregnancy, fetus, or child

Acute **Pain** r/t surgical intervention

Ineffective **Role** performance r/t inability to assume parenting role

Ineffective **Sexuality** pattern r/t self-esteem disturbance resulting from pregnancy loss and anxiety about future pregnancies

Chronic **Sorrow** r/t loss of a fetus or child

Spiritual distress r/t intense suffering from loss of child

Risk for deficient **Fluid** volume: Risk factor: blood loss

Risk for complicated **Grieving:** Risk factor: loss of pregnancy

Risk for **Infection:** Risk factor: retained products of conception

Risk for **Powerlessness:** Risk factor: situational crisis

Risk for ineffective **Relationship:** Risk factor: poor communication skills in dealing with the loss

Risk for **Spiritual** distress: Risk factor: intense suffering

Readiness for enhanced **Communication:** willingness to express feelings and thoughts about loss

Readiness for enhanced **Hope:** expresses desire to enhance hope

Readiness for enhanced **Spiritual** well-being: desire for acceptance of loss

PREGNANCY, NORMAL

Anxiety r/t unknown future, threat to self secondary to pain of labor

Disturbed **Body Image** r/t altered body function and appearance

Interrupted **Family** processes r/t developmental transition of pregnancy

Fatigue r/t increased energy demands

Fear r/t labor and delivery

Deficient **Knowledge** r/t primiparity

Nausea r/t hormonal changes of pregnancy

Imbalanced **Nutrition:** less than body requirements r/t growing fetus, nausea

Imbalanced **Nutrition:** more than body requirements r/t deficient knowledge regarding nutritional needs of pregnancy

Sleep deprivation r/t uncomfortable pregnancy state

Impaired **Urinary** elimination r/t frequency caused by increased pelvic pressure and hormonal stimulation

P

Risk for **Constipation:** Risk factor: pregnancy

Risk for **Sexual** dysfunction: Risk factors: altered body function, self-concept, body image with pregnancy

Readiness for enhanced **Childbearing** process: appropriate prenatal care

Readiness for enhanced family **Coping:** satisfying partner relationship, attention to gratification of needs, effective adaptation to developmental tasks of pregnancy

Readiness for enhanced **Family** processes: family adapts to change

Readiness for enhanced **Health** management: seeks information for prenatal self care

Readiness for enhanced **Nutrition:** desire for knowledge of appropriate nutrition during pregnancy

Readiness for enhanced **Parenting:** expresses willingness to enhance parenting skills

Readiness for enhanced **Relationship:** meeting developmental goals associated with pregnancy

Readiness for enhanced **Spiritual** well-being: new role as parent

See Discomforts of Pregnancy

PREMATURE DILATION OF THE CERVIX (INCOMPETENT CERVIX)

Ineffective **Activity** planning r/t unrealistic perception of events

Ineffective **Coping** r/t bed rest, threat to fetus

Deficient **Diversional** activity r/t bed rest

Fear r/t potential loss of infant

Grieving r/t potential loss of infant

Deficient **Knowledge** r/t treatment regimen, prognosis for pregnancy

Impaired physical **Mobility** r/t imposed bed rest to prevent preterm birth

Powerlessness r/t inability to control outcome of pregnancy

Ineffective **Role** performance r/t inability to continue usual patterns of responsibility

Situational low **Self-Esteem** r/t inability to complete normal pregnancy

Sexual dysfunction r/t fear of harm to fetus

Impaired **Social** interaction r/t bed rest

Risk for **Infection:** Risk factor: invasive procedures to prevent preterm birth

Risk for **Injury:** fetal: Risk factors: preterm birth, use of anesthetics

Risk for **Injury:** maternal: Risk factor: surgical procedures to prevent preterm birth (e.g., cerclage)

Risk for impaired **Resilience:** Risk factor: complication of pregnancy

Risk for **Spiritual** distress: Risk factor: physical/psychological stress

PREMATURE INFANT (CHILD)

Insufficient **Breast Milk** r/t ineffective sucking, latching on of the infant

Impaired **Gas** exchange r/t effects of cardiopulmonary insufficiency

Disorganized **Infant** behavior r/t prematurity

Insomnia r/t noisy and noxious intensive care environment

Neonatal **Jaundice** r/t infant experiences difficulty making transition to extrauterine life

Imbalanced **Nutrition:** less than body requirements r/t delayed or understimulated rooting reflex, easy fatigue during feeding, diminished endurance

Impaired **Swallowing** r/t decreased or absent gag reflex, fatigue

Ineffective **Thermoregulation** r/t large body surface/weight ratio, immaturity of thermal regulation, state of prematurity

Risk for delayed **Development:** Risk factor: prematurity

Risk for disproportionate **Growth:** Risk factor: prematurity

P

Risk for **Infection:** Risk factor: inadequate, immature, or undeveloped acquired immune response

Risk for **Injury:** Risk factors: prolonged mechanical ventilation, retinopathy of prematurity (ROP) secondary to 100% oxygen environment

Risk for neonatal **Jaundice:** Risk factor: late preterm birth

Readiness for enhanced organized **Infant** behavior: use of some self-regulatory measures

PREMATURE INFANT (PARENT)

Ineffective **Breastfeeding** r/t disrupted establishment of effective pattern secondary to prematurity or insufficient opportunities

Decisional Conflict r/t support system deficit, multiple sources of information

Compromised family **Coping** r/t disrupted family roles and disorganization, prolonged condition exhausting supportive capacity of significant persons

Grieving r/t loss of perfect child possibly leading to complicated grieving

Complicated **Grieving** (prolonged) r/t unresolved conflicts

Parental **Role** conflict r/t expressed concerns; expressed inability to care for child's physical, emotional, or developmental needs

Chronic **Sorrow** r/t threat of loss of a child, prolonged hospitalization

Spiritual distress r/t challenged belief or value systems regarding moral or ethical implications of treatment plans

Risk for impaired **Attachment:** Risk factors: separation, physical barriers, lack of privacy

Risk for disturbed **Maternal–Fetal** dyad: Risk factor: complication of pregnancy

Risk for **Powerlessness:** Risk factor: inability to control situation

Risk for impaired **Resilience:** Risk factor: premature infant

Risk for **Spiritual** distress: Risk factor: challenged belief or value systems regarding moral or ethical implications of treatment plans

Readiness for enhanced **Family** process: adaptation to change associated with premature infant

See Child with Chronic Condition; Hospitalized Child

PREMATURE RUPTURE OF MEMBRANES

Anxiety r/t threat to infant's health status

Disturbed **Body Image** r/t inability to carry pregnancy to term

Ineffective **Coping** r/t situational crisis

Grieving r/t potential loss of infant

Situational low **Self-Esteem** r/t inability to carry pregnancy to term

Risk for ineffective **Childbearing** process: Risk factor: complication of pregnancy

Risk for **Infection:** Risk factor: rupture of membranes

Risk for **Injury:** fetal: Risk factor: risk of premature birth

PREMENSTRUAL TENSION SYNDROME (PMS)

See PMS (Premenstrual Tension Syndrome)

PRENATAL CARE, NORMAL

Readiness for enhanced **Childbearing** process: appropriate prenatal lifestyle

Readiness for enhanced **Knowledge:** appropriate prenatal care

Readiness for enhanced **Spiritual** well-being: new role as parent

See Pregnancy, Normal

PRENATAL TESTING

Anxiety r/t unknown outcome, delayed test results

Acute **Pain** r/t invasive procedures

Risk for **Infection:** Risk factor: invasive procedures during amniocentesis or chorionic villus sampling

Risk for **Injury:** fetal r/t invasive procedures

PREOPERATIVE TEACHING

See Surgery, Preoperative Care

PRESSURE ULCER

Impaired bed **Mobility** r/t intolerance to activity, pain, cognitive impairment, depression, severe anxiety, severity of illness

Imbalanced **Nutrition:** less than body requirements r/t limited access to food, inability to absorb nutrients because of biological factors, anorexia

Acute **Pain** r/t tissue destruction, exposure of nerves

Impaired **Skin** integrity: stage I or II pressure ulcer r/t physical immobility, mechanical factors, altered circulation, skin irritants, excessive moisture

Impaired **Tissue** integrity: stage III or IV pressure ulcer r/t altered circulation, impaired physical mobility, excessive moisture

Risk for **Infection:** Risk factors: physical immobility, mechanical factors (shearing forces, pressure, restraint, altered circulation, skin irritants, excessive moisture, open wound)

Risk for **Pressure** ulcer (See **Pressure** ulcer, risk for, Section III)

PRETERM LABOR

Anxiety r/t threat to fetus, change in role functioning, change in environment and interaction patterns, use of tocolytic drugs

Ineffective **Coping** r/t situational crisis, preterm labor

Deficient **Diversional** activity r/t long-term hospitalization

Grieving r/t loss of idealized pregnancy, potential loss of fetus

Impaired **Home** maintenance r/t medical restrictions

Impaired physical **Mobility** r/t medically imposed restrictions

Ineffective **Role** performance r/t inability to carry out normal roles secondary to bed rest or hospitalization, change in expected course of pregnancy

Situational low **Self-Esteem** r/t threatened ability to carry pregnancy to term

Sexual dysfunction r/t actual or perceived limitation imposed by preterm labor and/or prescribed treatment, separation from partner because of hospitalization

Sleep deprivation r/t change in usual pattern secondary to contractions, hospitalization, treatment regimen

Impaired **Social** interaction r/t prolonged bed rest or hospitalization

Risk for **Injury:** fetal: Risk factors: premature birth, immature body systems

Risk for **Injury:** maternal: Risk factor: use of tocolytic drugs

Risk for **Powerlessness:** Risk factor: lack of control over preterm labor

Risk for **Vascular Trauma:** Risk factor: intravenous medication

Readiness for enhanced **Childbearing** process: appropriate prenatal lifestyle

Readiness for enhanced **Comfort:** expresses desire to enhance relaxation

Readiness for enhanced **Communication:** willingness to discuss thoughts and feelings about situation

PROBLEM-SOLVING DYSFUNCTION

Defensive **Coping** r/t situational crisis

Impaired emancipated **Decision-Making** r/t problem-solving dysfunction

Risk for chronic low **Self-Esteem:** Risk factor: repeated failures

Readiness for enhanced **Communication:** willing to share ideas with others

Readiness for enhanced **Relationship:** shares information and ideas between partners

P

Readiness for enhanced **Resilience**: identifies available resources

Readiness for enhanced **Spiritual** well-being: desires to draw on inner strength and find meaning and purpose to life

PROJECTION

Anxiety r/t threat to self-concept

Defensive **Coping** r/t inability to acknowledge that own behavior may be a problem, blaming others

Chronic low **Self-Esteem** r/t failure

Impaired **Social** interaction r/t self-concept disturbance, confrontational communication style

Risk for **Loneliness**: Risk factor: blaming others for problems

See Paranoid Personality Disorder

PROLAPSED UMBILICAL CORD

Fear r/t threat to fetus, impending surgery

Ineffective peripheral **Tissue Perfusion**: fetal r/t interruption in umbilical blood flow

Risk for ineffective **Cerebral** tissue perfusion: fetal: Risk factor: cord compression

Risk for **Injury**: maternal: Risk factor: emergency surgery

PROSTATECTOMY

See TURP (Transurethral Resection of the Prostate)

PROSTATIC HYPERTROPHY

Ineffective **Health** maintenance r/t deficient knowledge regarding self-care and prevention of complications

Sleep deprivation r/t nocturia

Urinary Retention r/t obstruction

Risk for **Infection**: Risk factors: urinary residual after voiding, bacterial invasion of bladder

See BPH (Benign Prostatic Hypertrophy)

PROSTATITIS

Impaired **Comfort** r/t inflammation

Ineffective **Health** maintenance r/t deficient knowledge regarding treatment

Urge urinary **Incontinence** r/t irritation of bladder

Ineffective **Protection** r/t depressed immune system

PRURITUS

Impaired **Comfort** r/t itching

Deficient **Knowledge** r/t methods to treat and prevent itching

Risk for impaired **Skin** integrity: Risk factor: scratching from pruritus

PSORIASIS

Disturbed **Body Image** r/t lesions on body

Impaired **Comfort** r/t irritated skin

Ineffective **Health** maintenance r/t deficient knowledge regarding treatment modalities

Powerlessness r/t lack of control over condition with frequent exacerbations and remissions

Impaired **Skin** integrity r/t lesions on body

PSYCHOSIS

Ineffective **Activity** planning r/t compromised ability to process information

Ineffective **Health** maintenance r/t cognitive impairment, ineffective individual and family coping

Self-Neglect r/t mental disorder

Impaired individual **Resilience** r/t psychological disorder

Situational low **Self-Esteem** r/t excessive use of defense mechanisms (e.g., projection, denial, rationalization)

Risk for disturbed personal **Identity**: Risk factor: psychosis

Impaired **Mood** regulation r/t psychosis

Risk for **Post-Trauma** syndrome: Risk factor: diminished ego strength

See Schizophrenia

PTCA (PERCUTANEOUS TRANSLUMINAL CORONARY ANGIOPLASTY)

See Angioplasty, Coronary

PTSD (POSTTRAUMATIC STRESS DISORDER)

Anxiety r/t exposure to internal or external cues that symbolize or resemble an aspect of the traumatic event

Chronic **Sorrow** r/t chronic disability (e.g., physical, mental)

Death **Anxiety** r/t psychological stress associated with traumatic event

Ineffective **Breathing** pattern r/t hyperventilation associated with anxiety

Ineffective **Coping** r/t extreme anxiety

Ineffective **Impulse** control r/t thinking of initial trauma experience

Insomnia r/t recurring nightmares

Post-Trauma syndrome r/t exposure to a traumatic event

Sleep deprivation r/t nightmares interrupting sleep associated with traumatic event

Spiritual distress r/t feelings of detachment or estrangement from others

Risk for impaired **Resilience:** Risk factor: chronicity of existing crisis

Risk for **Powerlessness:** Risk factors: flashbacks, reliving event

Risk for ineffective **Relationship:** Risk factor: stressful life events

Risk for self- or other-directed **Violence:** Risk factor: fear of self or others

Readiness for enhanced **Comfort:** expresses desire to enhance relaxation

Readiness for enhanced **Communication:** willingness to express feelings and thoughts

Readiness for enhanced **Spiritual** well-being: desire for harmony after stressful event

PULMONARY EDEMA

Anxiety r/t fear of suffocation

Ineffective **Airway** clearance r/t presence of tracheobronchial secretions

Decreased **Cardiac** output r/t increased preload, infective forward perfusion

Impaired **Gas** exchange r/t extravasation of extravascular fluid in lung tissues and alveoli

Ineffective **Health** maintenance r/t deficient knowledge regarding treatment regimen

Sleep deprivation r/t inability to breathe

Risk for acute **Confusion:** Risk factor: hypoxia

See Heart Failure

PULMONARY EMBOLISM

Anxiety r/t fear of suffocation

Decreased **Cardiac** output r/t right ventricular failure secondary to obstructed pulmonary artery

Fear r/t severe pain, possible death

Impaired **Gas** exchange r/t altered blood flow to alveoli secondary to embolus

Deficient **Knowledge** r/t activities to prevent embolism, self-care after diagnosis of embolism

Acute **Pain** r/t biological injury, lack of oxygen to cells

Ineffective peripheral **Tissue Perfusion** r/t deep vein thrombus formation

See Anticoagulant Therapy

PULMONARY STENOSIS

See Congenital Heart Disease/Cardiac Anomalies

PULSE DEFICIT

Risk for decreased **Cardiac** output r/t dysrhythmia

See Dysrhythmia

PULSE OXIMETRY

Readiness for enhanced **Knowledge:** information about treatment regimen

See Hypoxia

P

PULSE PRESSURE, INCREASED

See Intracranial Pressure, Increased

PULSE PRESSURE, NARROWED

See Shock, Hypovolemic

PULSES, ABSENT OR DIMINISHED PERIPHERAL

Ineffective peripheral **Tissue Perfusion** r/t interruption of arterial flow

Risk for **Peripheral Neurovascular** dysfunction: Risk factors: fractures, mechanical compression, orthopedic surgery trauma, immobilization, burns, vascular obstruction

PURPURA

See Clotting Disorder

PYELONEPHRITIS

Ineffective **Health** maintenance r/t deficient knowledge regarding self-care, treatment of disease, prevention of further urinary tract infections

Acute **Pain** r/t inflammation and irritation of urinary tract

Disturbed **Sleep** pattern r/t urinary frequency

Impaired **Urinary** elimination r/t irritation of urinary tract

Risk for ineffective **Renal** perfusion: Risk factor: infection

PYLORIC STENOSIS

Imbalanced **Nutrition:** less than body requirements r/t vomiting secondary to pyloric sphincter obstruction

Acute **Pain** r/t abdominal fullness

Risk for decreased **Fluid** volume: Risk factors: vomiting, dehydration

See Hospitalized Child

PYLOROMYOTOMY (PYLORIC STENOSIS REPAIR)

See Surgery, Perioperative Care; Surgery, Postoperative Care; Surgery, Preoperative Care

R

RA (RHEUMATOID ARTHRITIS)

See Rheumatoid Arthritis (RA)

RABIES

Ineffective **Health** maintenance r/t deficient knowledge regarding care of wound, isolation, and observation of infected animal

Acute **Pain** r/t multiple immunization injections

Risk for ineffective **Cerebral** tissue perfusion: Risk factor: rabies virus

RADIAL NERVE DYSFUNCTION

Acute **Pain** r/t trauma to hand or arm

See Neuropathy, Peripheral

RADIATION THERAPY

Activity intolerance r/t fatigue from possible anemia

Disturbed **Body Image** r/t change in appearance, hair loss

Diarrhea r/t irradiation effects

Fatigue r/t malnutrition from lack of appetite, nausea, and vomiting; side effect of radiation

Deficient **Knowledge** r/t what to expect with radiation therapy, how to do self-care

Nausea r/t side effects of radiation

Imbalanced **Nutrition:** less than body requirements r/t anorexia, nausea, vomiting, irradiation of areas of pharynx and esophagus

Impaired **Oral Mucous Membrane** r/t irradiation effects

Ineffective **Protection** r/t suppression of bone marrow

Risk for impaired **Oral Mucous Membranes:** Risk factor: radiation treatments

Risk for **Powerlessness:** Risk factors: medical treatment and possible side effects

Risk for impaired **Resilience:** Risk factor: radiation treatment

Risk for impaired **Skin** integrity: Risk factor: irradiation effects

Risk for **Spiritual** distress: Risk factors: radiation treatment, prognosis

RADICAL NECK DISSECTION

See Laryngectomy

RAGE

Risk-prone **Health** behavior r/t multiple stressors

Labile Emotional Control r/t psychiatric disorders and mood disorders

Impaired individual **Resilience** r/t poor impulse control

Stress overload r/t multiple coexisting stressors

Risk for **Self-Mutilation**: Risk factor: command hallucinations

Risk for **Suicide**: Risk factor: desire to kill self

Risk for other-directed **Violence**: Risk factors: panic state, manic excitement, organic brain syndrome

RAPE-TRAUMA SYNDROME

Rape-Trauma syndrome (See **Rape-Trauma** syndrome, Section III)

Chronic **Sorrow** r/t forced loss of virginity

Risk for ineffective **Childbearing** process r/t to trauma and violence

Risk for **Post-Trauma** syndrome: Risk factor: trauma or violence associated with rape

Risk for **Powerlessness**: Risk factor: inability to control thoughts about incident

Risk for ineffective **Relationship** r/t to trauma and violence

Risk for chronic low **Self-Esteem** r/t perceived lack of respect from others/feeling violated

Risk for **Spiritual** distress: Risk factor: forced loss of virginity

RASH

Impaired **Comfort** r/t pruritus

Impaired **Skin** integrity r/t mechanical trauma

Risk for **Infection**: Risk factors: traumatized tissue, broken skin

Risk for **Latex Allergy** response: Risk factor: allergy to products associated with latex

RATIONALIZATION

Defensive **Coping** r/t situational crisis, inability to accept blame for consequences of own behavior

Ineffective **Denial** r/t fear of consequences, actual or perceived loss

Impaired individual **Resilience** r/t psychological disturbance

Risk for **Post-Trauma** syndrome: Risk factor: survivor's role in event

Readiness for enhanced **Communication**: expresses desire to share thoughts and feelings

Readiness for enhanced **Spiritual** well-being: possibility of seeking harmony with self, others, higher power, God

RATS, RODENTS IN HOME

Impaired **Home** maintenance r/t lack of knowledge, insufficient finances

Risk for **Allergy** response r/t repeated exposure to environmental contamination

See Filthy Home Environment

RAYNAUD'S DISEASE

Deficient **Knowledge** r/t lack of information about disease process, possible complications, self-care needs regarding disease process and medication

Ineffective peripheral **Tissue Perfusion** r/t transient reduction of blood flow

Acute **Pain** r/t transient reduction in blood flow

R

RDS (RESPIRATORY DISTRESS SYNDROME)

See Respiratory Conditions of the Neonate

RECTAL FULLNESS

Chronic functional **Constipation** r/t decreased activity level, decreased fluid intake, inadequate fiber in diet, decreased peristalsis, side effects of antidepressant or antipsychotic therapy

Risk for chronic functional **Constipation:** Risk factor: habitual denial of or ignoring urge to defecate

RECTAL LUMP

See Hemorrhoids

RECTAL PAIN/BLEEDING

Chronic functional **Constipation** r/t pain on defecation

Deficient **Knowledge** r/t possible causes of rectal bleeding, pain, treatment modalities

Acute **Pain** r/t pressure of defecation

Risk for **Bleeding:** Risk factor: rectal disease

RECTAL SURGERY

See Hemorrhoidectomy

RECTOCELE REPAIR

Chronic functional **Constipation** r/t painful defecation

Ineffective **Health** maintenance r/t deficient knowledge of postoperative care of surgical site, dietary measures, exercise to prevent constipation

Acute **Pain** r/t surgical procedure

Urinary retention r/t edema from surgery

Risk for **Bleeding:** Risk factor: surgery

Risk for **Infection:** Risk factors: surgical procedure, possible contamination of area with feces

REFLEX INCONTINENCE

Reflex urinary **Incontinence** (See **Incontinence,** urinary, reflex, Section III)

REGRESSION

Anxiety r/t threat to or change in health status

Defensive **Coping** r/t denial of obvious problems, weaknesses

Self-Neglect r/t functional impairment

Powerlessness r/t health care environment

Impaired individual **Resilience** r/t psychological disturbance

Ineffective **Role** performance r/t powerlessness over health status

See Hospitalized Child; Separation Anxiety

REGRETFUL

Anxiety r/t situational or maturational crises

Death **Anxiety** r/t feelings of not having accomplished goals in life

Risk for **Spiritual** distress: Risk factor: inability to forgive

REHABILITATION

Ineffective **Coping** r/t loss of normal function

Impaired physical **Mobility** r/t injury, surgery, psychosocial condition warranting rehabilitation

Self-Care deficit: specify r/t impaired physical mobility

Risk for **Falls:** Risk factor: physical deconditioning

Readiness for enhanced **Comfort:** expresses desire to enhance feeling of comfort

Readiness for enhanced **Self-Concept:** accepts strengths and limitations

Readiness for enhanced **Health Management:** expresses desire to manage rehabilitation

RELATIONSHIP

Ineffective **Relationship** (See ineffective **Relationship,** Section III)

Readiness for enhanced **Relationship** (See Risk for enhanced **Relationship** see Section III)

RELAXATION TECHNIQUES

Anxiety r/t situational crisis

Readiness for enhanced **Comfort:** expresses desire to enhance relaxation

Readiness for enhanced **Health** management: desire to manage illness

Readiness for enhanced **Religiosity:** requests religious materials or experiences

Readiness for enhanced **Resilience:** desire to enhance resilience

Readiness for enhanced **Self-Concept:** willingness to enhance self-concept

Readiness for enhanced **Spiritual** well-being: seeking comfort from higher power

RELIGIOSITY

Impaired **Religiosity** (See **Religiosity,** impaired, Section III)

Risk for impaired **Religiosity** (See **Religiosity,** impaired, risk for, Section III)

Readiness for enhanced **Religiosity** (See **Religiosity,** readiness for enhanced, Section III)

RELIGIOUS CONCERNS

Spiritual distress r/t separation from religious or cultural ties

Risk for impaired **Religiosity:** Risk factors: ineffective support, coping, caregiving

Risk for **Spiritual** distress: Risk factor: physical or psychological stress

Readiness for enhanced **Spiritual** well-being: desire for increased spirituality

RELOCATION STRESS SYNDROME

Relocation stress syndrome (See **Relocation** stress syndrome, Section III)

Risk for **Relocation** stress syndrome (See **Relocation** stress syndrome, risk for, Section III)

RESPIRATORY ACIDOSIS

See Acidosis, Respiratory

RESPIRATORY CONDITIONS OF THE NEONATE (RESPIRATORY DISTRESS SYNDROME [RDS], MECONIUM ASPIRATION, DIAPHRAGMATIC HERNIA)

Ineffective **Airway** clearance r/t sequelae of attempts to breathe in utero resulting in meconium aspiration

Fatigue r/t increased energy requirements and metabolic demands

Impaired **Gas** exchange r/t decreased surfactant, immature lung tissue

Dysfunctional **Ventilator** weaning response r/t immature respiratory system

Risk for **Infection:** Risk factor: tissue destruction or irritation as a result of aspiration of meconium fluid

See Bronchopulmonary Dysplasia; Hospitalized Child; Premature Infant, Child

RESPIRATORY DISTRESS

See Dyspnea

RESPIRATORY DISTRESS SYNDROME (RDS)

See Respiratory Conditions of the Neonate

RESPIRATORY INFECTIONS, ACUTE CHILDHOOD (CROUP, EPIGLOTTITIS, PERTUSSIS, PNEUMONIA, RESPIRATORY SYNCYTIAL VIRUS)

Activity intolerance r/t generalized weakness, dyspnea, fatigue, poor oxygenation

Ineffective **Airway** clearance r/t excess tracheobronchial secretions

Ineffective **Breathing** pattern r/t inflamed bronchial passages, coughing

Fear r/t oxygen deprivation, difficulty breathing

Deficient **Fluid** volume r/t insensible losses (fever, diaphoresis), inadequate oral fluid intake

R

Impaired **Gas** exchange r/t insufficient oxygenation as a result of inflammation or edema of epiglottis, larynx, bronchial passages

Imbalanced **Nutrition:** less than body requirements r/t anorexia, fatigue, generalized weakness, poor sucking and breathing coordination, dyspnea

Ineffective **Thermoregulation** r/t infectious process

Risk for **Aspiration:** Risk factors: inability to coordinate breathing, coughing, sucking

Risk for **Infection:** transmission to others: Risk factor: virulent infectious organisms

Risk for **Injury** (to pregnant others): Risk factors: exposure to aerosolized medications (e.g., ribavirin, pentamidine), resultant potential fetal toxicity

Risk for **Suffocation:** Risk factors: inflammation of larynx, epiglottis

See Hospitalized Child

RESPIRATORY SYNCYTIAL VIRUS

See Respiratory Infections, Acute Childhood

RESTLESS LEG SYNDROME

Disturbed **Sleep** pattern r/t leg discomfort during sleep relieved by frequent leg movement

Chronic **Pain** r/t leg discomfort

See Stress

RETARDED GROWTH AND DEVELOPMENT

See Growth and Development Lag

RETCHING

Nausea r/t chemotherapy, postsurgical anesthesia, irritation to gastrointestinal system, stimulation of neuropharmacological mechanisms

Imbalanced **Nutrition:** less than body requirements r/t inability to ingest food

Risk for **Fatigue:** Risk factors: stress of retching, muscle contractions

RETINAL DETACHMENT

Anxiety r/t change in vision, threat of loss of vision

Deficient **Knowledge** r/t symptoms, need for early intervention to prevent permanent damage

Vision Loss r/t impaired visual acuity

Risk for impaired **Home** maintenance: Risk factors: postoperative care, activity limitations, care of affected eye

Risk for impaired **Resilience:** Risk factor: possible loss of vision

See Vision Impairment

RETINOPATHY, DIABETIC

See Diabetic Retinopathy

RETINOPATHY OF PREMATURITY (ROP)

Risk for **Injury:** Risk factors: prolonged mechanical ventilation, ROP secondary to 100% oxygen environment

See Retinal Detachment

RH FACTOR INCOMPATIBILITY

Anxiety r/t unknown outcome of pregnancy

Neonatal **Jaundice** r/t Rh factor incompatibility

Deficient **Knowledge** r/t treatment regimen from lack of experience with situation

Powerlessness r/t perceived lack of control over outcome of pregnancy

Risk for **Injury:** fetal: Risk factors: intrauterine destruction of red blood cells, transfusions

Risk for neonatal **Jaundice** r/t Rh factor incompatibility

Readiness for enhanced **Health** management: prenatal care, compliance with diagnostic and treatment regimen

RHABDOMYOLYSIS

Ineffective **Coping** r/t seriousness of condition

Impaired physical **Mobility** r/t myalgia and muscle weakness

Risk for deficient **Fluid** volume: Risk factor: reduced blood flow to kidneys

Risk for ineffective **Renal** perfusion: Risk factor: possible kidney failure from obstruction of kidney

Risk for **Shock:** Risk factor: hypovolemia

Readiness for enhanced **Health** management: seeks information to avoid condition

See Kidney Failure

RHEUMATIC FEVER

See Endocarditis

RHEUMATOID ARTHRITIS (RA)

Imbalanced **Nutrition:** less than body requirements r/t loss of appetite

Chronic **Pain** r/t joint inflammation

Risk for impaired **Resilience:** Risk factor: chronic, painful, progressive disease

See Arthritis; JRA (Juvenile Rheumatoid Arthritis)

RIB FRACTURE

Ineffective **Breathing** pattern r/t fractured ribs

Acute **Pain** r/t movement, deep breathing

Impaired **Gas** exchange r/t ventilation-perfusion imbalance, decreased depth of ventilation

RIDICULE OF OTHERS

Defensive **Coping** r/t situational crisis, psychological impairment, substance abuse

Risk for **Post-Trauma** syndrome: Risk factor: perception of event

RINGWORM OF BODY

Impaired **Comfort** r/t pruritus

Impaired **Skin** integrity r/t presence of macules associated with fungus

See Itching; Pruritus

RINGWORM OF NAILS

Disturbed **Body Image** r/t appearance of nails, removed nails

RINGWORM OF SCALP

Disturbed **Body Image** r/t possible hair loss (alopecia)

See Itching; Pruritus

ROACHES, INVASION OF HOME WITH

Impaired **Home** maintenance r/t lack of knowledge, insufficient finances

See Filthy Home Environment

ROLE PERFORMANCE, ALTERED

Ineffective **Role** performance (See **Role** performance, ineffective, Section III)

ROP (RETINOPATHY OF PREMATURITY)

See Retinopathy of Prematurity (ROP)

RSV (RESPIRATORY SYNCYTIAL VIRUS)

See Respiratory Infection, Acute Childhood

RUBELLA

See Communicable Diseases, Childhood

RUBOR OF EXTREMITIES

Ineffective peripheral **Tissue Perfusion** r/t interruption of arterial flow

See Peripheral Vascular Disease (PVD)

RUPTURED DISK

See Low Back Pain

S

SAD (SEASONAL AFFECTIVE DISORDER)

Readiness for enhanced **Resilience:** uses SAD lights during winter months

See Depression (Major Depressive Disorder)

SADNESS

Complicated **Grieving** r/t actual or perceived loss

S

Impaired **Mood** regulation r/t chronic illness (See **Mood** regulation, impaired, Section III)

Spiritual distress r/t intense suffering

Risk for **Powerlessness:** Risk factor: actual or perceived loss

Risk for **Spiritual** distress: Risk factor: loss of loved one

Readiness for enhanced **Communication:** willingness to share feelings and thoughts

Readiness for enhanced **Spiritual** well-being: desire for harmony after actual or perceived loss

See Depression (Major Depressive Disorder); Major Depressive Disorder

SAFE SEX

Readiness for enhanced **Health** management: takes appropriate precautions during sexual activity to keep from contracting sexually transmitted disease

See Sexuality, Adolescent; STD (Sexually Transmitted Disease)

SAFETY, CHILDHOOD

Deficient **Knowledge:** potential for enhanced health maintenance r/t parental knowledge and skill acquisition regarding appropriate safety measures

Risk for **Aspiration** (See **Aspiration**, risk for, Section III)

Risk for **Injury:** Risk factors: developmental age, altered home maintenance

Risk for impaired **Parenting:** Risk factors: lack of available and effective role model, lack of knowledge, misinformation from other family members (old wives' tales)

Risk for **Poisoning:** Risk factors: use of lead-based paint, presence of asbestos or radon gas, drugs not locked in cabinet, household products left in accessible area (bleach, detergent, drain cleaners, household cleaners), alcohol and perfume within reach of child, presence of poisonous plants, atmospheric pollutants

Risk for **Thermal** injury: Risk factor: inadequate supervision

Readiness for enhanced **Childbearing** process: expresses appropriate knowledge for care of child

SALMONELLA

Impaired **Home** maintenance r/t improper preparation or storage of food, lack of safety measures when caring for pet reptile

Risk for **Shock:** Risk factors: hypovolemia, diarrhea, sepsis

Readiness for enhanced **Health** management: avoiding improperly prepared or stored food, wearing gloves when handling pet reptiles or their feces

See Gastroenteritis; Gastroenteritis, Child

SALPINGECTOMY

Decisional Conflict r/t sterilization procedure

Grieving r/t possible loss from tubal pregnancy

Risk for impaired **Urinary** elimination: Risk factor: trauma to ureter during surgery

See Hysterectomy; Surgery, Perioperative Care; Surgery, Postoperative Care; Surgery, Preoperative Care

SARCOIDOSIS

Anxiety r/t change in health status

Impaired **Gas** exchange r/t ventilation-perfusion imbalance

Ineffective **Health** maintenance r/t deficient knowledge regarding home care and medication regimen

Acute **Pain** r/t possible disease affecting joints

Ineffective **Protection** r/t immune disorder

Risk for decreased **Cardiac** tissue perfusion: Risk factor: dysrhythmias

Risk for impaired **Skin** integrity: Risk factor: immunological disorder

SARS (SEVERE ACUTE RESPIRATORY SYNDROME)

Risk for **Infection:** Risk factor: increased environmental exposure (travelers in close proximity to infected persons, traveling when a fever is present)

Readiness for enhanced **Knowledge:** information regarding travel and precautions to avoid exposure to SARS

See Pneumonia

SBE (SELF-BREAST EXAMINATION)

Readiness for enhanced **Health** management: desires to have information about SBE

Readiness for enhanced **Knowledge:** self-breast examination

SCABIES

See Communicable Diseases, Childhood

SCARED

Anxiety r/t threat of death, threat to or change in health status

Death **Anxiety** r/t unresolved issues surrounding end-of-life decisions

Fear r/t hospitalization, real or imagined threat to own well-being

Impaired individual **Resilience** r/t violence

Readiness for enhanced **Communication:** willingness to share thoughts and feelings

SCHIZOPHRENIA

Ineffective **Activity** planning r/t compromised ability to process information

Anxiety r/t unconscious conflict with reality

Impaired verbal **Communication** r/t psychosis, disorientation, inaccurate perception, hallucinations, delusions

Ineffective **Coping** r/t inadequate support systems, unrealistic perceptions, inadequate coping skills, disturbed thought processes, impaired communication

Deficient **Diversional** activity r/t social isolation, possible regression

Interrupted **Family** processes r/t inability to express feelings, impaired communication

Fear r/t altered contact with reality

Ineffective **Health** maintenance r/t cognitive impairment, ineffective individual and family coping, lack of material resources

Ineffective family **Health** management r/t chronicity and unpredictability of condition

Impaired **Home** maintenance r/t impaired cognitive or emotional functioning, insufficient finances, inadequate support systems

Hopelessness r/t long-term stress from chronic mental illness

Disturbed personal **Identity** r/t psychiatric disorder

Impaired **Memory** r/t psychosocial condition

Imbalanced **Nutrition:** less than body requirements r/t fear of eating, lack of awareness of hunger, disinterest toward food

Impaired individual **Resilience** r/t psychological disorder

Self-Care deficit: specify r/t loss of contact with reality, impairment of perception

Self-Neglect r/t psychosis

Sleep deprivation r/t intrusive thoughts, nightmares

Impaired **Social** interaction r/t impaired communication patterns, self-concept disturbance, disturbed thought processes

Social isolation r/t lack of trust, regression, delusional thinking, repressed fears

Chronic **Sorrow** r/t chronic mental illness

Spiritual distress r/t loneliness, social alienation

Risk for **Caregiver Role Strain:** Risk factors: bizarre behavior of client, chronicity of condition

Risk for compromised **Human Dignity:** Risk factor: stigmatizing label

Risk for **Loneliness:** Risk factor: inability to interact socially

Risk for **Post-Trauma** syndrome: Risk factor: diminished ego strength

Risk for **Powerlessness:** Risk factor: intrusive, distorted thinking

S

Risk for impaired **Religiosity:** Risk factors: ineffective coping, lack of security

Risk for **Suicide:** Risk factor: psychiatric illness

Risk for self-directed **Violence:** Risk factors: lack of trust, panic, hallucinations, delusional thinking

Risk for other-directed **Violence:** Risk factor: psychotic disorder

Readiness for enhanced **Hope:** expresses desire to enhance interconnectedness with others and problem-solve to meet goals

Readiness for enhanced **Power:** expresses willingness to enhance participation in choices for daily living and health and enhance knowledge for participation in change

SCIATICA

See Neuropathy, Peripheral

SCOLIOSIS

Risk-prone **Health** behavior r/t lack of developmental maturity to comprehend long-term consequences of noncompliance with treatment procedures

Disturbed **Body Image** r/t use of therapeutic braces, postsurgery scars, restricted physical activity

Impaired **Comfort** r/t altered health status and body image

Impaired **Gas** exchange r/t restricted lung expansion as a result of severe presurgery curvature of spine, immobilization

Ineffective **Health** maintenance r/t deficient knowledge regarding treatment modalities, restrictions, home care, postoperative activities

Impaired physical **Mobility** r/t restricted movement, dyspnea caused by severe curvature of spine

Acute **Pain** r/t musculoskeletal restrictions, surgery, reambulation with cast or spinal rod

Impaired **Skin** integrity r/t braces, casts, surgical correction

Chronic **Sorrow** r/t chronic disability

Risk for **Infection:** Risk factor: surgical incision

Risk for **Perioperative Positioning** injury: Risk factor: prone position

Risk for impaired **Resilience:** Risk factor: chronic condition

Readiness for enhanced **Health** management: desires knowledge regarding treatment for condition

See Hospitalized Child; Maturational Issues, Adolescent

SEDENTARY LIFESTYLE

Activity intolerance r/t sedentary lifestyle

Sedentary lifestyle (See **Sedentary** lifestyle, Section III)

Obesity (See **Obesity,** Section III)

Overweight (See **Overweight,** Section III)

Risk for **Overweight** (See **Overweight,** Section III)

Risk for ineffective peripheral **Tissue Perfusion:** Risk factor: insufficient knowledge of aggravating factors (e.g., immobility, obesity)

Readiness for enhanced **Coping:** seeking knowledge of new strategies to adjust to sedentary lifestyle

SEIZURE DISORDERS, ADULT

Acute **Confusion** r/t postseizure state

Social isolation r/t unpredictability of seizures, community-imposed stigma

Risk for ineffective **Airway** clearance: Risk factor: accumulation of secretions during seizure

Risk for **Falls:** Risk factor: uncontrolled seizure activity

Risk for **Powerlessness:** Risk factor: possible seizure

Risk for impaired **Resilience:** Risk factor: chronic illness

Readiness for enhanced **Knowledge:** anticonvulsive therapy

Readiness for enhanced **Self-Care:** expresses desire to enhance knowledge and responsibility for self-care

See Epilepsy

SEIZURE DISORDERS, CHILDHOOD (EPILEPSY, FEBRILE SEIZURES, INFANTILE SPASMS)

Ineffective **Health** maintenance r/t lack of knowledge regarding anticonvulsive therapy, fever reduction (febrile seizures)

Social isolation r/t unpredictability of seizures, community-imposed stigma

Risk for ineffective **Airway** clearance: Risk factor: accumulation of secretions during seizure

Risk for delayed **Development:** Risk factors: effects of seizure disorder, parental overprotection

Risk for disproportionate **Growth:** Risk factors: congenital disorder, malnutrition

Risk for **Falls:** Risk factor: possible seizure

Risk for **Injury:** Risk factors: uncontrolled movements during seizure, falls, drowsiness caused by anticonvulsants

See Epilepsy

SELF-BREAST EXAMINATION (SBE)

See SBE (Self-Breast Examination)

SELF-CARE

Readiness for enhanced **Self-Care** (See **Self-Care,** readiness for enhanced, Section III)

SELF-CARE DEFICIT, BATHING

Bathing **Self-Care** deficit (See **Self-Care** deficit, bathing, Section III)

SELF-CARE DEFICIT, DRESSING

Dressing **Self-Care** deficit (See **Self-Care** deficit, dressing, Section III)

SELF-CARE DEFICIT, FEEDING

Feeding **Self-Care** deficit (See **Self-Care** deficit, feeding, Section III)

SELF-CARE DEFICIT, TOILETING

Toileting **Self-Care** deficit (See **Self-Care** deficit, toileting, Section III)

SELF-CONCEPT

Readiness for enhanced **Self-Concept** (See **Self-Concept,** readiness for enhanced, Section III)

SELF-DESTRUCTIVE BEHAVIOR

Post-Trauma syndrome r/t unresolved feelings from traumatic event

Risk for **Self-Mutilation:** Risk factors: feelings of depression, rejection, self-hatred, depersonalization; command hallucinations

Risk for **Suicide:** Risk factor: history of self-destructive behavior

Risk for self-directed **Violence:** Risk factors: panic state, history of child abuse, toxic reaction to medication

SELF-ESTEEM, CHRONIC LOW

Chronic low **Self-Esteem** (See **Self-Esteem,** low, chronic, Section III)

Risk for disturbed personal **Identity:** Risk factor: chronic low self-esteem

SELF-ESTEEM, SITUATIONAL LOW

Situational low **Self-Esteem** (See **Self-Esteem,** low, situational, Section III)

Risk for situational low **Self-Esteem** (See **Self-Esteem,** low, situational, risk for, Section III)

SELF-MUTILATION

Ineffective **Impulse** control r/t ineffective management of anxiety

Self-Mutilation (See **Self-Mutilation,** Section III)

Risk for **Self-Mutilation** (See **Self-Mutilation,** risk for, Section III)

SENILE DEMENTIA

Ineffective **Relationship** r/t cognitive changes in one partner

S

Sedentary lifestyle r/t lack of interest in movement

See Dementia

SEPARATION ANXIETY

Ineffective **Coping** r/t maturational and situational crises, vulnerability related to developmental age, hospitalization, separation from family and familiar surroundings, multiple caregivers

Insomnia r/t separation from significant others

Risk for impaired **Attachment:** Risk factor: separation

See Hospitalized Child

SEPSIS, CHILD

Impaired **Gas** exchange r/t pulmonary inflammation associated with disease process

Imbalanced **Nutrition:** less than body requirements r/t anorexia, generalized weakness, poor sucking reflex

Delayed **Surgical** recovery r/t presence of infection

Ineffective **Thermoregulation** r/t infectious process, septic shock

Ineffective peripheral **Tissue Perfusion** r/t arterial or venous blood flow exchange problems, septic shock

Risk for deficient **Fluid** volume: Risk factor: inflammation leading to decreased systemic vascular resistance

Risk for impaired **Skin** integrity: Risk factor: desquamation caused by disseminated intravascular coagulation

See Hospitalized Child; Premature Infant, Child

SEPTICEMIA

Imbalanced **Nutrition:** less than body requirements r/t anorexia, generalized weakness

Ineffective peripheral **Tissue Perfusion** r/t decreased systemic vascular resistance

Risk for deficient **Fluid** volume: Risk factors: vasodilation of peripheral vessels, leaking of capillaries

Risk for **Shock:** Risk factors: hypotension, hypovolemia

See Sepsis, Child; Shock, Septic

SEVERE ACUTE RESPIRATORY SYNDROME (SARS)

See SARS (Severe Acute Respiratory Syndrome); Pneumonia

SEXUAL DYSFUNCTION

Sexual dysfunction (See **Sexual** dysfunction, Section III)

Ineffective **Relationship** r/t reported sexual dissatisfaction between partners

Chronic **Sorrow** r/t loss of ideal sexual experience, altered relationships

Risk for chronic low **Self-Esteem**

See Erectile Dysfunction (ED)

SEXUALITY, ADOLESCENT

Disturbed **Body Image** r/t anxiety caused by unachieved developmental milestone (puberty) or deficient knowledge regarding reproductive maturation with expressed concerns regarding lack of growth of secondary sex characteristics

Impaired emancipated **Decision-Making:** sexual activity r/t undefined personal values or beliefs, multiple or divergent sources of information, lack of relevant information

Ineffective **Impulse** control r/t denial of consequences of actions

Deficient **Knowledge:** potential for enhanced health maintenance r/t multiple or divergent sources of information or lack of relevant information regarding sexual transmission of disease, contraception, prevention of toxic shock syndrome

See Maturational Issues, Adolescent

SEXUALITY PATTERN, INEFFECTIVE

Ineffective **Sexuality** pattern (See **Sexuality** pattern, ineffective, Section III)

SEXUALLY TRANSMITTED DISEASE (STD)

See STD (Sexually Transmitted Disease)

SHAKEN BABY SYNDROME

Decreased intracranial **Adaptive** capacity r/t brain injury

Impaired **Parenting** r/t stress, history of being abusive

Impaired individual **Resilience** r/t poor impulse control

Stress overload r/t intense repeated family stressors, family violence

Risk for other-directed **Violence:** Risk factors: history of violence against others, perinatal complications

See Child Abuse; Suspected Child Abuse and Neglect (SCAN), Child; Suspected Child Abuse and Neglect (SCAN), Parent

SHAKINESS

Anxiety r/t situational or maturational crisis, threat of death

SHAME

Situational low **Self-Esteem** r/t inability to deal with past traumatic events, blaming of self for events not in one's control

SHINGLES

Acute **Pain** r/t vesicular eruption along the nerves

Ineffective **Protection** r/t abnormal blood profiles

Social isolation r/t altered state of wellness, contagiousness of disease

Risk for **Infection:** Risk factor: tissue destruction

See Itching

SHIVERING

Impaired **Comfort** r/t altered health status

Fear r/t serious threat to health status

Hypothermia r/t exposure to cool environment

Ineffective **Thermoregulation** r/t serious infectious process resulting in immune response of fever

See Shock, Septic

SHOCK, CARDIOGENIC

Decreased **Cardiac** output r/t decreased myocardial contractility, dysrhythmia

SHOCK, HYPOVOLEMIC

Deficient **Fluid** volume r/t abnormal loss of fluid, trauma, third spacing

SHOCK, SEPTIC

Deficient **Fluid** volume r/t abnormal loss of intravascular fluid, pooling of blood in peripheral circulation, overwhelming inflammatory response

Ineffective **Protection** r/t inadequately functioning immune system

See Sepsis, Child; Septicemia

SHOULDER REPAIR

Self-Care deficit: bathing, dressing, feeding r/t immobilization of affected shoulder

Risk for **Perioperative Positioning** injury: Risk factor: immobility

See Surgery, Preoperative; Surgery, Perioperative; Surgery, Postoperative; Total Joint Replacement (Total Hip/Total Knee/Shoulder)

SICKLE CELL ANEMIA/CRISIS

Activity intolerance r/t fatigue, effects of chronic anemia

Deficient **Fluid** volume r/t decreased intake, increased fluid requirements during sickle cell crisis, decreased ability of kidneys to concentrate urine

Impaired physical **Mobility** r/t pain, fatigue

Acute **Pain** r/t viscous blood, tissue hypoxia

Ineffective peripheral **Tissue Perfusion** r/t effects of red cell sickling, infarction of tissues

S

Risk for decreased **Cardiac** tissue perfusion: Risk factors: effects of red cell sickling, infarction of tissues

Risk for disproportionate **Growth**: Risk factor: chronic illness

Risk for **Infection**: Risk factor: alterations in splenic function

Risk for impaired **Resilience**: Risk factor: chronic illness

Risk for ineffective cerebral **Tissue** perfusion: Risk factors: effects of red cell sickling, infarction of tissues

Risk for ineffective **Gastrointestinal** perfusion: Risk factors: coagulopathy, sickle cell anemia.

See Child with Chronic Condition; Hospitalized Child

SIDS (SUDDEN INFANT DEATH SYNDROME)

Anxiety: parental worry r/t life-threatening event

Interrupted **Family** processes r/t stress as a result of special care needs of infant with apnea

Grieving r/t potential loss of infant

Insomnia: parental/infant r/t home apnea monitoring

Deficient **Knowledge:** potential for enhanced health maintenance r/t knowledge or skill acquisition of cardiopulmonary resuscitation and home apnea monitoring

Impaired **Resilience** r/t sudden loss

Risk for **Sudden Infant Death** syndrome (See **Sudden Infant Death** syndrome, risk for, Section III)

Risk for **Powerlessness:** Risk factor: unanticipated life-threatening event

See Terminally Ill Child/Death of Child, Parent

SITTING PROBLEMS

Impaired **Sitting** (See **Sitting**, impaired, Section III)

SITUATIONAL CRISIS

Ineffective **Coping** r/t situational crisis

Interrupted **Family** processes r/t situational crisis

Risk for ineffective **Activity** planning: Risk factor: inability to process information

Risk for disturbed personal **Identity**: Risk factor: situational crisis

Readiness for enhanced **Communication:** willingness to share feelings and thoughts

Readiness for enhanced **Religiosity:** requests religious material and/or experiences

Readiness for enhanced **Resilience:** desire to enhance resilience

Readiness for enhanced **Spiritual** well-being: desire for harmony following crisis

SJS (STEVENS-JOHNSON SYNDROME)

See Stevens-Johnson Syndrome (SJS)

SKIN CANCER

Ineffective **Health** maintenance r/t deficient knowledge regarding self-care with skin cancer

Ineffective **Protection** r/t weakened immune system

Impaired **Tissue** integrity r/t abnormal cell growth in skin, treatment of skin cancer

Readiness for enhanced **Health** management: follows preventive measures

Readiness for enhanced **Knowledge:** self-care to prevent and treat skin cancer

SKIN DISORDERS

Impaired **Skin** integrity (See **Skin** integrity, impaired, Section III)

SKIN TURGOR, CHANGE IN ELASTICITY

Deficient **Fluid** volume r/t active fluid loss

S

SLEEP

Readiness for enhanced **Sleep** (See **Sleep**, readiness for enhanced, Section III)

SLEEP APNEA

Ineffective **Breathing** pattern r/t obesity, substance abuse, enlarged tonsils, smoking, or neurological pathology such as a brain tumor

SLEEP DEPRIVATION

Fatigue r/t lack of sleep

Sleep deprivation (See **Sleep** deprivation, Section III)

SLEEP PROBLEMS

Insomnia (See **Insomnia,** Section III)

SLEEP PATTERN, DISTURBED, PARENT/CHILD

Insomnia: child r/t anxiety or fear

Insomnia: parent r/t parental responsibilities, stress

See Suspected Child Abuse and Neglect (SCAN), Child; Suspected Child Abuse and Neglect (SCAN), Parent

SLURRING OF SPEECH

Impaired verbal **Communication** r/t decrease in circulation to brain, brain tumor, anatomical defect, cleft palate

Situational low **Self-Esteem** r/t speech impairment

See Communication Problems

SMALL BOWEL RESECTION

See Abdominal Surgery

SMELL, LOSS OF ABILITY TO

Risk for **Injury:** Risk factor: inability to detect gas fumes, smoke smells

See Anosmia

SMOKE INHALATION

Ineffective **Airway** clearance r/t smoke inhalation

Impaired **Gas** exchange r/t ventilation-perfusion imbalance

Risk for acute **Confusion:** Risk factor: decreased oxygen supply

Risk for **Infection:** Risk factors: inflammation, ineffective airway clearance, pneumonia

Risk for **Poisoning:** Risk factor: exposure to carbon monoxide

Readiness for enhanced **Health** management: functioning smoke detectors and carbon monoxide detectors in home and at work, escape route planned and reviewed

See Atelectasis; Burns; Pneumonia

SMOKING BEHAVIOR

Insufficient **Breast Milk** r/t smoking

Risk-prone **Health** behavior r/t smoking

Ineffective **Health** maintenance r/t denial of effects of smoking, lack of effective support for smoking withdrawal

Readiness for enhanced **Knowledge:** expresses interest in smoking cessation

Risk for dry **Eye:** Risk factor: smoking

Risk for ineffective peripheral **Tissue Perfusion:** Risk factor: effect of nicotine

Risk for **Thermal** injury: Risk factor: unsafe smoking behavior

SOCIAL INTERACTION, IMPAIRED

Impaired **Social** interaction (See **Social** interaction, impaired, Section III)

SOCIAL ISOLATION

Social isolation (See **Social** isolation, Section III)

SOCIOPATHIC PERSONALITY

See Antisocial Personality Disorder

SODIUM, DECREASE/INCREASE

See Hyponatremia; Hypernatremia

SOMATIZATION DISORDER

Anxiety r/t unresolved conflicts channeled into physical complaints or conditions

Ineffective **Coping** r/t lack of insight into underlying conflicts

S

Ineffective **Denial** r/t displaced psychological stress to physical symptoms

Nausea r/t anxiety

Chronic **Pain** r/t unexpressed anger, multiple physical disorders, depression

Impaired individual **Resilience** r/t possible psychological disorders

SORE NIPPLES, BREASTFEEDING

Ineffective **Breastfeeding** r/t deficient knowledge regarding correct feeding procedure

See Painful Breasts, Sore Nipples

SORE THROAT

Impaired **Comfort** r/t sore throat

Deficient **Knowledge** r/t treatment, relief of discomfort

Impaired **Oral Mucous Membrane** r/t inflammation or infection of oral cavity

Impaired **Swallowing** r/t irritation of oropharyngeal cavity

SORROW

Grieving r/t loss of significant person, object, or role

Chronic **Sorrow** (See **Sorrow**, chronic, Section III)

Readiness for enhanced **Communication**: expresses thoughts and feelings

Readiness for enhanced **Spiritual** well-being: desire to find purpose and meaning of loss

SPASTIC COLON

See IBS (Irritable Bowel Syndrome)

SPEECH DISORDERS

Anxiety r/t difficulty with communication

Impaired verbal **Communication** r/t anatomical defect, cleft palate, psychological barriers, decrease in circulation to brain

SPINA BIFIDA

See Neural Tube Defects

SPINAL CORD INJURY

Deficient **Diversional** activity r/t long-term hospitalization, frequent lengthy treatments

Fear r/t powerlessness over loss of body function

Complicated **Grieving** r/t loss of usual body function

Sedentary lifestyle r/t lack of resources or interest

Impaired wheelchair **Mobility** r/t neuromuscular impairment

Impaired **Standing** r/t spinal cord injury

Urinary Retention r/t inhibition of reflex arc

Risk for **Latex Allergy** response: Risk factor: continuous or intermittent catheterization

Risk for **Autonomic Dysreflexia**: Risk factors: bladder or bowel distention, skin irritation, deficient knowledge of patient and caregiver

Risk for ineffective **Breathing** pattern: Risk factor: neuromuscular impairment

Risk for **Infection**: Risk factors: chronic disease, stasis of body fluids

Risk for **Loneliness**: Risk factor: physical immobility

Risk for **Powerlessness**: Risk factor: loss of function

Risk for **Pressure** ulcer: Risk factor: immobility and decreased sensation

See Child with Chronic Condition; Hospitalized Child; Neural Tube Defects; Paralysis

SPINAL FUSION

Impaired bed **Mobility** r/t impaired ability to turn side to side while keeping spine in proper alignment

Impaired physical **Mobility** r/t musculoskeletal impairment associated with surgery, possible back brace

Readiness for enhanced **Knowledge:** expresses interest in information associated with surgery

See Acute Back; Back Pain; Scoliosis; Surgery, Preoperative Care; Surgery, Perioperative Care; Surgery, Postoperative Care

SPIRITUAL DISTRESS

Spiritual distress (See **Spiritual** distress, Section III)

Risk for chronic low **Self-Esteem:** Risk factor: unresolved spiritual issues

Risk for **Spiritual** distress (See **Spiritual** distress, risk for, Section III)

SPIRITUAL WELL-BEING

Readiness for enhanced **Spiritual** well-being (See **Spiritual** well-being, readiness for enhanced, Section III)

SPLENECTOMY

See Abdominal Surgery

SPRAINS

Acute **Pain** r/t physical injury

Impaired physical **Mobility** r/t injury

Impaired **Walking** r/t injury

STANDING PROBLEMS

Impaired **Standing** (see Impaired **Standing**, Section III)

STAPEDECTOMY

Hearing Loss r/t edema from surgery

Acute **Pain** r/t headache

Risk for **Falls:** Risk factor: dizziness

Risk for **Infection:** Risk factor: invasive procedure

STASIS ULCER

Impaired **Tissue** integrity r/t chronic venous congestion

Risk for **Infection:** Risk factor: open wound

See CHF (Congestive Heart Failure); Varicose Veins

STD (SEXUALLY TRANSMITTED DISEASE)

Impaired **Comfort** r/t infection

Fear r/t altered body function, risk for social isolation, fear of incurable illness

Ineffective **Health** maintenance r/t deficient knowledge regarding transmission, symptoms, treatment of STD

Ineffective **Sexuality** pattern r/t illness, altered body function, need for abstinence to heal

Social isolation r/t fear of contracting or spreading disease

Risk for **Infection:** spread of infection: Risk factor: lack of knowledge concerning transmission of disease

Readiness for enhanced **Knowledge:** seeks information regarding prevention and treatment of STDs

See Maturational Issues, Adolescent; PID (Pelvic Inflammatory Disease)

STEMI (ST-ELEVATION MYOCARDIAL INFARCTION)

See MI (Myocardial Infarction)

STENT (CORONARY ARTERY STENT)

Risk for **Injury:** Risk factor: complications associated with stent placement

Risk for decreased **Cardiac** tissue perfusion: Risk factor: possible restenosis

Risk for **Vascular Trauma:** Risk factors: insertion site, catheter width

Readiness for enhanced **Decision-Making:** expresses desire to enhance risk-benefit analysis, understanding and meaning of choices, and decisions regarding treatment

See Angioplasty, Coronary; Cardiac Catheterization

STERILIZATION SURGERY

Decisional Conflict r/t multiple or divergent sources of information, unclear personal values or beliefs

S

See Surgery, Preoperative Care; Surgery, Perioperative Care; Surgery, Postoperative Care; Tubal Ligation; Vasectomy

STERTOROUS RESPIRATIONS

Ineffective **Airway** clearance r/t pharyngeal obstruction

STEVENS-JOHNSON SYNDROME (SJS)

Impaired **Oral Mucous Membrane** r/t immunocompromised condition associated with allergic medication reaction

Acute **Pain** r/t painful skin lesions and painful mucosa lesions

Impaired **Skin** integrity r/t allergic medication reaction

Risk for deficient **Fluid** volume: Risk factors: factors affecting fluid needs (hypermetabolic state, fever), excessive losses through normal routes (vomiting and diarrhea)

Risk for **Infection:** Risk factor: sloughing skin

Risk for impaired **Liver** function: Risk factor: impaired immune response

STILLBIRTH

See Pregnancy Loss

STOMA

See Colostomy; Ileostomy

STOMATITIS

Impaired **Oral Mucous Membrane** r/t pathological conditions of oral cavity; side effects of chemotherapy

Risk for impaired **Oral Mucous Membranes** (See impaired **Oral Mucous Membranes**, risk for, Section III)

STONE, KIDNEY

See Kidney Stone

STOOL, HARD/DRY

Chronic functional **Constipation** r/t inadequate fluid intake, inadequate fiber intake, decreased activity level, decreased gastric motility

STRAINING WITH DEFECATION

Chronic functional **Constipation** r/t less than adequate fluid intake, less than adequate dietary intake

Risk for decreased **Cardiac** output: Risk factor: vagal stimulation with dysrhythmia resulting from Valsalva maneuver

STREP THROAT

Risk for **Infection:** Risk factor: exposure to pathogen

See Sore Throat

STRESS

Anxiety r/t feelings of helplessness, feelings of being threatened

Ineffective **Coping** r/t ineffective use of problem-solving process, feelings of apprehension or helplessness

Fear r/t powerlessness over feelings

Stress overload r/t intense or multiple stressors

Readiness for enhanced **Communication:** shows willingness to share thoughts and feelings

Readiness for enhanced **Spiritual** well-being: expresses desire for harmony and peace in stressful situation

See Anxiety

STRESS URINARY INCONTINENCE

Stress urinary **Incontinence** r/t degenerative change in pelvic muscles

STRIDOR

Ineffective **Airway** clearance r/t obstruction, tracheobronchial infection, trauma

STROKE

See CVA (Cerebrovascular Accident)

STUTTERING

Anxiety r/t impaired verbal communication

Impaired verbal **Communication** r/t anxiety, psychological problems

SUBARACHNOID HEMORRHAGE

Acute **Pain:** headache r/t irritation of meninges from blood, increased intracranial pressure

Risk for ineffective **Cerebral** tissue perfusion: Risk factor: bleeding from cerebral vessel

See Intracranial Pressure, Increased

SUBSTANCE ABUSE

Compromised family **Coping** r/t codependency issues

Defensive **Coping** r/t substance abuse

Disabled family **Coping** r/t differing coping styles between support persons

Ineffective **Coping** r/t use of substances to cope with life events

Ineffective **Denial** r/t refusal to acknowledge substance abuse problem

Dysfunctional **Family** processes r/t substance abuse

Deficient community **Health** r/t prevention and control of illegal substances in community

Ineffective **Impulse** control r/t addictive process

Ineffective **Relationship** r/t inability for well-balanced collaboration between partners

Insomnia r/t irritability, nightmares, tremors

Risk for impaired **Attachment:** Risk factor: substance abuse

Risk for disturbed personal **Identity:** Risk factor: ingestion/inhalation of toxic chemicals

Risk for chronic low **Self-Esteem:** Risk factors: perceived lack of respect from others, repeated failures, repeated negative reinforcement

Risk for **Thermal** injury: Risk factor: intoxication with drugs or alcohol

Risk for **Vascular Trauma:** Risk factor: chemical irritant self injected into veins

Risk for self-directed **Violence:** Risk factors: reactions to substances used, impulsive behavior, disorientation, impaired judgment

Risk for other-directed **Violence:** Risk factor: access to weapon

Readiness for enhanced **Coping:** seeking social support and knowledge of new strategies

Readiness for enhanced **Self-Concept:** accepting strengths and limitations

See Alcoholism; Drug Abuse; Maturational Issues, Adolescent

SUBSTANCE ABUSE, ADOLESCENT

See Alcohol Withdrawal; Maturational Issues, Adolescent; Substance Abuse

SUBSTANCE ABUSE IN PREGNANCY

Ineffective **Childbearing** process r/t substance abuse

Defensive **Coping** r/t denial of situation, differing value system

Ineffective **Health** management r/t addiction

Deficient **Knowledge** r/t lack of exposure to information regarding effects of substance abuse in pregnancy

Risk for impaired **Attachment:** Risk factors: substance abuse, inability of parent to meet infant's or own personal needs

Risk for **Infection:** Risk factors: intravenous drug use, lifestyle

Risk for **Injury:** fetal: Risk factor: effects of drugs on fetal growth and development

Risk for **Injury:** maternal: Risk factor: drug or alcohol use

Risk for impaired **Parenting:** Risk factor: lack of ability to meet infant's needs due to addiction with use of alcohol or drugs

See Alcoholism; Drug Abuse; Substance Abuse

S

SUCKING REFLEX

Effective **Breastfeeding** r/t regular and sustained sucking and swallowing at breast

SUDDEN INFANT DEATH SYNDROME (SIDS)

See SIDS (Sudden Infant Death Syndrome)

SUFFOCATION, RISK FOR

Risk for **Suffocation** (See **Suffocation**, risk for, Section III)

SUICIDE ATTEMPT

Risk-prone **Health** behavior r/t low self-efficacy

Ineffective **Coping** r/t anger, complicated grieving

Hopelessness r/t perceived or actual loss, substance abuse, low self-concept, inadequate support systems

Ineffective **Impulse** control r/t inability to modulate stress, anxiety

Post-Trauma syndrome r/t history of traumatic events, abuse, rape, incest, war, torture

Impaired individual **Resilience** r/t poor impulse control

Situational low **Self-Esteem** r/t guilt, inability to trust, feelings of worthlessness or rejection

Social isolation r/t inability to engage in satisfying personal relationships

Spiritual distress r/t hopelessness, despair

Risk for **Post-Trauma** syndrome: Risk factor: survivor's role in suicide attempt

Risk for **Suicide** (See **Suicide**, risk for, Section III)

Readiness for enhanced **Communication**: willingness to share thoughts and feelings

Readiness for enhanced **Spiritual** well-being: desire for harmony and inner strength to help redefine purpose for life

See Violent Behavior

SUPPORT SYSTEM, INADEQUATE

Readiness for enhanced family **Coping**: ability to adapt to tasks associated with care, support of significant other during health crisis

Readiness for enhanced **Family** processes: activities support the growth of family members

Readiness for enhanced **Parenting**: children or other dependent person(s) expressing satisfaction with home environment

SUPPRESSION OF LABOR

See Preterm Labor; Tocolytic Therapy

SURGERY, PERIOPERATIVE CARE

Risk for imbalanced **Fluid** volume: Risk factor: surgery

Risk for **Perioperative Hypothermia**: Risk factors: inadequate covering of client, cold surgical room

Risk for **Perioperative Positioning** injury: Risk factors: predisposing condition, prolonged surgery

SURGERY, POSTOPERATIVE CARE

Activity intolerance r/t pain, surgical procedure

Anxiety r/t change in health status, hospital environment

Deficient **Knowledge** r/t postoperative expectations, lifestyle changes

Nausea r/t manipulation of gastrointestinal tract, postsurgical anesthesia

Imbalanced **Nutrition:** less than body requirements r/t anorexia, nausea, vomiting, decreased peristalsis

Ineffective peripheral **Tissue Perfusion** r/t hypovolemia, circulatory stasis, obesity, prolonged immobility, decreased coughing, decreased deep breathing

Acute **Pain** r/t inflammation or injury in surgical area

Delayed **Surgical** recovery r/t extensive surgical procedure, postoperative surgical infection

Urinary retention r/t anesthesia, pain, fear, unfamiliar surroundings, client's position

Risk for **Bleeding:** Risk factor: surgical procedure

Risk for ineffective **Breathing** pattern: Risk factors: pain, location of incision, effects of anesthesia or opioids

Risk for **Constipation:** Risk factors: decreased activity, decreased food or fluid intake, anesthesia, pain medication

Risk for imbalanced **Fluid** volume: Risk factors: hypermetabolic state, fluid loss during surgery, presence of indwelling tubes, fluids used to distend organ structures being absorbed into body

Risk for **Infection:** Risk factors: invasive procedure, pain, anesthesia, location of incision, weakened cough as a result of aging

SURGERY, PREOPERATIVE CARE

Anxiety r/t threat to or change in health status, situational crisis, fear of the unknown

Insomnia r/t anxiety about upcoming surgery

Deficient **Knowledge** r/t preoperative procedures, postoperative expectations

Readiness for enhanced **Knowledge:** shows understanding of preoperative and postoperative expectations for self-care

SURGICAL RECOVERY, DELAYED

Delayed **Surgical** recovery (See **Surgical** recovery, delayed, Section III)

Risk for delayed **Surgical** recovery (See **Surgical** recovery, delayed, risk for, Section III)

SUSPECTED CHILD ABUSE AND NEGLECT (SCAN), CHILD

Ineffective **Activity** planning r/t lack of family support

Anxiety: child r/t threat of punishment for perceived wrongdoing

Deficient community **Health** r/t inadequate reporting and follow-up of SCAN

Disturbed personal **Identity** r/t dysfunctional family processes

Rape-Trauma syndrome r/t altered lifestyle because of abuse, changes in residence

Risk for impaired **Resilience:** Risk factor: adverse situation

Readiness for enhanced community **Coping:** obtaining resources to prevent child abuse, neglect

See Child Abuse; Hospitalized Child; Maturational Issues, Adolescent

SUSPECTED CHILD ABUSE AND NEGLECT (SCAN), PARENT

Disabled family **Coping** r/t dysfunctional family, underdeveloped nurturing parental role, lack of parental support systems or role models

Dysfunctional **Family** processes r/t inadequate coping skills

Ineffective **Health** maintenance r/t deficient knowledge of parenting skills as result of unachieved developmental tasks

Impaired **Home** maintenance r/t disorganization, parental dysfunction, neglect of safe and nurturing environment

Ineffective **Impulse** control r/t projection of anger, frustration onto child

Impaired **Parenting** r/t unrealistic expectations of child; lack of effective role model; unmet social, emotional, or maturational needs of parents; interruption in bonding process

Impaired individual **Resilience** r/t poor impulse control

Chronic low **Self-Esteem** r/t lack of successful parenting experiences

Risk for other-directed **Violence:** parent to child: Risk factors: inadequate coping mechanisms, unresolved stressors, unachieved maturational level by parent

S

SUSPICION

Disturbed personal **Identity** r/t psychiatric disorder

Powerlessness r/t repetitive paranoid thinking

Impaired **Social** interaction r/t disturbed thought processes, paranoid delusions, hallucinations

Risk for self-directed **Violence:** Risk factor: inability to trust

Risk for other-directed **Violence:** Risk factor: impulsiveness

SWALLOWING DIFFICULTIES

Impaired **Swallowing** (See **Swallowing,** impaired, Section III)

SWINE FLU (H1N1)

See Influenza

SYNCOPE

Anxiety r/t fear of falling

Impaired physical **Mobility** r/t fear of falling

Ineffective **Health** management r/t lack of knowledge in how to prevent syncope

Social isolation r/t fear of falling

Risk for decreased **Cardiac** output: Risk factor: dysrhythmia

Risk for **Falls:** Risk factor: syncope

Risk for **Injury:** Risk factors: altered sensory perception, transient loss of consciousness, risk for falls

Risk for ineffective **Cerebral** tissue perfusion: Risk factor: interruption of blood flow

SYPHILIS

See STD (Sexually Transmitted Disease)

SYSTEMIC LUPUS ERYTHEMATOSUS

See Lupus Erythematosus

T

T & A (TONSILLECTOMY AND ADENOIDECTOMY)

Ineffective **Airway** clearance r/t hesitation or reluctance to cough because of pain

Deficient **Knowledge:** potential for enhanced health maintenance r/t insufficient knowledge regarding postoperative nutritional and rest requirements, signs and symptoms of complications, positioning

Nausea r/t gastric irritation, pharmaceuticals, anesthesia

Acute **Pain** r/t surgical incision

Risk for **Aspiration:** Risk factors: postoperative drainage, impaired swallowing

Risk for deficient **Fluid** volume: Risk factors: decreased intake because of painful swallowing, effects of anesthesia (nausea, vomiting), hemorrhage

Risk for imbalanced **Nutrition:** less than body requirements: Risk factors: hesitation or reluctance to swallow

TACHYCARDIA

See Dysrhythmia

TACHYPNEA

Ineffective **Breathing** pattern r/t pain, anxiety, hypoxia

See cause of Tachypnea

TARDIVE DYSKINESIA

Ineffective **Health** management r/t complexity of therapeutic regimen or medication

Deficient **Knowledge** r/t cognitive limitation in assimilating information relating to side effects associated with neuroleptic medications

Risk for **Injury:** Risk factor: drug-induced abnormal body movements

TASTE ABNORMALITY

Frail Elderly syndrome r/t chronic illness

TB (PULMONARY TUBERCULOSIS)

Ineffective **Airway** clearance r/t increased secretions, excessive mucus

Ineffective **Breathing** pattern r/t decreased energy, fatigue

Fatigue r/t disease state

Impaired **Gas** exchange r/t disease process

Ineffective **Health** management r/t deficient knowledge of prevention and treatment regimen

Impaired **Home** maintenance management r/t client or family member with disease

Ineffective **Thermoregulation** r/t presence of infection

Risk for **Infection:** Risk factor: insufficient knowledge regarding avoidance of exposure to pathogens

Readiness for enhanced **Health** management: takes medications according to prescribed protocol for prevention and treatment

TBI (TRAUMATIC BRAIN INJURY)

Interrupted **Family** processes r/t traumatic injury to family member

Chronic **Sorrow** r/t change in health status and functional ability

Risk for **Post-Trauma** syndrome: Risk factor: perception of event causing TBI

Risk for impaired **Religiosity:** Risk factor: impaired physical mobility

Risk for impaired **Resilience:** Risk factor: crisis of injury

See Head Injury; Neurologic Disorders

TD (TRAVELER'S DIARRHEA)

Diarrhea r/t travel with exposure to different bacteria, viruses

Risk for deficient **Fluid** volume: Risk factors: excessive loss of fluids, diarrhea

Risk for **Infection:** Risk factor: insufficient knowledge regarding avoidance of exposure to pathogens (water supply, iced drinks, local cheeses, ice cream, undercooked meat, fish and shellfish, uncooked vegetables, unclean eating utensils, improper handwashing)

TEMPERATURE, DECREASED

Hypothermia r/t exposure to cold environment

TEMPERATURE, HIGH

Hyperthermia r/t neurological damage, disease condition with high temperature, excessive heat, inflammatory response

TEMPERATURE REGULATION, IMPAIRED

Ineffective **Thermoregulation** r/t trauma, illness, cerebral injury

TEN (TOXIC EPIDERMAL NECROLYSIS)

See Toxic Epidermal Necrolysis (TEN)

TENSION

Anxiety r/t threat to or change in health status, situational crisis

Readiness for enhanced **Communication:** expresses willingness to share feelings and thoughts

See Stress

TERMINALLY ILL ADULT

Death **Anxiety** r/t unresolved issues relating to death and dying

Risk for **Spiritual** distress: Risk factor: impending death

Readiness for enhanced **Religiosity:** requests religious material and/or experiences

Readiness for enhanced **Spiritual** well-being: desire to achieve harmony of mind, body, spirit

See Terminally Ill Child/Death of Child, Parent

TERMINALLY ILL CHILD, ADOLESCENT

Disturbed **Body Image** r/t effects of terminal disease, already critical feelings of group identity and self-image

T

Ineffective **Coping** r/t inability to establish personal and peer identity because of the threat of being different or not being healthy, inability to achieve maturational tasks

Impaired **Social** interaction r/t forced separation from peers

See Child with Chronic Condition; Hospitalized Child; Terminally Ill Child/Death of Child, Parent

TERMINALLY ILL CHILD, INFANT/TODDLER

Ineffective **Coping** r/t separation from parents and familiar environment from inability to understand dying process

See Child with Chronic Condition; Terminally Ill Child/Death of Child, Parent

TERMINALLY ILL CHILD, PRESCHOOL CHILD

Fear r/t perceived punishment, bodily harm, feelings of guilt caused by magical thinking (i.e., believing that thoughts cause events)

See Child with Chronic Condition; Terminally Ill Child/Death of Child, Parent

TERMINALLY ILL CHILD, SCHOOL-AGE CHILD/ PREADOLESCENT

Fear r/t perceived punishment, body mutilation, feelings of guilt

See Child with Chronic Condition; Terminally Ill Child/Death of Child, Parent

TERMINALLY ILL CHILD/DEATH OF CHILD, PARENT

Compromised family **Coping** r/t inability or unwillingness to discuss impending death and feelings with child or support child through terminal stages of illness

Decisional Conflict r/t continuation or discontinuation of treatment, do-not-resuscitate decision, ethical issues regarding organ donation

Ineffective **Denial** r/t complicated grieving

Interrupted **Family** processes r/t situational crisis

Grieving r/t death of child

Hopelessness r/t overwhelming stresses caused by terminal illness

Insomnia r/t grieving process

Impaired **Parenting** r/t risk for overprotection of surviving siblings

Powerlessness r/t inability to alter course of events

Impaired **Social** interaction r/t complicated grieving

Social isolation· imposed by others r/t feelings of inadequacy in providing support to grieving parents

Social isolation: self-imposed r/t unresolved grief, perceived inadequate parenting skills

Spiritual distress r/t sudden and unexpected death, prolonged suffering before death, questioning the death of youth, questioning the meaning of one's own existence

Risk for complicated **Grieving**: Risk factor: prolonged, unresolved, obstructed progression through stages of grief and mourning

Risk for impaired **Resilience**: Risk factor: impending death

Readiness for enhanced family **Coping**: impact of crisis on family values, priorities, goals, or relationships; expressed interest or desire to attach meaning to child's life and death

TETRALOGY OF FALLOT

See Congenital Heart Disease/Cardiac Anomalies

TETRAPLEGIA

Autonomic dysreflexia r/t bladder or bowel distention, skin irritation, infection, deficient knowledge of patient and caregiver

Grieving r/t loss of previous functioning

Powerlessness r/t inability to perform previous activities

Impaired **Sitting** r/t paralysis of extremities

Impaired spontaneous **Ventilation** r/t loss of innervation of respiratory muscles, respiratory muscle fatigue

Risk for **Aspiration:** Risk factor: inadequate ability to protect airway from neurological damage

Risk for **Infection:** Risk factor: urinary stasis

Risk for impaired **Skin** integrity: Risk factor: physical immobilization and decreased sensation

Risk for ineffective **Thermoregulation:** Risk factors: inability to move to increase temperature, possible presence of infection to increase temperature

THERMOREGULATION, INEFFECTIVE

Ineffective **Thermoregulation** (See **Thermoregulation,** ineffective, Section III)

THORACENTESIS

See Pleural Effusion

THORACOTOMY

Activity intolerance r/t pain, imbalance between oxygen supply and demand, presence of chest tubes

Ineffective **Airway** clearance r/t drowsiness, pain with breathing and coughing

Ineffective **Breathing** pattern r/t decreased energy, fatigue, pain

Deficient **Knowledge** r/t self-care, effective breathing exercises, pain relief

Acute **Pain** r/t surgical procedure, coughing, deep breathing

Risk for **Bleeding:** Risk factor: surgery

Risk for **Infection:** Risk factor: invasive procedure

Risk for **Injury:** Risk factor: disruption of closed-chest drainage system

Risk for **Perioperative Positioning** injury: Risk factors: lateral positioning, immobility

Risk for **Vascular Trauma:** Risk factors: chemical irritant, antibiotics

THOUGHT DISORDERS

See Schizophrenia

THROMBOCYTOPENIC PURPURA

See ITP (Idiopathic Thrombocytopenic Purpura)

THROMBOPHLEBITIS

See DVT

THYROIDECTOMY

Risk for ineffective **Airway** clearance r/t edema or hematoma formation, airway obstruction

Risk for impaired verbal **Communication:** Risk factors: edema, pain, vocal cord or laryngeal nerve damage

Risk for **Injury:** Risk factor: possible parathyroid damage or removal

See Surgery, Preoperative Care; Surgery, Perioperative Care; Surgery, Postoperative Care

TIA (TRANSIENT ISCHEMIC ATTACK)

Acute **Confusion** r/t hypoxia

Readiness for enhanced **Health** management: obtains knowledge regarding treatment prevention of inadequate oxygenation

See Syncope

TIC DISORDER

See Tourette's Syndrome (TS)

TINEA CAPITIS

Impaired **Comfort** r/t inflammation from skin irritation

See Ringworm of Scalp

TINEA CORPORIS

See Ringworm of Body

T

TINEA CRURIS
See Jock Itch; Itching; Pruritus

TINEA PEDIS
See Athlete's Foot; Itching; Pruritus

TINEA UNGUIUM (ONYCHOMYCOSIS)
See Ringworm of Nails

TINNITUS

Ineffective **Health** maintenance r/t deficient knowledge regarding self-care with tinnitus

Hearing Loss r/t ringing in ears obscuring hearing

TISSUE DAMAGE, CORNEAL

Risk for corneal **Injury** (See corneal **Injury**, risk for, Section III)

TISSUE DAMAGE, INTEGUMENTARY

Impaired **Tissue** integrity (See **Tissue** integrity, impaired, Section III)

Risk for impaired **Tissue** integrity (See **Tissue** integrity, impaired, risk for, Section III)

TISSUE PERFUSION, PERIPHERAL

Ineffective peripheral **Tissue Perfusion** (See **Tissue Perfusion**, peripheral, ineffective, Section III)

Risk for ineffective peripheral **Tissue Perfusion** (See **Tissue Perfusion**, peripheral, ineffective, risk for, Section III)

TOILETING PROBLEMS

Toileting **Self-Care** deficit r/t impaired transfer ability, impaired mobility status, intolerance of activity, neuromuscular impairment, cognitive impairment

Impaired **Transfer** ability r/t neuromuscular deficits

TOILET TRAINING

Deficient **Knowledge:** parent r/t signs of child's readiness for training

Risk for **Constipation:** Risk factor: withholding stool

Risk for **Infection:** Risk factor: withholding urination

TONSILLECTOMY AND ADENOIDECTOMY (T & A)
See T & A (Tonsillectomy and Adenoidectomy)

TOOTHACHE

Impaired **Dentition** r/t ineffective oral hygiene, barriers to self-care, economic barriers to professional care, nutritional deficits, lack of knowledge regarding dental health

Acute **Pain** r/t inflammation, infection

TOTAL ANOMALOUS PULMONARY VENOUS RETURN
See Congenital Heart Disease/Cardiac Anomalies

TOTAL JOINT REPLACEMENT (TOTAL HIP/TOTAL KNEE/ SHOULDER)

Disturbed **Body Image** r/t large scar, presence of prosthesis

Impaired physical **Mobility** r/t musculoskeletal impairment, surgery, prosthesis

Risk for **Injury:** neurovascular: Risk factors: altered peripheral tissue perfusion, impaired mobility, prosthesis

Risk for **Peripheral Neurovascular** dysfunction r/t immobilization, surgical procedure

Ineffective peripheral **Tissue** perfusion r/t surgery

See Surgery, Preoperative Care; Surgery, Perioperative Care; Surgery, Postoperative Care

TOTAL PARENTERAL NUTRITION (TPN)
See TPN (Total Parenteral Nutrition)

TOURETTE'S SYNDROME (TS)

Hopelessness r/t inability to control behavior

Impaired individual **Resilience** r/t uncontrollable behavior

Risk for situational low **Self-Esteem**: Risk factors: uncontrollable behavior, motor and phonic tics

See Attention Deficit Disorder

TOXEMIA

See PIH (Pregnancy-Induced Hypertension/Preeclampsia)

TOXIC EPIDERMAL NECROLYSIS (TEN) (ERYTHEMA MULTIFORME)

Death **Anxiety** r/t uncertainty of prognosis

See Stevens-Johnson Syndrome (SJS)

TPN (TOTAL PARENTERAL NUTRITION)

Imbalanced **Nutrition**: less than body requirements r/t inability to digest food or absorb nutrients as a result of biological or psychological factors

Risk for **Electrolyte** imbalance: Risk factor: need for regulation of electrolytes in TPN fluids

Risk for excess **Fluid** volume: Risk factor: rapid administration of TPN

Risk for unstable blood **Glucose** level: Risk factor: high glucose levels in TPN to be regulated according to blood glucose levels

Risk for **Infection**: Risk factors: concentrated glucose solution, invasive administration of fluids

Risk for **Vascular Trauma**: Risk factors: insertion site, length of treatment time

TRACHEOESOPHAGEAL FISTULA

Ineffective **Airway** clearance r/t aspiration of feeding because of inability to swallow

Imbalanced **Nutrition**: less than body requirements r/t difficulties swallowing

Risk for **Aspiration**: Risk factor: common passage of air and food

Risk for **Vascular Trauma**: Risk factors: venous medications, site

See Respiratory Conditions of the Neonate; Hospitalized Child

TRACHEOSTOMY

Ineffective **Airway** clearance r/t increased secretions, mucous plugs

Anxiety r/t impaired verbal communication, ineffective airway clearance

Disturbed **Body Image** r/t abnormal opening in neck

Impaired verbal **Communication** r/t presence of mechanical airway

Deficient **Knowledge** r/t self-care, home maintenance management

Acute **Pain** r/t edema, surgical procedure

Risk for **Aspiration**: Risk factor: presence of tracheostomy

Risk for **Bleeding**: Risk factor: surgical incision

Risk for **Infection**: Risk factors: invasive procedure, pooling of secretions

TRACTION AND CASTS

Constipation r/t immobility

Deficient **Diversional** activity r/t immobility

Impaired physical **Mobility** r/t imposed restrictions on activity because of bone or joint disease injury

Acute **Pain** r/t immobility, injury, or disease

Self-Care deficit: feeding, dressing, bathing, toileting r/t degree of impaired physical mobility, body area affected by traction or cast

Impaired **Transfer** ability r/t presence of traction, casts

Risk for **Disuse** syndrome: Risk factor: mechanical immobilization

See Casts

TRANSFER ABILITY

Impaired **Transfer** ability (See **Transfer** ability, impaired, Section III)

T

TRANSIENT ISCHEMIC ATTACK (TIA)

See TIA (Transient Ischemic Attack)

TRANSPOSITION OF GREAT VESSELS

See Congenital Heart Disease/Cardiac Anomalies

TRANSURETHRAL RESECTION OF THE PROSTATE (TURP)

See TURP (Transurethral Resection of the Prostate)

TRAUMA IN PREGNANCY

Anxiety r/t threat to self or fetus, unknown outcome

Deficient **Knowledge** r/t lack of exposure to situation

Acute **Pain** r/t trauma

Impaired **Skin** integrity r/t trauma

Risk for **Bleeding:** Risk factor: trauma

Risk for deficient **Fluid** volume: Risk factor: fluid loss

Risk for **Infection:** Risk factor: traumatized tissue

Risk for **Injury:** fetal: Risk factor: premature separation of placenta

Risk for disturbed **Maternal–Fetal** dyad: Risk factor: complication of pregnancy

TRAUMA, RISK FOR

Risk for **Trauma** (See **Trauma,** risk for, Section III)

TRAUMATIC BRAIN INJURY (TBI)

See TBI (Traumatic Brain Injury); Intracranial Pressure, Increased

TRAUMATIC EVENT

Post-Trauma syndrome r/t previously experienced trauma

TRAVELER'S DIARRHEA (TD)

See TD (Traveler's Diarrhea)

TREMBLING OF HANDS

Fear r/t threat to or change in health status, threat of death, situational crisis

TRICUSPID ATRESIA

See Congenital Heart Disease/Cardiac Anomalies

TRIGEMINAL NEURALGIA

Ineffective **Health** management r/t deficient knowledge regarding prevention of stimuli that trigger pain

Imbalanced **Nutrition:** less than body requirements r/t pain when chewing

Acute **Pain** r/t irritation of trigeminal nerve

Risk for corneal **Injury:** Risk factor: possible decreased corneal sensation

TRUNCUS ARTERIOSUS

See Congenital Heart Disease/Cardiac Anomalies

TS (TOURETTE'S SYNDROME)

See Tourette's Syndrome (TS)

TSE (TESTICULAR SELF-EXAMINATION)

Readiness for enhanced **Health** management: seeks information regarding self-examination

TUBAL LIGATION

Decisional Conflict r/t tubal sterilization

See Laparoscopy

TUBE FEEDING

Risk for **Aspiration:** Risk factors: improperly administered feeding, improper placement of tube, improper positioning of client during and after feeding, excessive residual feeding or lack of digestion, altered gag reflex

Risk for deficient **Fluid** volume: Risk factor: inadequate water administration with concentrated feeding

Risk for imbalanced **Nutrition:** less than body requirements: Risk factors: intolerance to tube feeding, inadequate calorie replacement to meet metabolic needs

TUBERCULOSIS (TB)

See TB (Pulmonary Tuberculosis)

TURP (TRANSURETHRAL RESECTION OF THE PROSTATE)

Deficient **Knowledge** r/t postoperative self-care, home maintenance management

Acute **Pain** r/t incision, irritation from catheter, bladder spasms, kidney infection

Urinary retention r/t obstruction of urethra or catheter with clots

Risk for **Bleeding:** Risk factor: surgery

Risk for deficient **Fluid** volume: Risk factors: fluid loss, possible bleeding

Risk for urge urinary **Incontinence:** Risk factor: edema from surgical procedure

Risk for **Infection:** Risk factors: invasive procedure, route for bacteria entry

ULCER, PEPTIC (DUODENAL OR GASTRIC)

Fatigue r/t loss of blood, chronic illness

Ineffective **Health** maintenance r/t lack of knowledge regarding health practices to prevent ulcer formation

Nausea r/t gastrointestinal irritation

Acute **Pain** r/t irritated mucosa from acid secretion

Risk for ineffective **Gastrointestinal** perfusion: Risk factor: ulcer

See GI Bleed (Gastrointestinal Bleeding)

ULCERATIVE COLITIS

See Inflammatory Bowel Disease (Child and Adult)

ULCERS, STASIS

See Stasis Ulcer

UNILATERAL NEGLECT OF ONE SIDE OF BODY

Unilateral Neglect (See **Unilateral Neglect,** Section III)

UNSANITARY LIVING CONDITIONS

Impaired **Home** maintenance r/t impaired cognitive or emotional functioning, lack of knowledge, insufficient finances, addiction

Risk for **Allergy** response: Risk factor: exposure to environmental contaminants

URGENCY TO URINATE

Urge urinary **Incontinence** (See **Incontinence,** urinary, urge, Section III)

Risk for urge urinary **Incontinence** (See **Incontinence,** urinary, urge, risk for, Section III)

URINARY CATHETER

Risk for urinary tract **Injury:** Risk factors: confused client, long-term use of catheter, large retention balloon or catheter, perirectal burn injured client

URINARY DIVERSION

See Ileal Conduit

URINARY ELIMINATION, IMPAIRED

Impaired **Urinary** elimination (See **Urinary** elimination, impaired, Section III)

URINARY INCONTINENCE

See Incontinence of Urine

URINARY RETENTION

Urinary Retention (See **Urinary Retention,** Section III)

URINARY TRACT INFECTION (UTI)

See UTI (Urinary Tract Infection)

UROLITHIASIS

See Kidney Stone

UTERINE ATONY IN LABOR

See Dystocia

U

UTERINE ATONY IN POSTPARTUM

See Postpartum Hemorrhage

UTERINE BLEEDING

See Hemorrhage; Postpartum Hemorrhage; Shock, Hypovolemic

UTI (URINARY TRACT INFECTION)

Ineffective **Health** maintenance r/t deficient knowledge regarding methods to treat and prevent UTIs, prolonged use of indwelling urinary catheter

Acute **Pain**: dysuria r/t inflammatory process in bladder

Impaired **Urinary** elimination: frequency r/t urinary tract infection

Risk for urge urinary **Incontinence**: Risk factor: hyperreflexia from cystitis

Risk for ineffective **Renal** perfusion: Risk factor: infection

V

VAD (VENTRICULAR ASSIST DEVICE)

See Ventricular Assist Device (VAD)

VAGINAL HYSTERECTOMY

Urinary retention r/t edema at surgical site

Risk for urge urinary **Incontinence**: Risk factors: edema, congestion of pelvic tissues

Risk for **Infection**: Risk factor: surgical site

Risk for **Perioperative Positioning** injury: Risk factor: lithotomy position

VAGINITIS

Impaired **Comfort** r/t pruritus, itching

Ineffective **Health** maintenance r/t deficient knowledge regarding self-care with vaginitis

Ineffective **Sexuality** pattern r/t abstinence during acute stage, pain

VAGOTOMY

See Abdominal Surgery

VALUE SYSTEM CONFLICT

Decisional Conflict r/t unclear personal values or beliefs

Spiritual distress r/t challenged value system

Readiness for enhanced **Spiritual** well-being: desire for harmony with self, others, higher power, God

VARICOSE VEINS

Ineffective **Health** maintenance r/t deficient knowledge regarding health care practices, prevention, treatment regimen

Chronic **Pain** r/t impaired circulation

Ineffective peripheral **Tissue Perfusion** r/t venous stasis

Risk for impaired **Tissue** integrity: Risk factor: altered peripheral tissue perfusion

VASCULAR DEMENTIA (FORMERLY CALLED MULTIINFARCT DEMENTIA)

See Dementia

VASCULAR OBSTRUCTION, PERIPHERAL

Anxiety r/t lack of circulation to body part

Acute **Pain** r/t vascular obstruction

Ineffective peripheral **Tissue Perfusion** r/t interruption of circulatory flow

Risk for **Peripheral Neurovascular** dysfunction: Risk factor: vascular obstruction

VASECTOMY

Decisional Conflict r/t surgery as method of permanent sterilization

VENEREAL DISEASE

See STD (Sexually Transmitted Disease)

VENTILATED CLIENT, MECHANICALLY

Ineffective **Airway** clearance r/t increased secretions, decreased cough and gag reflex

Ineffective **Breathing** pattern r/t decreased energy and fatigue as a result of possible altered nutrition: less than body requirements, neurological disease or damage

Impaired verbal **Communication** r/t presence of endotracheal tube, inability to phonate

Fear r/t inability to breathe on own, difficulty communicating

Impaired **Gas** exchange r/t ventilation-perfusion imbalance

Powerlessness r/t health treatment regimen

Social isolation r/t impaired mobility, ventilator dependence

Impaired spontaneous **Ventilation** r/t metabolic factors, respiratory muscle fatigue

Dysfunctional **Ventilatory** weaning response r/t psychological, situational, physiological factors

Risk for **Falls:** Risk factors: impaired mobility, decreased muscle strength

Risk for **Infection:** Risk factors: presence of endotracheal tube, pooled secretions

Risk for pressure **Ulcer:** Risk factor: decreased mobility

Risk for impaired **Resilience:** Risk factor: illness

See Child with Chronic Condition; Hospitalized Child; Respiratory Conditions of the Neonate

VENTRICULAR ASSIST DEVICE (VAD)

Anxiety r/t possible failure of device

Risk for **Infection:** Risk factor: device insertion site

Risk for **Vascular Trauma:** Risk factor: insertion site

Readiness for enhanced **Decision-Making:** expresses desire to enhance the understanding of the meaning of choices regarding implanting a ventricular assist device

See Open Heart Surgery

VENTRICULAR FIBRILLATION

See Dysrhythmia

VERTIGO

See Syncope

VIOLENT BEHAVIOR

Risk for other-directed **Violence** (See **Violence,** other-directed, risk for, Section III)

Risk for self-directed **Violence** (See **Violence,** self-directed, risk for, Section III)

VIRAL GASTROENTERITIS

Diarrhea r/t infectious process, Norovirus

Deficient **Fluid** volume r/t vomiting, diarrhea

Ineffective **Health** management r/t inadequate handwashing

See Gastroenteritis, Child

VISION IMPAIRMENT

Fear r/t loss of sight

Social isolation r/t altered state of wellness, inability to see

Vision Loss r/t impaired visual function; integration; reception; and or transmission

Risk for impaired **Resilience:** Risk factor: presence of new crisis

See Blindness; Cataracts; Glaucoma

VOMITING

Nausea r/t chemotherapy, postsurgical anesthesia, irritation to the gastrointestinal system, stimulation of neuropharmacological mechanisms

Imbalanced **Nutrition:** less than body requirements r/t inability to ingest food

Risk for **Electrolyte** imbalance: Risk factor: vomiting

VTE (VENOUS THROMBOEMBOLISM)

See DVT (Deep Vein Thrombosis)

V

W

WALKING IMPAIRMENT

Impaired **Walking** (See **Walking**, impaired, Section III)

WANDERING

Wandering (See **Wandering**, Section III)

WEAKNESS

Fatigue r/t decreased or increased metabolic energy production

Risk for **Falls:** Risk factor: weakness

WEIGHT GAIN

Overweight (See **Overweight**, Section III)

WEIGHT LOSS

Imbalanced **Nutrition:** less than body requirements r/t inability to ingest food because of biological, psychological, economic factors

WELLNESS-SEEKING BEHAVIOR

Readiness for enhanced **Health** management: expresses desire for increased control of health practice

WERNICKE-KORSAKOFF SYNDROME

See *Korsakoff's Syndrome*

WEST NILE VIRUS

See *Meningitis/Encephalitis*

WHEELCHAIR USE PROBLEMS

Impaired wheelchair **Mobility** (See **Mobility**, wheelchair, impaired, Section III)

WHEEZING

Ineffective **Airway** clearance r/t tracheobronchial obstructions, secretions

WILMS' TUMOR

Chronic functional **Constipation** r/t obstruction associated with presence of tumor

Acute **Pain** r/t pressure from tumor

See *Chemotherapy; Hospitalized Child; Radiation Therapy; Surgery, Preoperative Care; Surgery, Perioperative Care; Surgery, Postoperative Care*

WITHDRAWAL FROM ALCOHOL

See *Alcohol Withdrawal*

WITHDRAWAL FROM DRUGS

See *Drug Withdrawal*

WOUND DEBRIDEMENT

Acute **Pain** r/t debridement of wound

Impaired **Tissue** integrity r/t debridement, open wound

Risk for **Infection:** Risk factors: open wound, presence of bacteria

WOUND DEHISCENCE, EVISCERATION

Fear r/t client fear of body parts "falling out," surgical procedure not going as planned

Disturbed **Body Image** r/t change in body structure and wound appearance

Imbalanced **Nutrition:** less than body requirements r/t inability to digest nutrients, need for increased protein for healing

Risk for deficient **Fluid** volume: Risk factors: inability to ingest nutrients, obstruction, fluid loss

Risk for **Injury:** Risk factor: exposed abdominal contents

Risk for delayed **Surgical** recovery: Risk factors: separation of wound, exposure of abdominal contents

WOUND INFECTION

Disturbed **Body Image** r/t open wound

Imbalanced **Nutrition:** less than body requirements r/t biological factors, infection, fever

Ineffective **Thermoregulation** r/t infection in wound resulting in fever

Impaired **Tissue** integrity r/t wound, presence of infection

Risk for imbalanced **Fluid** volume: Risk factor: increased metabolic rate

Risk for **Infection:** spread of: Risk factor: imbalanced nutrition: less than body requirements

Risk for delayed **Surgical** recovery: Risk factor: presence of infection

WOUNDS, OPEN

See Lacerations

Guide to Planning Care

Section II is a listing of nursing diagnosis care plans according to NANDA-I. The care plans are arranged alphabetically by diagnostic concept.

MAKING AN ACCURATE NURSING DIAGNOSIS
Verify the accuracy of the previously suggested nursing diagnoses (from Section I) for the client. To do this:
- Read the definition for the suggested nursing diagnosis and determine if it sounds appropriate.
- Compare the Defining Characteristics with the symptoms that were identified from the client data collected.
- Compare the Risk Factors with the symptoms that were identified from the client data collected (if it is a "Risk for" Nursing Diagnosis, they do not have defining characteristics).

WRITING OUTCOMES, STATEMENTS, AND NURSING INTERVENTIONS
After selecting the appropriate nursing diagnosis, use this section to write outcomes and interventions by using the Client Outcomes/ Nursing Interventions as written.

Following these steps, you will be able to write a nursing care plan:
- Follow this care plan to administer nursing care to the client.
- Document all steps and evaluate and update the care plan as needed.

A   Activity intolerance

NANDA-I Definition

Insufficient physiological or psychological energy to endure or complete required or desired daily activities

Defining Characteristics

Abnormal blood pressure response to activity; abnormal heart rate response to activity; ECG change (e.g., arrhythmia, conduction abnormality, ischemia); exertional discomfort; exertional dyspnea; fatigue; generalized weakness

Related Factors (r/t)

Bed rest; generalized weakness; imbalance between oxygen supply/demand; immobility; sedentary lifestyle

Client Outcomes

Client Will (Specify Time Frame)

- Participate in prescribed physical activity with appropriate changes in heart rate, blood pressure, and breathing rate; maintain monitor patterns (rhythm and ST segment) within normal limits
- State symptoms of adverse effects of exercise and report onset of symptoms immediately
- Maintain normal skin color; skin is warm and dry with activity
- Verbalize an understanding of the need to gradually increase activity based on testing, tolerance, and symptoms
- Demonstrate increased tolerance to activity

Nursing Interventions

- Determine cause of Activity intolerance (see Related Factors) and determine whether cause is physical, psychological, or motivational.
- If mainly on bed rest, minimize cardiovascular deconditioning by positioning the client in an upright position several times daily if possible.
- Assess the client daily for appropriateness of activity and bed rest orders. Mobilize the client as soon as possible.
- If the client is mostly immobile, consider use of a transfer chair: a chair that becomes a stretcher.
- When appropriate, gradually increase activity, allowing the client to assist with positioning, transferring, and self-care as able. Progress the client from sitting in bed to dangling, to standing, to ambulation. Always have the client dangle at the bedside before standing to evaluate for postural hypotension.

• = Independent   ▲ = Collaborative

- When getting a client up, observe for symptoms of intolerance such as nausea, pallor, dizziness, visual dimming, and impaired consciousness, as well as changes in vital signs; manual blood pressure monitoring is best.
- If the client has symptoms of postural hypotension, such as dizziness, lightheadedness, or pallor, take precautions, such as dangling the client and applying leg compression stockings before the client stands.
- Perform range-of-motion (ROM) exercises if the client is unable to tolerate activity or is mostly immobile. See care plan for Risk for **Disuse** syndrome.
- Monitor and record the client's ability to tolerate activity: note pulse rate, blood pressure, respiratory pattern, dyspnea, use of accessory muscles, and skin color before, during, and after the activity. If the following signs and symptoms of cardiac decompensation develop, activity should be stopped immediately:
  o Onset of chest discomfort or pain
  o Dyspnea
  o Palpitations
  o Excessive fatigue
  o Lightheadedness, confusion, ataxia, pallor, cyanosis, nausea, or any peripheral circulatory insufficiency
  o Dysrhythmia
  o Exercise hypotension
  o Excessive rise in blood pressure
  o Inappropriate bradycardia
  o Increased heart rate
  o Decreased oxygen saturation
- ▲ Instruct the client to stop the activity immediately and report to the health care provider if the client is experiencing the following symptoms: new or worsened intensity or increased frequency of discomfort; tightness or pressure in chest, back, neck, jaw, shoulders, and/or arms; palpitations; dizziness; weakness; unusual and extreme fatigue; excessive air hunger.
- Observe and document skin integrity several times a day. Refer to the care plan Risk for impaired **Skin** integrity.
- Assess for constipation. If present, refer to care plan for **Constipation.**

• = Independent   ▲ = Collaborative

A

▲ Refer the client to physical therapy to help increase activity levels and strength.

▲ Consider a dietitian referral to assess nutritional needs related to **Activity** intolerance; provide nutrition as indicated. If the client is unable to eat food, use enteral or parenteral feedings as needed.

• Recognize that malnutrition causes significant morbidity due to the loss of lean body mass.

• Provide emotional support and encouragement to the client to gradually increase activity. Work with the client to set mutual goals that increase activity levels. Fear of breathlessness, pain, or falling may decrease willingness to increase activity.

▲ Observe for pain before activity. If possible, treat pain before activity and ensure that the client is not heavily sedated.

▲ Obtain any necessary assistive devices or equipment needed before ambulating the client (e.g., walkers, canes, crutches, portable oxygen).

▲ Use a gait walking belt when ambulating the client.

Activity Intolerance Due to Respiratory Disease

• If the client is able to walk and has chronic obstructive pulmonary disease (COPD), use the traditional 6-minute walk distance to evaluate ability to walk.

▲ Ensure that the chronic pulmonary client has oxygen saturation testing with exercise. Use supplemental oxygen to keep oxygen saturation 90% or above or as prescribed with activity.

• Monitor a respiratory client's response to activity by observing for symptoms of respiratory intolerance, such as increased dyspnea, loss of ability to control breathing rhythmically, use of accessory muscles, nasal flaring, appearance of facial distress, and skin tone changes such as pallor and cyanosis.

• Instruct and assist the client with COPD in using conscious, controlled breathing techniques during exercise, including pursed-lip breathing, and inspiratory muscle use.

▲ Evaluate the client's nutritional status. Refer to a dietitian if indicated. Use nutritional supplements to increase nutritional level if needed.

▲ For the client in the intensive care unit, consider mobilizing the client with passive exercise.

▲ Refer the COPD client to a pulmonary rehabilitation program.

• = Independent   ▲ = Collaborative

Activity Intolerance Due to Cardiovascular Disease
- If the client is able to walk and has heart failure, consider use of the 6-minute walk test to determine physical ability.
- Allow for periods of rest before and after planned exertion periods such as meals, baths, treatments, and physical activity.
- ▲ Refer to a heart failure program or cardiac rehabilitation program for education, evaluation, and guided support to increase activity and rebuild life.
- ▲ Refer to a community support program that includes support of significant others.
- See care plan for Decreased **Cardiac** output for further interventions.

Pediatric
- Focus interview questions toward exercise tolerance specifically including any history of asthma exacerbations.

Geriatric
- Slow the pace of care. Allow the client extra time to carry out physical activities.
- ▲ Assess for swaying, poor balance, weakness, and fear of falling while older clients stand/walk. Refer to physical therapy if appropriate. Refer to the care plan for Risk for **Falls** and Impaired **Walking.**
- ▲ Initiate ambulation by simply ambulating a patient a few steps from bed to chair, once a health care provider's out-of-bed order is obtained.
- ▲ Evaluate medications the client is taking to see if they could be causing **Activity** intolerance.
- ▲ If heart disease is causing **Activity** intolerance, refer the client for cardiac rehabilitation.
- ▲ Refer the disabled older client to physical therapy for functional training including gait training, stepping, and sit-to-stand exercises, or for strength training.

Home Care
- ▲ Begin discharge planning as soon as possible with the case manager or social worker to assess the need for home support systems and the need for community or home health services.
- ▲ Assess the home environment for factors that contribute to decreased activity tolerance such as stairs or distance to the bathroom. Refer the client for occupational therapy, if needed, to assist the client in restructuring the home and ADL patterns.

• = Independent   ▲ = Collaborative

A

▲ Refer the client for physical therapy for strength training and possible weight training to regain strength, increase endurance, and improve balance. If the client is homebound, the physical therapist can also initiate cardiac rehabilitation.

• Encourage progress with positive feedback.

• Teach the client/family the importance of and methods for setting priorities for activities, especially those having a high energy demand (e.g., home/family events). Instruct in realistic expectations.

• Encourage routine low-level exercise periods such as a daily short walk or chair exercises.

• Provide the client/family with resources such as senior centers, exercise classes, educational and recreational programs, and volunteer opportunities that can aid in promoting socialization and appropriate activity.

• Instruct the client and family in the importance of maintaining proper nutrition.

• Instruct the client in use of dietary supplements as indicated.

▲ Refer to medical social services as necessary to assist the family in adjusting to major changes in patterns of living because of **Activity** intolerance.

▲ Assess the need for long-term supports for optimal activity tolerance of priority activities (e.g., assistive devices, oxygen, medication, catheters, massage), especially for a hospice client. Evaluate intermittently.

▲ Refer to home health aide services to support the client and family through changing levels of activity tolerance. Introduce aide support early. Instruct the aide to promote independence in activity as tolerated.

• Allow terminally ill clients and their families to guide care. Control by the client or family respects their autonomy and promotes effective coping.

• Provide increased attention to comfort and dignity of the terminally ill client in care planning.

▲ Institute case management of frail elderly to support continued independent living.

Client/Family Teaching and Discharge Planning

• Instruct the client on techniques for avoiding **Activity** intolerance, such as controlled breathing techniques.

• = Independent   ▲ = Collaborative

- Teach the client techniques to decrease dizziness from postural hypotension when standing up.
- Help client with energy conservation and work simplification techniques in ADLs.
- Describe to the client the symptoms of **Activity** intolerance, including which symptoms to report to the physician.
- Explain to the client how to use assistive devices, oxygen, or medications before or during activity.
- Help the client set up an activity log to record exercise and exercise tolerance.

Risk for Activity intolerance
NANDA-I Definition
Vulnerable to insufficient physiological or psychological energy to endure or complete required or desired daily activities, which may compromise health
Risk Factors
Circulatory problems; history of previous intolerance; inexperience with an activity; physical deconditioning; respiratory condition
Client Outcomes, Nursing Interventions, and Client/Family Teaching and Discharge Planning
Refer to care plan for **Activity** intolerance.

Ineffective Activity planning
NANDA-I Definition
Inability to prepare for a set of actions fixed in time and under certain conditions
Defining Characteristics
Absence of plan; excessive anxiety about a task to be undertaken; insufficient organizational skills; insufficient resources (e.g., financial, social, knowledge); pattern of failure; pattern of procrastination; unmet goals for chosen activity; worry about a task to be undertaken
Related Factors
Flight behavior when faced with proposed solution; hedonism; insufficient information processing ability; insufficient social support; unrealistic perception of event; unrealistic perception of personal abilities

• = Independent   ▲ = Collaborative

Patient Outcomes

Patient Will (Specify Time Frame):

- Verbalize need for self-directed activity
- Choose the health care option that fits his or her lifestyle within an appropriate amount of time that allows enactment of the choice
- Describe how the chosen option fits into current lifestyle before or after the decision has been made
- Verbalize the need for a behavioral change to improve physical activity

Nursing Interventions

- Ask the client how he or she perceives the situation in order to gather his personal vision of the problem and how they envisage their self-involvement. Specify the goals.
  - ○ Identify the informational needs of the client: understanding of the client's state of health, supervision of client's treatment if he or she is receiving treatment, diet, and important telephone numbers.
  - ○ Tackle the client's fears and worries and encourage him to make a cognitive reconstruction. Use "desire thinking." Drill and repeat: "I can change false ideas that make me believe that I am unable to carry out (achieve) my plan."
- Client verbalizes need for behavioral change for improved physical activity.
- Encourage client to verbalize the need for physical activity to help reduce role overload.
- ▲ Determine as fairly as possible the success factors needed for the planning and success of the project: financial resources; the family situation; prior medical, psychiatric, and psychosocial conditions; material resources; and the ability to manage stress.

Pediatric

- Begin activity planning in preschool-aged children of working parents.
- Establish a contract.
- Provide support to the schools for physical activities in all venues of schools.

Geriatric

- Plan activities for older clients.
- Plan activities for older clients with impaired mental function.

• = Independent   ▲ = Collaborative

Multicultural
- Provide literature and information in the appropriate language for the client who speaks little to no English.
- Preplanning educational programs for the culturally diverse population needs to be developed.

Home Care
- Have a preplanned activity exercise for the home client with a debilitating musculoskeletal disease to help improve functional status.
- Assess the home environment for barriers that can impact the client's motivation to be a participant in the activity planned.
- For additional interventions, refer to care plans **Anxiety,** Readiness for enhanced family **Coping,** Readiness for enhanced **Decision-Making, Fear,** Readiness for enhanced **Hope,** Readiness for enhanced **Power,** Readiness for enhanced **Spiritual** well-being, and Readiness for enhanced **Health** management.

Risk for Ineffective Activity planning
NANDA-I Definition

Vulnerable to an inability to prepare for a set of actions fixed in time and under certain conditions, which may compromise health

Risk Factors

Flight behavior when faced with proposed solution; hedonism; insufficient information processing ability; insufficient social support; pattern of procrastination; unrealistic perception of event; unrealistic perception of personal abilities

Client Outcomes, Nursing Interventions, and Client/Family Teaching and Discharge Planning

Refer to ineffective **Activity** planning.

Ineffective Airway clearance
NANDA-I Definition

Inability to clear secretions or obstructions from the respiratory tract to maintain a clear airway

Defining Characteristics

Absent cough; adventitious breath sounds; alteration in respiratory pattern; alteration in respiratory rate; cyanosis; difficulty verbalizing; diminished breath sounds; dyspnea; excessive sputum; ineffective cough; orthopnea; restlessness; wide-eyed look

Related Factors (r/t)

Environmental

Exposure to smoke, secondhand smoke; smoking

Obstructed Airway

Airway spasm; chronic obstructive pulmonary disease; exudate in the alveoli; excessive mucus; foreign body in airway; hyperplasia of bronchial walls; presence of artificial airway; retained secretions

Physiological

Allergic airways; asthma; infection; neuromuscular impairment

Client Outcomes

Client Will (Specify Time Frame)

- Demonstrate effective coughing and clear breath sounds
- Maintain a patent airway at all times
- Explain methods useful to enhance secretion removal
- Explain the significance of changes in sputum to include color, character, amount, and odor
- Identify and avoid specific factors that inhibit effective airway clearance

Nursing Interventions

- Auscultate breath sounds every 1 to 4 hours.
- Monitor respiratory patterns, including rate, depth, and effort.
- Monitor blood gas values and pulse oxygen saturation levels as available. An oxygen saturation of less than 90% (normal: 95% to 100%) or a partial pressure of oxygen of less than 80 mm Hg (normal: 80 to 100 mm Hg) indicates significant oxygenation problems (Schultz, 2011).
- ▲ Administer oxygen as ordered. Position the client to optimize respiration (e.g., head of bed elevated 30 to 45 degrees).
- Help the client deep breathe and perform controlled coughing. Have the client inhale deeply, hold breath for several seconds, and cough two or three times with mouth open while tightening the upper abdominal muscles.
- If the client has obstructive lung disease, such as chronic obstructive pulmonary disease (COPD), cystic fibrosis, or bronchiectasis, consider helping the client use the forced expiratory technique, the "huff cough." The client does a series of coughs while saying the word "huff."

A

▲ Encourage the client to use an incentive spirometer. Recognize that controlled coughing and deep breathing may be just as effective as incentive spirometry (Gosselink et al, 2008).

• Encourage activity and ambulation as tolerated. If the client cannot be ambulated, turn the client from side to side at least every 2 hours. (See interventions for Impaired **Gas** exchange for further information on positioning a respiratory patient.)

• Encourage fluid intake of up to 2500 mL/day within cardiac or renal reserve.

▲ Administer medications such as bronchodilators or inhaled steroids as ordered. Watch for side effects such as tachycardia or anxiety with bronchodilators, or inflamed pharynx with inhaled steroids.

▲ Provide percussion, vibration, and oscillation as appropriate (Gosselink et al, 2008).

• Observe sputum, noting color, odor, and volume.

Critical Care

▲ In intubated patients, body positioning and mobilization may optimize airway secretion clearance. An early mobility and walking program can promote weaning from ventilator support as a patient's overall strength and endurance improve (Gosselink et al, 2008; Perme & Chandrashekar, 2009).

▲ An early mobility and walking program can promote weaning from ventilator support as a patient's overall strength and endurance improve (Gosselink et al, 2008; Perme & Chandrashekar, 2009).

• If the client is intubated and is stable, consider getting the client up to sit at the edge of the bed, transfer to a chair, or walk as appropriate, if an effective interdisciplinary team is developed to keep the client safe.

▲ If the client is intubated, consider use of kinetic therapy, using a kinetic bed that slowly moves the client with 40-degree turns.

• Reposition the client as needed. Use rotational or kinetic bed therapy in clients for whom side-to-side turning is contraindicated or difficult.

• When suctioning an endotracheal tube or tracheostomy tube for a client on a ventilator, do the following:
   ○ Explain the process of suctioning beforehand and ensure the client is not in pain or overly anxious.
   ○ Hyperoxygenate before and between endotracheal suction sessions.

• = Independent   ▲ = Collaborative

A

○ Suction for less than 15 seconds.
○ Use a closed, in-line suction system. Closed, in-line suctioning has minimal effects on heart rate, respiratory rate, tidal volume, and oxygen saturation (Chulay & Seckel, 2011; Seymour et al, 2009).
○ Avoid saline instillation during suctioning.
○ Document results of coughing and suctioning, particularly client tolerance and secretion characteristics such as color, odor, and volume (Chulay & Seckel, 2011).

Pediatric

* Educate parents about the risk factors for ineffective airway clearance such as foreign body ingestion and passive smoke exposure.
* See the care plan Risk for **Suffocation** for more interventions on choking.
* Educate children and parents on the importance of adherence to peak expiratory flow monitoring for asthma self-management.
* Educate parents and other caregivers that cough and cold medication bought over the counter are not safe for a child younger than 2 years unless specifically ordered by a health care provider.

Geriatric

* Encourage ambulation as tolerated without causing exhaustion.
* Actively encourage older adults to deep breathe and cough.
* Ensure adequate hydration within cardiac and renal reserves.

Home Care

* Some of the above interventions may be adapted for home care use.
▲ Begin discharge planning as soon as possible with case manager or social worker to assess need for home support systems, assistive devices, and community or home health services.
* Assess home environment for factors that exacerbate airway clearance problems (e.g., presence of allergens, lack of adequate humidity in air, poor air flow, stressful family relationships).
* Assess affective climate within family and family support system. Refer to care plan for **Caregiver Role Strain.**
* Refer to GOLD guidelines for management of home care and indications of hospital admission criteria. http://www.goldcopd.org/.
* When respiratory procedures are being implemented, explain equipment and procedures to family members and caregivers, and provide needed emotional support.

• = Independent   ▲ = Collaborative

A

- When electrically based equipment for respiratory support is being implemented, evaluate home environment for electrical safety, proper grounding, and so on. Ensure that notification is sent to the local utility company, the emergency medical team, and police and fire departments.
- Provide family with support for care of a client with chronic or terminal illness.
- Refer to care plans for **Anxiety** and **Powerlessness.**
- Instruct the client to avoid exposure to persons with upper respiratory infections, to avoid crowds of people, and to wash hands after each exposure to groups of people or public places.
▲ Determine client adherence to medical regimen. Instruct the client and family in importance of reporting effectiveness of current medications to health care provider.
- Teach the client when and how to use inhalant or nebulizer treatments at home.
- Teach the client/family importance of maintaining regimen and having "as-needed" drugs easily accessible at all times.
- Instruct the client and family in the importance of maintaining proper nutrition, adequate fluids, rest, and behavioral pacing for energy conservation and rehabilitation.
- Instruct in use of dietary supplements as indicated.
- Identify an emergency plan, including criteria for use.
▲ Refer for home health aide services for assistance with activities of daily living (ADLs).
▲ Assess family for role changes and coping skills. Refer to medical social services as necessary.
▲ For the client dying at home with a terminal illness, if the "death rattle" is present with gurgling, rattling, or crackling sounds in the airway with each breath, recognize that anticholinergic medications can often help control symptoms, if given early in the process.
▲ For the client with a death rattle, nursing care includes turning to mobilize secretions, keeping the head of the bed elevated for postural drainage of secretions, and avoiding suctioning.

Client/Family Teaching and Discharge Planning
▲ Teach the importance of not smoking. Refer to a smoking cessation program, and encourage clients who relapse to keep trying to quit. Ensure that the client receives appropriate medications to support smoking cessation from the primary health care provider.

• = Independent   ▲ = Collaborative

A

▲ Teach the client how to use a flutter clearance device if ordered, which vibrates to loosen mucus and gives positive pressure to keep airways open (Bhowmik et al, 2009; Gosselink et al, 2008).

▲ Teach the client how to use peak expiratory flow rate (PEFR) meter if ordered and when to seek medical attention if PEFR reading drops. Also teach how to use metered dose inhalers and self-administer inhaled corticosteroids as ordered following precautions to decrease side effects.

• Teach the client how to deep breathe and cough effectively.

• Teach the client/family to identify and avoid specific factors that exacerbate ineffective airway clearance, including known allergens and especially smoking (if relevant) or exposure to secondhand smoke.

• Educate the client and family about the significance of changes in sputum characteristics, including color, character, amount, and odor.

• Teach the client/family the importance of taking antibiotics as prescribed, consuming all tablets until the prescription has run out.

• Teach the family of the dying client in hospice with a death rattle that rarely are clients aware of the fluid that has accumulated, and help them find evidence of comfort in the client's nonverbal behavior (Hipp & Letizia, 2009; Fielding & Long 2014).

Risk for Allergy response
NANDA-I Definition

Vulnerable to exaggerated immune response or reaction to substances that may compromise health

Risk Factors

Allergy to insect sting; exposure to allergen (e.g., pharmaceutical agent); exposure to environmental allergen (e.g., dander, dust, mold, pollen); exposure to toxic chemical; food allergy (e.g., avocado, banana, chestnut, kiwi, peanut, shellfish, mushroom, tropical fruit); repeated exposure to allergen-producing environmental substance

Client Outcomes

Client Will (Specify Time Frame)

• State risk factors for allergies

• Demonstrate knowledge of plan to treat allergic reaction

• = Independent   ▲ = Collaborative

Nursing Interventions

- A careful history is important in detecting allergens and avoidance of allergen.
- Obtain a precise history of allergies, as well as medications taken and foods ingested before surgery.
- ▲ Teach the client about correct use of the injectable epinephrine and have the client do a return demonstration.
- ▲ Carefully assess the client for allergies. Below is information that is important for clients with allergies. Refer for immediate treatment if anaphylaxis is suspected.

Causes

Common allergens include animal dander; bee stings or stings from other insects; foods, especially nuts, fish, and shellfish; insect bites; medications; plants; pollens

Symptoms

Common symptoms of a mild allergic reaction include hives (especially over the neck and face), itching, nasal congestion, rashes, and watery, red eyes

Symptoms of a moderate or severe reaction include cramps or pain in the abdomen; chest discomfort or tightness; diarrhea; difficulty breathing; difficulty swallowing; dizziness or lightheadedness; fear or feeling of apprehension or anxiety; flushing or redness of the face; nausea and vomiting; palpitations; swelling of the face, eyes, or tongue; weakness; wheezing; unconsciousness

First Aid

For a mild to moderate reaction: Calm and reassure the person having the reaction, because anxiety can worsen symptoms.

1. Try to identify the allergen and have the person avoid further contact with it. If the allergic reaction is from a bee sting, scrape the stinger off the skin with something firm (e.g., fingernail or plastic credit card). Do not use tweezers; squeezing the stinger will release more venom.
2. Apply cool compresses and over-the-counter hydrocortisone cream for itchy rash.
3. Watch for signs of increasing distress.
4. Get medical help. For a mild reaction, a health care provider may recommend over-the-counter medications (e.g., antihistamines).

• = Independent   ▲ = Collaborative

A **For a severe allergic reaction (anaphylaxis):**

1. Check the person's airway, breathing, and circulation (the ABCs of Basic Life Support). A warning sign of dangerous throat swelling is a very hoarse or whispered voice, or coarse sounds when the person is breathing in air. If necessary, begin rescue breathing and cardiopulmonary resuscitation.
2. Call 911.
3. Calm and reassure the person.
4. If the allergic reaction is from a bee sting, scrape the stinger off the skin with something firm (e.g., fingernail or plastic credit card). Do not use tweezers; squeezing the stinger will release more venom.
5. If the person has emergency allergy medication on hand, help the person take or inject the medication. Avoid oral medication if the person is having difficulty breathing.
6. Take steps to prevent shock. Have the person lie flat, raise the person's feet about 12 inches, and cover him or her with a coat or blanket. Do NOT place the person in this position if a head, neck, back, or leg injury is suspected or if it causes discomfort.

Do NOT

- Do NOT assume that any allergy shots the person has already received will provide complete protection.
- Do NOT place a pillow under the person's head if he or she is having trouble breathing. This can block the airways.
- Do NOT give the person anything by mouth if the person is having trouble breathing.

When to Contact a Medical Professional

Call for immediate medical emergency assistance if:

- The person is having a severe allergic reaction—always call 911. Do not wait to see if the reaction is getting worse.
- The person has a history of severe allergic reactions (check for a medical ID tag).

Prevention

Avoid triggers such as foods and medications that have caused an allergic reaction (even a mild one) in the past. Ask detailed questions about ingredients when you are eating away from home. Carefully examine ingredient labels.

- If you have a child who is allergic to certain foods, introduce one new food at a time in small amounts so you can recognize an allergic reaction.

- People who know that they have had serious allergic reactions should wear a medical ID tag.
- Preoperative patients should be closely assessed for allergies to soybeans and eggs.
▲ If you have a history of serious allergic reactions, carry emergency medications (e.g., a chewable form of diphenhydramine and injectable epinephrine or a bee sting kit) according to your health care provider's instructions.
- Do not use your injectable epinephrine on anyone else. They may have a condition (e.g., a heart problem) that could be negatively affected by this drug.
▲ Refer the client for skin testing to confirm IgE-mediated allergic response.
- See care plans for **Latex Allergy** response and Risk for **Latex Allergy** response.

Pediatric

▲ Teach parents and children with allergies to peanuts and tree nuts to avoid them and to identify them.
▲ Teach parents and children with asthma about modifiable risk factors, which include allergy triggers.
▲ Counsel parents to limit infant exposure to traffic-related air pollution.
▲ Suspect FPIES (food protein-induced enterocolitis syndrome) in formula-fed infants with repetitive emesis, diarrhea, dehydration, and lethargy 1 to 5 hours after ingesting the offending food (the most common are cow's milk, soy, and rice). Remove the offending food.
▲ Children should be screened for seafood allergies and avoid seafood and any foods containing seafood if an allergy is detected.

Anxiety
NANDA-I Definition

Vague, uneasy feeling of discomfort or dread accompanied by an autonomic response (the source often nonspecific or unknown to the individual); a feeling of apprehension caused by anticipation of danger. It is an alerting sign that warns of impending danger and enables the individual to take measures to deal with threat

• = Independent   ▲ = Collaborative

Defining Characteristics

Behavioral

Decrease in productivity; extraneous movement; fidgeting; glancing about; hypervigilance; insomnia; poor eye contact; restlessness; scanning behavior; worry about change in life event

Affective

Anguish; apprehensiveness; distress; fear; feelings of inadequacy; helplessness; increase in wariness; irritability; jitteriness; overexcitement; rattled; regretful; self-focused; uncertain; worried

Physiological

Facial tension; hand tremors; increased perspiration; increased tension; shakiness; trembling; voice quivering

Sympathetic

Alteration in respiratory pattern; anorexia; brisk reflexes; cardiovascular excitation; diarrhea; dry mouth; facial flushing; heart palpitations; increase in blood pressure; increase in heart rate; increase in respiratory rate; pupil dilation; superficial vasoconstriction; twitching; weakness

Parasympathetic

Abdominal pain; alteration in sleep pattern; decrease in heart rate; decreased blood pressure; diarrhea; faintness; fatigue; nausea; tingling in extremities; urinary frequency; urinary hesitancy; urinary urgency

Cognitive

Alteration in attention; alteration in concentration; awareness of physiological symptoms; blocking of thoughts; confusion; decrease in perceptual field; diminished ability to learn; diminished ability to problem solve; fear; forgetfulness; preoccupation; rumination; tendency to blame others

Related Factors (r/t)

Conflict about life goals; exposure to toxin; family history of anxiety; heredity; interpersonal contagion; interpersonal transmission; major change (e.g., economic status, environment, health status, role function, role status); maturational crisis; situational crisis; stressors; substance abuse; threat of death; threat to current status; unmet needs; value conflict

Client Outcomes

Client Will (Specify Time Frame)

- Identify and verbalize symptoms of anxiety
- Identify, verbalize, and demonstrate techniques to control anxiety
- Verbalize absence of or decrease in subjective distress
- Have vital signs that reflect baseline or decreased sympathetic stimulation

• = Independent ▲ = Collaborative

A

- Have posture, facial expressions, gestures, and activity levels that reflect decreased distress
- Demonstrate improved concentration and accuracy of thoughts
- Demonstrate return of basic problem-solving skills
- Demonstrate increased external focus
- Demonstrate some ability to reassure self

Nursing Interventions

- Assess the client's level of anxiety and physical reactions to anxiety (e.g., tachycardia, tachypnea, nonverbal expressions of anxiety). Consider using the Hamilton Anxiety Scale, which grades 14 symptoms on a scale of 0 (not present) to 4 (very severe). Symptoms evaluated are mood, tension, fear, insomnia, concentration, worry, depressed mood, somatic complaints, and cardiovascular, respiratory, gastrointestinal, genitourinary, autonomic, and behavioral symptoms.
- Rule out withdrawal from alcohol, sedatives, or smoking as the cause of anxiety.
- Use empathy to encourage the client to interpret the anxiety symptoms as normal.
- If irrational thoughts or fears are present, offer the client accurate information and encourage him or her to talk about the meaning of the events contributing to the anxiety.
- Encourage the client to use positive self-talk.
- Intervene when possible to remove sources of anxiety.
- Explain all activities, procedures, and issues that involve the client; use nonmedical terms and calm, slow speech. Do this in advance of procedures when possible, and validate the client's understanding.
▲ Use massage therapy to reduce anxiety.
▲ Consider massage therapy for preoperative clients.
- Use therapeutic touch and healing touch techniques.
- Use guided imagery to decrease anxiety.
- Suggest yoga to the client.
- Provide clients with a means to listen to music of their choice or audiotapes.

Pediatric

- The above interventions may be adapted for the pediatric client.

Geriatric

▲ Monitor the client for depression. Use appropriate interventions and referrals.

• = Independent   ▲ = Collaborative

A

- Older adults report less worry than younger adults.
- Observe for adverse changes if antianxiety drugs are taken.
- Mindfulness meditation is successful in mediating anxiety.

Multicultural

- Assess for the presence of culture-bound anxiety states.
- Identify how anxiety is manifested in the culturally diverse client.
- For diverse clients experiencing preoperative anxiety, provide music of their choice.

Home Care

- The above interventions may be adapted for home care use.
- ▲ Assess for suicidal ideation. Implement emergency plan as indicated.
- Assess for influence of anxiety on medical regimen.
- Assess for presence of depression.
- Assist family to be supportive of the client in the face of anxiety symptoms.
- ▲ Consider referral for the prescription of antianxiety or antidepressant medications for clients who have panic disorder (PD) or other anxiety-related psychiatric disorders.
- ▲ Assist the client/family to institute medication regimen appropriately. Instruct in side effects, importance of taking medications as ordered, and effects to report immediately to health care provider.
- ▲ Refer for psychiatric home health care services for client reassurance and implementation of a therapeutic regimen.

Client/Family Teaching and Discharge Planning

- ▲ Teach use of appropriate community resources in emergency situations (e.g., suicidal thoughts), such as hotlines, emergency departments, law enforcement, and judicial systems.
- Teach the client/family the symptoms of anxiety.
- Teach the client techniques to self-manage anxiety.
- Teach the client to visualize or fantasize about the absence of anxiety or pain, successful experience of the situation, resolution of conflict, or outcome of procedure.
- Teach relationship between a healthy physical and emotional lifestyle and a realistic mental attitude.

• = Independent   ▲ = Collaborative

Death Anxiety

A

NANDA-I Definition

Vague uneasy feeling of discomfort or dread generated by perceptions of a real or imagined threat to one's existence

Defining Characteristics

Concern about strain on the caregiver; deep sadness; fear of developing terminal illness; fear of loss of mental abilities when dying; fear of pain related to dying; fear of premature death; fear of prolonged dying process; fear of suffering related to dying; fear of the dying process; negative thoughts related to death and dying; powerlessness; worried about the impact of one's death on significant other

Related Factors (r/t)

Anticipation of adverse consequences of anesthesia; anticipation of impact of death on others; anticipation of pain; anticipation of suffering; confronting the reality of terminal disease; discussions on topic of death; experiencing dying process; near-death experience; nonacceptance of own mortality; observations related to death; perceived imminence of death; uncertainty about encountering a higher power; uncertainty about life after death; uncertainty about the existence of a higher power; uncertainty of prognosis

Client Outcomes

Client Will (Specify Time Frame)

- State concerns about impact of death on others
- Express feelings associated with dying
- Seek help in dealing with feelings
- Discuss realistic goals
- Use prayer or other religious practice for comfort

Nursing Interventions

- ▲ Assess the psychosocial maturity of the individual.
- ▲ Assess clients for pain and provide pain relief measures.
- • Assess client for fears related to death.
- • Assist clients with life planning: consider and redefine main life goals, focus on areas of strength and/or goals that will provide satisfaction, adopt realistic goals, and recognize those that are impossible to achieve.
- • Assist clients with life review and reminiscence.
- • Provide music of the client's choosing.

• = Independent   ▲ = Collaborative

A

- Provide social support for families, understanding what is most important to families who are caring for clients at the end of life.
- Encourage clients to pray.

Geriatric

- Carefully assess older adults for issues regarding death anxiety.
- Provide back massage for clients who have anxiety regarding issues such as death.
- Refer to care plan for **Grieving**.

Multicultural

- Assist clients to identify with their culture and its values.
- Refer to care plans for **Anxiety** and **Grieving**.

Home Care

- The above interventions may be adapted for home care.
- Identify times and places when anxiety is greatest. Provide for psychological support at those times, using such strategies as personal contact, telephone contact, diversionary activities, or therapeutic self.
- Support religious beliefs; encourage the client to participate in services and activities of choice.
- ▲ Refer to medical social services or mental health services, including support groups as appropriate (e.g., anticipatory grieving groups from hospice, visiting volunteers of hospice).
- Encourage the client to verbalize feelings to family/caregivers, counselors, and self. Identify the client's preferences for end-of-life care; provide assistance in honoring preferences as much as practicable.
- ▲ Assist the client in making contact with death-related planning organizations, if appropriate, such as the Cremation Society and funeral homes.
- Refer to care plan for **Powerlessness**.

Client/Family Teaching and Discharge Planning

- Promote more effective communication to family members engaged in the caregiving role. Encourage them to talk to their loved one about areas of concern. Both caregivers and care receivers often avoid discussing areas of concern.
- Allow family members to be physically close to their dying loved one, giving them permission, instruction, and opportunities to touch. Keep family members informed.

• = Independent   ▲ = Collaborative

Risk for Aspiration

NANDA-I Definition

Vulnerable to entry of gastrointestinal secretions, oropharyngeal secretions, solids, or fluids to the tracheobronchial passages, which may compromise health

Risk Factors

Barrier to elevating upper body; decrease in gastrointestinal motility; decrease in level of consciousness; delayed gastric emptying; depressed gag reflex; enteral feedings; facial surgery; facial trauma; impaired ability to swallow; incompetent lower esophageal sphincter; increase in gastric residual; increase in intragastric pressure; ineffective cough; neck surgery; neck trauma; oral surgery; oral trauma; presence of oral/nasal tube (e.g., tracheal, feeding); treatment regimen; wired jaw

Client Outcomes

Client Will (Specify Time Frame)

- Maintain patent airway and clear lung sounds
- Swallow and digest oral, nasogastric, or gastric feeding without aspiration

Nursing Interventions

- Monitor respiratory rate, depth, and effort. Note any signs of aspiration such as dyspnea, cough, cyanosis, wheezing, hoarseness, foul-smelling sputum, or fever. If new onset of symptoms, perform oral suction and notify provider immediately.
- Auscultate lung sounds frequently and before and after feedings; note any new onset of crackles or wheezing.
- Take vital signs frequently, noting onset of a fever, increased respiratory rate, and increased heart rate.
- Before initiating oral feeding, check client's gag reflex and ability to swallow by feeling the laryngeal prominence as the client attempts to swallow (Rees, 2013). If client is having problems swallowing, see nursing interventions for Impaired **Swallowing.**
- If client needs to be fed, feed slowly and allow adequate time for chewing and swallowing.
- When feeding client, watch for signs of impaired swallowing or aspiration, including coughing, choking, and spitting food.
- Have suction machine available when feeding high-risk clients. If aspiration does occur, suction immediately. A client with aspiration needs immediate suctioning and may need further lifesaving

• = Independent ▲ = Collaborative

interventions such as intubation and mechanical ventilation (Rees, 2013).
- Keep the head of the bed (HOB) elevated at 30 to 45 degrees, preferably with the client sitting up in a chair at 90 degrees when feeding. Keep head elevated for an hour after eating.
- Note presence of nausea, vomiting, or diarrhea. Treat nausea promptly with antiemetics.
- If the client shows symptoms of nausea and vomiting, position on side.
- Assess the abdomen and listen to bowel sounds frequently, noting if they are decreased, absent, or hyperactive.
- Note new onset of abdominal distention or increased rigidity of abdomen.
- If client has a tracheostomy, ask for referral to speech pathologist for swallowing studies before attempting to feed.
- Provide meticulous oral care including brushing of teeth at least two times per day.
- Sedation agents can reduce cough and gag reflexes as well as interfere with the client's ability to manage oropharyngeal secretions.

Enteral Feedings
- Insert nasogastric feeding tube using the internal nares to distal-lower esophageal-sphincter distance, an updated version of the Hanson method. The ear-to-nose-to-xiphoid process is often inaccurate.
- Tape the feeding tube securely to the nose using a skin protectant under the tape.
- Check to make sure the initial nasogastric feeding tube placement was confirmed by x-ray, with the openings of the tube in the stomach, not the esophagus or lungs. This is especially important if a small-bore feeding tube is used, although larger tubes used for feedings or medication administration should be verified by radiography also.
- After radiographic verification of correct placement of the tube or the intestines, mark the tube's exit site clearly with tape or a permanent marker (Simons & Abdallah, 2012).
- Measure and record the length of the tube that is outside of the body at defined intervals to help ensure correct placement.

• = Independent   ▲ = Collaborative

A

- Note the placement of the tube on any chest or abdominal radiographs that are obtained for the client.
- Check the pH of the aspirate.
- Use a number of determinants for verification of correct placement before each feeding or every 4 hours if the client is on continuous feeding. Measure length of tube outside the body, and review recent x-ray results, check pH of aspirate if relevant, and characteristic appearance of aspirate. If findings do not ensure correct placement of the tube, obtain a radiograph to verify placement. Do not rely on the air insufflation method to assess correct tube placement.
- Follow unit policy regarding checking for gastric residual volume during continuous feedings or before feedings, and holding feedings if increased residual is present.
- Follow unit protocol regarding returning or discarding gastric residual volume. At this time there is not a definitive research base to guide practice.
- Do not use glucose testing to determine correct placement of enteral tube or to identify aspirated enteral feeding.
- Do not use blue dye to tint enteral feedings (Guenter, 2010).
- During enteral feedings, position client with HOB elevated 30 to 45 degrees (Bell, 2011; Schallom et al, 2015).
- Take actions to prevent inadvertent misconnections with enteral feeding tubes into intravenous (IV) lines or other harmful connections. Safety actions that should be taken to prevent misconnections include:
  - Trace tubing back to origin. Recheck connections at time of client transfer and at change of shift.
  - Label all tubing.
  - Use oral syringes for medications through the enteral feeding; **do not use IV syringes.**
  - Teach nonprofessional personnel "Do Not Reconnect" if a line becomes dislodged; rather, find the nurse instead of taking the chance of plugging the tube into the wrong place.

Critical Care

- Recognize that critically ill clients are at an increased risk for aspiration because of severe illness and interventions that compromise the gag reflex.
- Recognize that intolerance to feeding as defined by increased gastric residual is more common early in the feeding process.

• = Independent   ▲ = Collaborative

A **Geriatric**

- Carefully check older client's gag reflex and ability to swallow before feeding.
- Watch for signs of aspiration pneumonia in older adults with cerebrovascular accidents, even if there are no apparent signs of difficulty swallowing or of aspiration.
- Recognize that older adults with aspiration pneumonia have fewer symptoms than younger people; repeat cases of pneumonia in older adults are generally associated with aspiration (Eisenstadt, 2010).
- Use central nervous system depressants cautiously; older clients may have an increased incidence of aspiration with altered levels of consciousness.
- Keep an older, mostly bedridden client sitting upright for 45 minutes to 1 hour after meals.
- Recommend to families that enteral feedings may or may not be indicated for clients with advanced dementia. Instead, if possible use hand-feeding assistance, modified food consistency as needed, and feeding favorite foods for comfort (Sorrell, 2010).

Home Care

- The above interventions may be adapted for home care use.
- For clients at high risk for aspiration, obtain complete information from the discharging institution regarding institutional management.
- Assess the client and family for willingness and cognitive ability to learn and cope with swallowing, feeding, and related disorders.
- Assess caregiver understanding and reinforce teaching regarding positioning and assessment of the client for possible aspiration.
- Provide the client with emotional support in dealing with fears of aspiration.
- Establish emergency and contingency plans for care of the client.
- Have a speech and occupational therapist assess the client's swallowing ability and other physiological factors and recommend strategies for working with the client in the home (e.g., pureeing foods served to the client; providing adequate adaptive equipment for independence in eating).
- Obtain suction equipment for the home as necessary.
- Teach caregivers safe, effective use of suctioning devices. Inform the client and family that only individuals instructed in suctioning should perform the procedure.

• = Independent   ▲ = Collaborative

- Institute case management of frail elderly to support continued independent living.

Client/Family Teaching and Discharge Planning
- Teach the client and family signs of aspiration and precautions to prevent aspiration.
- Teach the client and family how to safely administer tube feeding.
- Teach the family about proper client positioning to facilitate feeding and reduce risk of aspiration.
- Verify client family/caregiver knowledge about feeding, aspiration precautions, and signs of aspiration.

Risk for impaired Attachment

NANDA-I Definition

Vulnerable to disruption of the interactive process between parent/significant other and child that fosters the development of a protective and nurturing reciprocal relationship

Risk Factors

Anxiety; child's illness prevents effective initiation of parental contact; disorganized infant behavior; inability of parent to meet personal needs; insufficient privacy; parental conflict resulting from disorganized infant behavior; parent-child separation; physical barrier (e.g., infant in isolette); prematurity; substance abuse

Client Outcomes

Parent(s)/Caregiver(s) Will (Specify Time Frame)
- Be willing to consider pumping breast milk (and storing appropriately) or breastfeeding, if feasible
- Demonstrate behaviors that indicate secure attachment to infant/child
- Provide a safe environment, free of physical hazards
- Provide nurturing environment sensitive to infant/child's need for nutrition/feeding, sleeping, comfort, and social play
- Read and respond contingently to infant/child's distress
- Support infant's self-regulation capabilities, intervening when needed
- Engage in mutually satisfying interactions that provide opportunities for attachment
- Give infant nurturing sensory experiences (e.g., holding, cuddling, stroking, rocking)
- Demonstrate an awareness of developmentally appropriate activities that are pleasurable, emotionally supportive, and growth fostering

• = Independent   ▲ = Collaborative

A

- Avoid physical and emotional abuse and/or neglect as retribution for parent's perception of infant/child's misbehavior
- State appropriate community resources and support services

Nursing Interventions

- Establish a trusting relationship with parent/caregiver.
- Support mothers of preterm infants in providing pumped breast milk to their babies until they are ready for oral feedings and transitioning from gavage to breast.
- Identify factors related to postpartum depression (PPD)/major depression and offer appropriate interventions/referrals.
- Identify eating disorders/comorbid factors related to depression and offer appropriate interventions/referrals.
- Nurture parents so that they in turn can nurture their infant/child.
- Offer parents opportunities to verbalize their childhood fears associated with attachment.
- Suggest journaling or scrapbooking as a way for parents of hospitalized infants to cope with stress and emotions.
- Offer parent-to-parent support to parents of infants in the neonatal intensive care unit (NICU).
- Encourage parents of hospitalized infants to "personalize the baby" by bringing in clothing, pictures of themselves, toys, and tapes of their voices.
- Encourage physical closeness using skin-to-skin experiences as appropriate.
- Plan ways for parents to interact/assist with infant/child caregiving.
- Educate parents about the importance of the infant-caregiver relationship as a foundation for the development of the infant's self-regulation capacities.
- Assist parents in developing new caregiving competencies and/or revising/extending old ones.
- Educate parents in reading/responding sensitively to their infant's unique "body language" (behavior cues) that communicate approach ("I'm ready to play"), avoidance/stress ("I'm unhappy. I need a change."), and self-calming ("I'm helping myself").
- Educate and support parents' ability to relieve infant/child's stress/distress.
- Guide parents in adapting their behaviors/activities with infant/child cues and changing needs.

• = Independent   ▲ = Collaborative

A

- Attend to both parents and infant/child to strengthen high-quality interactions.
- Assist parents with providing pleasurable sensory learning experiences (i.e., sight, sound, movement, touch, and body awareness).
- Encourage physical closeness using skin-to-skin experiences as appropriate.
- Encourage parents and caregivers to massage their infants and children.
- Identify mothers who may need assistance in enhancing maternal role attainment (MRA).
- Recognize that fathers, compared to mothers, may have different starting points in the attachment process in the NICU as nurses encourage parents to have early skin-to-skin contact.

Pediatric

- Recognize and support infant/child's capacity for self-regulation and intervene when appropriate.
- Provide lyrical, soothing music in nursery and home that is age-appropriate (i.e., corrected, in the case of premature infants) and contingent with state/behavioral cues.
- Recognize and support infant/child's attention capabilities.
- Encourage opportunities for mutually satisfying interactions between infant and parent.
- Encourage opportunities for physical closeness.

Multicultural

- Provide culturally sensitive parent support to non–English-speaking mothers and families.
- Discuss cultural norms with families to provide care that is appropriate for enhancing attachment with the infant/child.
- Promote the attachment process in women who have abused substances by providing a culturally based, women-centered treatment environment.
- Promote attachment process/development of maternal sensitivity in incarcerated women.
- Empower family members to draw on personal strengths in which multiple worldviews/values are recognized, incorporated, and negotiated.
- Encourage positive involvement and relationship development between children and fathers.

• = Independent　　　　▲ = Collaborative

A Home Care

- The above interventions may be adapted for home care use.
- Assess quality of interaction between parent and infant/child.
- Use "interaction coaching" (i.e., teaching mother to let the infant lead) so that the mother will match her interaction style to the baby's cues.
▲ Provide supportive care for infants and children whose parents have been deployed during wartime.
- Encourage custodial grandparents to utilize support groups available for caregivers of children.

Autonomic Dysreflexia

NANDA-I Definition

Life-threatening, uninhibited sympathetic response of the nervous system to a noxious stimulus after a spinal cord injury at T7 or above

Defining Characteristics

Blurred vision; bradycardia; chest pain; chilling; conjunctival congestion; diaphoresis (above the injury); headache (diffuse pain in different areas of the head and not confined to any nerve distribution area); Horner's syndrome; metallic taste in mouth; nasal congestion; pallor (below injury); paresthesia; paroxysmal hypertension; pilomotor reflex; red blotches on skin (above the injury); tachycardia

Related Factors

Bladder distention; bowel distention; insufficient caregiver knowledge of disease process; insufficient knowledge of disease process; skin irritation

Client Outcomes

Client Will (Specify Time Frame)

- Maintain normal vital signs
- Remain free of dysreflexia symptoms
- Explain symptoms, prevention, and treatment of dysreflexia

Nursing Interventions

- Monitor the client for symptoms of dysreflexia, particularly those with high-level and more extensive spinal cord injuries. See Defining Characteristics.
- Collaborate with providers and caregivers to identify the cause of dysreflexia. AD is triggered by a stimulus from below the level of injury. The most common triggers are distention of the bladder,

• = Independent   ▲ = Collaborative

A

kidney stones, kink in urinary catheter, urinary tract infection, fecal impaction, pressure ulcer, ingrown toenail, menstruation, hemorrhoids, invasive testing, and sexual intercourse (Cragg & Krassioukov, 2013; Wan & Krassioukov, 2014).

▲ If symptoms of dysreflexia are present, place client in high Fowler's position, remove all support hoses or binders, loosen clothing, and immediately determine the noxious stimulus causing the response. If blood pressure cannot be decreased within 1 minute, notify the provider emergently (i.e., STAT). To determine the stimulus for dysreflexia:

○ First, assess bladder function. Check for distention, and if present catheterize the client using an anesthetic jelly as a lubricant. Do not use the Valsalva maneuver or Crede's method to empty the bladder. Ensure existing catheter patency. Also assess for signs of urinary tract infection.

○ Second, assess bowel function. Numb the bowel area with a topical anesthetic as ordered and gently check for impaction.

○ Third, assess the skin, looking for any points of pressure and ingrown toenails.

▲ Initiate antihypertensive therapy as soon as ordered and monitor for cardiac dysrhythmias.

▲ Be careful not to increase noxious sensory stimuli during assessment for cause of AD. If numbing agent is ordered, use it on anus and 1 inch of rectum before attempting to remove a fecal impaction. If necessary to replace an obstructed catheter, use an anesthetic jelly as ordered during the insertion.

• Monitor vital signs every 3 to 5 minutes during acute event; continue to monitor vital signs after event is resolved (e.g., symptoms resolve and vital signs return to baseline, usually up to 2 hours post event).

• Watch for complications of dysreflexia, including signs of cerebral hemorrhage, seizures, cardiac dysfunction, or intraocular hemorrhage.

• Accurately and completely record any incidences of dysreflexia; especially note the precipitating stimuli.

• Use the following interventions to prevent dysreflexia:

○ Ensure that drainage from an indwelling catheter is good and that bladder is not distended. Assess the client frequently for signs and symptoms of urinary tract infection.

• = Independent   ▲ = Collaborative

A

- ○ Ensure a regular pattern of defecation to prevent fecal impaction.
- ○ Frequently change position of client to relieve pressure and prevent formation of pressure ulcers.
- ▲ If ordered, apply an anesthetic agent to any wound below the level of injury before performing wound care.
- ▲ Because episodes can recur, notify all health care team members of the possibility of a dysreflexia episode. All health care personnel working with the client should be aware of the condition and how to treat it.
- ▲ For female clients with spinal cord injury, assess the client for AD during menstrual cycle. If the client becomes pregnant, collaborate with obstetrical health care practitioners to monitor for signs and symptoms of dysreflexia.

Home Care

- • The above interventions may be adapted for home care use.
- • Provide the client and caregiver with written information on common causes of AD and initial treatment.
- • Provide resources to the client with any known proclivity toward dysreflexia to wear a medical alert bracelet and carry a medical alert wallet card when not in a safe environment (i.e., not with someone who knows client has the condition and can respond appropriately).
- ▲ Establish an emergency plan: obtain provider orders for medications to be used in situations in which first aid does not work and plans to identify potential stimuli.
- • When episode of dysreflexia is resolved, monitor blood pressure every 30 to 60 minutes for next 2 hours or admit to institution for observation.

Client/Family Teaching and Discharge Planning

- • Teach recognition of the earliest symptoms of dysreflexia, the actions that should be taken when they occur, and the need to obtain help immediately. Give client a written card describing signs and symptoms of AD and initial actions.
- • Teach steps to prevent dysreflexia episodes: care of bladder, bowel, and skin and prevention of other forms of noxious stimuli (e.g., not wearing clothing that is too tight, nail care). Discuss the potential impact of sexual intercourse and pregnancy on autonomic dysreflexia.

• = Independent   ▲ = Collaborative

Risk for Autonomic Dysreflexia

A

NANDA-I Definition

Vulnerable to life-threatening, uninhibited response of the sympathetic nervous system after spinal shock in an individual with spinal cord injury or lesion at T6 or above (has been demonstrated in clients with injuries at T7 and T8), which may compromise health

Risk Factors

Cardiopulmonary Stimuli

Deep vein thrombosis; pulmonary emboli

Gastrointestinal Stimuli

Bowel distention; constipation; difficult passage of feces; digital stimulation; enemas; esophageal reflux disease; fecal impaction; gallstones; gastric ulcer; gastrointestinal system pathology; hemorrhoids; suppositories

Musculoskeletal-Integumentary Stimuli

Cutaneous stimulations (e.g., pressure ulcer, ingrown toenail, dressings, burns, rash); fracture; heterotrophic bone; pressure over bony prominence; pressure over genitalia; range-of-motion exercises; spasm; sunburn; wound

Neurological Stimuli

Irritating stimuli below level of injury; painful stimuli below level of injury

Regulatory Stimuli

Extremes of environmental temperature; temperature fluctuations

Reproductive Stimuli

Ejaculation; labor and delivery period; menstruation; ovarian cyst; pregnancy; sexual intercourse

Situational Stimuli

Constrictive clothing (e.g., straps, stockings, shoes); pharmaceutical agent; positioning; substance withdrawal (e.g., narcotic, opiate); surgical procedure

Urological Stimuli

Bladder distention; bladder spasm; cystitis; detrusor sphincter dyssynergia; epididymitis; instrumentation; renal calculi; surgical procedure; urethritis; urinary catheterization; urinary tract infection

Client Outcomes, Nursing Interventions, and Client/Family Teaching and Discharge Planning

Refer to care plan for **Autonomic Dysreflexia**.

• = Independent   ▲ = Collaborative

Risk for Bleeding

B
NANDA-I Definition

Vulnerable to a decrease in blood volume, which may compromise health

Risk Factors

Aneurysm; circumcision; disseminated intravascular coagulopathy; gastro-intestinal condition (e.g., ulcer, polyps, varices); history of falls; impaired liver function (e.g., cirrhosis, hepatitis); inherent coagulopathy (e.g., thrombocytopenia); insufficient knowledge of bleeding precautions; post-partum complications (e.g., uterine atony, retained placenta); pregnancy complications (e.g., premature rupture of membranes, placenta previa/abruption, multiple gestations); trauma; treatment regimen

Client Outcomes

Client Will (Specify Time Frame)

- Discuss precautions to prevent bleeding complications
- Explain actions that should be taken if bleeding happens
- Maintain adherence to agreed upon anticoagulant medication and lab work regimens
- Monitor for signs and symptoms of bleeding
- Maintain a mean arterial pressure above 70 mm Hg, a heart rate between 60 and 100 bpm with a normal rhythm, and urine output greater than 0.5 mL/kg/hr
- Maintain warm, dry skin

Nursing Interventions

- Perform admission risk assessment for falls and for signs of bleeding. Safety precautions should be implemented for all at-risk clients.
- Monitor the client closely for hemorrhage, especially in those at increased risk for bleeding. Watch for any signs of bleeding, including bleeding of the gums; blood in sputum, emesis, urine, or stool; bleeding from a wound; bleeding into the skin with petechiae; and purpura.
- If bleeding develops, apply pressure over the site or appropriate artery as needed. Apply pressure dressing if indicated.
- ▲ Collaborate on an appropriate bleeding management plan, including nonpharmacological and pharmacological measures to stop bleeding based on the antithrombotic used.
- ▲ Monitor coagulation studies, including prothrombin time, INR, activated partial thromboplastin time (aPTT), fibrinogen, fibrin degradation/split products, and platelet counts as appropriate.

• = Independent   ▲ = Collaborative

- Assess vital signs at frequent intervals to assess for physiological evidence of bleeding, such as tachycardia, tachypnea, and hypotension. Symptoms may include dizziness, shortness of breath, and fatigue.
▲ Monitor all medications for potential to increase bleeding, including aspirin, NSAIDs, SSRIs, and complementary and alternative therapies such as coenzyme Q10 and ginger.

Consensus on Delivery of Inpatient Anticoagulant Therapy 2013

▲ **QSEN:** Systems-based process should be used for the management of inpatient anticoagulant therapy (Nutescu et al, 2013).
▲ **QSEN:** Multidisciplinary involvement that is accountable and provides leadership should be incorporated (Nutescu et al, 2013).
▲ **QSEN:** Seamless integration of anticoagulant system with all client resources including electronic health records (Nutescu et al, 2013; Villanueva et al, 2013).
▲ **QSEN:** Evidence-based standards, periodically reviewed, should be used to ensure appropriate use of anticoagulant therapies in all situations (Nutescu et al, 2013).
▲ **QSEN:** Competency-based education for all multidisciplinary personnel engaged in anticoagulant management (Nutescu et al, 2013).
▲ **QSEN:** Ensure safe and effective use of therapies during care transitions and discharge through appropriate client education (Nutescu et al, 2013).
▲ **QSEN:** Ensure safe care transitions and maintenance of prescribed anticoagulants (Nutescu et al, 2013).
▲ **QSEN:** Measure quality indicators and assess client outcomes with a focus on quality improvement (Nutescu et al, 2013).

Safety Guidelines for Anticoagulant Administration: Joint Commission National Patient Safety Goals

Follow approved protocol for anticoagulant administration:
- Use prepackaged medications and prefilled or premixed parenteral therapy as ordered
- Check laboratory tests (i.e., INR) before administration
- Use programmable pumps when using parenteral administration
- Ensure appropriate education for client/family and all staff concerning anticoagulants used
- Notify dietary services when warfarin is prescribed (to reduce vitamin K in diet)

• = Independent   ▲ = Collaborative

B

- Monitor for any symptoms of bleeding before administration.
- Anticoagulation therapy is complex.
▲ Before administering anticoagulants, assess the clotting profile of the client. If the client is on warfarin, assess the INR. Hold the medication if the INR is outside of the recommended parameters and notify the health care provider or advanced practice nurse.
▲ Recognize that vitamin K for vitamin K antagonists (e.g., warfarin, phenprocoumon, Sinthrome, and phenindione) may be given orally or intravenously as ordered for INR levels greater than 5. In some circumstances, pro-hemostatic therapies may be warranted (tranexamic acid, desmopressin, fresh frozen plasma, cryoprecipitate, platelet transfusion, fibrinogen concentrate, prothrombin complex concentrate, activated prothrombin complex concentrate, and/or recombinant factor VIIa) if serious or life-threatening bleeding occurs (Makris et al, 2013).
▲ Manage fluid resuscitation and volume expansion as ordered.
▲ Consider use of permissive hypotension and restrictive transfusion strategies when treating bleeding episodes.
▲ Consider discussing the coadministration of a proton-pump inhibitor alongside traditional NSAIDs, or with the use of a cyclo-oxygenase 2 inhibitor with the prescriber.
- Ensure adequate nurse staffing to provide a high level of surveillance capability.

Pediatric

▲ Recognize that prophylactic vitamin K administration should be used in neonates for vitamin K deficiency bleeding (VKDB).
▲ Recognize warning signs of VKDB, including minimal bleeds, evidence of cholestasis (icteric sclera, dark urine, irritability), and failure to thrive.
▲ Use caution in administering NSAIDs in children. Monitor children and adolescents for potential bleeding after trauma.
▲ Closely monitor children after cardiac surgery for excessive blood loss.

Client/Family Teaching and Discharge Planning

- Teach client and family or significant others about any anticoagulant medications prescribed, including when to take, how often to have lab tests done, signs of bleeding to report, dietary restrictions needed, and precautions to be followed. Instruct the client to report any adverse side effects to his or her health care provider.

- Instruct the client and family on disease process and rationale for care. When clients and their family members have sufficient understanding of their disease process they can participate more fully in care and healthy behaviors. Knowledge empowers clients and family members, allowing them to be active participants in their care.
- Provide client and family or significant others with both oral and written educational materials that meet the standards of client education and health literacy.

Disturbed Body Image

NANDA-I Definition

Confusion in mental picture of one's physical self

Defining Characteristics

Absence of body part; alteration in body function; alteration in body structure; alteration in view of one's body (e.g., appearance, structure, function); avoids looking at one's body; avoids touching one's body; behavior of acknowledging one's body; behavior of monitoring one's body; change in ability to estimate spatial relationship of body to environment; change in lifestyle; change in social involvement; depersonalization of body part by use of impersonal pronouns; depersonalization of loss by use of impersonal pronouns; emphasis on remaining strengths; extension of body boundary (e.g., includes external object); fear of reaction by others; focus on past appearance; focus on past function; focus on previous strength; heightened achievement; hiding of body part; negative feeling about body; nonverbal response to change in body (e.g., appearance, structure, function); nonverbal response to perceived change in body (e.g., appearance, structure, function); overexposure of body part; perceptions that reflect an altered view of one's body appearance; personalization of body part by name; personalization of loss by name; preoccupation with change; preoccupation with loss; refusal to acknowledge change; trauma to nonfunctioning body part

Related Factors (r/t)

Alteration in body function (due to, for example, anomaly, disease, medication, pregnancy, radiation, surgery, trauma); alteration in cognitive functioning; alteration in self perception; cultural incongruence; developmental transition; illness; impaired psychosocial functioning; injury; spiritual incongruence; surgical procedure; trauma; treatment regimen

• = Independent   ▲ = Collaborative

B

Client Outcomes

Client Will (Specify Time Frame)

- Demonstrate adaptation to changes in physical appearance or body function as evidenced by adjustment to lifestyle change
- Identify and change irrational beliefs and expectations regarding body size or function
- Recognize health-destructive behaviors and demonstrate willingness to adhere to treatments or methods that will promote health
- Verbalize congruence between body reality and body perception
- Describe, touch, or observe affected body part
- Demonstrate social involvement rather than avoidance and use adaptive coping and/or social skills
- Use cognitive strategies or other coping skills to improve perception of body image and enhance functioning
- Use strategies to enhance appearance (e.g., wig, clothing)

Nursing Interventions

- Incorporate psychosocial questions related to body image as part of nursing assessment to identify clients at risk for body image disturbance (e.g., body builders; cancer survivors; clients with eating disorders, burns, skin disorders, polycystic ovary disease; or those with stomas/ostomies/colostomies or other disfiguring conditions).
- ▲ Discuss treatment options and outcomes for women diagnosed with breast cancer. Be prepared to explore options of lumpectomy vs. mastectomy and the potential for reconstructive surgery. Include cosmetic and appliance options available to mitigate effects of mastectomy and/or chemotherapy, such as wigs and customized mastectomy bras.
- Discuss individual emphasis placed on body image before mastectomy. Be aware of increased psychosocial distress for women who maintain great emphasis on personal appearance.
- ▲ Assess for history of childhood maltreatment in clients suffering from body dissatisfaction, anorexia, or other eating disorders and make appropriate psychosocial referrals if indicated.
- ▲ Assess for body dysmorphic disorder (BDD) (pathological preoccupation with muscularity and leanness; occurs more often in males than in females), and refer to psychiatry or other appropriate provider.
- ▲ Determine if body image impairment is actual or perceived and extent to which it affects the social actions and behaviors through

• = Independent   ▲ = Collaborative

the use of assessment tools such as Assessment of the Attitudinal Component of Body Image in Children or the Measures of Body Satisfaction and Related Concepts in Adolescents and Adults.

- Assess for lipodystrophy (an abnormal redistribution of adipose tissue) in clients receiving antiretroviral therapy for HIV/AIDS. This condition is common and can be a source of distress to clients.
- Discuss expectations for weight loss and anticipated body changes with clients planning to undergo bariatric surgery for morbid obesity. Assist the client in identifying realistic goals.
- ▲ Use cognitive-behavioral therapy (CBT) to assist the client to express his emotions and feelings.
- Provide education and support for clients receiving treatments or medications that have the potential to alter body image. Discuss alternatives if available.
- Take cues from clients regarding their readiness to look at a wound (ask if the client has seen the wound yet) and use clients' questions or comments as way to teach about wound care and healing.
- ▲ Encourage clients to participate in regular aerobic and/or nonaerobic exercise when feasible.
- ▲ Provide client with a list of appropriate community support groups (e.g., Reach to Recovery, Ostomy Association).

Pediatric
Many of the above interventions are appropriate for the pediatric client.

- ▲ Refer parents of children with eating disorders to a support group.
- ▲ When caring for teenagers, be aware of the impact of acne vulgaris on quality of life. The impact was proportional to the severity of acne. Assess for symptoms of social withdrawal, limited eye contact, and expressions of low self-esteem. Educate teens on skin care and hygiene, and assist with referrals to a dermatologist when needed.
- ▲ Refer families of children with severe facial burns for psychosocial support.
- ▲ Assess family dynamics and refer parents of adolescents with anorexia or other eating disorders to professional family counseling if indicated.

Geriatric

- Focus on remaining abilities. Have client make a list of strengths. Encourage regular exercise for older adults.

• = Independent ▲ = Collaborative

B

Multicultural

- Assess for the influence of cultural beliefs, regional norms, and values on the client's body image.
- Acknowledge that body image disturbances can affect all individuals regardless of culture, race, or ethnicity.

Home Care

The above interventions may be adapted for home care use.

- Assess client's level of social support. Social support is one of the determinants of the client's recovery and emotional health.
- Assess family/caregiver level of acceptance of client's body changes.
- Encourage clients to discuss concerns related to sexuality and provide support or information as indicated. Many conditions that affect body image also affect sexuality.
- Teach all aspects of care. Involve clients and caregivers in self-care as soon as possible. Do this in stages if clients still have difficulty looking at or touching changed body part.

Client/Family Teaching and Discharge Planning

- Teach appropriate care of surgical site (e.g., mastectomy site, amputation site, ostomy site).
- Encourage significant others to offer support.
- ▲ Refer clients who are having difficulty with personal acceptance, personal and social body image disruption, sexual concerns, reduced self-care skills, and management of surgical complications to an interdisciplinary team or specialist (e.g., ostomy nurse) if available.

Insufficient Breast Milk

NANDA-I Definition

Low production of maternal breast milk

Defining Characteristics

Infant

Constipation; frequent crying; frequently seeks to suckle at breast; prolonged breastfeeding time; suckling time at breast appears unsatisfactory; voids small amounts of concentrated urine; weight gain less than 500 g in a month

Mother

Absence of milk production with nipple stimulation; delay in milk production; expresses breast milk less than prescribed volume

• = Independent   ▲ = Collaborative

B

Related Factors
Infant

Ineffective latching on to breast; ineffective sucking reflex; insufficient opportunity for suckling at the breast; insufficient suckling time at breast; rejection of breast

Mother

Alcohol consumption; insufficient fluid volume; malnutrition; pregnancy; smoking; treatment regimen

Client Outcomes
Client Will (Specify Time Frame)

- State knowledge of indicators of adequate milk supply
- State and demonstrate measures to ensure adequate milk supply

Nursing Interventions

- Provide lactation support at all phases of lactation (Neifert & Bunick, 2013; Nielsen et al, 2011).
- Initiate skin-to-skin contact at birth and undisturbed contact for the first hour following birth; the mother should be encouraged to watch the baby, not the clock.
- Encourage postpartum women to start breastfeeding based on infant need as early as possible and reduce formula use to increase breastfeeding frequency. Use nonnarcotic analgesics as early as possible.
- Provide suggestions for mothers on how to increase milk production and how to determine whether there is insufficient milk supply.
- Instruct mothers that breastfeeding frequency, sucking times, and amounts are variable and normal. Assist mothers in optimal milk removal frequency.
- ▲ Consider the use of medication for mothers of preterm infants with insufficient expressed breast milk.

Pediatric

- Provide individualized follow-up with extra home visits or outpatient visits for teen mothers within the first few days after hospital discharge and encourage schools to be more compatible with breastfeeding.

Multicultural

- Provide information and support to mothers on benefits of breastfeeding at antenatal visits.
- Refer to care plans Interrupted **Breastfeeding** and Readiness for enhanced **Breastfeeding** for additional interventions.

• = Independent   ▲ = Collaborative

Ineffective Breastfeeding

B

NANDA-I Definition

Difficulty providing milk to an infant or young child directly from the breasts, which may compromise nutritional status of the infant/child

Defining Characteristics

Inadequate infant stooling; infant arching at breast; infant crying at breast; infant crying within first hour after breastfeeding; infant fussing within 1 hour of breastfeeding; infant inability to latch on to maternal breast correctly; infant resisting latching on to breast; infant unresponsive to other comfort measures; insufficient infant weight gain; insufficient emptying of each breast per feeding; insufficient signs of oxytocin release; perceived inadequate milk supply; sore nipples persisting beyond first week; sustained infant weight loss; unsustained suckling at the breast

Related Factors (r/t)

Delayed lactogenesis II; inadequate milk supply; insufficient family support; insufficient opportunity for suckling at breast; insufficient parental knowledge regarding breastfeeding techniques; insufficient parental knowledge regarding importance of breastfeeding; interrupted breastfeeding; maternal ambivalence; maternal anxiety; maternal breast anomaly; maternal fatigue; maternal obesity; maternal pain; oropharyngeal defect; pacifier use; poor infant sucking reflex; prematurity; previous breast surgery; previous history of breastfeeding failure; short maternity leave; supplemental feedings with artificial nipple

Client Outcomes

Client Will (Specify Time Frame)

- Achieve effective breastfeeding (dyad)
- Verbalize/demonstrate techniques to manage breastfeeding problems (mother)
- Manifest signs of adequate intake at the breast (infant)
- Manifest positive self-esteem in relation to the infant feeding process (mother)
- Explain alternative method of infant feeding if unable to continue exclusive breastfeeding (mother)

Nursing Interventions

- Identify women with risk factors for lower breastfeeding initiation and continuation rates (lack of information, inadequate family and social support) as well as factors contributing to ineffective breastfeeding as early as possible in the perinatal experience.

• = Independent ▲ = Collaborative

B

- Provide time for clients to express expectations and concerns, and provide emotional support as needed.
- Encourage skin-to-skin holding, beginning immediately after delivery.
- Use valid and reliable tools to measure breastfeeding performance and to predict early discontinuance of breastfeeding whenever possible/feasible.
- Promote comfort and relaxation to reduce pain and anxiety.
- Avoid supplemental feedings.
- Teach mother to observe for infant behavioral cues and responses to breastfeeding.
▲ Provide necessary equipment/instruction/assistance for milk expression as needed.
▲ Provide referrals and resources: lactation consultants, nurse and peer support programs, community organizations, and written and electronic sources of information.
- See care plan for Readiness for enhanced **Breastfeeding.**

Multicultural
- Assess whether the client's cultural beliefs about breastfeeding are contributing to ineffective breastfeeding.
- Assess the influence of family support on the decision to continue or discontinue breastfeeding.
- Provide traditional ethnic foods for breastfeeding mothers.
- See care plan for Readiness for enhanced **Breastfeeding.**

Home Care
- The above interventions may be adapted for home care use.
- Provide anticipatory guidance in relation to home management of breastfeeding.
▲ Investigate availability of and refer to public health department, hospital home follow-up breastfeeding program, or other postdischarge support.
- See care plan for Risk for impaired **Attachment.**

Client/Family Teaching and Discharge Planning
- Instruct the client on maternal breastfeeding behaviors/techniques (preparation for, positioning, initiation of/promoting latch-on, burping, completion of session, and frequency of feeding). Consider use of a video.

• = Independent   ▲ = Collaborative

B

- Teach the client self-care measures for the breastfeeding woman (e.g., breast care, management of breast/nipple discomfort, nutrition/fluid, rest/activity).
- Provide information regarding infant cues and behaviors related to breastfeeding and appropriate maternal responses (e.g., cues that the infant is ready to feed, behaviors during feeding that contribute to effective breastfeeding, measures of infant feeding adequacy).
- Provide education to partner/family/significant others as needed.

Interrupted Breastfeeding

NANDA-I Definition

Break in the continuity of providing milk to an infant or young child directly from the breasts, which may compromise breastfeeding success and/or nutritional status of the infant/child.

Defining Characteristics

Nonexclusive breastfeeding

Related Factors (r/t)

Contraindications to breastfeeding (e.g., pharmaceutical agents); hospitalization of child; infant illness; maternal employment; maternal illness; maternal infant separation; need to abruptly wean infant; prematurity

Client Outcomes

Client Will (Specify Time Frame)

Infant
- Receive mother's breast milk if not contraindicated by maternal conditions (e.g., certain drugs, infections) or infant conditions (e.g., galactosemia)

Maternal
- Maintain lactation
- Achieve effective breastfeeding or satisfaction with the breastfeeding experience
- Demonstrate effective methods of breast milk collection and storage

Nursing Interventions

- Discuss and provide support for mother's desire/intention to begin or resume breastfeeding.
- Clarify that interruption in breastfeeding is truly necessary.
- Provide anticipatory guidance to the mother/family regarding potential duration of the interruption when possible/feasible.

• = Independent   ▲ = Collaborative

B

Reassure mother/family that measures to sustain or restart lactation and promote parent-infant attachment can make it possible to resume breastfeeding when the condition/situation requiring interruption is resolved.
- Reassure the mother/family that the infant will benefit from any amount of breast milk provided.
- Assess mother's concerns, and observe mother performing psychomotor skills (expression, storage, alternative feeding, skin to skin care, and/or breastfeeding) and assist as needed.
- Collaborate with mother/family/health care providers (as needed) to develop a plan for skin-to-skin contact.
- Collaborate with the mother/family/health care provider/employer (as needed) to develop a plan for expression/pumping of breast milk and/or infant feeding.
- Monitor for signs indicating infant's ability to breastfeed and interest in breastfeeding.
- Use supplementation only as medically indicated.
- Provide anticipatory guidance for common problems associated with interrupted breastfeeding (e.g., incomplete emptying of milk glands, diminishing milk supply, infant difficulty with resuming breastfeeding, or infant refusal of alternative feeding method).
▲ Initiate follow-up and make appropriate referrals.
- Assist the client to accept and learn an alternative method of infant feeding if effective breastfeeding is not achieved.
- See care plans for Readiness for enhanced **Breastfeeding** and Ineffective **Breastfeeding.**

Multicultural
- Teach culturally appropriate techniques for maintaining lactation.
- See care plans for Readiness for enhanced **Breastfeeding** and Ineffective **Breastfeeding.**

Home Care
- The above interventions may be adapted for home care use.

Client/Family Teaching and Discharge Planning
- Teach mother effective methods to express breast milk.
- Teach mother/parents about skin-to-skin care.
- Instruct mother on safe breast milk handling techniques.
- See care plans for Readiness for enhanced **Breastfeeding** and Ineffective **Breastfeeding.**

• = Independent   ▲ = Collaborative

Readiness for enhanced Breastfeeding

B

NANDA-I Definition

A pattern of providing milk to an infant or young child directly from the breasts, which may be strengthened

Defining Characteristics

Mother expresses desire to enhance ability to provide breast milk for child's nutritional needs; mother expresses desire to enhance ability to exclusively breastfeed

Client Outcomes

Client Will (Specify Time Frame)

- Maintain effective breastfeeding without supplementation with formula
- Maintain normal growth patterns (infant)
- Verbalize satisfaction with breastfeeding process (mother)

Nursing Interventions

- Encourage expectant mothers to learn about breastfeeding before and during pregnancy.
- Encourage and facilitate early skin-to-skin contact (position includes contact of the naked baby with the mother's bare chest).
- Encourage rooming-in and breastfeeding on demand.
- Monitor the breastfeeding process and identify opportunities to enhance knowledge and experience regarding breastfeeding.
- Give encouragement/positive feedback related to breastfeeding mother-infant interactions.
- Discuss prevention and treatment of common breastfeeding problems, such as nipple pain and/or trauma.
- Teach mother to observe for infant behavioral cues and responses to breastfeeding.
- Identify current support-person network and opportunities for continued breastfeeding support.
- Avoid supplemental bottle feedings and do not provide samples of formula on discharge.
- ▲ Provide follow-up contact; as available, provide home visits and/or peer counseling.

Multicultural

- Assess for the influence of cultural beliefs, norms, and values on current breastfeeding practices.

• = Independent   ▲ = Collaborative

B

Home Care
- The above interventions may be adapted for home care use.

Client/Family Teaching and Discharge Planning
- Include the partner and other family members in education about breastfeeding.
- Teach the client the importance of maternal nutrition.
- Teach mother about the infant's subtle hunger cues (e.g., rooting, sucking, mouthing, hand-to-mouth, hand-to-hand activity) and encourage her to breastfeed whenever signs are apparent.
- Review guidelines for frequency (at least every 2 to 3 hours, or 8 to 12 feedings per 24 hours) and duration (until suckling and swallowing slow down and satiety is reached) of feeding times.
- Provide information about common infant behaviors related to breastfeeding, and appropriate maternal responses.
▲ Provide referrals and resources: lactation consultants, nurse and peer support programs, community organizations, and written and electronic sources of information.

Ineffective Breathing pattern

NANDA-I Definition
Inspiration and/or expiration that does not provide adequate ventilation

Defining Characteristics
Abnormal breathing pattern (e.g., rate, rhythm, depth); altered chest excursion; bradypnea; decrease in expiratory pressure; decrease in inspiratory pressure; decrease in minute ventilation; decrease in vital capacity; dyspnea; increase in anterior-posterior chest diameter; nasal flaring; orthopnea; prolonged expiration phase; pursed-lip breathing; tachypnea; use of accessory muscles to breathe; use of three-point position

Related Factors (r/t)
Anxiety; body position that inhibits lung expansion; bony deformity; chest wall deformity; fatigue; chest wall deformity; fatigue; hyperventilation; hypoventilation syndrome; musculoskeletal impairment; neurological immaturity; neurological impairment (e.g., positive electroencephalogram, head trauma, seizure disorders); neuromuscular impairment; obesity; pain; respiratory muscle fatigue; spinal cord injury

• = Independent   ▲ = Collaborative

B

Client Outcomes

Client Will (Specify Time Frame)

- Demonstrate a breathing pattern that supports blood gas results within the client's normal parameters
- Report ability to breathe comfortably
- Demonstrate ability to perform pursed-lip breathing and controlled breathing
- Identify and avoid specific factors that exacerbate episodes of ineffective breathing patterns

Nursing Interventions

- Monitor respiratory rate, depth, and ease of respiration.
- Note pattern of respiration. If client is dyspneic, note what seems to cause the dyspnea, the way in which the client deals with the condition, and how the dyspnea resolves or gets worse.
- Note amount of anxiety associated with the dyspnea.
- Attempt to determine if client's dyspnea is physiological or psychological in cause.
- The rapidity of which the onset of dyspnea is noted is also an indicator of the severity of the pathological condition (Croucher, 2014).

Psychological Dyspnea—Hyperventilation

- Monitor for symptoms of hyperventilation including rapid respiratory rate, sighing breaths, lightheadedness, numbness and tingling of hands and feet, palpitations, and sometimes chest pain (Bickley & Szilagyi, 2012).
- Assess cause of hyperventilation by asking client about current emotions and psychological state.
- Ask the client to breathe with you to slow down respiratory rate. If client has chronic problems with hyperventilation, numbness and tingling in extremities, dizziness, and other signs of panic attacks, refer for counseling.

Physiological Dyspnea

- ▲ Ensure that client in acute dyspneic state has received any ordered medications, oxygen, and any other treatment needed.
- Note client description of the quality of breathing discomfort, such as chest tightness, air hunger, inability to breathe deeply, urge to breathe, starved for air, feeling of suffocation (Parshall et al, 2012).
- Note use of accessory muscles, nasal flaring, retractions, irritability, confusion, or lethargy.

• = Independent   ▲ = Collaborative

- Observe color of tongue, oral mucosa, and skin for signs of cyanosis.
- In central cyanosis, both the skin and mucous membranes are affected due to seriously impaired pulmonary function from unventilated or underventilated alveoli. Peripheral cyanosis (skin only) usually indicates vasoconstriction or obstruction to blood flow (Loscalzo, 2013).
- Auscultate breath sounds, noting decreased or absent sounds, crackles, or wheezes.
- Monitor oxygen saturation continuously using pulse oximetry. Note blood gas results as available.
- Using touch on the shoulder, coach the client to slow respiratory rate, demonstrating slower respirations, making eye contact with the client, and communicating in a calm, supportive fashion.
- Support the client in using pursed-lip and controlled breathing techniques.
- If the client is acutely dyspneic, consider having the client lean forward over a bedside table, resting elbows on the table if tolerated.
- Position the client in an upright or semi-Fowler's position. See nursing interventions for Impaired **Gas** exchange for further information on positioning.
- Administer oxygen as ordered.
- Increase client's activity to walking three times per day as tolerated. Assist the client to use oxygen during activity as needed. See nursing interventions for **Activity** intolerance. Walking 20 minutes per day is recommended for those unable to be in a structured program (GOLD, 2015)
- Schedule rest periods before and after activity.
- Evaluate the client's nutritional status. Refer to a dietitian if needed. Use nutritional supplements to increase nutritional level if needed.
- Provide small, frequent feedings.
- Offer a fan to move the air in the environment.
- Encourage the client to take deep breaths at prescribed intervals and do controlled coughing.
- Help the client with chronic respiratory disease to evaluate dyspnea experience to determine whether previous incidences of dyspnea were similar and to recognize that the client survived those incidences. Encourage the client to be self-reliant if possible, use problem-solving skills, and maximize use of social support.

• = Independent ▲ = Collaborative

B

- See Ineffective **Airway** clearance if client has a problem with increased respiratory secretions.
- ▲ Refer the client with COPD for pulmonary rehabilitation.

Geriatric

- Assess respiratory systems in older adults with the understanding that inspiratory muscles weaken, resulting in a slight barrel chest. Expiratory muscles work harder with use of accessory muscles (Martin-Plank, 2014).
- Encourage ambulation as tolerated.
- Encourage older clients to sit upright or stand and to avoid lying down for prolonged periods during the day.

Home Care

- The above interventions may be adapted for home care use.
- Work with the client to determine what strategies are most helpful during times of dyspnea. Educate and empower the client to self-manage the disease associated with impaired gas exchange.
- Assist the client and family with identifying other factors that precipitate or exacerbate episodes of ineffective breathing patterns (i.e., stress, allergens, stairs, activities that have high energy requirements).
- Assess client knowledge of and compliance with medication regimen.
- Refer the client for telemonitoring with a pulmonologist as appropriate, with use of an electronic spirometer or an electronic peak flowmeter.
- Teach the client and family the importance of maintaining the therapeutic regimen and having as-needed drugs easily accessible at all times.
- Provide the client with emotional support in dealing with symptoms of respiratory difficulty. Provide family with support for care of a client with chronic or terminal illness. Refer to care plan for **Anxiety.** When respiratory procedures (e.g., apneic monitoring for an infant) are being implemented, explain equipment and procedures to family members, and provide needed emotional support. When electrically based equipment for respiratory support is being implemented, evaluate home environment for electrical safety, such as proper grounding. Ensure that notification is sent to the local utility company, the emergency medical team, and police and fire departments.

• = Independent ▲ = Collaborative

- Refer to GOLD guidelines for management of home care and indications of hospital admission criteria.
- Support clients' efforts at self-care. Ensure they have all the information they need to participate in care.
- Identify an emergency plan including when to call your health care provider or 911. Refer to home health aide services as needed to support energy conservation.
- Institute case management of frail elderly to support continued independent living (Martin-Plank et al, 2014).

Client/Family Teaching and Discharge Planning
- Teach pursed-lip and controlled breathing techniques.
- Teach about dosage, actions, and side effects of medications.
- Using a pre-recorded tape, teach client progressive muscle relaxation techniques.
- Teach the client to identify and avoid specific factors that exacerbate ineffective breathing patterns, such as exposure to other sources of air pollution, especially smoking. If client smokes, refer to the smoking cessation section in the impaired **Gas** exchange care plan.

Decreased Cardiac output

NANDA-I Definition

Inadequate blood pumped by the heart to meet the metabolic demands of the body

Defining Characteristics

Altered Heart Rate/Rhythm

Bradycardia, electrocardiogram change (e.g., arrhythmia, conduction abnormality, ischemia)

Altered Preload

Decreased central venous pressure (CVP); decrease in pulmonary artery wedge pressure (PAWP); edema; fatigue; heart murmur; increase in CVP; increase in PAWP; jugular vein distention; weight gain

Altered Afterload

Abnormal skin color (e.g., pale, dusky, cyanosis); alteration in blood pressure; clammy skin; decrease in peripheral pulses; decrease in pulmonary vascular resistance (PVR); decrease in systemic vascular resistance (SVR); dyspnea; increase in PVR; increase in SVR; oliguria, prolonged capillary refill

• = Independent ▲ = Collaborative

Altered Contractility

Adventitious breath sounds; coughing; decreased cardiac index; decrease in ejection fraction; decrease in left ventricular stroke work index; decrease in stroke volume index; orthopnea; paroxysmal nocturnal dyspnea; presence of S3 heart sound; presence of S4 heart sound

Behavioral/Emotional

Anxiety; restlessness

Related Factors (r/t)

Alteration in heart rate; alteration in heart rhythm; altered afterload; altered contractility; altered preload; altered stroke volume

Client Outcomes

Client Will (Specify Time Frame)

- Demonstrate adequate cardiac output as evidenced by blood pressure, pulse rate and rhythm within normal parameters for client; strong peripheral pulses; maintained level of mentation, lack of chest discomfort or dyspnea, and adequate urinary output; an ability to tolerate activity without symptoms of dyspnea, syncope, or chest pain
- Remain free of side effects from the medications used to achieve adequate cardiac output
- Explain actions and precautions to prevent primary or secondary cardiac disease

Nursing Interventions

- Recognize primary characteristics of decreased cardiac output as fatigue, dyspnea, edema, orthopnea, paroxysmal nocturnal dyspnea, and increased CVP. Recognize secondary characteristics of decreased cardiac output as weight gain, hepatomegaly, jugular venous distention, palpitations, lung crackles, oliguria, coughing, clammy skin, and skin color changes.
- Monitor and report presence and degree of symptoms including dyspnea at rest or with reduced exercise capacity, orthopnea, paroxysmal nocturnal dyspnea, nocturnal cough, distended abdomen, fatigue, or weakness. Monitor and report signs including jugular vein distention, S3 gallop, rales, positive hepatojugular reflux, ascites, laterally displaced or pronounced point of maximal impact, heart murmurs, narrow pulse pressure, cool extremities, tachycardia with pulsus alternans, and irregular heartbeat.
- Monitor orthostatic blood pressures and daily weights.
- Recognize that decreased cardiac output can occur in a number of noncardiac disorders such as septic shock and hypovolemia. Expect

• = Independent   ▲ = Collaborative

C

variation in orders for differential diagnoses related to decreased cardiac output, because orders will be distinct to address the primary cause of the altered cardiac output.

- Obtain a thorough history.
- Monitor pulse oximetry and administer oxygen as needed per health care provider's order. Supplemental oxygen increases oxygen availability to the myocardium and can relieve symptoms of hypoxemia. Resting hypoxia or oxygen desaturation may indicate fluid overload or concurrent pulmonary disease.
- Place client in semi-Fowler's or high Fowler's position with legs down or in a position of comfort. Elevating the head of the bed and legs in down position may decrease the work of breathing and may also decrease venous return and preload.
- During acute events, ensure client remains on short-term bed rest or maintains activity level that does not compromise cardiac output.
- Provide a restful environment by minimizing controllable stressors and unnecessary disturbances. Reducing stressors decreases cardiac workload and oxygen demand.
- Apply graduated compression stockings or intermittent sequential pneumatic compression (ISPC) leg sleeves as ordered. Ensure proper fit by measuring accurately. Remove stocking at least twice a day, then reapply. Assess the condition of the extremities frequently. Graduated compression stockings may be contraindicated in clients with peripheral arterial disease (Kahn et al, 2012).
- Check blood pressure, pulse, and condition before administering cardiac medications such as angiotensin-converting enzyme inhibitors, angiotensin receptor blockers, digoxin, and beta-blockers. Notify health care provider if heart rate or blood pressure is low before holding medications. It is important that the nurse evaluate how well the client is tolerating current medications before administering cardiac medications; do not hold medications without health care provider input. The health care provider may decide to have medications administered even though the blood pressure or pulse rate has lowered.
- Observe for and report chest pain or discomfort; note location, radiation, severity, quality, duration, and associated manifestations such as nausea, indigestion, or diaphoresis; also note precipitating and relieving factors. Chest pain/discomfort may indicate an

C

inadequate blood supply to the heart, which can further compromise cardiac output.

▲ If chest pain is present, refer to the nursing interventions for Risk for decreased **Cardiac** tissue perfusion.

• Recognize the effect of sleep disordered breathing in HF and that sleep disorders are common in patients with HF (Yancy et al, 2013).

• Administer continuous positive airway pressure (CPAP) or supplemental oxygen at night as ordered for management of suspected or diagnosed sleep apnea.

• Closely monitor fluid intake, including intravenous lines. Maintain fluid restriction if ordered. In clients with decreased cardiac output, poorly functioning ventricles may not tolerate increased fluid volumes.

• Monitor intake and output (I&O). If client is acutely ill, measure hourly urine output and note decreases in output. Decreased cardiac output results in decreased perfusion of the kidneys, with a resulting decrease in urine output.

• Note results of initial diagnostic studies, including electrocardiography, echocardiography, and chest radiography.

• Note results of further diagnostic imaging studies such as radionuclide imaging, stress echocardiography, cardiac catheterization, or magnetic resonance imaging (MRI).

• Review laboratory data as needed including arterial blood gases, complete blood count, serum electrolytes (sodium, potassium, magnesium, calcium), blood urea nitrogen, creatinine, urinalysis, glucose, fasting lipid profile, liver function tests, thyroid stimulating hormone, B-type natriuretic peptide (BNP assay), or N-terminal pro-B-type natriuretic peptide (NTpro-BNP). Routine blood work can provide insight into the etiology of HF and extent of decompensation.

• Gradually increase activity when the client's condition is stabilized by encouraging slower-paced activities, or shorter periods of activity, with frequent rest periods following exercise prescription; observe for symptoms of intolerance. Take blood pressure and pulse before and after activity and note changes. Activity of the cardiac client should be closely monitored. See **Activity** intolerance.

• Serve small, frequent, sodium-restricted, low-saturated-fat meals. Sodium-restricted diets help decrease fluid volume excess. Low-saturated-fat diets help decrease atherosclerosis, which can cause

• = Independent   ▲ = Collaborative

coronary artery disease. Clients with cardiac disease tolerate smaller meals better because they require less cardiac output to digest (Hooper et al, 2012).

- Monitor bowel function. Provide stool softeners as ordered. Caution client not to strain when defecating. Decreased activity, pain medication, and diuretics can cause constipation.
- Weigh the client at the same time daily (after voiding). Daily weight is a good indicator of fluid balance. Use the same scale if possible when weighing clients for consistency. Increased weight and severity of symptoms can signal decreased cardiac function with retention of fluids.
- Provide influenza and pneumococcal vaccines as needed before client discharge for those who have yet to receive those inoculations (Centers for Disease Control, 2015).
- Assess for presence of anxiety and refer for treatment if present. See nursing interventions for **Anxiety** to facilitate reduction of anxiety in clients and family.
- Assess for presence of depression and refer for treatment if needed.
- Refer to a cardiac rehabilitation program for education and monitored exercise.
- Refer to an HF program for education, evaluation, and guided support to increase activity and rebuild quality of life. Support for the HF client should be patient-centered, culturally sensitive, and include family and social support.

Critically Ill

▲ Observe for symptoms of cardiogenic shock, including impaired mentation, hypotension, decreased peripheral pulses, cold and clammy skin, signs of pulmonary congestion, and decreased organ function. If present, notify health care provider immediately. Cardiogenic shock is a state of circulatory failure from loss of cardiac function associated with inadequate organ perfusion and a high mortality rate.

▲ If shock is present, monitor hemodynamic parameters for an increase in pulmonary wedge pressure, an increase in systemic vascular resistance, or a decrease in stroke volume, cardiac output, and cardiac index.

▲ Titrate inotropic and vasoactive medications within defined parameters to maintain contractility, preload, and afterload per health care provider's order. By following parameters, the nurse ensures

• = Independent ▲ = Collaborative

maintenance of a delicate balance of medications that stimulate the heart to increase contractility, while maintaining adequate perfusion of the body.

▲ Identify significant fluid overload and initiate intravenous diuretics as ordered. Monitor I&Os, daily weight, and vital signs, as well as signs and symptoms of congestion. Watch laboratory data, including serum electrolytes, creatinine, and urea nitrogen.

▲ When using pulmonary arterial catheter technology, be sure to appropriately level and zero the equipment, use minimal tubing, maintain system patency, perform square wave testing, position the client appropriately, and consider correlation to respiratory and cardiac cycles when assessing waveforms and integrating data into client assessment.

▲ Observe for worsening signs and symptoms of decreased cardiac output when using positive pressure ventilation.

▲ Recognize that clients with cardiogenic pulmonary edema may have noninvasive positive pressure ventilation ordered.

▲ Monitor client for signs and symptoms of fluid and electrolyte imbalance when clients are receiving ultrafiltration or continuous renal replacement therapy (CRRT). Clients with refractory HF may have ultrafiltration or CRRT ordered as a mechanical method to remove excess fluid volume.

• Recognize that hypoperfusion from low cardiac output can lead to altered mental status and decreased cognition.

• Recognize that clients with severe HF may undergo additional therapies, such as internal pacemaker or defibrillator placement, and/or placement of a ventricular assist device (VAD).

Geriatric

• Recognize that older clients may demonstrate fatigue and depression as signs of HF and decreased cardiac output.

▲ If the client has heart disease causing activity intolerance, refer for cardiac rehabilitation.

▲ Recognize that edema can present differently in the older population.

▲ Recognize that blood pressure control is beneficial for older clients to reduce the risk of worsening HF.

▲ Recognize that renal function is not always accurately represented by serum creatinine in the older population due to less muscle mass (Yancy et al, 2013).

• = Independent   ▲ = Collaborative

▲ Observe for side effects from cardiac medications. Older adults can have difficulty with metabolism and excretion of medications due to decreased function of the liver and kidneys; therefore, toxic side effects are more common.

▲ Older adults may require more frequent visits, closer monitoring of medication dose changes, and more gradual increases in medications, due to changes in the metabolism of medications and impaired renal function (Yancy et al, 2013).

▲ As older adults approach end of life, clinicians should help to facilitate a comprehensive plan of care that incorporates the patient and family's values, goals, and preferences (Allen et al, 2012).

Home Care

• Some of the above interventions may be adapted for home care use. Home care agencies may use specialized staff and methods to care for chronic HF clients.

• Assess for fatigue and weakness frequently. Assess home environment for safety, as well as resources/obstacles to energy conservation.

• Help family adapt daily living patterns to establish life changes that will maintain improved cardiac functioning in the client. Take the client's perspective into consideration and use a holistic approach in assessing and responding to client planning for the future.

• Assist client to recognize and exercise power in using self-care management to adjust to health change. Refer to care plan for **Powerlessness.**

▲ Refer to medical social services, cardiac rehabilitation, telemonitoring and case management as necessary for assistance with home-care, access to resources, and counseling about the impact of severe or chronic cardiac diseases.

▲ As the client chooses, refer to palliative care for care, which can begin earlier in the care of the HF client. Palliative care can be used to increase comfort and quality of life in the HF client before end-of-life care (Buck & Zambroski, 2012).

▲ If the client's condition warrants, refer to hospice.

Client/Family Teaching and Discharge Planning

• Begin discharge planning as soon as possible upon admission to the emergency department (ED), if appropriate, with a case manager or social worker to assess home support systems and the need for community or home health services.

• = Independent   ▲ = Collaborative

C

- Discharge education should be comprehensive, evidence based, culturally sensitive, and include both the client and family (Yancy et al, 2013).
- Teach client about any medications prescribed. Medication teaching includes the drug name, its purpose, administration instructions, such as taking it with or without food, and any side effects to be aware of. Instruct the client to report any adverse side effects to his/her health care provider.
- Teach the importance of performing and recording daily weights upon arising for the day, and to report weight gain. Ask if client has a scale at home; if not, assist in getting one.
- Teach the types and progression patterns of worsening heart failure symptoms, when to call a health care provider for help, and when to go to the hospital for urgent care (Yancy et al, 2013).
- Stress the importance of ceasing tobacco use.
▲ Individuals should be screened for electronic cigarette use (e-cigarette).
- Upon hospital discharge, educate clients about low-sodium, low-saturated-fat diet, with consideration to client education, literacy, and health literacy level.
- Instruct client and family on the importance of regular follow-up care with health care providers.
▲ Teach stress reduction (e.g., imagery, controlled breathing, and muscle relaxation techniques).
- Discuss advance directives with the HF client, including resuscitation preferences.
- Patients should be provided with education regarding the influenza vaccine and pneumococcal vaccine prior to discharge.
- Teach the importance of physical activity as tolerated.

Risk for decreased Cardiac output
NANDA-I Definition

Vulnerable to inadequate blood pumped by the heart to meet metabolic demands of the body, which may compromise health

Risk Factors

Alteration in heart rate; alteration in heart rhythm; alteration in afterload; altered contractility; altered preload; altered stroke volume

Client Outcomes, Nursing Interventions, and Client/Family Teaching and Discharge Planning

Refer to care plan for Decreased **Cardiac** output.

Risk for decreased Cardiac tissue perfusion

NANDA-I Definition

Vulnerable to a decrease in cardiac (coronary) circulation, which may compromise health

Risk Factors

Cardiac tamponade; cardiovascular surgery; coronary artery spasm; diabetes mellitus; family history of cardiovascular disease; hyperlipidemia; hypertension; hypovolemia; hypoxemia; hypoxia; increase in C-reactive protein; insufficient knowledge about modifiable risk factors (e.g., smoking, sedentary lifestyle, obesity); pharmaceutical agent; substance abuse

Client Outcomes

Client Will (Specify Time Frame)

- Maintain vital signs within normal range
- Retain an asymptomatic cardiac rhythm (have absence of arrhythmias, tachycardia, or bradycardia)
- Be free from chest and radiated discomfort as well as associated symptoms related to acute coronary syndromes (ACSs)
- Deny nausea and be free of vomiting
- Have skin that is dry and of normal temperature

Nursing Interventions

- Be aware that the primary cause of ACS—unstable angina (UA), non–ST-elevation myocardial infarction (NSTEMI), and ST-elevation myocardial infarction (STEMI)—is an imbalance between myocardial oxygen consumption and demand that is associated with partially or fully occlusive thrombus development in coronary arteries (Amsterdam et al, 2014).
- Assess for symptoms of coronary hypoperfusion and possible ACS, including chest discomfort (pressure, tightness, crushing, squeezing, dullness, or achiness), with or without radiation (or originating) in the retrosternum; back, neck, jaw, shoulder, or arm discomfort or

• = Independent   ▲ = Collaborative

C

numbness; shortness of breath (SOB); associated diaphoresis; abdominal pain; dizziness, lightheadedness, loss of consciousness, or unexplained fatigue; nausea or vomiting with chest discomfort, heartburn, or indigestion; associated anxiety.

- Consider atypical presentations of ACS for women, older adults, and individuals with diabetes mellitus, impaired renal function, and dementia.
- Review the client's medical, surgical, social, and familial history.
- Perform physical assessments for both CAD and noncoronary findings related to decreased coronary perfusion, including vital signs, pulse oximetry, equal blood pressure in both arms, heart rate, respiratory rate, and pulse oximetry. Check bilateral pulses for quality and regularity. Report tachycardia, bradycardia, hypotension or hypertension, pulsus alternans or pulsus paradoxus, tachypnea, or abnormal pulse oximetry reading. Assess cardiac rhythm for arrhythmias; skin and mucous membrane color, temperature, and dryness; and capillary refill. Assess neck veins for elevated central venous pressure, cyanosis, and pericardial or pleural friction rub. Examine client for cardiac S_4 gallop, new heart murmur, lung crackles, altered mentation, pain on abdominal palpation, decreased bowel sounds, or decreased urinary output.
- ▲ Administer supplemental oxygen as ordered and needed for clients presenting with ACS, respiratory distress, or other high-risk features of hypoxemia to maintain a Po_2 of at least 90%.
- ▲ Use continuous pulse oximetry as ordered.
- ▲ Insert one or more large-bore intravenous catheters to keep the vein open. Routinely assess saline locks for patency. Clients who come to the hospital with possible decrease in coronary perfusion or ACS may have intravenous fluids and medications ordered routinely or emergently to maintain or restore adequate cardiac function and rhythm.
- ▲ Observe the cardiac monitor for hemodynamically significant arrhythmias, ST depressions or elevations, T-wave inversions and/or q-waves as signs of ischemia or injury. Report abnormal findings.
- Have emergency equipment and defibrillation capability nearby and be prepared to defibrillate immediately if ventricular tachycardia with clinical deterioration or ventricular fibrillation occurs.

• = Independent ▲ = Collaborative

C

▲ Perform a 12-lead ECG as ordered, to be interpreted within 10 minutes of emergency department arrival and during episodes of chest discomfort or angina equivalent.

▲ Administer nonenteric coated aspirin as ordered, as soon as possible after presentation and for maintenance.

▲ Administer nitroglycerin tablets sublingually as ordered, every 5 minutes until the chest pain is resolved while also monitoring the blood pressure for hypotension, for a maximum of three doses as ordered. Administer nitroglycerin paste or intravenous preparations as ordered.

• Do not administer nitroglycerin preparations to individuals with hypotension, or individuals who have received phosphodiesterase type 5 inhibitors, such as sildenafil, tadalafil, or vardenafil, in the last 24 hours (48 hours for long-acting preparations).

▲ Administer morphine intravenously as ordered every 5 to 30 minutes until pain is relieved while monitoring blood pressure when nitroglycerin alone does not relieve chest discomfort.

▲ Assess and report abnormal lab work results of cardiac enzymes, specifically troponin I or T, B-type natriuretic peptide, chemistries, hematology, coagulation studies, arterial blood gases, finger stick blood sugar, elevated C-reactive protein, or drug screen.

• Assess for individual risk factors for coronary artery disease, such as hypertension, dyslipidemia, cigarette smoking, diabetes mellitus, or family history of heart disease. Other risk factors include sedentary lifestyle, obesity, or cocaine or amphetamine use. Note age and gender as risk factors.

▲ Administer additional heart medications as ordered, including beta blockers, calcium channel blockers, angiotensin-converting enzyme inhibitors, angiotensin II receptor blockers, aldosterone antagonists, antiplatelet agents, and anticoagulants. Always check blood pressure and pulse rate before administering these medications. If the blood pressure or pulse rate is low, contact the health care provider to establish whether the medication should be withheld. Also check platelet counts, renal function, and coagulation studies as ordered to assess proper effects of these agents.

▲ Administer lipid-lowering therapy as ordered.

▲ Prepare client with education, withholding of meals and/or medications, and intravenous access for early invasive therapy with

• = Independent   ▲ = Collaborative

C

cardiac catheterization, reperfusion therapy, and possible percutaneous coronary intervention in individuals with refractory angina or hemodynamic or electrical instability, and first medical contact to device time of less than 90 minutes if STEMI is suspected.

▲ Prepare clients with education, withholding of meals and/or medications, and intravenous access for noninvasive cardiac diagnostic procedures such as 2D echocardiogram, exercise or pharmacological stress test, and cardiac computed tomography scan as ordered.

▲ Request a referral to a cardiac rehabilitation program.

Geriatric

• Consider atypical presentations of possible ACS in older adults.

▲ Ask the prescriber about possible reduced dosage of medications for older clients, considering weight, creatinine clearance, and glomerular filtration rate.

• Consider issues such as quality of life, palliative care, end-of-life care, and differences in sociocultural aspects for clients and families when supporting them in decisions regarding aggressiveness of care. Ask about living wills, as well as medical and durable power of attorney.

Client/Family Teaching and Discharge Planning

▲ Client and family education regarding a multidisciplinary plan of care should start early. Special attention to client and family education should occur during transitions of care.

• Teach the client and family to call 911 for symptoms of new angina, existing angina unresponsive to rest and sublingual nitroglycerin tablets, or heart attack, or if an individual becomes unresponsive.

• Upon discharge, instruct clients about symptoms of ischemia, when to cease activity, when to use sublingual nitroglycerin, and when to call 911.

• Teach client about any medications prescribed. Medication teaching includes the drug name, its purpose, administration instructions such as taking it with or without food, and any side effects to be aware of. Instruct the client to report any adverse side effects to the health care provider.

• Upon hospital discharge, educate clients and significant others about discharge medications, including nitroglycerin sublingual tablets or spray, with written, easy-to-understand, culturally sensitive information.

• = Independent   ▲ = Collaborative

C

- Provide client education related to risk factors for decreased cardiac tissue perfusion, such as hypertension, hypercholesterolemia, diabetes mellitus, tobacco use, advanced age, and gender (female).
- Instruct the client on antiplatelet and anticoagulation therapy, and about signs of bleeding, need for ongoing medication compliance, and international normalized ratio monitoring.
- After discharge, continue education and support for client blood pressure and diabetes control, weight management, and resumption of physical activity.
▲ Clients should be provided with education regarding the influenza vaccine and pneumococcal vaccine before hospital discharge.
▲ Stress the importance of ceasing tobacco use.
▲ Individuals should be screened for electronic cigarette use (e-cigarette).
▲ Upon hospital discharge, educate clients about a low sodium, low saturated fat diet, with consideration to client education, literacy, and health literacy level.
- Teach the importance of physical activity.

Risk for impaired Cardiovascular function

NANDA-I Definition

Vulnerable to internal or external causes that can damage one or more vital organs and the circulatory system itself

Risk Factors

Age older than 65 years; diabetes mellitus; dyslipidemia; family history of cardiovascular disease; history of cardiovascular disease; hypertension; insufficient knowledge of modifiable risk factors; obesity; pharmaceutical agent; sedentary lifestyle; smoking

Client Outcomes, Nursing Interventions, and Client/Family Teaching and Discharge Planning

Refer to care plans for Decreased **Cardiac** output, Risk for decreased **Cardiac** tissue perfusion, and **Sedentary** lifestyle.

Caregiver Role Strain

NANDA-I Definition

Difficulty in performing family/significant other caregiver role

• = Independent   ▲ = Collaborative

Defining Characteristics

Caregiving Activities

Apprehension about future ability to provide care; apprehension about the future health of care receiver; apprehension about possible institutionalization of care receiver; apprehension about well-being of care receiver if unable to provide care; difficulty completing required tasks; difficulty performing required tasks; dysfunctional change in caregiving activities; preoccupation with care routine

Caregiver Health Status: Physiological

Cardiovascular disease; diabetes mellitus; fatigue; gastrointestinal distress; headache; hypertension; rash; weight change

Caregiver Health Status: Emotional

Alteration in sleep pattern; anger; depression; emotional vacillation; frustration; impatience; ineffective coping strategies; insufficient time to meet personal needs; nervousness; somatization; stressors

Caregiver Health Status: Socioeconomic

Changes in leisure activities; low work productivity; refusal of career advancement; social isolation

Caregiver-Care Receiver Relationship

Difficulty watching care receiver with illness; grieving of changes with care recipient; uncertainty about changes in relationship with care receiver

Family Processes

Concerns about family members; family conflict

Related Factors (r/t)

Care Recipient Health Status

Alteration in cognitive functioning; chronic illness; codependency; dependency; illness severity; increase in care needs; problematic behavior; psychiatric disorder; substance abuse; unpredictability of illness trajectory; unstable health condition

Caregiver Health Status

Alteration in cognitive functioning; codependency; ineffective coping strategies; insufficient fulfillment of others' expectations; insufficient fulfillment of self-expectations; physical conditions; substance abuse; unrealistic self-expectations

Caregiver-Care Receiver Relationship

Abusive relationship; care receiver's condition inhibits conversation; pattern of ineffective relationships; unrealistic care receiver expectations; violent relationship

• = Independent ▲ = Collaborative

C

Caregiving Activities

Around-the-clock care responsibilities; change in nature of care activities; complexity of care activities; duration of caregiving; excessive caregiving activities; recent discharge home with significant care needs; unpredictability of care situation

Family Processes

Pattern of family dysfunction; pattern of ineffective family coping

Resources

Caregiver not developmentally ready for caregiver role; difficulty accessing assistance; difficulty accessing community resources; difficulty accessing support; financial crisis (e.g., debt, insufficient finances); inexperience with caregiving; insufficient assistance; insufficient caregiver privacy; insufficient community resources (e.g., respite services, recreation, social support); insufficient emotional resilience; insufficient equipment for providing care; insufficient knowledge about community resources; insufficient physical environment for providing care; insufficient time; insufficient transportation

Socioeconomic

Alienation; competing role commitments; insufficient recreation; social isolation

Client Outcomes

Throughout the Care Situation, the Caregiver Will

- Feel supported by health care professionals, family, and friends; Report reduced or acceptable feelings of burden or distress; Take part in self-care activities to maintain own physical and psychological/emotional health; Identify resources available to help in giving care or to support the caregiver to give care; Verbalize mastery of the care situation; Feel confident and competent to provide care;
- Ask for help

Throughout the Care Situation, the Care Recipient Will

- Obtain quality and safe care

Nursing Interventions

- Regularly monitor signs of depression, anxiety, burden, and deteriorating physical health in the caregiver throughout the care situation, especially if the relationship is poor, the care recipient has cognitive or neuropsychiatric symptoms, there is little social support available, the caregiver becomes enmeshed in the care situation, or the caregiver is older, female, or has poor preexisting physical or

• = Independent   ▲ = Collaborative

emotional health. Refer to the care plan for **Hopelessness** when appropriate.

C

- Assess the impact of providing care on the caregiver's emotional health at regular intervals using a reliable and valid instrument such as the Caregiver Strain Risk Index, which was validated with caregivers of clients with diagnosed Parkinson's disease.
- Identify potential caregiver resources such as mastery, social support, optimism, and positive aspects of care.
- Screen for caregiver role strain at the onset of the care situation, at regular intervals throughout the care situation, and with changes in care recipient status and care transitions, including institutionalization.
- Watch for caregivers who become enmeshed in the care situation.
- Arrange for intervals of respite care for the caregiver; encourage use if available.
- Regularly monitor social support for the caregiver and help the caregiver identify and use appropriate support systems for varying times in the care situation.
- Encourage the caregiver to grieve over changes in the care recipient's condition and give the caregiver permission to share angry feelings in a safe environment. Refer to nursing interventions for **Grieving.**
- Help the caregiver find personal time to meet his or her needs, learn stress management techniques, schedule regular health screenings, and schedule regular respite time.
- Encourage the caregiver to talk about feelings, concerns, uncertainties, and fears. Support groups can be used to gain mutual and educational support.
- Observe for any evidence of caregiver or care recipient violence or abuse, particularly verbal abuse; if evidence is present, speak with the caregiver and care recipient separately.
- ▲ Involve the family in care transitions; use a multidisciplinary team to provide medical and social services for instruction and planning specific to the care situation.
- ▲ Encourage regular communication with the care recipient and with the health care team.
- Help caregiver assess his or her financial resources (services reimbursed by insurance, available support through community and

• = Independent   ▲ = Collaborative

religious organizations) and the impact of providing care on his or her financial status.

- Help the caregiver identify competing occupational demands and potential benefits to maintaining work as a way of providing normalcy. Guide caregivers to seek ways to maintain employment through mechanisms such as job sharing or decreasing hours at work.
- Help the caregiver problem solve to meet the care recipient's needs.

Geriatric

- Monitor the caregiver for psychological distress and signs of depression, especially if caring for a mentally impaired older adult or if there was an unsatisfactory marital relationship before caregiving.
- Assess the health of caregivers, particularly their control over chronic diseases, at regular intervals.
- Assess the presence of and use of social support and encourage the use of secondary caregivers with older caregivers.
- To improve the ability to provide safe care: provide skills training related to direct care, perform complex monitoring tasks, supervise and interpret client symptoms, assist with decision-making, assist with medication adherence, provide emotional support and comfort, and coordinate care.
- Teach symptom management techniques (assessment, potential causes, aggravating factors, potential alleviating factors, reassessment), particularly for fatigue, constipation, anorexia, and pain.

Multicultural

- Assess for the influence of cultural beliefs, norms, and values on the client's ability to modify health behavior.
- Despite the importance of cultural differences in perceptions of caregiver role strain, there are certain characteristics that are distressing to caregivers across multiple cultures.
- Persons with different cultural backgrounds may not perceive the provision of care with equal degrees of distress.
- Recognize that cultures often play a role in identifying who will be recognized as a family caregiver and form partnerships with those groups.
- Encourage spirituality as a source of support for coping.
- Assess for the presence of conflicting values within the culture.
- Recognize that different cultures value and use caregiving resources in different ways.

• = Independent   ▲ = Collaborative

C

Home Care

- Assess the client and caregiver at every visit for quality of relationship, and for the quality of caring that exists.
- Assess preexisting strengths and weaknesses the caregiver brings to the situation, as well as current responses, depression, and fatigue levels.
- ▲ Refer the client to home health aide services for assistance with activities of daily living and light housekeeping. Allow the caregiver to gain confidence in the respite provider.

Client/Family Teaching and Discharge Planning

- Identify client and caregiver factors that necessitate the use of formal home care services, that may affect provision of care, or that need to be addressed before the client can be safely discharged from home care.
- Collaborate with the caregiver and discuss the care needs of the client, disease processes, medications, and what to expect; use a variety of instructional techniques (e.g., explanations, demonstrations, visual aids) until the caregiver is able to express a degree of comfort with care delivery.
- Assess family caregiving skill. The identification of caregiver difficulty with any of a core set of processes highlights areas for intervention.
- Discharge care should be individualized to specific caregiver needs and care situations, and enable them to be prepared.
- Assess the caregiver's need for information such as information on symptom management, disease progression, specific skills, and available support.
- Teach the caregiver warning signs for burnout, depression, and anxiety. Help them identify a resource in case they begin to feel overwhelmed.
- Teach the caregiver methods for managing disruptive behavioral symptoms if present. Refer to the care plan for Chronic **Confusion.**
- Teach the caregiver how to provide the care needed and put a plan in place for monitoring the care provided.
- Provide ongoing support and evaluation of care skills as the care situation and care demands change.
- Provide information regarding the care recipient's diagnosis, treatment regimen, and expected course of illness.

• = Independent   ▲ = Collaborative

▲ Refer to counseling or support groups to assist in adjusting to the caregiver role and periodically evaluate not only the caregiver's emotional response to care but the safety of the care delivered to the care recipient.

C

Risk for Caregiver Role Strain
NANDA-I Definition
Vulnerable to difficulty in performing the family/significant other caregiver role, which may compromise health
Risk Factors
Alteration in cognitive functioning in care receiver; care receiver discharged home with significant needs; care receiver exhibits bizarre behavior; care receiver exhibits deviant behavior; caregiver health impairment; caregiver isolation; caregiver not developmentally ready for caregiver role; caregiver's competing role commitments; caregiving task complexity; codependency; congenital disorder; developmental delay; developmental delay of caregiver; excessive caregiving activities; exposure to violence; extended duration of caregiving required family isolation; female caregiver; illness severity of care receiver; inadequate physical environment for providing care; ineffective caregiver coping pattern; ineffective family adaptation; experience with caregiving; instability in care receiver's health; insufficient caregiver recreation; insufficient respite for caregiver; partner as caregiver; pattern of family dysfunction prior to the caregiving situation; pattern of ineffective relationship between caregiver and care receiver; prematurity; presence of abuse (e.g., physical, psychological, sexual); psychological disorder in caregiver; psychological disorder in care receiver; stressors; substance abuse; unpredictability of illness trajectory
Client Outcomes, Nursing Interventions, and Client/Family Teaching and Discharge Planning
Refer to care plan for **Caregiver Role Strain.**

Risk for ineffective Cerebral tissue perfusion
NANDA-I Definition
Vulnerable to a decrease in cerebral tissue circulation, which may compromise health

C

Risk Factors

Abnormal partial thromboplastin time; abnormal prothrombin time; akinetic left ventricular wall segment; aortic atherosclerosis; arterial dissection; atrial fibrillation; atrial myxoma; brain injury (e.g., cerebrovascular impairment, neurological illness, trauma, tumor); brain neoplasm; carotid stenosis; cerebral aneurysm; coagulopathy (e.g., sickle cell anemia); dilated cardiomyopathy; disseminated intravascular coagulopathy; embolism; hypercholesterolemia; hypertension; infective endocarditis; mechanical prosthetic valve; mitral stenosis; pharmaceutical agent; recent myocardial infarction; sick sinus syndrome; substance abuse; treatment regimen

Client Outcomes

Client Will (Specify Time Frame)

- State absence of headache
- Demonstrate appropriate orientation to person, place, time, and situation
- Demonstrate ability to follow simple commands
- Demonstrate equal bilateral motor strength
- Demonstrate adequate swallowing ability

Nursing Interventions

- To decrease risk of reduced cerebral perfusion related to stroke or transient ischemic attack:
  - Obtain a family history of hypertension and stroke to identify persons who may be at increased risk of stroke.
  - Monitor blood pressure (BP) regularly, because hypertension is a major risk factor for both ischemic and hemorrhagic stroke.
  - Teach hypertensive clients the importance of taking their health care provider-ordered antihypertensive agent to prevent stroke.
  - Stress smoking cessation at every encounter with clients, using multimodal techniques to aid in quitting, such as counseling, nicotine replacement, and oral smoking cessation medications.
  - Teach clients who experience a transient ischemic attack (TIA) that they are at increased risk for a stroke
  - Screen clients 65 years of age and older for atrial fibrillation with pulse assessment.
  - Call 911 or activate the rapid response team of a hospital immediately when clients display symptoms of stroke as determined by the Cincinnati Stroke Scale (F: facial drooping; A: arm drift on one side; S: speech slurred), being careful to note the time of symptom appearance. Additional symptoms of stroke

• = Independent   ▲ = Collaborative

include sudden numbness/weakness of face, arm, or leg, especially on one side; sudden confusion; trouble speaking or understanding; sudden difficulty seeing with one or both eyes; sudden trouble walking; dizziness; loss of balance or coordination; or sudden severe headache (National Stroke Association, 2012).

o Use clinical practice guidelines for glycemic control and BP targets to guide the care of clients with diabetes who have had a stroke or TIA.

o Maintain head of bed less than 30 degrees in the acute phase (<72 hours of symptom onset) of ischemic stroke.

o Head of bed may be elevated to sitting position without detrimental effect to cerebral blood flow in clients with ischemic stroke or subarachnoid hemorrhage at 72 hours after symptom onset.

o Administer oral nimodipine as prescribed by the health care provider after subarachnoid hemorrhagic strokes for 21 days.

▲ To decrease risk of reduced cerebral perfusion pressure (CPP): Cerebral perfusion pressure = Mean arterial pressure − Intracranial pressure (CPP = MAP − ICP): See care plan for Decreased **Intracranial** adaptive capacity.

o Maintain euvolemia.

▲ To treat decreased CPP:

o Clients with subarachnoid hemorrhagic stroke experiencing delayed cerebral ischemia, as evidenced by declining neurological exam, should undergo a trial of induced hypertension.

o Administer phenylephrine infusion to raise MAP per collaborative protocol.

Ineffective Childbearing process
NANDA-I Definition

Pregnancy and childbirth process and care of the newborn that does not match the environmental context, norms, and expectations

During Pregnancy

Inadequate prenatal care; inadequate prenatal lifestyle (e.g., elimination, exercise, nutrition, personal hygiene, sleep); inadequate preparation of newborn care items; inadequate preparation of the home environment; ineffective management of unpleasant symptoms in pregnancy; insufficient access of support system; insufficient respect for unborn baby; unrealistic birth plan

During Labor and Delivery

Decrease in proactivity during labor and delivery; inadequate lifestyle for stage of labor (e.g., elimination, exercise, nutrition, personal hygiene, sleep); inappropriate response to onset of labor; insufficient access or support system; insufficient attachment behavior

After Birth

Inadequate baby care techniques; inadequate postpartum lifestyle (e.g., elimination, exercise, nutrition, personal hygiene, sleep); inappropriate baby feeding techniques; inappropriate breast care; insufficient access of support system; insufficient attachment behavior; unsafe environment for infant

Related Factors

Domestic violence; inconsistent prenatal health visits; insufficient knowledge of childbearing process; inadequate maternal nutrition; insufficient parental role model; insufficient prenatal care; insufficient support system; low maternal confidence; maternal powerlessness; maternal psychological distress; substance abuse; unplanned pregnancy; unrealistic birth plan; unsafe environment; unwanted pregnancy

Client Outcomes

Client Will (Specify Time Frame)

Antepartum

- Obtain early prenatal care in the first trimester and maintain regular visits
- Obtain knowledge level needed for appropriate care of oneself during pregnancy including good nutrition and psychological health
- Understand the risks of substance abuse and resources available
- Feel empowered to seek social and spiritual support for emotional well-being during pregnancy
- Use support systems for labor and emotional support
- Develop a realistic birth plan, taking into account any high-risk pregnancy issues
- Understand the labor and delivery process and comfort measures to manage labor pain

Postpartum

- Use a safe environment for self and infant
- Obtain knowledge to provide appropriate newborn care and postpartum care of self
- Obtain knowledge to develop appropriate bonding and parenting skills

• = Independent ▲ = Collaborative

Nursing Interventions

- Encourage early prenatal care and regular prenatal visits.
- ▲ Identify any high-risk factors that may require additional surveillance, such as preterm labor, hypertensive disorders of pregnancy, diabetes, depression, other chronic medical conditions, presence of fetal anomalies, or other high-risk factors.
- ▲ Assess and screen for signs and symptoms of depression during pregnancy and in the postpartal period including history of depression or postpartum depression, poor prenatal care, poor weight gain, hygiene issues, sleep problems, substance abuse, and preterm labor. If depression is present, refer for behavioral-cognitive counseling and/or medication (postpartum period only). Both counseling and medication are considered relatively equal to help with depression.
- ▲ Observe for signs of alcohol use, and counsel women to stop drinking during pregnancy. Give appropriate referral for treatment if needed.
- ▲ Obtain a smoking history, and counsel women to stop smoking for the safety of the baby. Give appropriate referral to smoking cessation program if needed.
- ▲ Monitor for substance abuse with recreational drugs. Refer to drug treatment program as needed. Refer opiate-dependent women to methadone clinics to improve maternal and fetal pregnancy outcomes.
- ▲ Monitor for psychosocial issues including lack of social support system, loneliness, depression, lack of confidence, maternal powerlessness, domestic violence, and socioeconomic problems.
- ▲ Monitor for signs of domestic violence. Refer to a community program for abused women that provides safe shelter as needed.
- Provide antenatal education to increase the woman's knowledge needed to make informed choices during pregnancy, labor, and delivery and to promote a healthy lifestyle.
- Encourage expectant parents to prepare a realistic birth plan in order to prepare for the physical and emotional aspects of the birth process and to plan ahead for how they want various situations handled.
- Encourage good nutritional intake during pregnancy to facilitate proper growth and development of the fetus. Women should consume an additional 300 calories per day during pregnancy, take a multi-micronutrient supplement containing at least 400 µg folic acid, and achieve a total weight gain of 25 to 30 lb.

• = Independent   ▲ = Collaborative

Multicultural
▲ Provide for a translator if needed.

C

▲ Provide depression screening for clients of all ethnicities.
• Perform a cultural assessment and provide obstetrical care that is culturally appropriate to ensure a safe and satisfying childbearing experience.

Readiness for enhanced Childbearing process

NANDA-I Definition

A pattern of preparing for and maintaining a healthy pregnancy, childbirth process, and care of newborn for ensuring well-being that can be strengthened

Defining Characteristics

During Pregnancy

Expresses desire to enhance knowledge of childbearing process; expresses desire to enhance management of unpleasant pregnancy symptoms; expresses desire to enhance prenatal lifestyle (e.g., elimination, exercise, nutrition, personal hygiene, sleep); expresses desire to enhance preparation for newborn

During Labor and Delivery

Expresses desire to enhance lifestyle appropriate for stage of labor (e.g., elimination, exercise, nutrition, personal hygiene, sleep); expresses desire to enhance proactivity during labor and delivery

After Birth

Expresses desire to enhance attachment behavior; expresses desire to enhance baby care techniques; expresses desire to enhance baby feeding techniques; expresses desire to enhance breast care; expresses desire to enhance environmental safety for the baby; expresses desire to enhance postpartum lifestyle (e.g., elimination, exercise, nutrition, personal hygiene, sleep); expresses desire to enhance use of support system

Client Outcomes

Client Will (Specify Time Frame)

During Pregnancy
• State importance of frequent prenatal care/education
• State knowledge of anatomic, physiological, psychological changes with pregnancy

• = Independent   ▲ = Collaborative

- Report appropriate lifestyle choices prenatal: Activity and exercise/ healthy nutritional practices

During Labor and Delivery
- Report appropriate lifestyle choices during labor
- State knowledge of birthing options, signs and symptoms of labor, and effective labor techniques

After Birth
- Report appropriate lifestyle choices postpartum
- State normal physical sensations following delivery
- State knowledge of recommended nutrient intake, strategies to balance activity and rest, appropriate exercise, time frame for resumption of sexual activity, strategies to manage stress
- List strategies to bond with infant
- State knowledge of proper handling and positioning of infant/infant safety
- State knowledge of feeding technique and bathing of infant

Nursing Interventions

Refer to care plans: Risk for impaired **Attachment**; Readiness for enhanced **Breastfeeding**; Readiness for enhanced family **Coping**; Readiness for enhanced **Family** processes; Risk for disproportionate **Growth**; Readiness for enhanced **Nutrition**; Readiness for enhanced **Parenting**; Ineffective **Role** performance.

Prenatal Care

▲ Ensure that pregnant clients have an adequate diet and take multi-micronutrient supplements containing at least 400 micrograms of folic acid during pregnancy.
- Encourage pregnant clients to include enriched cereal grain products in their diets.
- Assess smoking status of pregnant clients and offer effective smoking-cessation interventions.
- Also see Risk for disturbed **Maternal–Fetal** dyad for USDHHS guidelines.
▲ Assess for signs of depression and make appropriate referral: inadequate weight gain, underutilization of prenatal care, increased substance use, and premature birth. Past personal or family history of depression, single, poor health functioning, and alcohol use.
- Discuss breastfeeding with a pregnant client, including all the benefits both to the infant and the mother.

• = Independent ▲ = Collaborative

Intrapartal Care

- Encourage psychosocial support during labor, especially by the father of the baby or the woman's mother if possible.
- Consider using aromatherapy during labor.
- Provide massage and relaxation techniques during labor.
- Offer the client in labor a clear liquid diet and water if allowed.

Multicultural

Prenatal

- Assess the client's beliefs and concerns about prenatal care. Provide culturally appropriate prenatal care for clients.
- ▲ Refer the client to a centering pregnancy group (8 to 10 women of similar gestational age receive group prenatal care after initial obstetrical visit) or group prenatal care.

Intrapartal

- Assess client's beliefs and concerns about labor. Consider the client's culture when assisting in labor and delivery.

Postpartal

- Assess client's beliefs and concerns about the postpartum period. Provide culturally appropriate health and nutrition information and guidance on contemporary postpartum practices and take away common misconceptions about traditional dietary and health behaviors (e.g., fruit and vegetables should be restricted because of cold nature). Encourage a balanced diet and discourage unhealthy hygiene taboos.

Home Care

Prenatal

- ▲ Involve pregnant drug users in drug treatment programs that include coordinated interventions in several areas: drug use, infectious diseases, mental health, personal and social welfare, and gynecological/obstetric care.

Postpartal

- Provide video conferencing to support new parents.
- Consider reflexology for postpartum women to improve sleep quality.

Client/Family Teaching and Discharge Planning

Prenatal

- Provide dietary and lifestyle counseling as part of prenatal care to pregnant women.

• = Independent   ▲ = Collaborative

- Provide the following information in parenting classes via DVD and Internet: support mechanisms, information and antenatal education, breastfeeding, practical baby care, and relationship changes. Include fathers in the parenting classes.
- Provide group prenatal care to families in the military.

Postpartal

- Encourage physical activity in postpartum women, after being cleared by health care provider; provide telephone counseling, teach postpartum women that exercise may reduce anxiety and depression, encourage to download phone apps that help track exercise like Fitbit or Pedometer Master.
▲ Provide breastfeeding mothers contact information for a lactation consultant, phone numbers and website information for La Leche League (http://www.lalecheleague.org), and local breastfeeding support groups.
- Teach mothers of young children principles of a healthy lifestyle: substitute foods high in saturated fat with foods moderate in polyunsaturated fatty acids (PUFAs) such as avocados, tuna, walnuts, and olive oil. Include lean protein, fruits and vegetables, and complex carbohydrates. It is also important to increase physical activity.

Risk for ineffective Childbearing process

NANDA-I Definition

Vulnerable to not matching environmental context, norms, and expectations of pregnancy, childbirth process, and the care of the newborn

Risk Factors

Domestic violence; inconsistent prenatal health visits; insufficient cognitive readiness for parenting; insufficient knowledge of childbearing process; inadequate maternal nutrition; insufficient parental role model; insufficient prenatal care; insufficient support system; low maternal confidence; maternal powerlessness; maternal psychological distress; substance abuse; unplanned pregnancy; unrealistic birth plan; unwanted pregnancy

Client Outcomes, Nursing Interventions, and Client/Family Teaching and Discharge Planning

Refer to care plan for Ineffective **Childbearing** process.

• = Independent   ▲ = Collaborative

C

Impaired Comfort

NANDA-I Definition

Perceived lack of ease, relief, and transcendence in physical, psychospiritual, environmental, cultural, and/or social dimensions

Defining Characteristics

Alteration in sleep pattern; anxiety; crying; discontent with situation; distressing symptoms; fear; feeling cold; feeling hot; feeling of discomfort; feeling of hunger; inability to relax; irritability; itching; moaning; restlessness; sighing; uneasy in situation

Related Factors (r/t)

Illness-related symptoms; insufficient environmental control; insufficient privacy; insufficient resources (e.g., financial, social, knowledge); insufficient situational control; noxious environmental stimuli; treatment regimen

Client Will (Specify Time Frame)

- Provide evidence for improved comfort compared to baseline
- Identify strategies, with or without significant others, to improve and/or maintain acceptable comfort level
- Perform appropriate interventions, with or without significant others, as needed to improve and/or maintain acceptable comfort level
- Evaluate the effectiveness of strategies to maintain and/or reach an acceptable comfort level
- Maintain an acceptable level of comfort when possible

Nursing Interventions

- Assess client's understanding of ranking his or her comfort level.
- Ask about client's current level of comfort. This is the first step in helping clients achieve improved comfort.
- Comfort is a holistic state under which pain management is included.
- Assist clients to understand how to rate their current state of holistic comfort, using the institution's preferred method of documentation.
- Enhance feelings of trust between the client and the health care provider. To attain the highest comfort level, clients must be able to trust their nurse.
- Manipulate the environment as necessary to improve comfort.
- Encourage early mobilization and provide routine position changes. Range of motion and weight bearing decrease physical discomforts and disability associated with bed rest.

• = Independent   ▲ = Collaborative

- Provide simple massage. Massage has many therapeutic effects, including improved relaxation, circulation, and well-being.
- Provide healing touch, which is well suited for clients who cannot tolerate more stimulating interventions.
- Use empathy as a response to a client's negative emotions.
- Encourage clients to use relaxation techniques to reduce pain, anxiety, depression, and fatigue.

Geriatric
- Use hand massage for older adults. Most older adults respond well to touch and the health care provider's presence. Lines of communication open naturally during hand massage.
- Discomfort from cold can be treated with warmed blankets. There are physiological dangers associated with hypothermia.
- Use complementary therapies such as doll therapy in clients with dementia to increase comfort and reduce stress.
- Address any unmet physical, psychological, emotional, spiritual, and environmental needs when attempting to mediate the behavior of an older client with dementia.
- Provide simple massage.

Multicultural
- Identify and clarify cultural language used to describe pain and other discomforts. Expressions of pain and discomfort vary across cultures.
- Assess skin for ashy or yellow-brown appearance.
- Use soap sparingly if the skin is dry. Black skin tends to be dry, and soap exacerbates this condition.
- Encourage and allow clients to practice their own cultural beliefs and recognize the impact that different cultures have on a client's belief about health care, comforting measures, and decision-making.
- Assess for cultural and religious beliefs when providing care.

Client/Family Teaching and Discharge Planning
- Teach techniques to use when the client is uncomfortable, including relaxation techniques, guided imagery, hand massage, and music therapy.
- At end of life, the dying client is comforted by having a companion.
- Instruct the client and family about prescribed medications and complementary therapies that improve comfort (Kolcaba, 2003).

• = Independent ▲ = Collaborative

C

- Teach the client to follow up with the health care provider if discomfort persists. There are many avenues for enhancing comfort (Kolcaba, 2003).
- Encourage clients to use the Internet as a means of providing education to complement medical care for those who may be homebound or unable to attend face-to-face education.

Mental Health

- Encourage clients to use guided imagery techniques. Guided imagery helps distract clients from stressful situations and facilitates relaxation.
- Provide psychospiritual support and a comforting environment to enhance comfort during emotional crises.
- When nurses attend to the comfort of perioperative clients, the clients' sense of hope for a full recovery increases.
- Providing music and verbal relaxation therapy enhances holistic comfort by reducing anxiety.
- Caregivers should not hesitate to use humor when caring for their clients.

Readiness for enhanced Comfort

NANDA-I Definition

A pattern of ease, relief, and transcendence in physical, psychospiritual, environmental, and/or social dimensions that is sufficient for well-being and can be strengthened

Defining Characteristics

Expresses desire to enhance comfort; expresses desire to enhance feelings of contentment; expresses desire to enhance relaxation; expresses desire to enhance resolution of complaints

Client Outcomes

Client Will (Specify Time Frame)

- Assess current level of comfort as acceptable
- Express the need to achieve an enhanced level of comfort
- Identify strategies to enhance comfort
- Perform appropriate interventions as needed for increased comfort
- Evaluate the effectiveness of interventions at regular intervals
- Maintain an enhanced level of comfort when possible

• = Independent   ▲ = Collaborative

C

Nursing Interventions

- Assess clients' comfort needs and current level of comfort in various contexts, as outlined in Kolcaba's (2003) Comfort theory and practice: physical, psychospiritual, sociocultural, and environmental.
- Educate clients about the various contexts of comfort and help them understand that enhanced comfort is a desirable, positive, and achievable goal.
- Enhance feelings of trust between the client and the health care provider in order to maintain an effective and therapeutic relationship.
- Maintain an open and effective communication with clients and keep them informed about their health, their plan of care, and their environment.
- Implement comfort rounds that regularly assess for clients' comfort needs.
- Collaborate with other health care professionals, such as health care providers, pharmacists, social workers, chaplains, occupational and physical therapists, dietitians, among others, in planning interventions that address comfort needs in various contexts: physical, psychospiritual, sociocultural, and environmental.
- Educate clients about and encourage the use of various integrative therapies and modalities to provide options that enhance comfort, beyond the traditional plan of care. Institute of Medicine (IOM) and PAINS—Examples of such modalities are listed below:
  - Therapeutic massage and touch therapy.
  - Guided imagery.
  - Mindfulness and mindfulness-based interventions such as mindfulness-based stress reduction (MBSR), mantra repetition (silent repetition of a sacred word), mindfulness meditation, and mindful breathing and walking, among others. Since the original research by Kabat-Zinn, founder of MBSR, and colleagues established the effectiveness of mindfulness in helping clients manage chronic pain and improving body image and other symptoms, including anxiety and depression (Kabat-Zinn, Lipworth, & Burney, 1985), mindfulness-based interventions have been used to promote physical and psychospiritual comfort.
  - Energy therapy or biofield therapy such as healing touch, therapeutic touch, and reiki. Biofield therapy seems to be

• = Independent   ▲ = Collaborative

C

promising in promoting comfort and relaxation, but more sound and systematic research is needed to build a strong body of evidence.
- ○ Acupuncture and auricular acupuncture.
- ○ Aromatherapy.
- ○ Music.
- ○ Other mind-body therapies.
- Foster and instill hope in clients whenever possible. See the care plan for **Hopelessness.**
- Provide opportunities for and enhance spiritual care activities. The need for comfort and reassurance may be perceived as spiritual needs. To meet these needs, nurses engaged in interaction when they comforted and assured clients. Participants also identified absolution as a spiritual need, and there is evidence that forgiveness may bring one feelings of joy, peace, and elation, and a sense of renewed self-worth (Narayanasomy et al, 2004). Individuals who practiced spiritual meditation were found to have a greater increase in pain tolerance (Wachholtz & Pargament, 2008).
- ▲ Enhance social support and family involvement.
- ▲ Encourage clients to use health information technology (HIT) as needed. Client services can now include management of medications, symptoms, emotional support, health education, and health information (Moody, 2005).
- Evaluate the effectiveness of all interventions at regular intervals and adjust therapies as necessary. It is important for nurses to determine comfort and pain management goals because comfort goals will change with circumstances. Ask questions and ask them frequently, such as, "How is your comfort?" Establish guidelines for frequency of assessment and document responses, noting whether goals are being met (Kolcaba, 2003).

Geriatric
- Refer to above interventions for geriatric interventions.

Pediatric
- Assess and evaluate child's level of comfort at frequent intervals. Comfort needs should be individually assessed and planned for. With assessment of pain in children, it is best to use input from the parents or a primary care provider. Use only accepted scales for standardized pain assessment (Remke & Chrastek, 2007).

C

- Skin-to-skin contact (SSC) and selection of the most effective method improves the comfort of newborns during routine blood draws.
- Adjust the environment as needed to enhance comfort. Environmental comfort measures include maintaining orderliness; quiet; minimizing furniture; special attention to temperature, light and sound, color, and landscape (Kolcaba & DeMarco, 2005).
- Encourage parental presence whenever possible. The same basic principles for managing pain in adults and children apply to neonates. In addition to other comfort measures, parental presence should be encouraged whenever possible (Pasero, 2004).
- Promote use of alternative comforting strategies such as positioning, presence, massage, spiritual care, music therapy, art therapy, and story-telling to enhance comfort when needed. In addition to oral sucrose, other comfort measures should be used to alleviate pain such as swaddling, skin-to-skin contact with mother, nursing, rocking, and holding (Pasero, 2004).
- Support the child's spirituality.

Multicultural

- Identify cultural beliefs, values, lifestyles, practices, and problem-solving strategies when assessing clients. Cultural sensitivity must always be a component of pain assessment. The nurse must remember that pain expression will vary among clients and that variation must also be acknowledged within cultures (Andrews & Boyle, 2003).
- Enhance cultural knowledge by actively seeking out information regarding different cultural and ethnic groups. Recognize the impact of culture on communication styles and techniques. Communication and culture are closely intertwined, and communication is the way culture is transmitted and preserved. It influences how feelings are expressed, decisions are made, and what verbal and nonverbal expressions are acceptable.
- Provide culturally competent care to clients from different cultural groups. Cultural competency requires health care providers to act appropriately in the context of daily interactions with people who are different from themselves. Health care providers need to honor and respect the beliefs, interpersonal styles, attitudes, and behaviors of others. This level of cultural awareness requires health care providers

• = Independent ▲ = Collaborative

to refrain from forming stereotypes and judgments based on one's own cultural framework (Institute of Medicine, 2002).

Home Care

- The nursing interventions described for Readiness for enhanced **Comfort** may be used with clients in the home care setting. When needed, adaptations can be made to meet the needs of specific clients, families, and communities.
- ▲ Make appropriate referrals to other organizations or health care providers as needed to enhance comfort. Referrals should have merit and be practical, timely, individualized, coordinated, and mutually agreed upon by all involved (Hunt, 2005).
- ▲ Promote an interdisciplinary approach to home care. Members of the interdisciplinary team who provide specialized care to enhance comfort can include the health care provider, physical therapist, occupational therapist, nutritionist, music therapist, and social worker, among others (Stanhope & Lancaster, 2006).
- Evaluate regularly if enhanced comfort is attainable in the home care setting. Home health agencies monitor client outcomes closely. Evaluation is an ongoing process and is essential for the provision of quality care (Stanhope & Lancaster, 2006).
- Use music therapy at home.

Client/Family Teaching and Discharge Planning

- Teach client how to regularly assess levels of comfort.
- Instruct client that a variety of interventions may be needed at any given time to enhance comfort.
- Help clients understand that enhanced comfort is an achievable goal.
- Teach techniques to enhance comfort as needed.
- ▲ When needed, empower clients to seek out other health professionals as members of the interdisciplinary team to assist with comforting measures and techniques.
- Encourage self-care activities and continued self-evaluation of achieved comfort levels to ensure enhanced comfort is maintained.

Readiness for enhanced Communication

NANDA-I Definition

A pattern of exchanging information and ideas with others that can be strengthened

• = Independent ▲ = Collaborative

C

Defining Characteristics

Expresses desire to enhance communication

Client Outcomes

Client Will (Specify Time Frame)

- Express willingness to enhance communication
- Demonstrate ability to speak or write a language
- Form words, phrases, and language
- Express thoughts and feelings
- Use and interpret nonverbal cues appropriately
- Express satisfaction with ability to share information and ideas with others

Nursing Interventions

- Establish a therapeutic nurse-client relationship: provide appropriate education for the client, demonstrate caring by being present to the client.
- Assess the client's readiness to communicate, using an individualized approach, and avoid making assumptions regarding the client's preferred communication method.
- Assess the client's literacy level so information can be tailored accordingly.
- Use these practical guidelines to assist in communication: Listen attentively and provide a comfortable environment for communicating; slow down and listen to the client's story; use augmentative and alternative communication methods (e.g., lip reading, communication boards, writing, body language, and computer/electronic communication devices) as appropriate; repeat instructions if necessary; limit the amount of information given; have the client "teach back" to confirm understanding; avoid asking, "Do you understand?"; be respectful, caring, and sensitive.
- ▲ Use interdisciplinary collaboration to ensure continuity of enhanced communication.
- ▲ Refer couples in maladjusted relationships for psychosocial intervention and social support to strengthen communication; consider nurse specialists.
- Consider using music to enhance communication between a client who is dying and his or her family.
- Encourage clients with aphasia to sing.
- See care plan for Impaired verbal **Communication.**

• = Independent   ▲ = Collaborative

Pediatric

* All individuals involved in the care and everyday life of children with learning difficulties need to have a collaborative approach to communication.
* See care plan for Impaired verbal **Communication**.

Geriatric

▲ Assess for hearing and vision impairments, and make appropriate referrals for hearing aids.
* Use touch if culturally acceptable when communicating with older clients and their families.
* Consider singing during caregiving of clients with dementia.
* See care plan for Impaired verbal **Communication**.

Multicultural

* See care plan for Impaired verbal **Communication**.

Home Care

* The interventions described previously may be used in home care.
* See care plan for Impaired verbal **Communication**.

Client/Family Teaching and Discharge Planning

* See care plan for Impaired verbal **Communication**.

Impaired verbal Communication

NANDA-I Definition

Decreased, delayed, or absent ability to receive, process, transmit, and/or use a system of symbols

Defining Characteristics

Absence of eye contact; difficulty comprehending communication; difficulty expressing thoughts verbally (e.g., aphasia, dysphasia, apraxia, dyslexia); difficulty forming sentences; difficulty forming words (e.g., aphonia, dyslalia, dysarthria); difficulty in selective attending; difficulty in use of body expressions; difficulty in use of facial expressions; difficulty maintaining communication; difficulty speaking; difficulty verbalizing; disoriented to person; disoriented to place; disoriented to time; does not speak; dyspnea; inability to speak; inability to speak language of caregiver; inability to use body expressions; inability to use facial expressions; inappropriate verbalization; partial visual deficit; refusal to speak; slurred speech stuttering; total visual deficit

• = Independent   ▲ = Collaborative

Related Factors (r/t)

Absence of significant other; alteration in development; alteration in perception; alteration in self concept; central nervous system impairment; cultural incongruence; emotional disturbance; environmental barrier; insufficient information; insufficient stimuli; low self-esteem; oropharyngeal defect; physical barrier (e.g., tracheostomy, intubation); physiological condition (e.g., brain tumor, decreased circulation to brain, weakened musculoskeletal system); psychotic disorder; treatment regimen; vulnerability

Client Outcomes

Client Will (Specify Time Frame)

- Use effective communication techniques
- Use alternative methods of communication effectively
- Demonstrate congruency of verbal and nonverbal behavior
- Demonstrate understanding even if not able to speak
- Express desire for social interactions

Nursing Interventions

- Use a comprehensive nursing assessment to determine the language spoken, cultural considerations, literacy level, cognitive level, and use of glasses and/or hearing aids.
- Determine client's own perception of communication difficulties and potential solutions when possible.
- Involve a familiar person when attempting to communicate with a client who has difficulty with communication, if accepted by the client.
- Listen carefully. Validate verbal and nonverbal expressions particularly when dealing with pain and use appropriate scales for pain when appropriate.
- Use appropriate scales to assess communication and behavior in clients who are nonvocal and mechanically ventilated.
- Use therapeutic communication techniques: speak in a well-modulated voice, use simple communication, maintain eye contact at the client's level, get the client's attention before speaking, and show concern for the client.
- Avoid ignoring the client with verbal impairment; be engaged and provide meaningful responses to client concerns. Place call light or bell within reach of client who cannot verbally call for help.
- Use touch as appropriate.
- Use presence: spend time with the client, allow time for responses, and make the call light readily available.

• = Independent   ▲ = Collaborative

- Explain all health care procedures.
- Be persistent in deciphering what the client is saying, and do not pretend to understand when the message is unclear.
- Use an individualized and creative multidisciplinary approach to augmentative and alternative communication (AAC) assistance and other interventions.
- Use consistent nursing staff for those with communication impairments.
▲ Consult communication specialists from various disciplines as appropriate. Speech language pathologists, audiologists, and interpreters provide comprehensive communication assistance for those with impaired communication.
▲ When the client is having difficulty communicating, assess and refer for audiology consultation for hearing loss. Suspect hearing loss when:
  ○ Client frequently complains that people mumble, claims that others' speech is not clear, or client hears only parts of conversations.
  ○ Client often asks people to repeat what they said.
  ○ Client's friends or relatives state that client doesn't seem to hear very well, or plays the television or radio too loudly.
  ○ Client does not laugh at jokes due to missing too much of the story.
  ○ Client needs to ask others about the details of a meeting that the client attended.
  ○ Client cannot hear the doorbell or the telephone.
  ○ Client finds it easier to understand others when facing them, especially in a noisy environment.
- People with hearing loss do not hear sounds clearly. The loss may range from hearing speech sounds faintly or in a distorted way to profound deafness (American Academy of Audiology, 2011).
- When communicating with a client with a hearing loss:
  ○ Obtain client's attention before speaking and face toward his or her unaffected side or better ear while allowing client to see speaker's face at a reasonably close distance; use gestures as appropriate to aid in communication.
  ○ Provide sufficient light and do not stand in front of window. Remove masks if safe to do so, or use see-through masks. Information on see-through masks: www.amphl.org.

○ Reduce background noise whenever possible.
○ Do not raise voice or over-enunciate.
○ Avoid making assumptions about the communication choice of those with hearing loss or voice impairments.
○ Encourage physical activity among those with hearing loss.

Pediatric

• Observe behavioral communication cues in infants.
• Identify and define at least two new forms of socially acceptable communication alternatives that may be used by children with significant disabilities.
• Teach children with severe disabilities functional communication skills.
▲ Refer children with primary speech and language delay/disorder for speech and language therapy interventions.

Geriatric

• Carefully assess all clients for hearing difficulty using an audiometer. Healthy People 2020 encourages early identification of people with hearing loss (Healthy People 2020, 2014).
• Avoid use of "elderspeak."
• Initiate communication with the client with dementia, and give client time to respond. The responsibility to use a creative approach and take the time to listen and understand clients who have dementia lies with the clinician (Jootun & McGhee, 2011).
• Encourage the client to wear hearing aids, if appropriate.
• Facilitate communication through reminiscing with memory boxes that contain objects, photographs, and writings that have meaning for the client. Reminiscence stimulates memories, thus improving communication (Swann, 2013).
• Continue to find means to communicate even with those who are completely nonverbal.

Multicultural

• Nurses should become more sensitive to the meaning of a culture's nonverbal communication modes, such as eye contact, facial expression, touching, and body language.
• Assess for the influence of cultural beliefs, norms, and values on the client's communication process.
• Assess personal space needs, acceptable communication styles, acceptable body language, interpretation of eye contact, perception of

• = Independent   ▲ = Collaborative

C

touch, and use of paraverbal modes when communicating with the
client.
• Assess for how language barriers contribute to health disparities
among ethnic and racial minorities.
• Although touch is generally beneficial, there may be times when it
may not be advisable due to cultural considerations.
• Modify and tailor the communication approach in keeping with the
client's particular culture.
• Use reminiscence therapy as a language intervention.
• The Office of Minority Health of the U.S. Department of Health
and Human Services standards on culturally and linguistically
appropriate services (CLAS) in health care should be used as
needed.

Home Care
The interventions described previously may be adapted for home care use.

Client/Family Teaching and Discharge Planning
▲ Refer the client to a speech-language pathologist (SLP) or
audiologist. Audiological assessment quantifies and qualifies hearing
in terms of the degree of hearing loss, the type of hearing loss, and
the configuration of the hearing loss. Once a particular hearing loss
has been identified, a treatment and management plan can be put
into place by an SLP (Baumgartner et al, 2008).
▲ Teach the client and family techniques to increase communication,
including the use of communication devices and tactile touch.
Incorporate multidisciplinary recommendations. The nurse plays a
critical role in individualized communication assessment as clients
transition from hospital to home (Cerantola & Happ, 2012).

Acute Confusion
NANDA-I Definition
Abrupt onset of reversible disturbances of consciousness, attention, cognition, and perception that develop over a short period of time

Defining Characteristics
Agitation; alteration in cognitive functioning; alteration in level of consciousness; alteration in psychomotor functioning; hallucinations; inability to initiate goal-directed behavior; inability to initiate purposeful behavior; insufficient follow-through with goal-directed behavior; insufficient following-through with purposeful behavior; misperception; restlessness

• = Independent   ▲ = Collaborative

Related Factors (r/t)

Age >60 years; alteration in sleep-wake cycle; delirium; dementia; substance abuse; polypharmacy

Client Outcomes

C

Client Will (Specify Time Frame)

- Demonstrate restoration of cognitive status to baseline
- Be oriented to time, place, and person
- Demonstrate appropriate motor behavior
- Maintain functional capacity

Nursing Interventions

- Recognize that delirium is characterized by an acute onset, a fluctuating course, inattention, and disordered thinking.
- Identify the three distinct types of delirium: hyperactive (easy to recognize), hypoactive (commonly missed), and mixed (the most commonly occurring) (Downing et al, 2013).
- Hyperactive: delirium characterized by restlessness, agitation, irritability, hypervigilance, hallucinations, and delusions; client may be combative or may attempt to remove tubes, lines
  - Hypoactive: delirium characterized by decreased motor activity, decreased vocalization, detachment, apathy, lethargy, somnolence, reduced awareness of surroundings, and confusion
  - Mixed: delirium characterized by the client fluctuating between periods of hyperactivity and agitation and hypoactivity and sedation.
- Obtain an accurate history and perform a mental status examination that includes the following assessment:
  - History from a reliable source that documents an acute and fluctuating change in cognitive function, attention, and behavior from baseline
  - Cognition as evidenced by level of consciousness; orientation to time, person, and place; thought process (thinking may be disorganized, distorted, fragmented, slow, or accelerated with delirium; conversation may be irrelevant or rambling); and content (perceptual disturbances such as visual, auditory, or tactile delusions or hallucinations)
  - Level of attention (may be decreased or may fluctuate with delirium; may be unable to focus, shift, or sustain attention; may be easily distracted or may be hypervigilant)

• = Independent   ▲ = Collaborative

C

○ Behavior characteristics and level of psychomotor behavior (activity may be increased or decreased and may include restlessness, finger tapping, picking at bedclothes, changing position frequently, spastic movements or tremors, or decreased psychomotor activity such as sluggishness, staring into space, remaining in the same position for prolonged periods)

○ Level of consciousness (may be easily aroused, lethargic, drowsy, difficult to arouse, unarousable, hyperalert, easily startled, overly sensitive to stimuli)

○ Mood and affect (may be paranoid or fearful with delirium; may have rapid mood swings)

○ Insight and judgment (may be impaired)

○ Memory (recent and immediate memory is impaired with delirium; unable to register new information)

○ Language (may have rapid, rambling, slurred, incoherent speech)

○ Altered sleep-wake cycle (insomnia, excessive daytime sleepiness)

• Assess the client's behavior and cognition systematically and continually throughout the day and night; use a validated tool to assess presence of delirium, such as the Confusion Assessment Method (CAM) or Delirium Observation Screening Scale (DOS).

• Recognize that delirium may be superimposed on dementia; the nurse must be aware of the client's baseline cognitive function.

• Identify predisposing factors that may precede the development of delirium: dementia, cognitive impairment, functional impairment, visual impairment, alcohol misuse, multiple comorbidities, severe illness, history of transient ischemic attack or stroke, depression, history of delirium, and advanced age (older than 70).

• Identify precipitating factors that may precede the development of delirium, especially for individuals with predisposing factors: use of restraints, indwelling bladder catheter, metabolic disturbances, polypharmacy, pain, infection, dehydration, blood loss, constipation, electrolyte imbalances, immobility, general anesthesia, hospital admission for fractures or hip surgery, anticholinergic medications, anxiety, sleep deprivation, lack of use of vision and/or hearing aids, and environmental factors.

▲ Assess for and report possible physiological alterations (e.g., sepsis, hypoglycemia, hypoxia, hypotension, infection, changes in temperature, fluid and electrolyte imbalance, and use of medications with known cognitive and psychotropic side effects).

• = Independent ▲ = Collaborative

C

- ○ Treat the underlying risk factors or the causes of delirium in collaboration with the health care team: establish/maintain normal fluid and electrolyte balance, normal body temperature, normal oxygenation (if the client experiences low oxygen saturation, deliver supplemental oxygen), normal blood glucose levels, and normal blood pressure, and address malnutrition and anemia.
▲ Conduct a medication review and eliminate unnecessary medications; potentially inappropriate medications for older adults at risk for delirium include anticholinergics, benzodiazepines, corticosteroids, H_2 receptor antagonists, sedative hypnotics, tricyclic antidepressants (American Geriatrics Society, 2012).
  - ○ Communicate client status, cognition, and behavioral manifestations to all necessary health care providers.
  - ○ Monitor for any trends occurring in these manifestations, including laboratory tests.
- Identify, evaluate, and treat pain quickly and adequately (see care plans for Acute **Pain** or Chronic **Pain**).
- Promote regulation of bowel and bladder function; use bladder scanning to identify retention; avoid prolonged insertion of urinary catheters, and remove catheters as soon as possible.
- Ensure adequate nutritional and fluid intake.
- Promote early mobilization and rehabilitation in a progressive manner.
- Promote continuity of care; avoid frequent changes in staff and surroundings.
- Plan care that allows for an appropriate sleep-wake cycle. Refer to the care plan for **Sleep** deprivation.
- Facilitate appropriate sensory input by having clients use aids (e.g., glasses, hearing aids, dentures) as needed; check for impacted ear wax.
- Modulate sensory exposure; eliminate excessive noise; use appropriate lighting based on the time of day; establish a calm environment.
- Provide cognitive stimulation through conversation about current events, viewpoints, and relationships and encourage reminiscence or word games.
- Provide reality orientation, including identifying self by name at each encounter with the client, calling the client by his or her preferred

• = Independent   ▲ = Collaborative

name, and the gentle use of orientation techniques; when reorientation is not effective, use distraction.

C

- Provide clocks and calendars; update dry erase white boards each shift; encourage family to visit regularly and to bring familiar objects from home, such as family photos or an afghan; and gently correct misperceptions.
- Use gentle, caring communication; provide reassurance of safety; give simple explanations of procedures.
- Provide supportive nursing care, including meeting basic needs such as feeding, regular toileting, and ensuring adequate hydration; closely observe behaviors that provide clues to what might be distressing the client. Delirious clients are unable to care for themselves due to their confusion (Rubin et al, 2011).

▲ Recognize that delirium is frequently treated with antipsychotic medications or sedatives; if there is no other way to keep the client safe, administer these medications cautiously, as ordered, while monitoring for medication side effects.

- ○ For clients nearing the end of life, for whom delirium may be irreversible, focus on relief of symptoms by increasing supervision, reducing invasive lines and devices that restrict movement, keeping the bed in low position, and placing mats on the floor; support of family, caregivers, and the health care team is also of prime importance.
- ○ Choose the appropriate medication and consider the type and reversibility of the delirium; titrate the medication to control the symptoms and minimize side effects.

Critical Care

- Recognize admission risk factors for delirium.
- Obtain an accurate history regarding cognitive impairment and mental health, including history of anxiety and depression, alcohol use, medication use, chronic pain, and use of benzodiazepines.
- Assess level of arousal using the Richmond Agitation Sedation Scale; clients receiving a score of −5 to −4 are comatose and unable to be assessed for delirium.
- Assess for pain every 2 to 3 hours or more frequently as needed with a standardized assessment tool, which includes either a numerical rating scale or one with behavioral indicators, such as the Behavioral Pain Scale (BPS) or Critical Care Pain Observation Tool (CPOT).

• = Independent   ▲ = Collaborative

▲ Incorporate the Awakening and Breathing Coordination, Delirium Monitoring and Management, and Early Mobility (ABCDE) ICU delirium and weakness prevention bundle in conjunction with the interdisciplinary team.

   o Assess safety of and implement a spontaneous awakening trial (SAT) using an established protocol.
   o Assess safety of and implement a spontaneous breathing trial (SBT).
   o Assess sedation and agitation level using a valid and reliable tool; titrate sedation to target sedation level.
   o Screen for delirium using a reliable and valid monitoring tool once per shift or more often if delirium is present, and recognize that hypoactive delirium is the form most often present in the ICU; communicate and discuss results with the interdisciplinary team.
   o Assess safety to begin mobilization; collaborate with physical therapy (PT), occupational therapy (OT), and respiratory therapy (RT) to implement an early mobility plan using a progressive approach.

• Encourage visits from families and educate families about delirium if it occurs.
• Promote uninterrupted sleep by grouping cares at night to avoid sleep interruption, offering eye mask, soft music, and earplugs; optimizing room temperature; reduce noise and light after 10 PM; prevent excessive daytime napping.

Geriatric
• The interventions described previously are relevant to the geriatric client.
• Reorient high-risk clients frequently, answer questions, discuss concerns; use a white board, clock, watch, and calendar; encourage family members to bring familiar objects from home such as family photos or afghan to assist with orientation.
• Provide cognitive stimulation by discussing current events, reading the newspaper, promoting reminiscence, or using games.
• Promote use of glasses, assistive hearing devices, hearing aids, and dentures.
• Provide feeding assistance as needed. See care plan for Imbalanced **Nutrition:** less than body requirements.

• = Independent   ▲ = Collaborative

C

- ▲ Determine whether the client is adequately nourished; watch for protein-calorie malnutrition. Consult with health care provider or dietitian as needed.
- Promote adequate hydration; keep a glass of water within easy reach of the client and offer fluids frequently.
- Avoid use of restraints; remove all nonessential equipment such as telemetry, blood pressure cuffs, catheters, and intravenous lines as soon as possible.
- Evaluate all medications for potential to cause or exacerbate delirium; potentially inappropriate medications for older adults at risk for delirium include tricyclic antidepressants, anticholinergics, antipsychotics, benzodiazepines, corticosteroids, H_2 receptor antagonists, and sedative hypnotics.
- Assess pain frequently and treat pain with the lowest dose of regularly scheduled medication as well as with nonpharmacologic approaches; use client self-report or a validated behavioral pain scale to assess pain accurately.
- ▲ Assess risk for falls and implement fall prevention strategies.
- Recognize that delirium may be superimposed on dementia; determine client's baseline cognitive status.
- ▲ Determine whether the client is nourished; watch for protein-calorie malnutrition. Consult with health care provider or dietitian as needed.
- Explain hospital routines and procedures slowly and in simple terms; repeat information as necessary.
- Provide continuity of care when possible; avoid room changes; encourage frequent visits from family members or significant others.
- Educate family members about delirium assessment and strategies to use to prevent and lessen delirium; use the Family Confusion Assessment Method (FAM-CAM) assessment tool to solicit accurate information from caregivers regarding the presence of delirium.
- If clients know that they are not thinking clearly, acknowledge the concern. Fear is frequently experienced by people with delirium.

Home Care

- The interventions described previously are relevant to home care use. Assess and monitor for acute changes in cognition and behavior.

• = Independent   ▲ = Collaborative

- Recognize that delirium is reversible but can become chronic if untreated in a multidisciplinary fashion; the client may be discharged from the hospital to home care in a state of undiagnosed delirium.
- Avoid preconceptions about the source of acute confusion; assess each occurrence on the basis of available evidence.
▲ Institute case management of frail elderly clients to support continued independent living if possible once delirium has resolved.

Client/Family Teaching and Discharge Planning

▲ Teach the family to recognize signs of early confusion and to seek medical help.
- Counsel the client and family regarding the management of delirium and its sequelae. Increased care requirements at discharge may be needed for clients who have experienced delirium; frailty and delirium can lead to functional decline and institutionalization (Quinlan et al, 2011).

Chronic Confusion

NANDA-I Definition

Irreversible, long-standing, and/or progressive deterioration of intellect and personality characterized by decreased ability to interpret environmental stimuli; decreased capacity for intellectual thought processes; manifested by disturbances of memory, orientation, and behavior

Defining Characteristics

Alteration in interpretation; alteration in personality; alteration in response to stimuli; alteration in short-term memory; impaired social functioning; chronic cognitive impairment; normal level of consciousness; organic brain disorder; progressive alteration in cognitive impairment

Related Factors (r/t)

Alzheimer's disease; cerebrovascular accident; Korsakoff's psychosis; multi-infarct dementia

Client Outcomes

Client Will (Specify Time Frame)

- Remain content and free from harm
- Function at maximal cognitive level
- Participate in activities of daily living at the maximum of functional ability
- Have minimal episodes of agitation (agitation occurs in up to 70% of clients with dementia)

• = Independent   ▲ = Collaborative

Nursing Interventions

C

- Determine the client's cognitive level using a screening tool such as the Mini-Mental State Exam (MMSE), Mini-Cog (includes a three-item recall and clock drawing test), or Montreal Cognitive Assessment.

▲ In clients who are complaining of memory loss, assess for depression, alcohol use, medication use, problems with sleep, and nutrition status.

▲ Recognize that pharmacological treatment to slow the progression of Alzheimer's disease is most effective when used early in the course of the disease.

- If the client is hospitalized, gather information about the client's preadmission cognitive functioning, daily routines and care, and decision-making capacity. Establishing continuity of care lessens risk for hospitalized clients. Informed consent may create a dilemma; decision-making capacity will vary depending on the degree of cognitive impairment (Weitzel et al, 2011).

- Assess the client for signs of depression: anxiety, sadness, irritability, agitation, somatic complaints, tension, loss of concentration, insomnia, poor appetite, apathy, flat affect, and withdrawn behavior.

- Assess the client for anxiety if he or she reports worry regarding physical or cognitive health; reports feelings of being anxious, short of breath, or dizzy; or exhibits behaviors such as restlessness, irritability, sensitivity to noise, motor tension, fatigue, or disturbed sleep. The Rating Anxiety in Dementia (RAID) scale may be used; this may require caregiver input. Recognize that anxiety is common in dementia, is often undiagnosed, and may significantly impact quality of life.

▲ Recognize that clients with Alzheimer's disease may experience neuropsychiatric symptoms such as apathy, anxiety and depression, delusions, disinhibition, euphoria, hallucinations, agitation, including verbal/vocal behavior, and aggression; nonpharmacological interventions for management should be attempted first.

- Obtain information about the client's life history, interests, routines, needs, and preferences from the family or significant others; collaborate with family members to engage in reminiscence.

- Begin each interaction with the client by gaining and maintaining eye contact, identifying yourself, and calling the client by name.

• = Independent   ▲ = Collaborative

Approach the client with a caring, accepting, and empathetic attitude, and speak calmly and slowly.

- To enhance communication, use a calm approach, avoid distractions, show interest, keep communication simple, give clear choices and one-step instructions, give the client time with word finding, use repetition and rephrasing, and use gestures, prompts, and cues or visual aids. Listen attentively to understand nonverbal messages, and engage in topics of interest to the client.
- Engage the client in scheduled activities that relate to past interests, experiences, and hobbies and are matched to current preferences and abilities.
- Promote regular exercise.
- Provide opportunities for contact with nature or nature-based stimuli, such as facilitating time spent outdoors or indoor gardening.
- Provide animal-assisted therapy to enhance the care environment.
- Break down self-care tasks into simple steps, giving one direction at a time. For example, instead of saying, "Take a shower," say to the client, "Please follow me. Sit down on the bed. Take off your shoes. Now take off your socks." Use gestures when giving directions; allow for adequate time and model the desired action if needed or possible.
- Promote engagement in individual client routines and facilitate success by keeping frequently used items in a visible and consistent location.
- Use reminiscence and life review therapeutic interventions for clients in the early to middle stages of dementia; ask questions about the client's past activities and important events and experiences from the past while using photographs, videos, artifacts, music, newspaper clippings, or multimedia technology to stimulate memories.
- Engage clients in the middle to late stages of dementia in creative expression through the use of Time Slips story-telling groups or through person-centered art activities.
- If the client is verbally agitated (repetitive verbalizations, complaints, moaning, muttering, threats, screaming), assess for and address unsatisfied basic needs or environmental factors that may be addressed, and redirect the individual.

• = Independent ▲ = Collaborative

C

- Assist clients in wayfinding, monitoring them so that they do not get lost in unfamiliar settings; place cues and familiar objects in the environment.
- For clients who wander, refer to the **Wandering** care plan.
- Promote sleep by promoting daytime activity, creating a restful sleep environment, decreasing waking, and promoting quiet.
- Provide activities for the client, such as folding, sorting, or stacking activities; arranging flowers; or other hobbies or routines the individual enjoyed before the onset of dementia.
- Anticipate and assess for physical stressors such as fatigue, hunger, thirst, constipation, urinary symptoms, and pain.
- ▲ If the client becomes increasingly confused and/or agitated, perform the following steps:
  - ○ Assess the client for physiological causes, including acute hypoxia, pain, medication effects, malnutrition, and infections such as urinary tract infection, fatigue, electrolyte disturbances, and constipation.
  - ○ Assess for psychological causes, including changes in the environment, caregiver, or routine; demands to perform beyond capacity; or multiple competing stimuli, including discomfort. Encourage communication by addressing the client in a calm, gentle tone of voice and by using appropriate body language, facial expressions, and gestures.
  - ○ Use music as a nonpharmacological approach to managing agitation. Identify the client's music preferences; interview family members if necessary.
  - ○ In clients with agitated behaviors, rather than confronting the client, decrease stimuli in the environment or provide gentle stimulation through diversional activities such as quiet music, looking through a photo album with a staff member, or providing the client with textured items to handle.
  - ○ If clients with dementia become more agitated, assess for pain.
- ▲ Avoid using restraints if possible.
- ▲ Use as-needed or low-dose regular dosing of psychotropic or antianxiety drugs only as a last resort; start with the lowest possible dose.
- ▲ Avoid the use of anticholinergic medications such as diphenhydramine. Anticholinergic medications have a high

• = Independent   ▲ = Collaborative

side-effect profile that includes disorientation, urinary retention, and excessive drowsiness, especially in those with decreased cognition.

- For interventions on bathing, refer to the geriatric interventions in the care plan for Bathing **Self-Care** deficit.
- For care of early dementia clients with primarily symptoms of memory loss, see the care plan for Impaired **Memory**.
- For clients nearing the end of life, consider a hospice referral.
- For care of clients with self-care deficits, see the appropriate care plan (Feeding **Self-Care** deficit; Dressing **Self-Care** deficit; Toileting **Self-Care** deficit).

Geriatric

NOTE: All interventions are appropriate for geriatric clients.

Multicultural

- Assess for the influence of cultural beliefs, norms, and values on the family's or caregiver's understanding of chronic confusion or dementia; assist the family or caregiver in identifying barriers that would prevent the use of social services or other supportive services that could help reduce the impact of caregiving and refer to social services or other supportive services.
- Inform the client's family or caregiver of the meaning of and reasons for common behavior observed in clients with dementia.

Home Care

NOTE: Keeping the client as independent as possible is important. Because community-based care is usually less structured than institutional care, in the home setting the goal of maintaining safety for the client takes on primary importance.

- The interventions described previously may be adapted for home care use.
- Provide information to the family and home care client regarding advance directives.
- Assess the client's memory and executive function deficits before assuming the inability to make any medical decisions; driving capacity and financial capacity should be assessed for clients with mild cognitive impairment.
- Assess the home for safety features and client needs for assistive devices. Refer to the interventions for Feeding **Self-Care** deficit; Dressing **Self-Care** deficit; and Bathing **Self-Care** deficit as needed.
- Promote cognitive stimulation and memory training exercises for individuals in the early stages of dementia.

• = Independent ▲ = Collaborative

C

- Provide education and support to the family regarding effective communication, home safety, fall prevention, engagement in meaningful activities, ways to manage cognitive and behavioral changes, and comprehensive health care including screening for depression; be prepared to offer support and information to family members who live at a distance as well.
- Use familiar aspects of the environment (smells, music, foods, pictures) to cue the client, capitalizing on habit to remind the client of activities in which the client can participate.
- Instruct the caregiver to provide a balanced activity schedule that does not stress the client or deprive him or her of stimulation; avoid sustained low- or high-stimulation activity.
- Encourage the caregiver to plan leisure activities that promote cognitive and physical stimulation.
- ▲ If the client will require extensive supervision on an ongoing basis, evaluate the client for adult day health care programs. Refer the family to medical social services to assist with this process if necessary.
- Encourage the family to include the client in family activities when possible. Reinforce the use of therapeutic communication guidelines (see Client/Family Teaching and Discharge Planning) and sensitivity to the number of people present. Assess family caregivers for caregiver stress, loneliness, and depression. Refer to the care plan for **Caregiver Role Strain.**
- ▲ Refer the client to medical social services as necessary to evaluate financial resources and initiate benefits, and to facilitate access to health care providers and community-based organizations such as support groups and training programs for caregivers.
- ▲ Institute case management for frail elderly clients to support continued independent living.

Client/Family Teaching and Discharge Planning

- In the client's early stages of dementia, provide the caregiver with information on illness processes, needed care, available services, role changes, and importance of advance directives discussion; facilitate family cohesion.
- Teach the family communication strategies, personal care techniques, mobility enhancement, prevention, recognition and management of anxiety and depression, strategies for handling challenging behaviors and legal and financial considerations.

• = Independent   ▲ = Collaborative

- Discuss with the family what to expect as the dementia progresses.
- ▲ Counsel the family about resources available regarding end-of-life decisions and legal concerns.
- ▲ Inform the family that as dementia progresses, hospice care may be available in the home or nursing home in the terminal stages to help the caregiver.

Risk for acute Confusion
NANDA-I Definition

Vulnerable to reversible disturbances of consciousness, attention, cognition, and perception that develop over a short period of time, which may compromise health

Risk Factors

Age ≥ 60 years; alteration in cognitive functioning; alteration in sleep-wake cycle; dehydration; dementia; history of cerebral vascular accident; impaired metabolic functioning (e.g., azotemia, decreased hemoglobin, electrolyte imbalance, increase in blood urea nitrogen/creatinine); impaired mobility; inappropriate use of restraints; infection; male gender; malnutrition; pain; pharmaceutical agent; sensory deprivation; substance abuse; urinary retention

Client Outcomes, Nursing Interventions, and Client/Family Teaching and Discharge Planning

Refer to care plan for Acute **Confusion.**

Constipation
NANDA-I Definition

Decrease in normal frequency of defecation accompanied by difficult or incomplete passage of stool and/or passage of excessively hard, dry stool

Defining Characteristics

Abdominal pain; abdominal tenderness with palpable muscle resistance; abdominal tenderness without palpable muscle resistance; anorexia; atypical presentations in older adults (e.g., change in mental status, urinary incontinence, unexplained falls, elevated body temperature); borborygmi; bright red blood with stool; change in bowel pattern; decrease in stool frequency; decrease in stool volume; distended abdomen; fatigue; hard, formed stool; headache; hyperactive bowel sounds; hypoactive bowel sounds; inability to defecate; increase in intra-abdominal pressure; indigestion; liquid stool; pain with defecation; palpable abdominal mass; palpable rectal mass; percussed abdominal dullness; rectal fullness; rectal pressure; severe flatus; soft, paste-like stool in rectum; straining with defecation; vomiting

Related Factors

Functional

Abdominal muscle weakness; average daily physical activity is less than recommended for gender and age; habitually ignores urge to defecate; inadequate toileting habits; irregular defecation habits; recent environmental change

Mechanical

Electrolyte imbalance; hemorrhoids; Hirschsprung's disease; neurological impairment (e.g., positive electroencephalogram, head trauma, seizure disorders); obesity; postsurgical bowel obstruction; pregnancy; prostate enlargement; rectal abscess; rectal anal fissures; rectal anal stricture; rectal prolapse; rectal ulcer; rectocele; tumors

Pharmacological

Laxative abuse; pharmaceutical agent

Physiological

Decrease in gastrointestinal motility; dehydration; eating habit change (e.g., foods, eating times); inadequate dentition; inadequate oral hygiene; insufficient dietary habits; insufficient fiber intake; insufficient fluid intake

Psychological

Confusion; depression; emotional disturbance

Client Outcomes

Client Will (Specify Time Frame)

Maintain passage of soft, formed stool every 1 to 3 days without straining; State relief from discomfort of constipation; Identify measures that prevent or treat constipation

Nursing Interventions

- Introduce yourself to the client and any companions, and inform them of your role. Introducing yourself to a client helps establish and develop a therapeutic relationship that recognizes the person within the client and forms the basis for building trust upon which to base the provision of care (Howatson-Jones, 2012).
- Gain consent to carry out care before proceeding further with the assessment. Clients have the right of autonomy both legally and

C

morally and therefore should be fully involved in the decision-making process (Avery, 2013).

- Wash hands using a recognized technique.
- Assess usual pattern of defecation and establish the extent of the constipation problem.
  - ○ Bowel habits: time of day; amount and frequency of stool; consistency of stool (using the Bristol Stool Scale); bleeding/passing mucus on defecation; history of bowel habits and/or laxative use
  - ○ Lifestyle assessment: fiber content in diet; daily fluid intake; exercise patterns; personal remedies for constipation; recently stopped smoking; alcohol consumption/recreational drug use
  - ○ Past medical history: obstetrical/gynecological/urological history and surgeries; diseases that affect bowel motility; bleeding/passing mucous on defecation; current medications
  - ○ Emotional influences: anxiety and depression; long-term defecation issues; stress
- Assess usual pattern of defecation, including time of day, amount and frequency of stool, consistency of stool; history of bowel habits or laxative use; diet, including fiber and fluid intake; exercise patterns; personal remedies for constipation; obstetrical/gynecological history; surgeries; diseases that affect bowel motility; alterations in perianal sensation; present bowel regimen. Individual bowel habits vary, and clients with constipation experience a variety of symptoms (Spinzi et al, 2009; Kyle 2011a).
- Consider emotional influences (e.g., depression and anxiety) on defecation. Emotions influence gastrointestinal function, possibly because control of both emotions and gastrointestinal function is located in the limbic system of the brain. Difficulties with defecation often begin in childhood (e.g., during toilet training), and constipation is also associated with sexual and physical abuse, depression, and anxiety (Whitehead et al, 2009).
- Complete a physical examination (palpation for abdominal distention, percussion for dullness, and auscultation for bowel sounds). A physical examination provides positive and negative findings and may provide the diagnosis without the need for further testing. It may also reveal unsuspected findings or confirm normality (Rhoads & Murphy-Jensen, 2014).

• = Independent   ▲ = Collaborative

C

- Encourage the client or family to keep a 7-day diary of bowel habits to include time of day, length of time spent on the toilet, consistency, amount and frequency of stool, and any straining (using the Bristol Stool Scale).
- Encourage the client or family to keep a 7-day diary of lifestyle issues in relation to bowel habits to include fluid consumption, fiber content in diet, usual bowel stimulus, and exercise regimen.
- Use the Bristol Stool Scale to assess stool consistency.
▲ Review the client's current medications.
- Discuss with clients already taking opioids (temporarily or long term) that constipation is a common side effect. Advise them to contact their health care provider for a prescription of an appropriate laxative.
▲ Recognize that opioids cause constipation. If the client is receiving temporary opioids (e.g., for acute postoperative pain), request an order for routine stool softeners from the primary care provider, monitor bowel movements, and request a laxative for the client if constipation develops. If the client is receiving around-the-clock opiates (e.g., for palliative care), request an order for Senokot-S and institute a bowel regimen.
▲ If the client is terminally ill and is receiving around-the-clock opioids for palliative care, speak with the prescribing health care provider about ordering methylnaltrexone, a drug that blocks opioid effects on the gastrointestinal tract without interfering with analgesia.
- If new onset of constipation, determine whether the client has recently stopped smoking.
- Palpate for abdominal distention, percuss for dullness, and auscultate bowel sounds.
▲ Check for impaction; if present, perform digital removal of stool per the health care provider's order. An impaction is hard stool that is too large to move through the sphincter and must be removed manually. Clients with neurogenic bowel dysfunction (e.g., spinal cord injury) commonly require manual evacuation of stool (Coggrave & Norton, 2010).
▲ Advise a fiber intake of 18 to 25 g daily and suggest foodstuffs high in fiber.
- Add fiber gradually to the diet to decrease bloating and flatus.

• = Independent   ▲ = Collaborative

- Use a mixture of bran cereal, applesauce, and prune juice; begin administration in small amounts and gradually increase amount. Keep refrigerated. Always check with the primary care provider before initiating this intervention. It is important that the client also ingest sufficient fluids.
- Provide prune or prune juice daily. Each 100 g of prunes contains about 6 g of fiber, 15 g of sorbitol, and 184 mg of polyphenol; all have laxative effects (Attaluri et al, 2011).
- Advise a fluid intake of 1.5 to 2 L of fluid per day (ideally, 6 to 8 glasses of water), unless contraindicated by comorbidities, such as kidney or heart disease.
▲ If the client is uncomfortable or in pain due to constipation or has acute or chronic constipation that does not respond to increased fiber, fluid, activity, and appropriate toileting, refer the client to the primary care provider for an evaluation of bowel function and health status.
- Encourage physical activity within the client's current ability to mobilize. Encourage turning and changing position in bed if immobile. For clients with reduced mobility, encourage knee to chest raises, waist twists, and stretching the arms away from the body. For fully mobile clients, encourage walking and swimming.
- Demonstrate the use of gentle external abdominal massage, using aromatherapy oils, following the direction of colon activity.
- Recommend clients establish a regular elimination routine. If required, assist clients to the bathroom at the same time every day, being mindful of the need for privacy (closing of bathroom doors).
- Provide privacy for defecation. If not contraindicated, help the client to the bathroom and close the door.
- Help clients onto a bedside commode or toilet so they can either squat or lean forward while sitting. Recognize that it is difficult to impossible to defecate in the lying supine position. Sitting upright allows gravity to aid defecation.
- Educate the client how to adopt the best posture for defecation. Keep knees slightly higher than hips, keep feet flat on the floor, and lean forward putting elbows onto knees.
- Teach clients of the importance of responding promptly to the urge to defecate.

• = Independent   ▲ = Collaborative

- Consider the use of laxatives, suppositories, enemas, and bowel irrigation as required if other more natural interventions are not effective.

C

- Discourage the use of long-term laxatives and enemas and advise clients to gradually reduce their use if taken regularly.

Geriatric

- Assess older adults for the presence of factors that contribute to constipation, including dietary fiber and fluid intake (less than 1.5 L/day), physical activity, use of constipating medications, and diseases that are associated with constipation.
- Explain the importance of adequate fiber intake, fluid intake, activity, and established toileting routines to ensure soft, formed stool.
- Determine the client's perception of normal bowel elimination and laxative use; promote adherence to a regular schedule.
- Explain why straining (Valsalva maneuver) should be avoided.
- Respond quickly to the client's call for assistance with toileting.
- Offer food, fluids, activity, and toileting opportunities to older clients who are cognitively impaired.
- Avoid regular use of enemas in older adults.
- ▲ Use opioids cautiously. Opioids cause constipation (Davies et al, 2008).
- Position the client on the toilet or commode and place a small footstool under the feet. Placing a small footstool helps the client assume a squatting posture to facilitate defecation.

Home Care

- The interventions described previously may be adapted for home care use.
- Take complaints seriously and evaluate claims of constipation in a matter-of-fact manner. Continued constipation can lead to bowel obstruction, a medical emergency. Use of a matter-of-fact manner will limit positive reinforcement of the behavior if actual constipation does not exist. Refer to the care plan for Perceived **Constipation**.
- Assess the self-care management activities the client is already using.
- Offer the following treatment recommendations:
- ▲ Acknowledge the client's life-long experience of bowel function; respect beliefs, attitudes, and preferences, and avoid patronizing responses.

• = Independent   ▲ = Collaborative

▲ Make available comprehensive, useful written information about constipation and possible solutions.

▲ Make available empathetic and accessible professional care to provide treatment and advice; a multidisciplinary approach (including health care provider, nurse, and pharmacist) should be used.

▲ Institute a bowel management program.

▲ Consider affordability when suggesting solutions to constipation; discuss cost-effective strategies.

▲ Discuss a range of solutions to constipation and allow the client to choose the preferred options.

▲ Have orders in place for a suppository and enema as the need may occur. As part of a bowel management program, suppositories or enemas may become necessary.

• Although the use of a bedside commode may be necessitated by the client's condition, allow the client to use the toilet in the bathroom when possible and provide assistance.

• In older clients, routinely advise consumption of fluids, fruits, and vegetables as part of the diet, and ambulation if the client is able. Introduce a bowel management program at the first sign of constipation. Constipation is a major problem for terminally ill or hospice clients, who may need very high doses of opioids for pain management (Sykes, 2006).

▲ Refer for consideration of the use of polyethylene glycol 3350 (PEG-3350) for constipation.

• Advise the client against attempting to remove impacted feces on his or her own.

• When using a bowel program, establish a pattern that is very regular and allows the client to be part of the family unit. Regularity of the program promotes psychological and/or physiological readiness to evacuate stool. Families of home care clients often cannot proceed with normal daily activities until bowel programs are complete.

Client/Family Teaching and Discharge Planning

• Instruct the client on normal bowel function and the need for adequate fluid and fiber intake, activity, and a defined toileting pattern in a bowel program.

• Encourage the client to heed defecation warning signs and develop a regular schedule of defecation by using a stimulus such as a warm drink or prune juice.

• = Independent   ▲ = Collaborative

- Encourage the client to avoid long-term use of laxatives and enemas and to gradually withdraw from their use if they are used regularly.
- If not contraindicated, teach the client how to do bent-leg sit-ups to increase abdominal tone; also encourage the client to contract the abdominal muscles frequently throughout the day. Help the client develop a daily exercise program to increase peristalsis.
- Provide client with comprehensive written information about constipation and its management.
- ▲ Collaborate with members of the interprofessional team to provide treatment and advice to clients and caregivers. Team working is a central process in health care organizations. It increases the capacity of teams to absorb and develop new knowledge, which will improve client health and well-being (Ortega et al, 2013).
- Formalize all advice by providing a bowel management program reiterating the mechanism of normal bowel function and the need for adequate fluid and fiber intake, physical activity, and a defined toileting pattern in an agreed bowel program.
- Document all care and advice given in a factual and comprehensive manner.

Chronic functional Constipation
NANDA-I Definition

Infrequent or difficult evacuation of feces, which has been present for at least 3 of the prior 12 months

Defining Characteristics

Abdominal distention; adult: presence of ≥2 of the following symptoms on Rome III classification system; lumpy or hard stools in ≥25% defecations; straining during ≥25% of defecations; sensation of incomplete evacuation for ≥25% of defecations; sensation of anorectal obstruction/blockage for ≥25% of defecations; manual maneuvers to facilitate ≥25% of defecations (digital manipulation, pelvic floor support); ≤3 evacuations per week; child: ≤4 years; presence of ≥2 criteria on Roman III pediatric classification system for ≥1 month; ≤2 defecations per week; ≥1 episode of fecal incontinence per week; stool retentive posturing; painful or hard bowel movements; presence of large fecal mass in the rectum; large-diameter stools that may obstruct the toilet; child: ≥4 years: presence of ≥2 criteria on Roman III pediatric classification system for ≥2 months; ≤2 defecations per week; ≥1 episode of fecal incontinence per week; stool

• = Independent   ▲ = Collaborative

retentive posturing; painful or hard bowel movements; presence of large fecal mass in the rectum; large-diameter stools that may obstruct the toilet; fecal impaction; fecal incontinence (in children); leakage of stool with digital stimulation; pain with defecation; palpable abdominal mass; positive fecal occult blood test; prolonged straining; type 1 or 2 on Bristol Stool Chart; amyloidosis; anal fissure; anal stricture; autonomic neuropathy; cerebral vascular accident; chronic intestinal pseudo-obstruction; chronic renal insufficiency; colorectal cancer; dehydration; dementia; depression; dermatomyositis; diabetes mellitus; diet disproportionally high in protein and fat; extraintestinal mass; failure to thrive; habitually ignores urge to defecate; hemorrhoids; Hirschsprung's disease; hypercalcemia; hypothyroidism; impaired mobility; inflammatory bowel disease; insufficient dietary intake; insufficient fluid intake; ischemic stenosis; low caloric intake; low-fiber diet; multiple sclerosis; myotonic dystrophy; panhypopituitarism; paraplegia; Parkinson's disease; pelvic floor dysfunction; perineal damage; pharmaceutical agent; polypharmacy; porphyria; postinflammatory stenosis; pregnancy; proctitis; scleroderma; sedentary lifestyle; slow colon transit time; spinal cord injury; surgical stenosis

Client Outcomes

Client Will (Specify Time Frame)

- Maintain passage of soft, formed stool every 1 to 3 days without straining
- State relief from discomfort of constipation
- Identify measures that prevent or treat constipation

Nursing Interventions

All Client Ages

- Introduce yourself to the client and anyone accompanying him or her and inform them of your role. Introducing yourself to a client helps establish and develop a therapeutic relationship that recognizes the person within the client and forms the basis for building trust on which to base the provision of care (Howatson-Jones et al, 2012).
- Gain consent to carry out care before proceeding further with the assessment. Clients have the right of autonomy both legally and morally and therefore should be fully involved in the decision-making process (Avery, 2013)
- Wash hands using a recognized technique. Strict hand-hygiene regimens significantly reduce the incidence of methicillin-resistant *Staphylococcus aureus* and *Clostridium difficile* (Health Protection Agency, 2013).

• = Independent ▲ = Collaborative

C

- Assess usual pattern of defecation and establish the extent of the constipation problem to include:
  - Bowel habits
    - Time of day
    - Amount and frequency of stool
    - Consistency of stool (using the Bristol Stool Scale)
    - Bleeding/passing mucus on defecation
    - History of bowel habits and/or laxative use
    - Assess children younger than 4 years using the Rome III pediatric classification (for at least 1 month)
    - Assess children older than age 4 years using the Rome III pediatric classification (for at least 2 months)
    - Assess adults using the Rome III classification
  - Lifestyle assessment
    - Fiber content in diet
    - Daily fluid intake
    - Exercise patterns
    - Personal remedies for constipation
    - Recently stopped smoking
    - Alcohol consumption/recreational drug use
    - Personal habits related to defecation
  - Past medical history
    - Obstetrical/gynecological/urological history and surgeries
    - Existing anatomical anomalies (e.g., anal fissures, anal strictures, and hemorrhoids)
    - Diseases that affect bowel motility (e.g., colorectal cancer, chronic intestinal pseudo-obstruction, and Hirschsprung's disease)
    - Bleeding/passing mucus on defecation
    - Current medications
    - Established algorithms and guidelines recommend that secondary pathology and causes of constipation are identified and firstly excluded before moving on to assessment of diet and lifestyle issues (Tack et al, 2011)
  - Emotional influences
    - Anxiety and depression
    - Long-term defecation issues
    - Stress

• = Independent   ▲ = Collaborative

C

- Complete a physical assessment (palpation for abdominal distention, percussion for dullness, auscultation for bowel sounds, observation for anal fissures, anal strictures, and hemorrhoids).
- Encourage the client or family to keep a 7-day diary of bowel habits to include time of day, length of time spent on the toilet, consistency, amount and frequency of stool, and any straining (using the Bristol Stool Scale).
- Encourage the client or family to keep a 7-day diary of lifestyle issues in relation to bowel habits to include fluid consumption, fiber content in diet, usual bowel stimulus, and exercise regime.
- Actively encourage the use of reward/star charts with children when establishing regular bowel routines.
- Discuss with clients already taking opioids (temporarily or long term) that constipation is a common side effect. Advise the client to contact their primary health care provider for a prescription of an appropriate laxative.
- Advise a fiber intake of 18 to 25 g of fiber daily and suggest foodstuffs to facilitate this diet (e.g., prune juice, leafy green vegetables, wholemeal bread and pasta).
- Advise a fluid intake of 1.5 to 2 L of fluid per day (ideally, 6 to 8 glasses of water), unless this is contraindicated by comorbidities such as renal or heart disease.
- Encourage physical activity within the client's current ability to mobilize. Encourage turning and changing position in bed if immobile. For reduced mobility clients, encourage knee to chest raises, waist twists, and stretching the arms away from the body. For fully mobile clients, encourage walking and swimming.
- Demonstrate the use of gentle external abdominal massage, using aromatherapy oils, following the direction of colon activity.
- Recommend clients establish a regular elimination routine. If required, assist clients to the bathroom at the same time every day, being mindful of the need for privacy (closing of bathroom doors).
- Educate the client how to adopt the best posture for defecation: keep knees slightly higher than hips, keep feet flat on the floor and lean forward, putting elbows onto knees.
- Consider the teaching of biofeedback therapy to encourage a "new normal" bowel routine for clients to adopt.

• = Independent ▲ = Collaborative

C

- Teach clients of the need to respond promptly to the defecation urge.
- Consider the use of laxatives, suppositories, enemas, and bowel irrigation as required when other more natural interventions are not effective.
- Discourage the use of long-term laxatives and enemas, and advise clients to gradually reduce their use if taken regularly.
- Provide client with comprehensive written information about constipation and its management.
- Provide written instructions for children about taking their medication and about how the bowel works.
- Liaise with members of the interprofessional team as appropriate to provide treatment and advice to clients and caregivers.
- Educate the client on the mechanism of normal bowel function and the need for adequate fluid and fiber intake, physical activity, and a defined toileting pattern in an agreed-upon bowel management program.
- Document all care and advice given in a factual and comprehensive manner.

Perceived Constipation

NANDA-I Definition

Self-diagnosis of constipation combined with abuse of laxatives, enemas, and/or suppositories to ensure a daily bowel movement

Defining Characteristics

Enema abuse; expects a daily bowel movement; expects a daily bowel movement at the same time every day; laxative abuse; suppository abuse

Related Factors

Cultural health believes; family health beliefs; impaired thought process

Client Outcomes

Client Will (Specify Time Frame)

- Regularly defecate soft, formed stool without use of aids
- Explain the need to decrease or eliminate the use of stimulant laxatives, suppositories, and enemas
- Identify alternatives to stimulant laxatives, enemas, and suppositories for ensuring defecation
- Explain that defecation does not have to occur every day

• = Independent   ▲ = Collaborative

Nursing Interventions

- Introduce yourself to the client and any companions, and inform them of your role.
- Gain consent before proceeding further with the assessment.
- Wash hands using a recognized technique.
- Assess usual pattern of defecation and establish the extent of the perceived constipation problem to include:
  - ○ Bowel Habits
    - ○ Time of day
    - ○ Amount and frequency of stool
    - ○ Consistency of stool (using the Bristol Stool Scale)
    - ○ Bleeding/passing mucus on defecation
    - ○ Patient history of bowel habits and/or laxative use
    - ○ Family history of bowel habits and/or laxative use
  - ○ Lifestyle Assessment
    - ○ Fiber content in diet
    - ○ Daily fluid intake
    - ○ Exercise patterns
    - ○ Personal remedies for constipation
    - ○ Cultural remedies for constipation
    - ○ Recently stopped smoking
    - ○ Alcohol consumption/recreational drug use
  - ○ Past Medical History
    - ○ Obstetrical/gynecological/urological history and surgeries
    - ○ Diseases that affect bowel motility
    - ○ Bleeding/passing mucus on defecation
    - ○ Current medications
  - ○ Emotional Influences
    - ○ Anxiety and depression/psychological disorders
    - ○ History of eating disorders
    - ○ History of physical and/or sexual abuse
    - ○ Long-term defecation issues
    - ○ Stress
- Encourage the client or family to keep a 7-day diary of bowel habits to include time of day, length of time spent on the toilet, consistency, amount and frequency of stool, and any straining (using the Bristol Stool Scale).

• = Independent   ▲ = Collaborative

C

- Encourage the client or family to keep a 7-day diary of lifestyle issues in relation to bowel habits to include fluid consumption, fiber content in diet, usual bowel stimulus, and exercise regimen.
- Educate the client that it is not necessary to have a daily bowel movement.
- Encourage the client to record use of laxatives, suppositories, or enemas, and suggest replacing them with an increase in fluid and fiber intake.
- Advise a fiber intake of 18 to 25 g daily and suggest foodstuffs high in fiber (e.g., prune juice, leafy green vegetables, wholemeal bread and pasta).
- Advise a fluid intake of 1.5 to 2 L of fluid per day (ideally, 6 to 8 glasses of water), unless contraindicated by comorbidities, such as kidney or heart disease.
- Obtain a referral to a dietitian for analysis of the client's diet and fluid intake to provide strategies to improve diet and nutrition.
- Encourage physical activity within the client's current ability to mobilize. Encourage turning and changing position in bed if immobile. For clients with reduced mobility, encourage knee to chest raises, waist twists, and stretching the arms away from the body. For fully mobile clients, encourage walking and swimming.
- Demonstrate the use of gentle external abdominal massage, using aromatherapy oils, following the direction of colon activity.
- Recommend clients establish a regular elimination routine. If required, assist clients to the bathroom at the same time every day, being mindful of the need for privacy (closing of bathroom doors).
- Observe for the presence of an eating disorder and the use of laxatives to control or decrease weight; refer for counseling if needed.
- Observe family cultural patterns related to eating and bowel habits. Cultural patterns may control bowel habits.

Client/Family Teaching and Discharge Planning

- Provide education to the client on ways to adopt the best posture for defecation. Keep knees slightly higher than hips, keep feet flat on the floor, and lean forward putting elbows onto knees.
- Teach clients of the importance of responding promptly to the urge to defecate.
- Discourage the use of long-term laxatives and enemas and explain the potential harmful effects of the continual use of defecation aids such as laxatives and enemas.

• = Independent   ▲ = Collaborative

- Advise clients to gradually reduce their use of laxatives, if taken regularly, which may take months to achieve.
- Provide client with comprehensive written information about constipation and its management.
- Collaborate with members of the interprofessional team to provide treatment and advice to clients and caregivers.
- Formalize all advice by providing a bowel management program, reiterating the mechanism of normal bowel function and the need for adequate fluid and fiber intake, physical activity, and a defined toileting pattern in an agreed bowel program.
- Document all care and advice given in a factual and comprehensive manner.

Risk for Constipation
NANDA-I Definition
Vulnerable to a decrease in normal frequency of defecation accompanied by difficult or incomplete passage of stool, which may compromise health

Risk Factors
Functional
Abdominal weakness; average daily physical activity is less than recommended for gender and age; habitually ignores urge to defecate; inadequate toileting habits; irregular defecation habits; recent environmental change

Psychological
Confusion; depression; emotional disturbance

Physiological
Decrease in gastrointestinal motility; dehydration; eating habit change (e.g., foods, eating times); inadequate dentition; inadequate oral hygiene; insufficient dietary habits; insufficient fiber intake; insufficient fluid intake

Pharmacological
Iron salts; laxative abuse; pharmaceutical agent

Mechanical
Electrolyte imbalance; hemorrhoids; Hirschsprung's disease; neurological impairment (e.g., positive electroencephalogram, head trauma, seizure disorders); obesity; postsurgical obstruction; pregnancy; prostate enlargement; rectal abscess; rectal anal fissures; rectal anal stricture; rectal prolapse; rectal ulcer; rectocele; tumor

• = Independent   ▲ = Collaborative

Client Outcomes, Nursing Interventions, and Client/Family Teaching and Discharge Planning

Refer to care plans for **Constipation.**

Risk for chronic functional Constipation

NANDA-I Definition

Vulnerable to infrequent or difficult evacuation of feces, which has occurred in nearly 3 of the prior 12 months, which may compromise health

Risk Factors

Aluminum-containing antacids; antiepileptics; antihypertensives; anti-Parkinsonian agents (anticholinergic or dopaminergic); calcium-channel antagonists; chronic intestinal pseudo-obstruction; decreased food intake; dehydration; depression; diet proportionally high in protein and fat; diuretics; failure to thrive; habitual ignoring of urge to defecate; impaired mobility; low-fiber diet; insufficient fluid intake; inactive lifestyle; iron preparations; low caloric intake; nonsteroidal anti-inflammatories; opioids; polypharmacy; slow colon transit time; tricyclic antidepressants

Client Outcomes, Nursing Interventions, and Client/Family Teaching and Discharge Planning

Refer to care plan for Chronic functional **Constipation.**

Contamination

NANDA-I Definition

Exposure to environmental contaminants in doses sufficient to cause adverse health effects

Defining Characteristics

Pesticides

Dermatological effects of pesticide exposure; gastrointestinal effects of pesticide exposure; neurological effects of pesticide exposure; pulmonary effects of pesticide exposure; renal effects of pesticide exposure

Chemicals

Dermatological effects of chemical exposure; gastrointestinal effects of chemical exposure; immunological effects of chemical exposure; neurological effects of chemical exposure; pulmonary effects of chemical exposure; renal effects of chemical exposure

• = Independent ▲ = Collaborative

Biologicals

Dermatological effects of exposure to biological; gastrointestinal effects of biological exposure; neurological effects of biological exposure; pulmonary effects of biological exposure; renal effects of biological exposure

Pollution

Neurological effects of pollution exposure; pulmonary effects of pollution exposure

Waste

Dermatological effects of waste exposure; gastrointestinal effects of waste exposure; hepatic effects of waste exposure; pulmonary effects of waste exposure

Radiation

Exposure to radioactive material; genetic effects of radiation exposure; immunological effects of radiation exposure; neurological effects of radiation exposure; oncological effects of radiation exposure

Related Factors (r/t)

External

Carpeted flooring; chemical contamination of food; chemical contamination of water; economically disadvantaged; exposure to areas with high contaminant level; exposure to atmospheric pollutants; exposure to bioterrorism; exposure to disaster (natural or man-made); exposure to radiation; flaking, peeling surface in presence of young children (e.g., paint, plaster); household hygiene practices; inadequate breakdown of contaminant; inadequate municipal services (e.g., trash removal, sewage treatment facilities); inadequate protective clothing; inappropriate use of protective clothing; ingestion of contaminated material (e.g., radioactive, food, water); personal hygiene practices; playing where environmental contaminants are used; unprotected exposure to chemical (e.g., arsenic); use of environmental contaminants in the home; use of noxious material in insufficiently ventilated area (e.g., lacquer, paint); use of noxious material without effective protection (e.g., lacquer, paint)

Internal

Age (e.g., children <5 years, older adults); concomitant exposure; developmental characteristics of children; extremes of age; female gender; gestational age during exposure; inadequate nutrition; preexisting disease; pregnancy; previous exposure to contaminant; smoking

• = Independent   ▲ = Collaborative

C

Client Outcomes

Client Will (Specify Time Frame)

- Have minimal health effects associated with contamination
- Cooperate with appropriate decontamination protocol
- Participate in appropriate isolation precautions

Community Will (Specify Time Frame)

- Use health surveillance data system to monitor for contamination incidents
- Use disaster plan to evacuate and triage affected members
- Have minimal health effects associated with contamination
- Employ measures to reduce household environmental risks

Nursing Interventions

▲ Help individuals cope with contamination incident by doing the following:

- ○ Use groups that have survived terrorist attacks as useful resource for victims
- ○ Provide accurate information on risks involved, preventive measures, use of antibiotics and vaccines
- ○ Assist to deal with feelings of fear, vulnerability, and grief
- ○ Encourage individuals to talk to others about their fears
- ○ Assist victims to think positively and to move toward the future

- Triage, stabilize, transport, and treat affected community members.
- Prioritize mental health care for highly vulnerable risk groups or those with special needs (deeply affected groups, women, older persons, children and adolescents, displaced persons—especially those living in shelters, persons with preexisting mental health disorders [including those living in institutions]) (Pan American Health Organization, 2012).
- Collaborate with other agencies (local health department, emergency medical service [EMS], state and federal agencies). Use approved procedures for decontamination of persons, clothing, and equipment. Use appropriate isolation precautions: universal, airborne, droplet, and contact isolation.
- Monitor individual for therapeutic effects, side effects, and compliance with post-exposure drug therapy. Drug therapy may extend over a long period of time and requires monitoring for compliance as well as for therapeutic and side effects (Veenema, 2013).

• = Independent   ▲ = Collaborative

C

- Perform effective hand washing before and after handling medical charts, entering case notes, touching clients, and performing procedures, especially in intensive care unit environments.
- Prevent cross contamination by systematically disinfecting stethoscopes (diaphragm and tubing) after each use.
- Complete proper hand washing after touching the client's privacy curtain and before touching the client.

Geriatric
- Help the client identify age-related factors that may affect response to contamination incidents.
- Advise older adults to follow public notices related to drinking water. Encourage older adults to receive influenza vaccination when it is available, beginning as early as late August and continuing through the end of February. Instruct older adults with special needs or chronic conditions to plan for emergencies and keep medications, prescriptions, and special devices on hand (Federal Emergency Management Agency, 2014).

Pediatric
- Provide environmental health hazard information.
- Reduce risks from exposure to environmental contaminants by identifying the ages and life stages of children.
- Screen newly arrived immigrant and refugee children for elevated blood lead levels secondary to lead hazards in older housing.
- Be aware that the risk for lead exposure is much higher in many of the countries from which children are adopted than in the United States (CDC, 2014c).
- Use the latest reference level of 5 µg/dL to identify children and environments associated with lead-exposure hazards.

Multicultural
- Ask about use of imported or culture-specific products that contain lead, such as greta and azarcon (Hispanic folk medicine for upset stomach and diarrhea), ghasard (Indian folk medicine tonic), and ba-baw-san (Chinese herbal remedy).
- Nurses need to consider the cultural and social factors that impact access to and understanding of the health care system, particularly for groups such as migrant workers who do not have consistent health care providers.

• = Independent   ▲ = Collaborative

C

Home Care

- Assess current environmental stressors and identify community resources.
- Recognize that relocated and unemployed individuals/families are at risk for psychological distress.
- Support policy and program initiatives that provide emergency mental health services following large-scale contamination events.
- Instruct community members concerned about lead in drinking water from plumbing pipes and fixtures to have the water tested by calling the EPA drinking water hotline at 800-426-4791.
- Educate community members to reduce exposure to lead by inquiring about lead-based paint before buying a home or renting an apartment built before 1978; Federal law requires disclosure of known information about lead-based paint (EPA, 2014).
- Instruct individuals and families that food contamination occurs through a variety of mechanisms and that food safety is associated with proper washing of hands and utensils, prompt refrigeration of food, and cooking foods at the correct temperature.

Client/Family Teaching and Discharge Planning

- Provide truthful information to the person or family affected.
- Discuss signs and symptoms of contamination.
- Explain decontamination protocols.
- Explain need for isolation procedures.
- Emphasize the importance of pre- and post-exposure treatment of contamination.
- Provide parents with actionable information to reduce environmental contamination in the home.

Risk for Contamination

NANDA-I Definition

Vulnerable to exposure to environmental contaminants, which may compromise health

Risk Factors

External

Carpeted flooring; chemical contamination of food; chemical contamination of water; economically disadvantaged; exposure to areas with high contaminant level; exposure to atmospheric pollutants; exposure to bioterrorism; exposure to disaster (natural or man-made); exposure to radiation;

• = Independent   ▲ = Collaborative

flaking, peeling surface in presence of young children (e.g., paint, plaster); inadequate breakdown of contaminant; inadequate household hygiene practices; inadequate municipal services (e.g., trash removal, sewage treatment facilities); inadequate personal hygiene practices; inadequate protective clothing; inappropriate use of protective clothing; playing where environmental contaminants are used; unprotected exposure to chemical (e.g., arsenic); unprotected exposure to heavy metal (e.g., chromium, lead); use of environmental contaminant in the home; use of noxious material (e.g., lacquer, paint) insufficiently ventilated area; use of noxious material (e.g., lacquer, paint) without effective protection

Internal

Concomitant exposure; developmental characteristics of children; extremes of age; female gender; gestational age during exposure; inadequate nutrition; preexisting disease; pregnancy; previous exposure to contaminant; smoking

Client Outcomes, Nursing Interventions, and Client/Family Teaching and Discharge Planning

Refer to care plans for **Contamination.**

Risk for adverse reaction to iodinated Contrast Media

NANDA-I Definition

Vulnerable to noxious or unintended reaction associated with the use of iodinated contrast media that can occur within 7 days after contrast agent injection, which may compromise health

Risk Factors

Anxiety; chronic illness; concurrent use of pharmaceutical agents (e.g., beta blockers, interleukin-2, metformin nephrotoxins); contrast media precipitates adverse event (e.g., iodine concentration, viscosity, ion toxicity); dehydration; extremes of age; fragile vein (e.g., chemotherapy/radiation in limb to be injected, indwelling line for more than 24 hours, axillary lymph node dissection in limb to be injected, distal intravenous [IV] access site); generalized debilitation; history of allergy; history of previous adverse effect from iodinated contrast media; unconsciousness

Client Outcomes

Client Will (Specify Time Frame):

- Maintain normal blood urea nitrogen and serum creatinine levels
- Maintain urine output of 0.5 mL/kg/hr
- Maintain serum electrolytes (K^+, PO_4, Na^+) within normal limits

• = Independent ▲ = Collaborative

C

Nursing Interventions

Recognize that iodinated contrast media can be harmful to clients in a number of ways, including onset of contrast-induced nephropathy, allergic reactions to the dye, and damage to veins and vascular access devices.

Contrast-Induced Nephropathy (CIN)

Protect clients from contrast media–induced nephropathy by taking the following actions:

▲ Assess clients for low body mass index (BMI) or history of heart failure. Low BMI and heart failure are risk factors for CIN (Balemans et al, 2012).

▲ In nondiabetic clients with acute coronary syndrome, assess for presence of hyperglycemia on admission and report to health care provider. "[Index] admission high blood glucose in acute coronary syndrome patients not known to be diabetic is associated with increased incidence of contrast induced nephropathy after percutaneous coronary intervention" (Islam et al, 2013).

• Identify clients who have had multiple doses of iodinated contrast media in less than 24 hours and report to health care provider.

• Notify the health care provider and the radiology staff if the client has preexisting renal disease.

▲ Ensure that clients having diagnostic testing with contrast are well hydrated with isotonic IV fluids as ordered before and after the examination.

▲ Verify that a baseline serum creatinine has been drawn from clients at risk for CIN.

• Recognize that many clients with decreased renal function are not aware of their health status and that a questionnaire checklist administered before testing may not be satisfactory to determine which clients with impaired renal function should receive contrast media carefully or which are not candidates for testing utilizing contrast media.

• Be vigilant for signs of CIN in clients who have cancer.

• Monitor the client carefully for symptoms of hypovolemia following use of contrast media, including measuring intake and output, obtaining blood pressure measurements, and assessing for new onset of postural hypotension with dizziness.

• = Independent   ▲ = Collaborative

C

▲ Monitor for and report signs of acute kidney injury for 48 hours following iodinated contrast administration in clients at risk: absolute serum creatinine increase ≥ 0.3 mg/dL, percentage increase in serum creatinine $\geq 50\%$, or urine output reduced to ≤ 0.5 mL/kg/hr for at least 6 hours.

Allergic Reaction to Contrast Media

▲ Discuss premedication with steroids or diphenhydramine with health care provider for clients who have had previous reactions to contrast media.

▲ Monitor carefully for symptoms of a reaction, which can be mild, moderate, or severe. Report all symptoms to primary care provider because symptoms can advance rapidly from mild to severe.
  ○ *Mild reactions:* Urticaria, pruritus, rhinorrhea, nausea, emesis, diaphoresis, coughing, dizziness
  ○ *Moderate reactions:* Persistent emesis, widespread urticaria, headache, edema of the face, laryngeal edema, mild dyspnea, palpitations, tachycardia/bradycardia, hypertension, abdominal cramps
  ○ *Severe reactions:* Severe bronchospasm, severe arrhythmias, severe hypotension, pulmonary edema, laryngeal edema, seizures, syncope, death (Wilson, 2011)

Vein Damage and Damage to Vascular Access Devices

• Recognize that only vascular access devices labeled "power injectable" can be used to administer power-injected contrast media. These include a power port, a power PICC line, and a power central venous catheter (Radiology and Biomedical Imaging, 2014).

• Reduce the risk of vein and vascular access device damage with the following:
  ○ Maintain constant communication with the client during the injection. Discontinue the injection if the client reports pain or the sensation of swelling at the injection site.
  ○ Be vigilant in clients at increased risk of extravasation.
  ○ Assess for venous backflow before injecting contrast.
  ○ Directly monitor and palpate the venipuncture site during the first 15 seconds of injection.

• After diagnostic testing using contrast media given intravenously, inspect the IV site used for administration for possible problems, such as extravasation or development of compartment syndrome

• = Independent　　　　　▲ = Collaborative

with excessive amounts of contrast pushed into the tissues under pressure.

C

Geriatric

• Screen the older client thoroughly before diagnostic testing utilizing contrast media.

Compromised family Coping

NANDA-I Definition

A usually supportive primary person (family member, significant other, or close friend) provides insufficient, ineffective, or compromised support, comfort, assistance, or encouragement that may be needed by the client to manage or master adaptive tasks related to his or her health challenge

Defining Characteristics

Assistive behaviors by support person produce unsatisfactory results; client complaint about support person's response to health problems; client concern about support person's response to health problem; limitation in communication between support person and client; protective behavior by support person incongruent with client's abilities; protective behavior by support person incongruent with client's need for autonomy; support person reports inadequate understanding that interferes with effective behaviors; support person reports insufficient knowledge that interferes with effective behaviors; support person reports preoccupation with own reaction to client's need; support person withdraws from client

Related Factors (r/t)

Coexisting situations affecting the support person; developmental crises experienced by support person; exhaustion of support person's capacity; family disorganization; family role change; insufficient information available to support person; insufficient reciprocal support; insufficient support given by client to support person; insufficient understanding of information by support person; misinformation obtained by support person; preoccupation by support person with concern outside of family; prolonged disease that exhausts capacity of support person; situational crisis faced by support person

Client Outcomes

Family/Significant Person Will (Specify Time Frame)

• Verbalize internal resources to help deal with the situation
• Verbalize knowledge and understanding of illness, disability, or disease

• = Independent ▲ = Collaborative

- Provide support and assistance as needed
- Identify need for and seek outside support

Nursing Interventions

C

- Assess the strengths and deficiencies of the family system.
- Establish rapport with families by providing accurate communication.
- Assist family members to recognize the need for help and teach them how to ask for it.
- Encourage expression of positive thoughts and emotions to help reduce stress.
- Encourage family members to verbalize feelings. Spend time with them, sit down and make eye contact, and offer coffee and other nourishment.
- Incorporate family variables, including dyadic adjustment, into assessment protocols and intervention strategies.
- Provide privacy during family visits. If possible, maintain flexible visiting hours to accommodate more frequent family visits. If possible, arrange staff assignments so the same staff members have contact with the family. Familiarize other staff members with the situation in the absence of the usual staff member. Providing privacy, maintaining flexible hours, and arranging consistent staff assignments reduces stress, enhances communication, and facilitates the building of trust.
- Provide education to clients regarding active coping strategies to use in situations involving chronic illnesses.
- Use evidence-based tools to assess for post-intensive care syndrome (e.g., anxiety, acute stress disorder, posttraumatic stress, depression, and complicated grief) in families who have experienced a critical illness.
- Refer the family with ill family members to appropriate resources for assistance as indicated (e.g., counseling, psychotherapy, financial assistance, or spiritual support).

Pediatric

- Provide screening for postpartum depression (PPD) during the prenatal period and during the 6-week postpartum check-up to identify symptoms of depression in mothers.
- ▲ Consider medication management and psychosocial interventions, including individual therapy, group therapy, support groups, and brief psychotherapy.

• = Independent   ▲ = Collaborative

C

- ▲ Use preventive strategies, such as screening, psychoeducation, postpartum debriefing, and companionship in the delivery room (e.g., community volunteer).
- Provide educational and psychosocial interventions, such as coping skills training, in treatment for families and their adolescents who have diabetes.
- Provide readily available resources to support parents of children with autism and their families.
- Provide family-centered care during neonatal intensive care to encourage family members to play an active role in providing emotional, social, and developmental support.
- Provide evidence-based psychological therapies for parents with children with chronic conditions.
- Assist with fostering co-parenting alliances in fragile families.
- Provide options for home-based interventions when severe childhood illnesses make it difficult for children and families to participate in interventions.

Geriatric
- ▲ Perform a holistic assessment of all needs of informal spousal caregivers.
- ▲ Provide caregivers with options for Internet-based support strategies to enhance coping.
- Assist in finding transportation to enable family members to visit.
- Assist informal caregivers with reducing unmet needs by helping them obtain the information and education necessary for caring for an older adult with a chronic health condition.

Multicultural
- Acknowledge racial/ethnic differences at the onset of care.
- Assess for the influence of cultural beliefs, norms, and values on the individual/family/community's perceptions of coping.
- Use valid and culturally competent assessment tools and procedures when working with families with different racial/ethnic backgrounds.
- Provide culturally relevant interventions by understanding and using treatment strategies that are acceptable and effective for a particular culture.
- Provide opportunities for families to discuss spirituality.
- Determine how the family's cultural context impacts their decisions in regard to managing and coping with a child's illness; recognize and validate the cultural context.

• = Independent   ▲ = Collaborative

Home Care

- The interventions described previously may be adapted for home care use.
- Assess the reason behind the breakdown of family coping.
- During the time of compromised coping, increase visits to ensure the safety of the client, support of the family, and reassurance regarding expectations for prognosis as appropriate.
- ▲ Assess the needs of the caregiver in the home, and intervene to meet needs as appropriate; explore all available resources that may be used to provide adequate home care (e.g., parish nursing as an effective adjunct, home health aide services to relieve the caregiver's fatigue).
- ▲ Encourage caregivers to attend to their own physical, mental, and spiritual health, and give more specific information about the client's needs and ways to meet them.
- ▲ Refer the family to medical social services for evaluation and supportive counseling. Serve as an advocate, mentor, and role model for caregiving; provide written information for the care needed by the client.
- ▲ A positive approach and caring by the nurse and concrete task definition and assignment reinforce positive coping strategies and allow caregivers to feel less guilty when tasks are delegated to multiple caregivers.
- ▲ When a terminal illness is the precipitating factor for ineffective coping, offer hospice services and support groups as possible resources.
- Encourage the client and family to discuss changes in daily functioning and routines created by the client's illness, and validate discomfort resulting from changes. Support positive individual and family coping efforts. If compromised family coping interferes with the ability to support the client's treatment plan, refer for psychiatric home health care services for family counseling and/or Internet-based behavioral interventions.

Client/Family Teaching and Discharge Planning

- Assess for and address grief issues that arise in the process, including anticipatory grief.
- ▲ Refer women with breast cancer and their family caregivers to support groups, including social network sites and online communities, to provide assistance with daily coping.

• = Independent   ▲ = Collaborative

C

- Promote individual and family relaxation and stress-reduction strategies.
- ▲ Refer parents to support and education groups to provide opportunities for parents to access support, learn new parenting skills, and ultimately, optimize their relationships with their children after divorce.
- Provide Internet-based resources, including online social networking groups, to enhance social support, bonding, and coping for caregivers.

Defensive Coping

NANDA-I Definition

Repeated projection of falsely positive self-evaluation based on a self-protective pattern that defends against underlying perceived threats to positive self-regard

Defining Characteristics

Alteration in reality testing; denial of problems; denial of weaknesses; difficulty establishing relationships; difficulty maintaining relationships; grandiosity; hostile laughter; hypersensitivity to a discourtesy; hypersensitivity to criticism; insufficient follow-through with treatment; insufficient participation in treatment; projection of blame; projection of responsibility; rationalization of failures; reality distortion; ridicule of others; superior attitude toward others

Related Factors

Conflict between self-perception and value system; fear of failure; fear of humiliation; fear of repercussions; insufficient confidence in others; insufficient resilience; insufficient self-confidence; insufficient support system; uncertainty; unrealistic self-expectations

Client Outcomes

Client Will (Specify Time Frame)

- Acknowledge need for change in coping style
- Accept responsibility for own behavior
- Establish realistic goals with validation from caregivers
- Solicit caregiver validation in decision-making

• = Independent   ▲ = Collaborative

Nursing Interventions

- Assess for possible symptoms associated with defensive coping: depressive symptoms, excessive self-focused attention, negativism and anxiety, hypertension, posttraumatic stress disorder (e.g., exposure to terrorism), unjust world beliefs.
▲ Use cognitive behavioral interventions.
- Ask appropriate questions to assess whether denial (defensive coping) is being used in association with health problems including alcoholism, myocardial infarction (MI), or rheumatoid arthritis.
- Promote interventions with multisensory stimulation environments.
- Empower the client/caregiver's self-knowledge.

Geriatric

▲ Identify problems with alcohol in older adults with the appropriate tools and make suitable referrals.
- Encourage exercise for positive coping.
- Stimulate individual reminiscence therapy.
- Stimulate group reminiscence therapy.

Multicultural

- Acknowledge racial/ethnic differences at the onset of care.
- Assess an individual's sociocultural backgrounds in teaching self-management and self-regulation.
- Encourage the client to use spiritual coping mechanisms such as faith and prayer.
- Encourage spirituality as a source of support for coping.

Home Care

▲ Refer the client for programs that teach coping skills.

Client/Family Teaching and Discharge Planning

- Teach coping skills to clients and caregivers.
- Teach reflexive and expressive writing to address emotions.

Disabled family Coping

NANDA-I Definition

Behavior of primary person (family member, significant other, or close friend) that disables his or her capacities and/or the client's capacities to effectively address tasks essential to either person's adaptation to the health challenge

• = Independent   ▲ = Collaborative

C

Defining Characteristics

Abandonment; aggression; agitation; carrying on usual routines without regard for client's needs; client's development of dependence; depression; desertion; disregarding client's needs; distortion of reality regarding client's health problem; family behaviors that are detrimental to well-being; hostility; impaired individualization; impaired restructuring of a meaningful life for self; intolerance; neglectful care of client in regard to basic human needs; neglectful care of client in regard to illness treatment; neglectful relationships with other family members; prolonged overconcern for client; psychosomaticism; rejection; taking on illness signs of client

Related Factors (r/t)

Arbitrary handling of family's resistance to treatment; dissonant coping styles for dealing with adaptive tasks by the significant person and client; dissonant coping styles among significant people; highly ambivalent family relationships; significant person with chronically unexpressed feelings (e.g., guilt, anxiety, hostility, despair)

Client Outcomes

Family/Significant Person Will (Specify Time Frame)

- Identify normal family routines that will need to be adapted
- Participate positively in the client's care within the limits of his or her abilities
- Identify responses that may be harmful
- Acknowledge and accept the need for assistance with circumstances
- Identify appropriate activities for affected family member

Nursing Interventions

- Families dealing with life-changing illnesses should be involved with the management process from the outset of treatment. Education and counseling should be provided early and repeatedly as learning and coping needs are reassessed. Caregivers should be invited to attend therapy sessions at an early stage.
- Assess coping strategies of both the client and the spouse when managing women with breast cancer and men with prostate cancer.
- ▲ Health care practitioners should be prepared to give specific information to families regarding the trajectory of a terminal illness.
- Nurses caring for clients with terminal cancer should recognize the need to treat family caregivers as "pseudopatients."
- Provide psychosocial intervention for parents dealing with a child who is suffering from a serious illness. Allow time for parents to

• = Independent   ▲ = Collaborative

express feelings. Recognize and validate parent's feelings of anxiety, depression, and stress.
- Assess social support of family members caring for survivors of traumatic brain injuries. Facilitate realistic expectations about caregiving.
- Assist families to identify physical and mental health effects of caregiving.
- Assist family members to find professional assistance for primary stressors such as financial issues, insurance coverage, or communicating with professionals.
- Handle dysfunctional family dynamics in an open, transparent, and professional way. Remain neutral when dealing with family conflicts and avoid involvement in long-term prior conflicts.
- Respect and promote the spiritual needs of the client and family.

Pediatric
- Siblings of sick children should be considered at risk for emotional disturbances until a full assessment of the family and social support circumstances proves otherwise.
- Assist parents and children suffering from chronic illness to develop accommodative coping skills (adapting to stressors rather than attempting to change the stressors).
- Assess educational level of parents of ill children and construct parent teaching to address educational attainment.
- Assess parents of children with chronic illness for depression.
- Recognize predictors of anger in adolescents: anxiety, depression, exposure to violence, and trait anger.

Geriatric
- Assess family members who are caring for clients in long-term care facilities for compassion fatigue: symptoms include the inability to disengage from the suffering of the loved one, a growing feeling of hopelessness or despair, sadness or grief, and inattention to personal care or outside responsibilities. Encourage family members to attend to their own physical, emotional, and social needs. Develop relationships of trust with family caregivers, providing them with a sense of confidence in the level of care their loved ones will be receiving in their absence. Promote therapeutic relationships with family members who are assisting with care, allowing for sharing of concerns and emotions.
- Be aware of age-related deterioration in coping skills.

C

Multicultural
- Health care professionals working with African American adolescents who are coping with parental cancer should be sensitive to the potential for post-traumatic growth.

Home Care
The interventions described previously may be adapted for home care use.
- Assess for strain in family caregivers.

Client/Family Teaching and Discharge Planning
- Involve the client and family in the planning of care as often as possible; mutual goal setting is considered part of "client safety." Major changes in the fifth annual issuance of National Patient Safety Goals include home care, assisted living, and disease-specific care programs in 2009. An expectation is to "encourage patients' active involvement in their own care as a patient safety strategy" (The Joint Commission, 2009).
- Recognize that family decision-makers may need additional psychosocial support services.
- Educate family members regarding stress management techniques including massage and alternative therapies.

Ineffective Coping
NANDA-I Definition
Inability to form a valid appraisal of the stressors, inadequate choices of practiced responses, and/or inability to use available resources

Defining Characteristics
Alteration in concentration; alteration in sleep pattern; change in communication pattern; destructive behavior toward others; destructive behavior toward self; difficulty organizing information; fatigue; frequent illness; inability to ask for help; inability to attend to information; inability to deal with a situation; inability to meet basic needs; inability to meet role expectation; ineffective coping strategies; insufficient access of social support; insufficient goal-directed behavior; insufficient problem resolution; insufficient problem-solving skills; risk-taking behavior; substance abuse

Related Factors
Gender differences in coping strategies; high degree of threat; inability to conserve adaptive energies; inaccurate threat appraisal; inadequate confidence in ability to deal with a situation; inadequate opportunity to prepare for stressor; inadequate resources; ineffective tension-release strategies;

• = Independent   ▲ = Collaborative

insufficient sense of control; insufficient social support; maturational crisis; situational crisis; uncertainty

Client Outcomes

Client Will (Specify Time Frame)

- Use effective coping strategies
- Use behaviors to decrease stress
- Remain free of destructive behavior toward self or others
- Report decrease in physical symptoms of stress
- Report increase in psychological comfort
- Seek help from a health care professional as appropriate

Nursing Interventions

- Observe for contributing factors of ineffective coping such as poor self-concept, grief, lack of problem-solving skills, lack of support, recent change in life situation, maturational or situational crises.
- Use verbal and nonverbal therapeutic communication approaches including empathy, active listening, and confrontation to encourage the client and family to express emotions such as sadness, guilt, and anger (within appropriate limits); verbalize fears and concerns; and set goals.
- Encourage the client to describe previous stressors and the coping mechanisms used.
- Provide opportunities for the client to discuss the meaning the situation might have for the client.
- Assist the client to set realistic goals and identify personal skills and knowledge.
- Provide information regarding care before care is given.
- Discuss changes with the client before making them.
- Provide mental and physical activities within the client's ability (e.g., reading, television, radio, crafts, outings, movies, dinners out, social gatherings, exercise, sports, games).
- Discuss the client's and family's power to change a situation or the need to accept a situation.
- Offer instruction regarding alternative coping strategies.
- Encourage use of spiritual resources as desired.
- Encourage use of social support resources.
- ▲ Refer for additional or more intensive therapies as needed.

Pediatric

- Monitor the client's risk of harming self or others and intervene appropriately.

• = Independent   ▲ = Collaborative

C

- Monitor adolescents for exposure to community violence.
- Support adolescent and children's individual coping styles.
- Encourage social support, religion-based coping, and moderate aerobic exercise as appropriate.

Geriatric

▲ Assess and report possible physiological alterations (e.g., sepsis, hypoglycemia, hypotension, infection, changes in temperature, fluid and electrolyte imbalances, and use of medications with known cognitive and psychotropic side effects).
- Screen for elder neglect or other forms of elder mistreatment.
- Encourage the client to make choices (as appropriate) and participate in planning care and scheduled activities.
- Target selected coping mechanisms for older persons based on client features, use, and preferences.
- Increase and mobilize support available to older persons by encouraging a variety of mechanisms involving family, friends, peers, and health care providers.
- Actively listen to complaints and concerns.
- Engage the client in reminiscence.

Multicultural

- Assess for the influence of cultural beliefs, norms, and values on the client's perceptions of effective coping.
- Assess the influence of fatalism and/or passivity on the client's coping behavior.
- Assess for intergenerational family problems that can overwhelm coping abilities.
- Negotiate with the client with regard to the aspects of coping behavior that will need to be modified.
- Encourage moderate aerobic exercise or other forms of physical activity (as appropriate).
- Identify which family members the client can count on for support.
- Support the inner resources that clients use for coping.
- Use an empowerment framework to redefine coping strategies.

Home Care

- The interventions described previously may be adapted for home care use.
- Discuss preferred coping strategies of family caregivers.
- Encourage the client to participate knowingly in their care. Refer to the care plan for **Powerlessness.**

• = Independent   ▲ = Collaborative

▲ Refer the client and family to support groups.
▲ If monitoring medication use, contract with the client or solicit assistance from a responsible caregiver.
▲ Institute case management for frail elderly clients to support continued independent living.

Client/Family Teaching and Discharge Planning

• Teach the client to problem solve. Have the client define the problem and cause, and list the advantages and disadvantages of the options.
• Teach relaxation techniques.
• Work closely with the client to develop appropriate educational tools that address individualized needs.
▲ Teach the client about available community resources (e.g., therapists, ministers, counselors, self-help groups).

Ineffective community Coping

NANDA-I Definition

A pattern of community activities for adaptation and problem solving that is unsatisfactory for meeting the demands or needs of the community

Defining Characteristics

Community does not meet expectations of its members; deficient community participation; elevated community illness rate; excessive community conflict; excessive stress; high incidence of community problems (e.g., homicides, vandalism, terrorism, robbery, abuse, unemployment, poverty, militancy, mental illness); perceived community powerlessness; perceived community vulnerability

Related Factors

Exposure to disaster (natural or man-made); history of disaster (e.g., natural, man-made); inadequate resources for problem solving; insufficient community resources (e.g., respite, recreation, social support); nonexistent community systems

Community Outcomes

A Broad Range of Community Members Will (Specify Time Frame)

• Participate in community actions to improve power resources
• Develop improved communication among community members
• Participate in problem solving
• Demonstrate cohesiveness in problem solving
• Develop new strategies for problem solving
• Express power to deal with change and manage problems

• = Independent   ▲ = Collaborative

Nursing Interventions

NOTE: The diagnosis of Ineffective **Coping** does not apply and should not be used when stress is being imposed by external sources or circumstances. If the community is a victim of circumstances, using the nursing diagnosis Ineffective **Coping** is equivalent to blaming the victim. See the care plan for Readiness for enhanced community **Coping.**

▲ Establish a collaborative partnership with the community (see the care plan for Readiness for enhanced community **Coping** for additional references).
• Assist the community with team building.
• Participate with community members in the identification of stressors and assessment of distress; for example, observe and participate in faith-based organizations that want to improve community stress management.
▲ Identify the health services and information resources that are currently available in the community.
▲ Consult with community mediation services, for example, the National Association of Community Mediation.
• Work with community members to increase awareness of ineffective coping behaviors (e.g., conflicts that prevent community members from working together, anger and hate that paralyze the community, health risk behaviors of adolescents).
• Provide support to the community and help community members identify and mobilize additional supports.
• Advocate for the community in multiple arenas (e.g., television, newspapers, and governmental agencies).
• Write grant proposals to help community members obtain funds for programs that reduce stress or improve coping.
• Work with members of the community to identify and develop coping strategies that promote a sense of power (e.g., obtaining sources for funding, collaborating with other communities).
• Protect children from exposure to community conflicts.

Multicultural

• Acknowledge the stressors unique to racial/ethnic communities.
• Identify community strengths with community members.
• Work with members of the community to prioritize and target health goals specific to the community.

• = Independent   ▲ = Collaborative

- Establish and sustain partnerships with key individuals within
  communities when developing and implementing programs.
- Use mentoring strategies for community members.
- Use community church settings as a forum for advocacy, teaching,
  and program implementation.

Community Teaching
- Teach strategies for stress management.
- Explain the relationship between enhancing power resources and
  coping.

Readiness for enhanced Coping

NANDA-I Definition

A pattern of cognitive and behavioral efforts to manage demands related
to well-being, which can be strengthened

Defining Characteristics

Awareness of possible environmental change; expresses desire to enhance
knowledge of stress management strategies; expresses desire to enhance
management of stressors; expresses desire to enhance social support;
expresses desire to enhance use of emotion-oriented strategies; expresses
desire to enhance use of problem-oriented strategies; expresses desire to
enhance use of spiritual resources

Client Outcomes

Client Will (Specify Time Frame)
- Acknowledge personal power
- State awareness of possible environmental changes that may contribute
  to decreased coping
- State that stressors are manageable
- Seek new effective coping strategies
- Seek social support for problems associated with coping
- Demonstrate ability to cope, using a broad range of coping strategies
- Use spiritual support of personal choice

Nursing Interventions

- Assess and support positive psychological strengths, that is, hope,
  optimism, self-efficacy, resiliency, and social support.
- Be physically and emotionally present for the client while using a
  variety of therapeutic communication techniques.

• = Independent ▲ = Collaborative

- Empower the client to set realistic goals and to engage in problem solving.
- Encourage expression of positive thoughts and emotions.
- Encourage the client to use spiritual coping mechanisms such as faith and prayer.
- Encourage the client to visit favorite natural settings or to have access to a window or pictures and sounds of nature.
- Help the client with serious and chronic conditions such as depression, cancer diagnosis, and chemotherapy treatment to maintain social support networks or assist in building new ones.
▲ Refer women facing diagnostic and curative breast cancer surgery for psychosocial support.
▲ Refer for cognitive-behavioral therapy (CBT) to enhance coping skills. Refer to the care plans for Readiness for enhanced **Communication** and Readiness for enhanced **Spiritual** well-being.

Pediatric

- Encourage children and adolescents to engage in diversional activities and exercise to promote self-esteem, enhance coping, and prevent behavioral and other physical and psychosocial problems.
- Encourage families of children with chronic illness to try additional coping strategies.

Geriatric

- Encourage active, meaning-based coping strategies for older adults with chronic illness.
- Consider the use of Web-based and technological resources for older adults in the community.
- Refer the older client to self-help support groups that address health, psychosocial, and/or social support.
▲ Refer the client with Alzheimer's disease who is terminally ill to hospice.

Multicultural

- Assess an individual's sociocultural backgrounds to identify factors that support coping.
- Encourage spirituality as a source of support for coping.
- Facilitate positive ethnocultural identity to enhance coping.
- Foster intergenerational support. Refer to the care plan for Ineffective **Coping.**

• = Independent ▲ = Collaborative

Home Care

- The interventions described previously may be adapted for home care use.
- Engage both clients and their caregivers as a dyad.
- Provide an Internet-based health coach to encourage self-management for clients with chronic conditions such as depression, impaired mobility, and chronic pain.
- Refer the client to mutual health support groups.
- Refer prostate cancer clients and their spouses to family programs that include family-based interventions of communication, hope, coping, uncertainty, and symptom management.
- ▲ Refer combat veterans and service members directly involved in combat as well as those providing support to combatants, including nurses for mental health services.

Client/Family Teaching and Discharge Planning

- Teach the client about available community resources (e.g., therapists, ministers, counselors, self-help groups, family education groups).
- Teach caregivers using a variety of interventions that contribute to coping.
- Teach expressive writing, journaling, and education about emotions.

Readiness for enhanced community Coping

NANDA-I Definition

A pattern of community activities for adaptation and problem solving for meeting the demands or needs of the community, which can be strengthened

Defining Characteristics

Expresses desire to enhance availability of community recreation programs; expresses desire to enhance availability of community relaxation programs; expresses desire to enhance communication among community members; expresses desire to enhance communication between aggregates and larger community; expresses desire to enhance community planning for predictable stressors; expresses desire to enhance community resources for managing stressors; expresses desire to enhance community responsibility for stress management; expresses desire to enhance problem solving for identified issue

• = Independent   ▲ = Collaborative

C

Community Outcomes

Community Will (Specify Time Frame)
- Develop enhanced coping strategies
- Maintain effective coping strategies for management of stress

Nursing Interventions

NOTE: Interventions depend on the specific aspects of community coping that can be enhanced (e.g., planning for stress management, communication, development of community power, community perceptions of stress, community coping strategies).

- Describe the roles of community/public health nurses in working with healthy communities.
- Help the community obtain funds for additional programs, or identify resources to assist in the funding of additional programs.
- Encourage positive attitudes toward the community through the media and other sources.
- Help community members collaborate with one another for power enhancement and coping skills.
- Assist community members with cognitive skills and habits of mind for problem solving. Teach critical thinking and strategizing skills to help open lines of communication and facilitate participation.
- Demonstrate optimum use of power resources.
- Reduce poverty whenever possible.
- ▲ Collaborate with community members to improve educational levels within the community.

Multicultural
- Refer to care plan for Ineffective community **Coping**.

Client/Family Teaching and Discharge Planning
- Review coping skills, power for coping, and the use of power resources.

Readiness for enhanced family Coping

NANDA-I Definition

A pattern of management of adaptive tasks by primary person (family member, significant other, or close friend) involved with the client's health change, which can be strengthened

• = Independent   ▲ = Collaborative

Defining Characteristics

Expresses desire to acknowledge growth impact of crisis; expresses desire to choose experiences that optimize wellness; expresses desire to enhance connection with others who have experienced a similar situation; expresses desire to enhance enrichment of lifestyle; expresses desire to enhance health promotion

Client Outcomes

Client Will (Specify Time Frame):

State a plan indicating coping strengths, abilities, and resources as well as areas for growth and change; Perform tasks and engage resources needed for growth and change; Evaluate changes and continually reevaluate plan for continued growth

Nursing Interventions

▲ Assess the structure, resources, and coping abilities of families and use these assessments in selecting interventions and formulating care plans.

▲ Acknowledge, assess, and support the spiritual needs and resources of families and clients.

▲ Establish rapport with families and empower their decision-making through effective, accurate, and empathic communication.

▲ Provide family members with educational and skill-building interventions to alleviate caregiving stress and to facilitate adherence to prescribed plans of care.

▲ Develop, provide, and encourage family members to use counseling services and interventions.

▲ Identify and refer to support programs that discuss experiences and challenges similar to those faced by the family (e.g., cancer support groups).

▲ Incorporate the use of emerging technologies to increase the reach of interventions to support family coping.

▲ Refer to Compromised family **Coping** for additional interventions.

Pediatric

▲ Identify and assess the management styles of families and facilitate the use of more effective ways of coping with childhood illness.

▲ Provide educational and supportive interventions for families caring for children with illness and disability.

Geriatric

▲ Encourage family caregivers to participate in counseling and support groups.

• = Independent   ▲ = Collaborative

▲ Provide educational and therapeutic interventions caregivers that focus on knowledge and skill building to family.

Multicultural

▲ Acknowledge and understand the importance of cultural influences in families and ensure that assessments and assessment tools account for such cultural differences.

▲ Understand and incorporate cultural differences into interventions to enhance the impact of family interventions.

Readiness for enhanced Decision-Making

NANDA-I Definition

A pattern of choosing a course of action for meeting short- and long-term health-related goals, which can be strengthened

Defining Characteristics

Expresses desire to enhance congruency of decisions with sociocultural goal; expresses desire to enhance congruency of decisions with sociocultural values; expresses desire to enhance congruency of decisions with goal; expresses desire to enhance congruency of decisions with values; expresses desire to enhance decision-making; expresses desire to enhance risk-benefit analysis of decisions; expresses desire to enhance understanding of choices for decision-making; expresses desire to enhance understanding of meaning of choices; expresses desire to enhance use of reliable evidence for decisions

Client Outcomes

Client Will (Specify Time Frame)

- Review treatment options with providers
- Ask questions about the benefits and risks of treatment options
- Communicate decisions about treatment options to providers in relation to personal preferences, values, and goals

Nursing Interventions

- Support and encourage clients and their representatives to engage in health care decisions.
- Respect personal preferences, values, needs, and rights.
- Determine the degree of participation desired by the client.
- Provide information that is appropriate, relevant, and timely.

• = Independent   ▲ = Collaborative

D

- Determine the health literacy of clients and their representatives before helping with decision-making.
- Tailor information to the specific needs of individual clients, according to principles of health literacy.
- Motivate clients to be as independent as possible in decision-making.
- Identify the client's level of choice in decision-making.
- Focus on the positive aspects of decision-making rather than the decisional conflicts.
- Design educational interventions for decision support.
- Acknowledge the complexity of everyday self-care decisions related to self-management of chronic illnesses.

Geriatric
- The above interventions may be adapted for geriatric use.
- Facilitate collaborative decision-making.

Multicultural
- Use existing decision aids for particular types of decisions or develop decision aids as indicated.

Home Care
- The above interventions may be adapted for home care use.
- Develop clinical practice guidelines that include shared decision-making.

Impaired emancipated Decision-Making

NANDA-I Definition

A process of choosing a health care decision that does not include personal knowledge and/or consideration of social norms, or does not occur in a flexible environment resulting in decisional dissatisfaction

Defining Characteristics

Delay in enacting chosen health care option; distress when listening to others' opinion; excessive concern about what others think is the best decision; excessive fear of what others think about a decision; feeling constrained in describing own opinion; inability to choose a health care option that best fits current lifestyle; limited verbalization about health care option in others' presence

• = Independent   ▲ = Collaborative

Related Factors

Decrease in understanding of all available health care options; inability to adequately verbalize perceptions about health care options; inadequate time to discuss health care options; insufficient privacy to openly discuss health care options; limited decision-making experience; traditional hierarchical family; traditional hierarchical health care system

Client Outcomes

Client Will (Specify Time Frame)

- Verbalize option outcomes freely before making a health care decision
- Freely verbalize own opinion with health care providers before making a health care decision
- Choose the health care option that fits his or her lifestyle within an appropriate amount of time that allows enactment of the choice
- Describe how the chosen option fits into his or her current lifestyle before or after the decision has been made
- Verbalizes appropriate concern about others' opinions before making the health care choice
- Remains stress-free when listening to others' opinions before making the health care choice
- Arrives at a decision in a timely manner

Nursing Interventions

- Assess client's readiness to openly discussing the decision-making process.
- Use active listening in a nonjudgmental manner to provide the client with a flexible decision-making environment. Use anticipatory guidance by proactively providing the client with information.
- Establish a purposeful provider-client relationship.
- ▲ Refer to counseling as needed.
- Provide decision-making support.
- Provide a flexible environment by encouraging others to accept client's choice.
- Encourage the client to use personal knowledge as part of the decision-making process to increase decisional satisfaction.

Pediatric

- When able, involve client in health care decision-making when possible.
- Provide parental information in the decision-making process.

• = Independent   ▲ = Collaborative

Critical Care
- Enhance client decision-making in the critical care setting.
Geriatric
- Include geriatric clients in the decisional process.
- Include family in the decision-making process when needed.
Multicultural
- Consider cultural influences on decision-making.
Home Care
- Use open communication to assist clients to develop health care plans to which they can adhere.

Readiness for enhanced emancipated Decision-Making

NANDA-I Definition

A process of choosing a health care decision that includes personal knowledge and/or consideration of social norms, which can be strengthened

Defining Characteristics

Expresses desire to enhance ability to choose health care options that best fit current lifestyle; expresses desire to enhance ability to enact chosen health care option; expresses desire to enhance ability to understand all available health care options; expresses desire to enhance ability to verbalize own opinion without constraint; expresses desire to enhance comfort to verbalize health care options in the presence of others; expresses desire to enhance confidence in decision-making; expresses desire to enhance confidence to discuss health care options openly; expresses desire to enhance decision making; expresses desire to enhance privacy to discuss health care options

Client Outcomes

Client Will (Specify Time Frame)
- Verbalize option of outcomes freely before making a health care decision
- Freely verbalize own opinion with health care providers before making a health care decision
- Choose the health care option that best fits his or her lifestyle within an appropriate amount of time that allows enactment of the choice
- Describe how the chosen option fits into his or her current lifestyle before or after the decision has been made

• = Independent ▲ = Collaborative

- Verbalizes appropriate concern about others' opinions before making the health care choice
- Remains stress-free when listening to others' opinions before making the health care choice
- Arrives at a decision in a timely manner

Nursing Interventions

- Assess client's readiness to choose through active listening.
- Use anticipatory guidance by proactively providing the client with information. (Refer to Impaired emancipated **Decision-Making**.)
- Establish a purposeful provider-client relationship.
- ▲ Include interdisciplinary health care professionals as needed to increase knowledge of chosen option.
- Provide decision-making support. (Refer to Impaired emancipated **Decision-Making**.)
- Continue to provide a flexible environment for client to enact choice.
- Encourage the client to use personal knowledge as part of the decision-making process to increase decisional satisfaction.

Pediatric

- Understand interventions that parents prefer when in the decision-making process.

Multicultural

- Use open communication to assist clients to develop health care plans to which they can adhere.

Home Care

- Optimize self-care personal knowledge for home care.
- Refer to care plan for Impaired emancipated **Decision-Making** for additional interventions for pediatric, critical care, geriatric, and multicultural care.

Risk for impaired emancipated Decision-Making

NANDA-I Definition

Vulnerable to the process of choosing a health care decision that does not include personal knowledge and/or considerations of social norms, or does not occur in a flexible environment, resulting in decisional satisfaction

Risk Factors

Inadequate time to discuss health care options; insufficient confidence to openly discuss health care options; insufficient information regarding

• = Independent   ▲ = Collaborative

health care options; insufficient privacy to openly discuss health care options; insufficient self-confidence in decision-making; limited decision-making experience; traditional hierarchical family; traditional hierarchical health care systems

D

Client Outcomes

Client Will (Specify Time Frame)

- Verbalize option outcomes freely before making a health care decision in a private setting with whom he or she feels comfortable
- Freely verbalize own opinion with health care providers before making a health care decision
- Discuss how options fit or hinder his or her lifestyle within an appropriate amount of time that allows enactment of the choice
- Discuss concerns about others' opinions before making the health care choice
- Decrease stress about others' opinions by placing options in perspective through informational resources
- Discuss the time frame in which the decision needs to be made

Nursing Interventions

- Assess client's vulnerability for an impaired decision-making process.
- Assess the client's experience with decision-making.
- Recognize traditional hierarchical family and health care systems.
- Provide privacy to discuss health care options.
- Allow the client time to choose.
- ▲ Understand primary care providers' role in the decision-making process.
- Provide informational resources.
- Provide encouragement so clients increase their confidence in the decision-making process.

Pediatric

- Understand the parent/guardian's vulnerability when making health care decisions for their children.
- Understand adolescent decision-making processes.
- Refer to care plan Impaired emancipated **Decision-Making** for additional interventions for critical, geriatric, multicultural, and home care.

• = Independent   ▲ = Collaborative

D

Decisional Conflict

NANDA-I Definition

Uncertainty about course of action to be taken when choice among competing actions involves risk, loss, or challenge to values and beliefs

Defining Characteristics

Delay in decision-making; distress while attempting a decision; physical sign of distress (e.g., increase in heart rate, restlessness); physical sign of tension; questioning of moral principle while attempting a decision; questioning of moral rule while attempting a decision; questioning of moral values while attempting a decision; questioning of personal beliefs while attempting a decision; questioning of personal values while attempting a decision; recognizes undesired consequences of actions being considered; self-focused; uncertainty about choices; vacillating among choices

Related Factors (r/t)

Conflict with moral obligation; conflicting information sources; inexperience with decision-making; insufficient information; insufficient support system; interference in decision-making; moral principle supports mutually inconsistent actions; moral rule supports mutually inconsistent actions; moral value supports mutually inconsistent actions; perceived threat to value system; unclear personal beliefs; unclear personal values

Client Outcomes

Client Will (Specify Time Frame)

- State the advantages and disadvantages of choices
- Share fears and concerns regarding choices and responses of others
- Seek resources and information necessary for making an informed choice
- Make an informed choice

Nursing Interventions

- Observe for factors causing or contributing to conflict (e.g., value conflicts, fear of outcome, poor problem-solving skills).
- Provide emotional support.
- Use decision aids or computer-based decision aids to assist clients in making decisions.
- Initiate health teaching and referrals when needed.
- Facilitate communication between the client and family members regarding the final decision; offer support to the person actually making the decision.

• = Independent   ▲ = Collaborative

D

Geriatric
- Carefully assess clients with dementia regarding ability to make decisions.
- Support previous wishes for clients with dementia.
- Discuss the purpose of advance directives such as a living will or medical power of attorney.

Multicultural
- Assess for the influence of cultural beliefs, norms, and values on the client's decision-making conflict.
- Provide support for client's decision-making.
- Use cross-cultural decision aids when possible to enhance an informed decision-making process.

Home Care
- The interventions described previously may be adapted for home care use.
- ▲ Before providing any home care, assess the client plan for advance directives (living will and power of attorney). If a plan exists, place a copy in the client file. If no plan exists, offer information on advance directives according to agency policy. Refer for assistance in completing advance directives as necessary. Do not witness a living will.
- Assess the client and family for consensus (or lack thereof) regarding the issue in conflict.
- Refer to care plan for **Anxiety** as indicated.

Client/Family Teaching and Discharge Planning
- Instruct the client and family members to provide advance directives in the following areas:
  - ○ Person to contact in an emergency
  - ○ Preference (if any) to die at home or in the hospital
  - ○ Desire to initiate advanced directives, such as a living will or medical power of attorney
  - ○ Desire to donate an organ
  - ○ Funeral arrangements (i.e., burial, cremation)
- Inform the family of treatment options; encourage and defend self-determination.
- Recognize and allow the client to discuss the selection of complementary therapies available, such as spiritual support, relaxation, imagery, exercise, lifestyle changes, diet (e.g., macrobiotic, vegetarian), and nutritional supplementation.

• = Independent   ▲ = Collaborative

▲ Provide the Physician Orders for Life-Sustaining Treatment (POLST) form for clients and families faced with end-of-life choices across the health care continuum.

D

Ineffective Denial
NANDA-I Definition

Conscious or unconscious attempt to disavow the knowledge or meaning of an event to reduce anxiety and/or fear, leading to the detriment of health

Defining Characteristics

Delays seeking health care; denies fear of death; denies fear of invalidism; displaces fear of impact of the condition; displaces source of symptoms; does not admit impact of disease on life; does not perceive relevance of danger; does not perceive relevance of symptoms; inappropriate affect; minimizes symptoms; refusal of health care; use of dismissive gestures when speaking of distressing event; use of dismissive comments when speaking of distressing event; use of treatment not advised by health care professional

Related Factors (r/t)

Anxiety; excessive stress; fear of death; fear of loss of autonomy; fear of separation; ineffective coping strategies; insufficient emotional support; insufficient sense of control; perceived inadequacy in dealing with strong emotions; threat of unpleasant reality

Client Outcomes

Client Will (Specify Time Frame)

- Seek out appropriate health care attention when needed
- Use home remedies only when appropriate
- Display appropriate affect and verbalize fears
- Actively engage in treatment program related to identified "substance" of abuse
- Remain substance-free
- Demonstrate alternate adaptive coping mechanism

Nursing Interventions

- Assess the client's and family's understanding of the illness, the treatments, and expected outcomes.
- Allow client time for adjustment to his/her situation.
- Aid the client in making choices regarding treatment and actively involve him or her in the decision-making process.

• = Independent ▲ = Collaborative

- Allow the client to express and use denial as a coping mechanism if appropriate to treatment.
- Support the client's spiritual coping measures.
- Develop a trusting, therapeutic relationship with the client/family.
- Assist the client in using existing and additional sources of support.
- Refer to care plans for Defensive **Coping** and Dysfunctional **Family** processes.

Geriatric

- Allow the client to explain his/her concepts of their health care needs, then use reality-focused techniques whenever possible to provide feedback.
- Encourage communication among family members.
- Recognize denial and be aware that grieving may prolong denial.

Multicultural

- Assess for the influence of cultural beliefs, norms, and values involved in the client's understanding of and ability to acknowledge health status.
- Discuss with the client those aspects of his/her health behavior/ lifestyle that will remain unchanged by health status and those aspects of health behavior that need to be modified to improve health status.
- Assess the role of fatalism in the client's ability to acknowledge health status.

Home Care

- Previously mentioned interventions may be adapted for home care utilization.
- Observe family interaction and roles. Refer the client/family for follow-up if prolonged denial is a risk.
- Encourage communication between family members, particularly when dealing with the loss of a significant person.

Client/Family Teaching and Discharge Planning

- Instruct client and family to recognize the signs and symptoms of recurring illness and the appropriate responses to alteration in client's health status.
- Consider the client's belief in and use of complementary therapies in self-managing his/her disease.
- Teach family members that denial may continue throughout the adjustment to treatment and they should not be confrontational.
- ▲ Inform family of available community support resources.

• = Independent   ▲ = Collaborative

Impaired Dentition

NANDA-I Definition

Disruption in tooth development/eruption patterns or structural integrity of individual teeth

Defining Characteristics

Abraded teeth; absence of teeth; dental caries; enamel discoloration; erosion of enamel; excessive oral calculus; excessive oral plaque; facial asymmetry; halitosis; incomplete tooth eruption for age; loose tooth; malocclusion; premature loss of primary teeth; root caries; tooth fracture; tooth misalignment; toothache

Related Factors (r/t)

Barriers to self-care; bruxism; chronic vomiting; difficulty accessing dental care; economically disadvantaged; excessive intake of fluoride; excessive use of abrasive oral cleaning agents; genetic predisposition; habitual use of staining substance (e.g., coffee, red wine, tea, tobacco); insufficient dietary habits; insufficient knowledge of dental health; insufficient oral hygiene; malnutrition; oral temperature sensitivity; pharmaceutical agent

Client Outcomes

Client Will (Specify Time Frame)

- Have clean teeth, healthy pink gums
- Be free of halitosis
- Explain how to perform oral care
- Demonstrate ability to masticate foods without difficulty
- State free of pain in mouth

Nursing Interventions

▲ Inspect oral cavity/teeth at least once daily and note any discoloration, presence of debris, amount of plaque buildup, presence of lesions such as white lesions or patches, edema, or bleeding, and intactness of teeth. Refer to a dentist or periodontist as appropriate.

- If the client is free of bleeding disorders and is able to swallow, encourage the client to brush teeth with a soft toothbrush using fluoride-containing toothpaste at least two times per day. Do not use foam swabs or lemon glycerin swabs to clean the teeth.
- Encourage the client to floss the teeth at least once per day if free of a bleeding disorder, or if the client is unable, floss the teeth for the client.
- Use a rotation-oscillation power toothbrush for removal of dental plaque.

• = Independent   ▲ = Collaborative

- Determine the client's mental status and manual dexterity; if the client is unable to care for self, nursing personnel must provide dental hygiene. The nursing diagnosis Bathing **Self-Care** deficit is then applicable.
- If the client is unable to brush own teeth, follow this procedure:
  1. Position the client sitting upright or on side.
  2. Use a soft bristle baby toothbrush.
  3. Use fluoride toothpaste and tap water or saline as a solution.
  4. Brush teeth in an up-and-down manner.
  5. Suction as needed.
- Monitor the client's nutritional and fluid status to determine if adequate. Recommend the client eat a balanced diet and limit between-meal snacks.
- Recommend the client stop or at least decrease intake of soft drinks.
- Instruct the client with halitosis to clean the tongue when performing oral hygiene. Brush tongue with a tongue scraper or toothbrush and follow with a mouth rinse.
- Determine the client's usual method of oral care. Whenever possible, build on the client's existing knowledge base and current practices to develop an individualized plan of care.
- Tell the client to direct the toothbrush at a 45-degree angle toward the tooth surfaces, not horizontally (ADA, 2015).
- Use an antimicrobial mouthwash as ordered or tap water or saline only for a mouth rinse. Avoid the use of hydrogen peroxide or alcohol-based mouthwashes.
- ▲ Recommend client see a dentist at prescribed intervals, generally two times per year if teeth are in satisfactory condition.
- ▲ If there are any signs of bleeding when the teeth are brushed, refer the client to a dentist or, if obvious signs of inflamed gums, a periodontist. Bleeding along with halitosis is associated with gingivitis. If platelet numbers are decreased, or if the client is edentulous, use moistened Toothettes or a specially made very soft toothbrush for oral care.
- Recognize that good dental care/oral care can be effective in preventing hospital-acquired (or extended care–acquired) pneumonia.
- Provide scrupulous dental care to critically ill clients, including ventilated clients to prevent ventilator-associated pneumonia.
- If teeth are nonfunctional for chewing, modification of oral intake (e.g., edentulous diet, soft diet) may be necessary. The nursing

• = Independent   ▲ = Collaborative

diagnosis Imbalanced **Nutrition:** less than body requirements may apply.
- If the client is unable to swallow, keep suction nearby when providing oral care.
- See care plan for Impaired **Oral Mucous Membrane.**

Pregnant Client
- Encourage the expectant mother to eat a healthy, balanced diet that is rich in calcium. The teeth usually start to form in the gums during the second trimester of pregnancy.
- Advise the pregnant mother not to smoke.
- Advise the expectant mother to practice good care of her teeth, to protect her child's teeth once born.

Infant Oral Hygiene
- Gently wipe baby's gums with a clean washcloth or sterile gauze at least once a day.
- Never allow the child to fall asleep with a bottle containing milk, formula, fruit juice, or sweetened liquids. If the child needs a comforter between regular feedings, at night, or during naps, fill a bottle with cool water or give the child a clean pacifier recommended by the dentist or health care provider. Never give child a pacifier dipped in any sweet liquid. Avoid filling child's bottle with liquids such as sugar water and soft drinks.
▲ When multiple teeth appear, brush with small toothbrush with small (pea-size) amount of fluoride toothpaste. Recommend that child either use a fluoride gel or fluoride varnish.
- Advise parents to begin dental visits at 1 year of age.

Older Children
▲ Encourage the family to talk with the dentist about dental sealants, which can help prevent cavities in permanent teeth.
- Teach to brush teeth twice a day.
- Recommend the child use dental floss to help prevent gum disease. The dentist will give guidelines on when to start using floss.
- Recommend to parents that they not permit the child to smoke or chew tobacco, and stress the importance of setting a good example by not using tobacco products themselves.
- Recommend the child drink fluoridated water when possible. Fluoride in drinking water is one of several available fluoride resources.
- Recommend the child use toothpaste containing fluoride.

• = Independent   ▲ = Collaborative

Geriatric

- Provide dentists with accurate medication history to avoid drug interactions and client harm. If the client is taking anticoagulants, the INR should be reviewed before providing dental care.
- Help clients brush own teeth, or provide dental care after breakfast and before bed every day.
- If the client has dementia or delirium and exhibits care-resistant behavior such as fighting, biting, or refusing care, use the following method:
  1. Ensure client is in a quiet environment such as own bathroom, sitting or standing at the sink to prime memory for appropriate actions.
  2. Approach the client at eye level within his/her range of vision.
  3. Approach with a smile, and begin conversation with a touch of the hand and gradually move up.
  4. Use mirror-mirror technique, standing behind the client, and brush and floss teeth.
  5. Use respectful adult speech, not elderspeak/sing-song voice, calling "deary," "honey," or the like.
  6. Promote self-care when client brushes own teeth if possible.
  7. Use distractors when needed, singing, talking, reminiscing, or use of a teddy bear.
- ▲ Ensure that dentures are removed and cleaned regularly, preferably after every meal and before bedtime. Soak dentures at night in cold water. Dentures left in the mouth at night impede circulation to the palate and predispose the client to oral lesions.
- ▲ Support other caregivers providing oral hygiene. Physical and cognitive impairment in older adults can interfere with the client's ability to perform oral hygiene, and oral hygiene should be provided by a caregiver. If no caregiver is available, the client is prone to dental problems such as dental caries, tooth abscess, tooth fracture, and gingival and periodontal disease.

Multicultural

- Assess for the influence of cultural beliefs, norms, and values on the client's understanding of dental care.
- Assess for barriers to access to dental care, such as lack of insurance.

• = Independent   ▲ = Collaborative

D

Home Care

- Assess client patterns for daily and professional dental care and related patterns (e.g., smoking, nail biting). Assess for environmental influences on dental status (e.g., fluoride).
- Assess client facilities and financial resources for providing dental care.
- Request dietary log from the client, adding column for type of food (i.e., soft, pureed, regular).
- Observe a typical meal to assess first-hand the impact of impaired dentition on nutrition.
- Assist the client with accessing financial or other resources to support optimum dental and nutritional status.

Client/Family Teaching and Discharge Planning

- Teach how to inspect the oral cavity and monitor for problems with the teeth and gums.
- Teach how to implement a personal plan of dental hygiene, including appropriate brushing of teeth and tongue and use of dental floss. Utilize motivational interviewing to facilitate increased compliance in dental care.
- Advise the clients to change their toothbrush every 3 to 4 months, because after that toothbrushes are less effective in removing plaque and are a source of bacterial contamination of the mouth and teeth (ADA, 2015).
- Teach the client the value of having an optimal fluoride concentration in drinking water, and to brush teeth twice daily with toothpaste containing fluoride.
- Teach clients of all ages the need to decrease intake of sugary foods and to brush teeth regularly.
- Inform individuals who are considering tongue piercing of the potential complications such as chipping and cracking of teeth and possible trauma to the gingiva. If piercing is done, teach the client how to care for the wound and prevent complications.

Risk for delayed Development

NANDA-I Definition

Vulnerable to delay of 25% or more in one or more of the areas of social or self-regulatory behavior, or in cognitive, language, gross, or fine motor skills, which may compromise health

• = Independent   ▲ = Collaborative

Risk Factors
Prenatal
Economically disadvantaged; endocrine disorder; functional illiteracy; genetic disorder; infection; inadequate nutrition; insufficient prenatal care; late-term prenatal care; maternal age ≤15 years; maternal age ≥35 years; substance abuse; unplanned pregnancy; unwanted pregnancy

Individual
Behavior disorder (e.g., attention deficit, oppositional defiant); brain injury (e.g., abuse, accident, hemorrhage, shaken baby syndrome); chronic illness; congenital disorder; failure to thrive; genetic disorder; hearing impairment; history of adoption; inadequate nutrition; involvement with the foster care system; lead poisoning; natural disaster; positive drug screen; prematurity; recurrent otitis media; seizure disorder; substance abuse; technology dependence (e.g., ventilator, augmentative communication); treatment regimen; visual impairment.

Environmental
Economically disadvantaged; exposure to violence

Caregiver
Learning disabilities; mental health issue (e.g., depression, psychosis, personality disorder, substance abuse); presence of abuse (e.g., physical, psychological, sexual)

Client Outcomes
Client/Parents/Primary Caregiver Will (Specify Time Frame)
- Infant/Child/Adolescent will achieve expected milestones in all areas of development (physical, cognitive, and psychosocial)
- Parent/Caregiver will verbalize understanding of potential impediments to normal development and demonstrate actions or environmental/lifestyle changes necessary to provide appropriate care in a safe, nurturing environment

Nursing Interventions
Preconception/Pregnancy
- Assess for alcohol/drug use during pregnancy. Expectant mothers should be instructed that no amount of alcohol consumption is safe during pregnancy.
- Be aware of state legislation requiring mandatory reporting of maternal prenatal drug use. Be aware that mandatory reporting may further hamper prenatal care in that drug-addicted mothers may delay or defer care for fear of legal action.

• = Independent   ▲ = Collaborative

D

- Advise expectant mothers to stop smoking and assist with methods of smoking cessation.
- Recommend that women of childbearing age take 400 mcg of folic acid daily in order to reduce the risk of neural tube defects.

Neonate/Infant

- Encourage mother/baby interactions when caring for premature infants.
- Assess infant iron status and encourage iron supplementation for deficient infants.
- ▲ Support early advanced developmental screening tests for male infants who are born prematurely or are medically fragile at birth.
- ▲ Encourage caution regarding use of glucocorticoids in premature and term infants.
- ▲ Be aware that socioeconomic factors are predictive of delayed infant development (physical and cognitive) and encourage continued screening along with follow-up care for these infants. Arrange appropriate social services referrals.
- ▲ Make arrangements for close follow-up monitoring of opioid-exposed infants.

Toddler/Preschooler/School Age

- Provide support and education to parents of toddlers with developmental disabilities (i.e., Down syndrome, cerebral palsy).
- Encourage parents of toddlers to obtain age-appropriate developmental screenings to detect early problems.
- Toddlers who are underweight should be offered solid foods first rather than juices.
- Teach parents the importance of avoiding lead-based paints in the home as well as other sources of lead in the environment.
- ▲ Discuss advantages of early speech-language intervention with parents of toddlers having delayed development in communication.
- Educate parents on the importance of providing oral care for children with mild/moderate disabilities. Parents may need to assume the responsibility of toothbrushing for the child.
- ▲ Encourage mothers with postpartum depression to seek assistance and support as appropriate to ensure normal development of their children.
- Teach new mothers the importance of breastfeeding.

Multicultural

- Recognize cultural risks associated with higher infant mortality.

• = Independent   ▲ = Collaborative

Diarrhea

NANDA-I Definition

Passage of loose, unformed stools

Defining Characteristics

Abdominal pain; bowel urgency; cramping; hyperactive bowel sounds; loose liquid stools >3 in 24 hours

Related Factors

Physiological

Gastrointestinal inflammation; gastrointestinal irritation; infection; malabsorption; parasite

Psychological

Anxiety; increase in stress level

Situational

Enteral feedings; exposure to contaminant; exposure to toxin; laxative abuse; substance abuse; travel; treatment regimen

Client Outcomes

Client Will (Specify Time Frame)

- Defecate formed, soft stool every 1 to 3 days
- Maintain the perirectal area free of irritation
- State relief from cramping and less or no diarrhea
- Explain cause of diarrhea and rationale for treatment
- Maintain good skin turgor and weight at usual level
- Have negative stool cultures

Nursing Interventions

- Assess pattern of defecation or have the client keep a diary that includes the following: time of day defecation occurs; usual stimulus for defecation; consistency, amount, and frequency of stool; type of, amount of, and time food consumed; fluid intake; history of bowel habits and laxative use; diet; exercise patterns; obstetrical/gynecological, medical, and surgical histories; medications; alterations in perianal sensations; and present bowel regimen.
- Recommend use of standardized tool to consistently assess, quantify, and then treat diarrhea.
- Inspect, auscultate, palpate, and percuss the abdomen, in that order.
- ▲ Use an evidence-based bowel management protocol that includes identifying and treating the cause of the diarrhea, obtaining a stool specimen if infectious etiology is suspected, evaluate current medications and osmolality of enteral feedings, assess and treat

• = Independent   ▲ = Collaborative

D

hydration status of client, review and stop ordered and/or over-the-counter laxatives, provide good skin care and apply barrier creams to prevent skin irritation from diarrhea, and evaluate need for antidiarrheal agents and possible fecal containment device with provider.

▲ Identify cause of diarrhea if possible based on history (e.g., infection; gastrointestinal inflammation; medication effect; malnutrition or malabsorption; laxative abuse; osmotic enteral feedings; anxiety; stress).

▲ Testing for diarrhea may consist of laboratory work such as a complete blood count with differential and blood cultures if the client is febrile. Also obtain stool specimens as ordered, to either rule out or diagnose an infectious process (e.g., ova and parasites, *Clostridium difficile* infection, bacterial cultures for food poisoning).

▲ Consider the possibility of *C. difficile* infection if the client has any of the following: watery diarrhea, low-grade fever, abdominal cramps, history of antibiotic therapy, history of gastrointestinal tract surgery, and if the client is taking medications that reduce gastric acid, including proton-pump inhibitors (PPIs).

• Use standard precautions when caring for clients with diarrhea to prevent spread of infectious diarrhea; use gloves and handwashing. *C. difficile* and viruses causing diarrhea have been shown to be highly contagious.

▲ Antibiotic stewardship is an important aspect in prevention of *C. difficile* infections. If the client has diarrhea associated with antibiotic therapy, consult with the health care provider regarding the use of probiotics, such as yogurt with active cultures, to treat diarrhea, or probiotic dietary supplements; or preferably use probiotics to prevent diarrhea when first beginning antibiotic therapy.

▲ If a probiotic is ordered, administer it with food. Recommend that it be taken through the antibiotic course and 10 to 14 days afterward.

▲ Recognize that *C. difficile* can commonly recur and that reculturing of stool is often required before initiating retreatment.

• Have the client complete a diet diary for 7 days and monitor the intake of high fructose corn syrup and fructose sweeteners in relation to onset of diarrhea symptoms. If diarrhea is associated with fructose ingestion, intake should be limited or eliminated.

• = Independent   ▲ = Collaborative

▲ If the client has infectious diarrhea, consider avoiding use of medications that slow peristalsis.

• Assess for dehydration by observing skin turgor over sternum and inspecting for longitudinal furrows of the tongue. Watch for excessive thirst, fever, dizziness, lightheadedness, palpitations, excessive cramping, bloody stools, hypotension, and symptoms of shock.

• Refer to care plans for Deficient **Fluid** volume and Risk for **Electrolyte** imbalance if appropriate.

▲ If the client has frequent or chronic diarrhea, consider suggesting use of dietary fiber after consultation with a nutritionist and/or provider.

▲ If diarrhea is chronic and there is evidence of malnutrition, consult with the provider for a dietary consult and possible nutrition supplementation to maintain nutrition while the gastrointestinal system heals (Change & Huang, 2013).

• Encourage the client to eat small, frequent meals, eating foods that are easy to digest at first (e.g., bananas, crackers, pretzels, rice, potatoes, clear soups, applesauce), but switch to a regular diet as soon as tolerated. Also recommend avoiding milk products, foods high in fiber, and caffeine (dark sodas, tea, coffee, chocolate).

• Provide a readily available bathroom, commode, or bedpan.

• Thoroughly cleanse and dry the perianal and perineal skin daily and as needed using a cleanser capable of stool removal. Apply skin moisture barrier cream as needed. Refer to perirectal skin care in the care plan for Bowel **Incontinence.**

▲ If the client has enteral tube feedings and diarrhea, consider infusion rate, position of feeding tube, tonicity of formula, possible formula contamination, and excessive intake of hyperosmolar medications, such as sorbitol commonly found in the liquid version of medications (Makic et al, 2011; Chang et al, 2013). Consider changing the formula to a lower osmolarity, lactose-free, or high-fiber feeding.

• Avoid administering bolus enteral feedings into the small bowel.

▲ Dilute liquid medications before administration through the enteral tube and flush the enteral feeding tube with sufficient water before and after medication administration.

• Teach clients with cancer the types of diarrhea they may encounter, emphasizing not only chemotherapy- and radiation-induced diarrhea, but also *C. difficile,* along with associated signs and symptoms, and treatments. For chemotherapy-induced diarrhea (CID) and radiation-induced diarrhea (RID), review rationale for pharmacological interventions, along with soluble fiber and probiotic supplements. Consult a registered dietitian to assist with recommendations to alleviate diarrhea, decrease dehydration, and maintain nutritional status.

▲ Acute traveler's diarrhea is the most common illness affecting individuals traveling to, usually, low-income regions of the world.

Pediatric

▲ Assess for mild or moderate signs of dehydration with both acute and persistent diarrhea: mild (increased thirst and dry mouth or tongue); moderate (decreased urination; no wet diapers for 3+ hours; feeling of weakness/lightheadedness, irritability, or listlessness; few or no tears when crying) (Pye, 2011). Refer to primary care provider for treatment.

▲ Recommend that parents give the child oral rehydration fluids to drink in the amounts specified by the health care provider, especially during the first 4 to 6 hours to replace lost fluid. Once the child is rehydrated, an orally administered maintenance solution should be used along with food. Continue even if child vomits.

• Recommend the mother resume breastfeeding as soon as possible.

• Recommend parents avoid giving the child flat soda, fruit juices, gelatin dessert, or instant fruit drink.

• Recommend parents give children foods with complex carbohydrates, such as potatoes, rice, bread, cereal, yogurt, fruits, and vegetables. Avoid fatty foods, foods high in simple sugars, and milk products.

▲ Recommend rotavirus vaccine within the child's vaccination schedule.

Geriatric

▲ Evaluate medications the client is taking. Recognize that many medications can result in diarrhea, including digitalis, propranolol, angiotensin-converting enzyme inhibitors, histamine-receptor antagonists, nonsteroidal anti-inflammatory drugs, anticholinergic agents, oral hypoglycemia agents, and antibiotics, among others.

▲ Monitor the client closely to detect whether an impaction is causing diarrhea; remove impaction as ordered. Clients with fecal impaction commonly experience leakage of mucus or liquid stool from the rectum, rectal irritation, distention, and impaired anal sensation (Meiner, 2010).

• = Independent   ▲ = Collaborative

▲ Seek medical attention if diarrhea is severe or persists for more than 24 hours, or if the client has history of dehydration or electrolyte disturbances, such as lassitude, weakness, or prostration.

• Provide emotional support for clients who are having trouble controlling unpredictable episodes of diarrhea. Diarrhea can be a great source of embarrassment to older clients and can lead to social isolation and a feeling of powerlessness.

D

Home Care

Previously mentioned interventions may be adapted for home care use to keep the client well hydrated.

• Assess the home for general sanitation and methods of food preparation. Reinforce principles of sanitation for food handling.

• Assess for methods of handling soiled laundry if the client is bed bound or has been incontinent. Instruct or reinforce universal precautions with family and bloodborne pathogen precautions with agency caregivers.

• When assessing medication history, include over-the-counter (OTC) drugs, both general and those currently being used to treat the diarrhea. Instruct clients not to mix OTC medications when self-treating.

• Evaluate current medications for indication that specific interventions are warranted.

▲ Evaluate the need for a home health aide or homemaker service referral. Caregiver may need support for maintaining client cleanliness to prevent skin breakdown.

• Evaluate the need for durable medical equipment in the home. The client may need a bedside commode, call bell, or raised toilet seat to facilitate prompt toileting.

Client/Family Teaching and Discharge Planning

• Encourage avoidance of coffee, spices, milk products, and foods that irritate or stimulate the gastrointestinal tract. A list of dietary items that may irritate the gastrointestinal track and trigger diarrhea is available at www.iffgd.org/site/gi-disorders/functional-gi-disorders/diarrhea/nutrition.

• Teach appropriate method of taking ordered antidiarrheal medications; explain side effects.

• Explain how to prevent the spread of infectious diarrhea (e.g., careful handwashing, appropriate handling and storage of food, and thoroughly cleaning the bathroom and kitchen).

• = Independent   ▲ = Collaborative

D

- Help the client to determine stressors and set up an appropriate stress reduction plan, if stress is the cause of diarrhea.
- Teach signs and symptoms of dehydration and electrolyte imbalance.
- Teach perirectal skin care.
▲ Consider teaching clients about complementary therapies, such as probiotics, after consultation with primary care provider.

Risk for Disuse syndrome

NANDA-I Definition

Vulnerable to deterioration of body systems as the result of prescribed or unavoidable musculoskeletal inactivity, which may compromise health

Risk Factors

Alteration in level of consciousness; mechanical immobility; pain; paralysis; prescribed immobility

Client Outcomes

Client Will (Specify Time Frame)

- Maintain full range of motion in joints
- Maintain intact skin, good peripheral blood flow, and normal pulmonary function
- Maintain normal bowel and bladder function
- Express feelings about imposed immobility
- Explain methods to prevent complications of immobility

Nursing Interventions

- When client's condition is stable, screen for mobility skills in the following order: (1) bed mobility; (2) supported and unsupported sitting; (3) transition movements such as sit to stand, sitting down, and transfers; (4) standing and walking activities. Use a tool such as the Assessment Criteria and Care Plan for Safe Patient Handling and Movement (Sedlak et al, 2009) or the Banner Mobility Assessment Tool for Nurses (2014).
- Assess the level of assistance needed by the client and express in terms of amount of effort expended by the person assisting the client. The range is as follows: total assist, meaning client performs 0% to 25% of task and, if client requires the help of more than one caregiver, it is referred to as a dependent transfer; maximum assist, meaning client gives 25% of effort while caregiver performs majority of the work; moderate assist, meaning client gives 50% of effort;

• = Independent ▲ = Collaborative

minimal assist, meaning client gives 75% of effort; contact guard assist, meaning no physical assist is given but caregiver is physically touching client for steadying, guiding, or in case of loss of balance; stand by assist, meaning caregiver's hands are up and ready in case needed; supervision, meaning supervision of task is needed even if at a distance; modified independent, meaning client needs assistive device or extra time to accomplish task; independent, meaning client is able to complete task safely without instruction or assistance.

▲ Request a referral to a physical therapist as needed so that client's range of motion, muscle strength, balance, coordination, and endurance can be part of the initial evaluation.

• Incorporate bed exercises such as flexing and extending feet and quadriceps or use of Thera-Bands for upper extremities into nursing care to help maintain muscle strength and tone (Koenig et al, 2012).

▲ If not contraindicated by the client's condition, obtain a referral to physical therapy for use of tilt table to help determine the cause of syncope.

• Perform range of motion exercises for all possible joints at least twice daily; perform passive or active range of motion exercises as appropriate.

• Use specialized boots to prevent pressure ulcers on the heels and footdrop; remove boots twice daily to provide foot care.

• When positioning a client on the side, tilt client 30 degrees or less while lying on side.

• Assess skin condition at least daily and more frequently if needed. Use a risk assessment tool such the Braden Scale or the Norton Scale to predict the risk of developing pressure ulcers.

• Discuss with staff and management a "safe handling" policy that may include a "no lift" policy.

• Turn clients at high risk for pressure/shear/friction frequently. Turn clients at least every 2 to 4 hours on a pressure-reducing mattress/every 2 hours on standard foam mattress.

• Provide the client with a pressure-relieving horizontal support surface. For further interventions on skin care, refer to the care plan for Impaired **Skin** integrity.

• Help the client out of bed as soon as he or she is able.

• When getting the client up after bed rest, do so slowly and watch for signs of postural (orthostatic) hypotension, tachycardia, nausea,

diaphoresis, or syncope. Take the blood pressure with the client lying, sitting, and standing, waiting 2 minutes between each reading.
- Obtain assistive devices such as braces, crutches, or canes to help the client reach and maintain as much mobility as possible.
▲ Apply graduated compression stockings as ordered. Ensure proper fit by measuring accurately. Remove the stockings at least twice a day, in the morning with the bath and in the evening to assess the condition of the extremity, then reapply. Knee length is preferred rather than thigh length.
- Observe for signs of VTE, including pain, tenderness, and swelling in the calf and thigh. Also observe for new onset of breathlessness.
- Have the client cough and deep breathe or use incentive spirometry every 2 hours while awake.
- Monitor respiratory functions, noting breath sounds and respiratory rate. Percuss for new onset of dullness in lungs.
- Note bowel function daily. Provide increased fluids, fiber, and natural laxatives such as prune juice as needed.
- Increase fluid intake to 2000 mL/day within the client's cardiac and renal reserve.
- Encourage intake of a balanced diet with adequate amounts of fiber and protein.

Critical Care

▲ Recognize that the client who has been in an intensive care environment may develop a neuromuscular dysfunction acquired in the absence of causative factors other than the underlying critical illness and its treatment, resulting in extreme weakness (Stevens et al, 2009). The client may need a workup to determine the cause before satisfactory ambulation can begin.
▲ Consider use of a continuous lateral rotation therapy bed.
▲ For the stable client in the intensive care unit, consider mobilizing the client in a four-phase method from dangling at the side of the bed to walking if there is sufficient knowledgeable staff available to protect the client from harm.

Geriatric

- Get the client out of bed as early possible and ambulate frequently after consultation with the health care provider.
- Use the Exercise Assessment and Screening for You (EASY), which was developed to identify benefits of exercise and to assist older

adults to select safe and effective exercises. This tool decreases barriers to exercise.

▲ Refer the client to physical therapy for resistance strength exercise training.

• Monitor for signs of depression: flat affect, poor appetite, insomnia, many somatic complaints.

• Keep careful track of bowel function in older adults; do not allow the client to become constipated.

Home Care

• Some of the previous interventions may be adapted for home care use.

▲ Begin discharge planning as soon as possible with case manager or social worker to assess need for home support systems and community or home health services.

▲ Become oriented to all programs of care for the client before discharge from institutional care.

▲ Confirm the immediate availability of all necessary assistive devices for home.

• Perform complete physical assessment and recent history at initial home visit.

▲ Refer to physical and occupational therapies for immediate evaluations of the client's potential for independence and functioning in the home setting and for follow-up care.

• Allow the client to have as much input and control of the plan of care as possible.

• Assess knowledge of all care with caregivers. Review as necessary.

▲ Support the family of the client in assumption of caregiver activities. Refer for home health aide services for assistance and respite as appropriate. Refer to medical social services as appropriate.

▲ Institute case management of frail elderly to support continued independent living, if possible in the home environment.

Client/Family Teaching and Discharge Planning

• Teach client/family how to perform range-of-motion exercises in bed if not contraindicated; this is referred to as a Home Exercise Program.

• Teach the family how to turn and position the client and provide all care necessary.

NOTE: Nursing diagnoses that are commonly relevant when the client is on bed rest include **Constipation,** risk for Impaired **Skin** integrity, Disturbed **Sleep** pattern, **Frail Elderly** syndrome, and **Powerlessness.**

D

Deficient Diversional activity
NANDA-I Definition
Decreased stimulation from (or interest or engagement in) recreational or leisure activities
Defining Characteristics
Boredom; current setting does not allow engagement in activity
Related Factors (r/t)
Insufficient diversional activity; extremes of age; prolonged hospitalization; prolonged institutionalization
Client Outcomes
Client Will (Specify Time Frame)
- Engage in personally satisfying diversional activities
Nursing Interventions
- Observe for signs of deficient diversional activity: restlessness, unhappy facial expression, and statements of boredom and discontent.
- Observe ability to engage in activities that require good vision and use of hands.
- Discuss activities that are interesting and feasible in the present environment with clients.
- Encourage the client to share feelings about situation of inactivity.
- Encourage the client to participate in any available social or recreational opportunities in the health care environment.
- Encourage a mix of physical and mental activities if possible (e.g., crafts, crossword puzzles).
- Provide videos and/or DVDs of movies for recreation and distraction.
- Provide magazines and books of interest.
- Provide books on CD and CD player, and electronic versions of books for listening or reading as available.
- Set up a puzzle in a community space, or provide individual puzzles as desired.
- Provide access to a portable computer so that the client can access email and the Internet. Give client a list of interesting websites,

• = Independent   ▲ = Collaborative

D

including games and directions on how to perform Web searches if needed.

- Help client find a support group for the appropriate condition on the Internet if interested.
▲ Arrange animal-assisted therapy if desired, with a dog, cat, or bird for the client to care for and interact with.
- Encourage the client to schedule visitors so that they are not all present at once or at inconvenient times.
- If clients are able to write, help them keep journals or engage them in opportunities for creative writing in a group; if clients are unable to write, have them record thoughts on tape or on videotape.
▲ Request recreational or art therapist to assist with activities.
▲ Refer to occupational therapy. Provide a change in scenery; get the client out of the room as possible.
- Help the client to experience nature through looking at a nature scene from a window or walking through a garden if possible.
- Structure the environment as needed to promote optimal comfort and sensory diversity (e.g., have family bring in posters, banners, or photos; change lighting; change arrangement of furniture).
- Work with family or music therapist to provide music that is enjoyable to the client.
- Structure the client's schedule around personal wishes for time of care, relaxation, and participation in fun activities.
- Spend time with the client when possible, giving the client full attention and being present in the moment, or arrange for a friendly visitor.

Pediatric

▲ Request an order for a child life specialist or, if not available, a play therapist for children.
- Promote a referral to a music therapist.
- Consider art therapy for children living with chronic illness who have activity restrictions.
- Provide opportunities for children to connect with family and friends through technology.
- Provide activities such as video projects and use of computer-based support groups for children, such as Starbright World, a computer network where teenagers interact virtually, sharing their experiences and escaping hospital routines (www.starbrightworld.org).

• = Independent   ▲ = Collaborative

- Provide animal-assisted therapy for hospitalized children.
- Provide computer games and virtual reality experiences for children, which can be used as distraction techniques during venipuncture, wound care, or other procedures.

Geriatric

- Assess the interests of older adults and the types of activities that they enjoy; encourage creative expression such as storytelling, drama, dance, art, writing, or music.
- If the client is able, arrange for him or her to attend group senior citizen activities.
- Promote activity for older adults through the use of exergames (video games combined with exercise).
- Encourage involvement in dance.
- Encourage involvement in gardening.
- Encourage clients to use their ability to help others by volunteering.
- Provide an environment that promotes activity (e.g., one that has adequate lighting for crafts, large-print books, and adequate acoustics).
- Balance effortful activities with restful activities.
- Provide tai chi as an activity.
- Provide opportunities for storytelling and life review.
- ▲ Use reminiscence therapy in conjunction with the expression of emotions. Refer to a reminiscence group if available.
- Arrange for intergenerational volunteering for individuals with mild to moderate dementia.
- Use the Eden Alternative for older adults; bring in appropriate plants for the older client to care for and animals such as birds, fish, dogs, and cats as appropriate for the client and children to visit.
- For clients who love gardening but who may have difficulty being outside, bring in seeds, soil, and pots for indoor gardening experiences. Use seeds such as sunflower, pumpkin, and zinnia that grow rapidly.
- For clients with depressive symptoms, facilitate regular music listening.
- For hospitalized clients with cognitive impairment, engage the assistance of volunteers to provide diversional activities.
- For clients in assisted-living facilities, provide leisure educational programs and pleasant dining experiences.

• = Independent   ▲ = Collaborative

- For clients who are interested in reading and writing, promote book or writing groups, journaling, or creative or expressive writing.
- Prescribe activities to engage passive dementia clients based on their former interests and hobbies.
- Initiate opportunities for creative expression such as a TimeSlips storytelling group or Memories in the Making project to foster meaningful activities for clients with dementia.

Home Care

- Many of the previously listed interventions may be administered in the home setting.
- Explore with the client previous interests; consider related activities that are within the client's capabilities.
- ▲ Assess the client for depression. Refer for mental health services as indicated.
- Assess the family's ability to respond to the client's psychosocial needs for stimulation. Assist as able.
- ▲ Refer to occupational therapy.
- Introduce (or continue) friendly volunteer visitors if the client is willing and able to have the company. If transportation is an issue or if the client does not want visitors in the home, consider alternatives (e.g., telephone contacts, computer messaging).
- For clients who are interested and capable, suggest involvement in a community gardening experience.
- If the client is approaching the end of life and is interested, assist in making a videotape, audiotape, or memory book for family members with treasured stories, memoirs, pictures, and video clips.

Client/Family Teaching and Discharge Planning

- Work with the client and family on learning diversional activities in which the client is interested (e.g., knitting, hooking rugs, writing memoirs).
- If the client is in isolation, give the client complete information on why isolation is needed and how it should be accomplished, especially guidelines for visitors; provide diversional activities and encourage visitation.

• = Independent　　　　▲ = Collaborative

Risk for Electrolyte imbalance
NANDA-I Definition

Vulnerable to changes in serum electrolyte levels, which may compromise health

Risk Factors

Compromised regulatory mechanism; diarrhea; endocrine regulatory dysfunction; fluid imbalance (e.g., glucose intolerance; increase in IGF-1, androgen, DHEA, and cortisol); excessive fluid volume; insufficient fluid volume; renal dysfunction; treatment regimen; vomiting

Client Outcomes

Client Will (Specify Time Frame)

- Maintain a normal sinus heart rhythm with a regular rate
- Have a decrease in edema
- Maintain an absence of muscle cramping
- Maintain normal serum potassium, sodium, calcium, and phosphorus
- Maintain normal serum pH

Nursing Interventions

▲ Monitor vital signs at least three times a day, or more frequently as needed. Notify health care provider of significant deviation from baseline.

▲ Monitor cardiac rate and rhythm. Report changes to provider.

• Monitor intake and output and daily weights using a consistent scale.

• Monitor for abdominal distention and discomfort.

• Monitor the client's respiratory status and muscle strength.

• Assess cardiac status and neurological alterations.

▲ Review laboratory data as ordered and report deviations to provider.

• Review the client's medical and surgical history for possible causes of altered electrolytes.

▲ Complete pain assessment. Assess and document the onset, intensity, character, location, duration, aggravating factors, and relieving factors. Notify the provider for any increase in pain or discomfort or if comfort measures are not effective.

▲ Monitor the effects of ordered medications such as diuretics and heart medications.

▲ Administer parenteral fluids as ordered and monitor their effects.

Geriatric

• Monitor electrolyte levels carefully, including sodium levels and potassium levels, with both increased and decreased levels possible.

• = Independent   ▲ = Collaborative

Client/Family Teaching and Discharge Planning
- Teach client/family the signs of low potassium and the risk factors.
- Teach client/family the signs of high potassium and the risk factors.
- Teach client/family the signs of low sodium and the risk factors.
- Teach client/family the signs of high sodium and the risk factors.
- Teach client/family the importance of hydration during exercise. Dehydration occurs when the amount of water leaving the body is greater than the amount consumed.
- Teach client/family the warning signs of dehydration. Early signs of dehydration include thirst and decreased urine output. As dehydration increases, symptoms may include dry mouth, muscle cramps, nausea and vomiting, lightheadedness, and orthostatic hypotension.
- Teach client about any medications prescribed. Medication teaching includes the drug name, its purpose, administration instructions such as taking it with or without food, and any side effects to be aware of.
▲ Instruct the client to report any adverse medication side effects to his/her health care provider.

Labile Emotional Control

NANDA-I Definition

Uncontrollable outbursts of exaggerated and involuntary emotional expression

Defining Characteristics

Absence of eye contact; difficulty in use of facial expressions; embarrassment regarding emotional expression; excessive crying without feeling sadness; excessive laughing without feeling happiness; expression of emotion incongruent with triggering factor; involuntary crying; involuntary laughing; tearfulness; uncontrollable crying; uncontrollable laughing; withdrawal from occupational situation; withdrawal from social situation

Related Factors

Alteration in self-esteem; brain injury; emotional disturbance; fatigue; functional impairment; insufficient knowledge about symptom control; insufficient knowledge of disease; insufficient muscle strength; mood disorder; musculoskeletal impairment; pharmaceutical agent; physical disability; psychiatric disorder; social distress; stressors; substance abuse

• = Independent ▲ = Collaborative

Client Outcomes

Client Will (Specify Time Frame)

- Improve coping strategies
- Improve knowledge about disease process, signs and symptoms, triggers, symptom control
- Employ mechanisms to control impulses and ask for help when feeling impulses
- Improve feelings of dignity
- Enhance and improve response to social and environmental stimuli

Nursing Interventions

- Provide progressive relaxation exercise techniques.
- Offer instruction regarding alternative coping strategies such as mindfulness and breath awareness.
- Use the Pathological Laughter and Crying Scale (PLACS) to identify pathological laughing and crying or related disorders (e.g., IEED, PBA).
- Consider using cognitive-behavioral therapy.

Multicultural, Home Care

- The above interventions may be adapted for multicultural and home care.

Client/Family Teaching and Discharge Planning

- Inform client and family about the emotional lability and talk with them about how to cope with the situation.
- Use verbal and nonverbal therapeutic communication approaches including empathy, active listening, and confrontation to encourage the client and family to express emotions such as sadness, guilt, and anger (within appropriate limits); verbalize fears and concerns; and set goals.
- Provide psychoeducation for stress-related variables to client and family.

Risk for dry Eye

NANDA-I Definition

Vulnerable to eye discomfort or damage to the cornea and conjunctiva due to reduced quantity or quality of tears to moisten the eye, which may compromise health

• = Independent   ▲ = Collaborative

Risk Factors

Aging; autoimmune diseases (e.g., rheumatoid arthritis, diabetes mellitus, thyroid disease); contact lens wearer; environmental factor (e.g., air conditioning, excessive wind, sunlight exposure, air pollution, low humidity); female gender; history of allergy; hormonal change; lifestyle choice (e.g., smoking, caffeine use, prolonged reading); mechanical ventilation; neurological lesions with sensory or motor reflex loss (e.g., lagophthalmos, lack of spontaneous blink reflex); ocular surface damage; treatment regimen; vitamin A deficiency

Client Outcomes

Client Will (Specify Time Frame)

- State eyes are comfortable with no itching, burning, or dryness
- Have corneal surface that is intact and without injury
- Demonstrate self-administration of eye drops if ordered
- State vision is clear

Nursing Interventions

▲ Assess for symptoms of dry eyes, such as "irritation, tearing, burning, stinging, dry or foreign body sensation, mild itching, photophobia, blurry vision, contact lens intolerance, redness, mucus discharge, increased frequency of blinking, eye fatigue, diurnal fluctuation, symptoms that worsen later in the day" (American Academy of Ophthalmology [AAO], 2013).

▲ If symptoms are present, refer client to an ophthalmologist for diagnosis and treatment.

▲ Administer ordered eye drops.

- Consider use of eyeglass side shields or moisture chambers.

▲ Watch for symptoms of blepharitis including crusting and irritation at the base of the lashes and adjacent redness of the eyelid, which may accompany dry eye; refer for treatment as needed.

▲ Discuss use of caffeine with client's health care provider.

Geriatric

- Recognize that symptoms of dry eye are more common in menopausal women and geriatric clients.

Critical Care

▲ Provide regular cleaning of the eyes, lubricating eye drops and ointments, and consultation with an ophthalmologist if infection is suspected in clients in the intensive care unit (ICU).

- Avoid using adhesive tape to keep eyes closed in sedated patients.

• = Independent   ▲ = Collaborative

F

Client/Family Teaching and Discharge Planning

- Teach client conditions that can exacerbate dry eye symptoms.
- Teach client good eye hygiene:
  - ○ Apply warm compresses for 10-minute intervals using a clean cloth and water that has been boiled and cooled (or sterile water).
  - ○ Gently massage around eyelids.
  - ○ Gently clean eyelids to remove excess oil, crusts, and bacteria. Use a few drops of baby shampoo in water that has been boiled and cooled, or in sterile water.
- Teach clients methods to decrease problems with dry eye including the following:
  - ○ Avoid drafty (e.g., ceiling fans) and low-humidity environments.
  - ○ Avoid smoking and exposure to second-hand smoke.
- ▲ Discuss avoidance of offending medications with health care provider.
- Drink plenty of water to keep well hydrated.
- Teach client to lower the computer screen to below eye level and to blink more frequently.
- ▲ Teach client to consult with the health care provider regarding use of omega-3 supplements to decrease dry eye.
- Teach client using eye drops how to self-administer eye drops.
- Warn clients with dry eyes that driving at night can be dangerous.

Risk for Falls

NANDA-I Definition

Vulnerable to increased susceptibility to falling, which may cause physical harm and compromise health

Risk Factors

Adults

Age ≥65 years; history of falls; living alone; lower limb prosthesis; use of assistive device (e.g., walker, cane, wheelchair)

Children

Absence of stairway gate; absence of window guard; age ≤2 years; inadequate supervision; insufficient automobile restraints; male gender when <1 year of age

Cognitive

Alteration in cognitive functioning

• = Independent   ▲ = Collaborative

Environment

Cluttered environment; exposure to unsafe weather-related condition (e.g., wet floors, ice); insufficient lighting; insufficient antislip material in bathroom; unfamiliar setting; use of restraints; use of throw rugs

Pharmaceutical Agents

Alcohol consumption; pharmaceutical agent

Physiological

Acute illness; alteration in blood glucose level; anemia; arthritis; condition affecting the foot; decrease in lower extremity strength; diarrhea; difficulty with gait; faintness when extending neck; faintness when turning neck; hearing impairment; impaired balance; impaired mobility; incontinence; neoplasm; neuropathy; orthostatic hypotension; postoperative recovery period; proprioceptive deficit; sleeplessness; urinary urgency; vascular disease; visual impairment

Client Outcomes

Client Will (Specify Time Frame):

- Remain free of falls
- Change environment to minimize the incidence of falls
- Explain methods to prevent injury

Nursing Interventions

- Safety Guidelines. Complete a fall-risk assessment for older adults in acute care using a valid and reliable tool such as the Hendrich II Model. Recognize that risk factors for falling include recent history of falls, fear of falling, confusion, depression, altered elimination patterns, cardiovascular/respiratory disease impairing perfusion or oxygenation, postural hypotension, dizziness or vertigo, primary cancer diagnosis, and altered mobility (Gray-Miceli, 2008).
- Screen all clients for balance and mobility skills (supine to sit, sitting supported and unsupported, sit to stand, standing, walking and turning around, transferring, stooping to floor and recovering, and sitting down). Use tools such as the Balance Scale by Tinetti or the Get Up and Go Scale.
- Recognize that when people attend to another task while walking, such as carrying a cup of water, clothing, or supplies, they are more likely to fall.
- Carefully assist a mostly immobile client up. Be sure to lock the bed and wheelchair and have sufficient personnel to protect the client from falls. When rising from a lying position, have the client change

• = Independent   ▲ = Collaborative

positions slowly, dangle legs, and stand next to the bed before walking to prevent orthostatic hypotension.
* Use a "high-risk fall" armband/bracelet and fall risk room sign to alert staff for increased vigilance and mobility assistance.
▲ Evaluate the client's medications to determine whether medications increase the risk of falling; consult with health care provider regarding the client's need for medication if appropriate.
* Orient the client to environment. Place the call light within reach and show how to call for assistance; answer call light promptly.
* Use one-fourth to one-half–length side rails only, and maintain bed in a low position. Ensure that wheels are locked on bed and commode. Keep dim light in room at night.
* Routinely assist the client with toileting on his or her own schedule. Take the client to bathroom on awakening and before bedtime (McCarter-Bayer et al, 2005; Goodwin et al, 2014). Keep the path to the bathroom clear, label the bathroom, and leave the door open.
▲ Avoid use of restraints if possible. Obtain health care provider's order if restraints are deemed necessary, and use the least restrictive device.
* In place of restraints, use the following:
  ○ Well-staffed and educated nursing personnel with frequent client contact with careful consideration during shift changes
  ○ Nursing units designed to care for clients with cognitive or functional impairments
  ○ Nonskid footwear, sneakers preferable
  ○ Adequate lighting, night-light in bathroom
  ○ Frequent toileting
  ○ Frequently assess need for invasive devices, tubes, intravenous (IV) access
  ○ Hide tubes with bandages to prevent pulling of tubes
  ○ Consider alternative IV placement site to prevent pulling out IV line
  ○ Alarm systems with ankle, above-the-knee, or wrist sensors
  ○ Bed or wheelchair alarms
  ○ Wedge cushions on chairs to prevent slipping
  ○ Increased observation of the client
  ○ Locked doors to unit
  ○ Low or very low height beds

• = Independent ▲ = Collaborative

 ○ Border-defining pillow/mattress to remind the client to stay in bed
- If the client has an acute change in mental status (delirium), recognize that the cause is usually physiological and is a medical emergency. Consider possible causes for delirium. Consult with the health care provider immediately. See interventions for Acute **Confusion.**
- If the client has chronic confusion due to dementia, implement individualized strategies to enhance communication. See interventions for Chronic **Confusion.**
- Ask family to stay with the client to assist with activities of daily living and prevent the client from accidentally falling or pulling out tubes.
▲ If the client is unsteady on his/her feet, have two nursing staff members alongside when walking the client. Use facility-approved mobility devices to assist with client ambulation (e.g., gait belts, walkers). Consider referral to physical therapy for gait training and strengthening.
- Place a fall-prone client in a room that is near the nurses' station.
- Help clients sit in a stable chair with arm rests. Avoid use of wheelchairs except for transportation as needed.
- Avoid use of wheelchairs as much as possible because they can serve as a restraint device. Most people in wheelchairs do not move.
▲ Refer to physical therapy or other programs for exercise programs that target strength, balance, flexibility, or endurance.

Geriatric
- Assess ability to move using the Hendrich II Fall Risk Model, which includes the Get Up and Go test. Ask the client to rise from a sitting position, walk 10 feet, turn, and return to the chair to sit.
- Complete a fall risk assessment for older adults in acute care using a valid and reliable tool such as the Hendrich II Fall Risk Model.
▲ If new onset of falling, assess for lab abnormalities and signs and symptoms of infection and dehydration, and check blood pressure and pulse rate with client in supine, sitting, and standing positions for hypotension and orthostatic hypotension. If the client has borderline high blood pressure, the risk of falling due to administration of antihypertensives may outweigh the benefits of the antihypertensive medication. Discuss with the health care provider on a client-to-client basis.

  • = Independent   ▲ = Collaborative

F

- Complete a fear-of-falling assessment for older adults. This includes measuring fear of falling, or the level of concern about falling, and falls self-efficacy, the degree of confidence a person has in performing common activities of daily living without falling. Fear of falling may be measured by a single-item question asking about the presence of fear of falling or rating severity of fear of falling on a 1-4 Likert scale as is commonly done in studies. Falls self-efficacy may be measured using a valid and reliable tool such as the Falls Efficacy Scale-International (Yardley et al, 2005; Greenberg, 2011).
- Encourage the client to wear glasses and use walking aids when ambulating.
- If the client experiences dizziness because of orthostatic hypotension when getting up, teach methods to decrease dizziness, such as rising slowly, remaining seated several minutes before standing, flexing feet upward several times while sitting, sitting down immediately if feeling dizzy, and trying to have someone present when standing.
▲ If the client is experiencing syncope, determine symptoms that occur before syncope, and note medications that the client is taking. Refer for medical care. The circumstances surrounding syncope often suggest the cause.
▲ Observe client for signs of anemia, and refer to health care provider for testing if appropriate.
- Evaluate client for chronic alcohol intake, as well as mental health and neurological function.
▲ Refer to physical therapy for strength training, using free weights or machines, and suggest participation in exercise programs.
▲ If an older woman has symptoms of urge incontinence, refer to a urologist or nurse specialist in incontinence for evaluation and ensure the path to the bathroom is well lit and free of obstructions.
▲ New evidence-based guidelines for preventing falls in older adults were published by the American Geriatrics Society (AGS) and British Geriatrics Society (BGS) collaboratively and specify recommendations for all clinical settings. The new recommendations include screening and assessment, as well as interventions. Examples of interventions include (1) exercise for balance and for gait and strength training, such as tai chi or physical therapy; (2) environmental adaptation to reduce fall risk factors in the home and in daily activities; (3) cataract surgery when indicated; (4) medication reduction with particular attention to medications that affect the

• = Independent   ▲ = Collaborative

brain such as sleeping medications and antidepressants; (5) assessment and treatment of postural hypotension; (6) identification and appropriate treatment of foot problems; (7) vitamin D supplementation for those with vitamin D (American Geriatrics Society, 2011).

Home Care

- Some of the above interventions may be adapted for home care use.
- Implement evidence-based fall prevention practices in community settings and home health care programs for older adults (Fortinsky et al, 2008).
- If the client was identified as a fall risk in the hospital, recognize that there is a high incidence of falls after discharge, and use all measures possible to reduce the incidence of falls.
- ▲ If delirium is present, assess for cause of delirium and/or falls with the use of an interprofessional team. Consult with the health care provider immediately. Assess and monitor for acute changes in cognition and behavior.
- Assess home environment for threats to safety including clutter, slippery floors, scatter rugs, and other potential hazards. Additionally, assess external environment (e.g., uneven pavement, unleveled stairs/steps).
- ▲ Institute a home-based, nurse-delivered exercise program to reduce falls or refer to physical therapy services for client and family education of safe transfers and ambulation and for strengthening exercises for the client (Grabiner, 2013).
- ▲ Instruct the client and family or caregivers on how to correct identified hazards for those with visual impairment. Refer to physical and occupational therapy services for assistance if needed.
- ▲ Use a multifactorial assessment along with interventions targeted to the identified risk factors. Key components of the interventions include evaluating need for all medications, balance, gait and strength training, use of strategies to deal with postural hypotension if present, home safety evaluation with needed modifications, and any needed cardiovascular treatment.
- Encourage the client to eat a balanced diet, with particular inclusion of vitamin D and calcium.
- If the client lives alone or spends a lot of time alone, teach the client what to do if he/she falls and cannot get up, and make sure he/she has a personal emergency response system or a mobile phone that is

• = Independent   ▲ = Collaborative

available from the floor (Tinetti, 2003). If the client is at risk for falls, use a gait belt and additional persons when ambulating.

- Ensure appropriate nonglare lighting in the home. Ask the client to install indoor strip or "runway" type of lighting to baseboards to help clients balance. Install motion-sensitive lighting that turns on automatically when the client gets out of bed to go to the bathroom.
- Have the client wear supportive, low-heeled shoes with good traction when ambulating. Avoid use of slip-on footwear. Wear appropriate footwear in inclement weather.
- Provide a signaling device for clients who wander or are at risk for falls.
- Provide medical identification bracelet for clients at risk for injury from dementia, diabetes, seizures, or other medical disorders.
- Suggest a tai chi class designed for older adults and selected clients who have sufficient balance to participate.

Client/Family Teaching and Discharge Planning

- Safety Guidelines. Teach the client and family about the fall reduction measures that are being used to prevent falls (The Joint Commission, 2009).
- Teach the client how to safely ambulate at home, including using safety measures such as hand rails in bathroom and avoiding carrying things or performing other tasks while walking.
- Teach the client the importance of maintaining a regular exercise program. If the client is afraid of falling while walking outside, suggest he/she walk the length of a local mall.

Dysfunctional Family processes
NANDA-I Definition

Psychosocial, spiritual, and physiological functions of the family unit are chronically disorganized, which leads to conflict, denial of problems, resistance to change, ineffective problem solving, and a series of self-perpetuating crises

Defining Characteristics

Behavioral

Agitation; alteration in concentration; blaming; broken promises; chaos; complicated grieving; conflict avoidance; contradictory communication pattern; controlling communication pattern; criticizing; decrease in

• = Independent ▲ = Collaborative

physical contact; denial of problems; dependency; difficulty having fun; difficulty with intimate relationships; difficulty with life cycle transitions; disturbances in academic performance in children; enabling substance use pattern; escalating conflict; failure to accomplish developmental tasks; harsh self-judgment; immaturity; inability to accept a wide range of feelings; inability to accept help; inability to adapt to change; inability to deal constructively with traumatic experiences; inability to express wide range of feelings; inability to meet the emotional needs of its members; inability to meet the security needs of its members; inability to meet the spiritual needs of its members; inability to receive help appropriately; inappropriate anger expression; ineffective communication skills; insufficient knowledge about substance abuse; insufficient problem-solving skills; lying; manipulation; nicotine addiction; orientation favors tension relief rather than goal attainment; paradoxical communication pattern; power struggles; rationalization; refusal to get help; seeking of affirmation; seeking of approval; self-blame; social isolation; special occasions centered on substance use; stress-related physical illnesses; substance abuse; unreliable behavior; verbal abuse of children; verbal abuse of parent; verbal abuse of partner

Feelings

Abandonment; anger; anxiety; confuses love and pity; confusion; depression; dissatisfaction; distress; embarrassment; emotional isolation; failure; fear; feeling different from others; feeling misunderstood; feeling unloved; frustration; guilt; hopelessness; hostility; hurt; insecurity; lack of identity; lingering resentment; loneliness; loss; mistrust; moodiness; powerlessness; rejection; reports feeling misunderstood; repressed emotions; responsibility for substance abuser's behavior; suppressed rage; shame; tension; unhappiness; vulnerability; worthlessness

Roles and Relationships

Change in role function; chronic family problems; closed communication systems; conflict between partners; deterioration in family relationships; diminished ability of family members to relate to each other for mutual growth and maturation; disrupted family rituals; disrupted family roles; disturbance in family dynamics; economically disadvantaged; family denial; inconsistent parenting; ineffective communication with partner; insufficient cohesiveness; insufficient family respect for autonomy of its members; insufficient family respect for individuality of its members; insufficient relationship skills; intimacy dysfunction; neglect of obligation to family member; pattern of rejection; perceived insufficient parental support; triangulating family relationships

• = Independent   ▲ = Collaborative

Related Factors (r/t)

Addictive personality; biological factors; family history of resistance to treatment; family history of substance abuse; genetic predisposition to substance abuse; ineffective coping skills; insufficient problem-solving skills; substance abuse

Client Outcomes

Family/Client Will (Specify Time Frame)

* State one way that alcoholism has affected the health of the family
* Identify three healthy coping behaviors that family members can employ to facilitate a shift toward improved family functioning
* Identify one Al-Anon meeting from Al-Anon meeting schedule that family members express a desire to attend
* Attend different types of meetings (lead, big book, discussion, beginner's meeting) to find a good match and commit to attending that group regularly

Nursing Interventions

* Refer to care plans for Ineffective **Denial** and Defensive **Coping** for additional interventions.
* ▲ Behavioral screening and intervention (BSI) should be integrated into all health care settings. Different terminology has evolved for screening, intervention, and referral for various behavioral issues. The five A's—ask, advise, assess, assist, and arrange—apply to tobacco use. SBIRT (screening, brief intervention, and referral to treatment) pertains to alcohol and drug use.
* Screen clients for at-risk drinking during routine primary care visits and before surgery using the Alcohol Use Disorders Identification Test (AUDIT).
* Provide brief education and individual counseling as a routine part of primary care.
* Refer for family therapy.
* ▲ Refer for possible use of medications to control alcohol dependence.

Pediatric

* ▲ Encourage early intervention when parental depression, childhood exposure to conflict and violence, and childhood experience with abuse and neglect co-exist with parental substance abuse, their children are more likely to engage in increased teacher-rated unfavorable student behavioral problems.
* ▲ Consider the Community Reinforcement Approach (CRA) that encourages clients to become progressively involved in alternative

• = Independent   ▲ = Collaborative

non–substance-related pleasant social activities and to work on enhancing the enjoyment they receive within the "community" of their family and job.
▲ Educate family members about available educational and support programs and encourage no/limited alcohol use in the home.
• Encourage adolescents to attend a 12-step program.
• Provide a school-based drug-prevention program to junior high students.

Geriatric
• Include assessment of possible alcohol abuse when assessing older family members.

Multicultural
• Acknowledge racial/ethnic differences at the onset of care.
• Use a family-centered approach when working with Latino, Asian American, African American, and Native American clients.
• Some less-acculturated Latino families may be unwilling to discuss family issues with health care providers until they perceive a close personal relationship with the provider.
• Work with families in a way that incorporates cultural elements.

Home Care
NOTE: In the community setting, alcoholism as cause of dysfunctional family processes must be considered in two categories: (1) when the client suffers personally from the illness, and (2) when a significant other suffers from the illness, that is, the client is not the active alcoholic but may depend on the alcoholic for caregiving. The following considerations apply to both situations with appropriate adaptation for the circumstances.
• The previous interventions may be adapted for home care use.
• Work with family members to support a sense of valued fit on their part; include them in treatment planning and identify the importance of their roles in the client's care. At the same time, encourage their pursuit of positive outside activities that enhance their sense of belonging.
• Educate client and family regarding the interactions of alcohol use with medications and the therapeutic regimen.
• Alcoholism is a family disease.
▲ Refer for psychiatric home health care services for client reassurance and implementation of therapeutic regimen.

• = Independent   ▲ = Collaborative

▲ Consider use of a smartphone-based intervention for alcohol use disorders.

Client/Family Teaching and Discharge Planning

• Suggest the client complete a confidential Internet self-screening test for identification of problems and suggestions for treatment if a problem with alcohol is suspected. Many tools are available.
• Provide education for family.
• Facilitate participation in mutual help groups (MHGs).

F

Interrupted Family processes

NANDA-I Definition

Change in family relationships and/or functioning

Defining Characteristics

Alteration in availability for affective responsiveness; alteration in family conflict resolution; alteration in family satisfaction; alteration in intimacy; alteration in participation for problem solving; assigned tasks change; change in communication pattern; change in somatization; change in stress reduction behavior; changes in expressions of conflict with community resources; changes in expressions of isolation from community resources; changes in participation for decision-making; changes in relationship pattern; decrease in available emotional support; decrease in mutual support; ineffective task completion; power alliance change; ritual change

Related Factors (r/t)

Alteration in family finances; change in family social status; changes in interaction with community; developmental crisis; developmental transition; power shift among family members; shift in family roles; shift in health status of a family member; situational crisis; situational transition

Client Outcomes

Family/Client Will (Specify Time Frame)

• Express feelings (family)
• Identify ways to cope effectively and use appropriate support systems (family)
• Treat impaired family member as normally as possible to avoid over-dependence (family)
• Meet physical, psychosocial, and spiritual needs of members or seek appropriate assistance (family)

• = Independent   ▲ = Collaborative

- Demonstrate knowledge of illness or injury, treatment modalities, and prognosis (family)
- Participate in the development of the plan of care to the best of ability (significant person)

Nursing Interventions

- Motivate family members to speak openly about illnesses, keeping in mind the importance of ethnic origin.
- Recognize informal roles in medical decision-making by family members.
- Acknowledge the range of emotions and feelings that may be experienced when the health status of a family member changes.
- Encourage family members to list their personal strengths and available resources.
- Establish relationships among clients, their families, and health care professionals.
- Encourage family to visit the client; adjust visiting hours to accommodate family's schedule.
- Allow and encourage family members to assist in the client's treatment.
- Support family members during emotional and conflict situations in the clinical setting.
- Refer to the care plan Readiness for enhanced **Family** processes for additional interventions.

Pediatric

- Carefully assess potential for reunifying children placed in foster care with their birth parents.
- Provide parents with both general information and professional support by family-centered early childhood intervention services to their families.
- Encourage and support parents/family to assist in client's care.
- ▲ Refer parents and other primary caregivers to a mindfulness-based stress reduction (MBSR) program.

Geriatric

- Encourage family members to be involved in the care of relatives who are in residential care settings.
- Support group problem solving among family caregivers and include the older member.
- ▲ Refer family for counseling with a psychotherapist who is knowledgeable about gerontology.

• = Independent   ▲ = Collaborative

F

- Refer to care plan for Readiness for enhanced **Family** processes for additional interventions.

Multicultural

- Refer to the care plan Readiness for enhanced **Family** processes for additional interventions.

Home Care

- The nursing interventions described in the care plan for Compromised family **Coping** should be used in the home environment with adaptations as necessary.
- Encourage family members to find meaning in a serious illness.

Client/Family Teaching and Discharge Planning

- Refer to Client/Family Teaching and Discharge Planning in Compromised family **Coping** and Readiness for enhanced family **Coping** for suggestions that may be used with minor adaptations.

Readiness for enhanced Family processes

NANDA-I Definition

A pattern of family functioning to support the well-being of family members, which can be strengthened

Defining Characteristics

Expresses desire to enhance balance between autonomy and cohesiveness; expresses desire to enhance communication pattern; expresses desire to enhance energy level of family to support activities of daily living; expresses desire to enhance family adaptation to change; expresses desire to enhance family dynamics; expresses desire to enhance family resilience; expresses desire to enhance growth of family members; expresses desire to enhance interdependence with community; expresses desire to enhance maintenance of boundaries between family members; expresses desire to enhance respect for family members; expresses desire to enhance safety of family members.

Client Outcomes

Family/Client Will (Specify Time Frame)

- Identify ways to cope effectively and use appropriate support systems (family)
- Meet physical, psychosocial, and spiritual needs of members or seek appropriate assistance (family)

• = Independent   ▲ = Collaborative

- Demonstrate knowledge of potential environmental, lifestyle, and genetic risks to health and use appropriate measures to decrease possibility of risk (family)
- Focus on wellness, disease prevention, and maintenance (family and individual)
- Seek balance among exercise, work, leisure, rest, and nutrition (family and individual)

F

Nursing Interventions

- Assess the family's stress level and coping abilities during the initial nursing assessment.
- Consider the use of family-centered theory as the conceptual foundation to help guide interventions.
- Use family-centered care and role modeling for holistic care of families.
- Discuss with family members and identify the perceptions of the health care experience.
- Support family needs, strengths, and resourcefulness through family interviews.
- Spend time with family members; allow them to verbalize their feelings.
- Encourage family members to find meaning in a serious illness.
- Provide family-centered care to explore and use all available resources appropriate for the situation (e.g., counseling, social services, self-help groups, pastoral care).
- Consider focus groups to provide insight to family perceptions of illness and/or disease prevention.

Pediatric

- Provide a parenting class series based on individual and couple changes in meaning and identity, roles and relationships, and interaction during the transition to parenthood. Address mother and father roles, infant communication abilities, and patterns of the first 3 months of life in a mutually enjoyable, possibility focused manner.
- Encourage families with adolescents to have family meals.
- ▲ Consider the use of adventure therapy for adolescents with cancer.

Geriatric

- Carefully listen to residents and family members in the long-term care facility.
- Support caregivers' awareness of the positive effects of their contribution to the well-being of parents.

• = Independent   ▲ = Collaborative

- Teach family members about the impact of developmental events (e.g., retirement, death, change in health status, and household composition).
- Encourage social networks; social integration; social engagement and Internet social networking with friends, children, and relatives of older adults.

F

Multicultural

- Assess for the influence of cultural beliefs, norms, and values on the family's perceptions of normal functioning.
- Identify and acknowledge the stresses unique to racial/ethnic families.
- With the client's consent, facilitate a group meeting for family members to discuss how the family is functioning.
- Facilitate modeling and role playing for the client and family regarding healthy ways to start a discussion about the client's prognosis.
- Encourage family mealtimes.

Home Care

- The previous nursing interventions should be used in the home environment with adaptations as necessary.
- ▲ Encourage virtual support groups to family caregivers.

Client/Family Teaching and Discharge Planning

- Refer to Client/Family Teaching and Discharge Planning for readiness for enhanced family **Coping** for suggestions that may be used with minor adaptations.

Fatigue

NANDA-I Definition

An overwhelming, sustained sense of exhaustion and decreased capacity for physical and mental work at the usual level

Defining Characteristics

Alteration in concentration; alteration in libido; disinterest in surroundings; drowsiness; guilt about difficulty maintaining responsibilities; impaired ability to maintain usual physical activity; impaired ability to maintain usual routines; increase in physical symptoms; increase in rest requirement; ineffective role performance; insufficient energy; introspection; lethargy; listlessness; nonrestorative sleep pattern (due to caregiver responsibilities, parenting practices, sleep partner); tiredness

• = Independent   ▲ = Collaborative

Related Factors (r/t)

Anxiety; depression; environmental barrier (e.g., ambient noise, daylight/darkness exposure, ambient temperature/humidity, unfamiliar setting); increase in physical exertion; malnutrition; negative life event; nonstimulating lifestyle; occupational demands (e.g., shift work, high level of activity, stress); physical deconditioning; physiological condition (e.g., anemia, pregnancy, disease); sleep deprivation; stressors

Client Outcomes

Client Will (Specify Time Frame)

- Identify potential etiology of fatigue
- Identify potential factors that aggravate and relieve fatigue
- Describe ways to assess and track patterns of fatigue over set periods of time (e.g., a few days, a week, a month)
- Describe ways in which fatigue affects the ability to accomplish goals and activities of daily living (ADLs)
- Verbalize increased energy and improved vitality
- Explain energy conservation plan to offset fatigue
- Explain energy restoration plan to offset fatigue

Nursing Interventions

- Assess severity of fatigue on a scale of 0 to 10 (average fatigue, worst and best levels); assess frequency of fatigue (number of days per week and time of day), activities, and symptoms associated with increased fatigue (e.g., pain), ability to perform ADLs and instrumental ADLs, interference with social and role function, times of increased energy, ability to concentrate, mood, usual pattern of physical activity, and typical sleep cycles. Consider use of an instrument such as the Profile of Mood State Short Form Fatigue Subscale, the Multidimensional Assessment of Fatigue, the Lee Fatigue Scale, the Multidimensional Fatigue Inventory, the HIV-Related Fatigue Scale, or the Brief Fatigue Inventory, Short Form Vitality Subscale, Piper Fatigue Scale, Chalder Fatigue Scale, or Nottingham of Chronic Illness Therapy Fatigue Scale.
- Evaluate adequacy of nutrition and sleep hygiene (napping throughout the day, inability to fall asleep or stay asleep). Encourage the client to get adequate rest, limit naps (particularly in the late afternoon or evening), use a routine sleep/wake schedule, plan and prioritize for daily activities as tolerated, allow exposure to sunlight during daytime hours by going outside or opening shades and curtains in the home, use relaxation techniques before bedtime such

---

• = Independent   ▲ = Collaborative

as meditation, music therapy, or guided imagery (Kwekkeboom et al, 2010), avoid caffeine in the late afternoon or evening, and eat a well-balanced diet that includes fresh fruits, vegetables, and lean meats. Refer to Imbalanced **Nutrition:** less than body requirements or **Insomnia** if appropriate.

F

- Evaluate fluid status and assess for dehydration. Encourage drinking at least eight glasses of water a day. Avoid caffeine, which can cause further dehydration.

▲ Collaborate with the primary care provider to identify physiological and/or psychological causes of fatigue that could be treated, such as anemia, pain, electrolyte imbalance (e.g., altered potassium levels), thyroid disorders, arthritis, depression, sleep disturbances (insomnia/sleep deprivation), acute or chronic infection, medication use or side effects, alcohol use/abuse, metabolic disorders (diabetes), or a preexisting comorbidity or disease (multiple sclerosis, cancer or cancer treatment, respiratory disease, fibromyalgia, cardiac disease, renal disease or renal replacement therapy, Parkinson's disease) (Berger et al, 2012; Connolly et al, 2013).

▲ Work with the primary care provider to determine if the client has chronic fatigue syndrome, paying attention to risk factors in particular populations.

- Encourage the client to express feelings, attribution of cause and behaviors about fatigue, including potential causes of fatigue, and possible interventions to alleviate fatigue. Such interventions could include setting small, easily achieved short-term goals and developing energy management techniques; use active listening techniques to help identify sources of hope. Assess client's level of motivation and willingness to adopt new behaviors that can improve symptoms of fatigue (Connolly et al, 2013).

- Encourage the client to keep a journal of activities that contribute to symptoms of fatigue, patterns of symptoms across days/weeks/months, and feelings, including how fatigue affects the client's normal daily activities and roles.

- Help the client identify sources of support and essential and nonessential tasks to determine which tasks can be delegated to whom. Give the client permission to limit social and role demands if needed (e.g., switch to part-time employment, hire cleaning service).

▲ Collaborate with the primary care provider regarding the appropriateness of referrals to physical therapy for carefully

• = Independent   ▲ = Collaborative

monitored aerobic exercise program and possible physical aids, such as a walker or cane if client has a disability requiring such support. Occupational therapy may also be indicated (Connolly et al, 2013).

- Encourage the client to try complementary and alternative therapy such as guided imagery, massage therapy, mindfulness, and acupressure.

▲ Refer the client to diagnosis-appropriate support groups such as the National Chronic Fatigue Syndrome Association, Multiple Sclerosis Association, or cancer fatigue websites such as the Oncology Nurses Association (http://www.ons.org) or the National Comprehensive Cancer Network.

▲ For a person with cardiac disease, recognize that fatigue is common after a myocardial infarction, CHF, or chronic cardiac insufficiency. Refer to cardiac rehabilitation for carefully prescribed and monitored exercise program.

- If fatigue is associated with cancer or cancer-related treatment, assess for other symptoms that may enhance fatigue (e.g., pain, insomnia, anemia, emotional distress, electrolyte imbalance [nausea, vomiting, diarrhea], or depression).

▲ Collaborate with primary care provider to identify attentional fatigue, which may manifest itself as the inability to direct attention necessary to perform usual activities. Attentional fatigue is associated with sleep disturbances, depressive symptoms, anxiety, and psychosocial stressors and can lead to irrational decision-making, inability to plan goals, and inability to control emotions or social interactions (Merriman et al, 2013).

▲ Collaborate with primary care providers to identify potential pharmacological treatment for fatigue.

Geriatric

- Evaluate fatigue in geriatric clients routinely, particularly in clients with limited physical function and lower levels of social support. Chronic conditions related to age can contribute to fatigue in the geriatric client, such as cancer, anemia, multiple medication usage and side effects, depression, insomnia (Naeim et al, 2014), nutritional deficiencies, electrolyte imbalance, and comorbidities involving multiple organ dysfunction (Giacalone et al, 2013).

- Review medications to determine possible side effects or interaction effects that could cause fatigue.

• = Independent   ▲ = Collaborative

- Review comorbid conditions that may contribute to fatigue, such as congestive heart failure, pulmonary disease, cardiac disease, arthritis, obesity, anemia, depression, insomnia, and cancer.
- Identify recent losses; monitor for depression or loneliness as a possible contributing factor to fatigue.
- Review other symptoms the client may be experiencing. Fatigue is often associated with other symptom clusters such as depression and sleep disturbances.
▲ Review medications for side effects. Certain medications (e.g., diuretics with associated loss of potassium, antihypertensives, antihistamines, pain medications [Rich & Nienaber, 2014], anticonvulsants [Siniscalchi et al, 2013], chemotherapeutic agents [Koornstra et al, 2014], psychiatric medications [Koornstra et al, 2014], and corticosteroids [Koornstra et al, 2014]) may cause fatigue, particularly in older adults.

Home Care

The above interventions may be adapted for home care use.

- Assess the client's history and current patterns of fatigue as they relate to the home environment and environmental and behavioral triggers of increased fatigue.
▲ Encourage planned exercise regimens or physical activities such as walking or light aerobic exercises. This activity can be organized in the home or in a setting such as senior centers or wellness facilities.
▲ Refer to occupational and/or physical therapy if substantial intervention is needed to assist the client in adapting to home and daily patterns.
- For clients receiving chemotherapy, intervene to:
  ○ Relieve symptom distress (anxiety, nausea and vomiting, diarrhea, lack of appetite, emotional distress, difficulty sleeping)
  ○ Encourage as much physical activity as possible with a specific regimen
  ○ Support a positive attitude for the future and reduce uncertainty by being sure clients know expectations and treatment expectations
  ○ Support adequate recovery time between treatments
- Teach the client and family the importance of and methods for setting priorities for activities, especially those with high energy demand (e.g., home or family events). Instruct in realistic expectations and behavioral pacing.

• = Independent   ▲ = Collaborative

- Assess effect of fatigue on the client's relatedness; recognize that the client's fatigue affects the whole family. Initiate the following interventions:
  - ○ Avoid dismissing reports of fatigue; validate the client's experience and foster hope for eventual treatment, if not resolution, of the fatigue.
  - ○ Identify with the client ways in which he or she continues to be a valued part of his or her social environment.
  - ○ Identify with the client ways in which he or she continues to participate in equitable exchange with others.
  - ○ Encourage the client to maintain regular family routines (e.g., meals, sleep patterns) as much as possible.
  - ○ Initiate cognitive restructuring to refute the client's guilt-producing and negative thought patterns.
  - ○ Assess and intervene with family's and friends' contributions to guilt-inducing self-talk.
  - ○ Work with the client to inoculate against the negative thinking of others.
  - ○ Explore family life and demands to identify accommodations.
  - ○ Support the client's efforts at limit setting on the demands of others.
  - ○ Assist the client to move toward a state of parallelism by working to identify and relieve sources of physical or emotional discomfort. Degree of involvement, limited by fatigue, need not be changed.
- ▲ Refer for family therapy in the event the client's fatigue interferes with normal family functioning.

Client/Family Teaching and Discharge Planning

- Help client to reframe cognitively; share information about fatigue and how to live with it, including need for positive self-talk.
- Teach strategies for energy conservation (e.g., sitting instead of standing during showering, storing items at waist level).
- Teach the client to carry a pocket calendar, make lists of required activities, and post reminders around the house. Attentional fatigue is associated with sleep disturbances, depressive symptoms, anxiety, and psychosocial stressors and can lead to irrational decision-making, inability to plan goals, and inability to control emotions or social interactions (Merriman et al, 2013).

• = Independent   ▲ = Collaborative

- Teach the importance of following a healthy lifestyle with adequate nutrition, fluids, and rest; pain relief; insomnia correction; and appropriate exercise to decrease fatigue (i.e., energy restoration).
- See **Hopelessness** care plan if appropriate.

F

Fear

NANDA-I Definition

Response to perceived threat that is consciously recognized as a danger

Defining Characteristics

Apprehensiveness; decrease in self-assurance; excitedness; feeling of dread; feeling of fear; feeling of pain; feeling of terror; feeling of alarm; increase in blood pressure; increase in tension; jitteriness; muscle tension; nausea; pallor; pupil dilation; vomiting

Cognitive

Decrease in learning ability; decrease in problem-solving ability; decrease in productivity; identifies object of fear; stimulus believed to be a threat

Behaviors

Attack behaviors; avoidance behaviors; focus narrowed to the source of fear; impulsiveness; increase in alertness

Physiological

Anorexia; change in physiological response (e.g., blood pressure, heart rate, respiratory rate, oxygen saturation, and end-tidal CO_2); diarrhea; dry mouth; dyspnea; fatigue; increase in perspiration; increase in respiratory rate

Related Factors (r/t)

Innate releasing mechanism to external stimuli (e.g., neurotransmitters); innate response to stimuli (e.g., sudden noise, height); language barrier; learned response; phobic stimulus; sensory deficit (e.g., visual, hearing); separation from support system; unfamiliar setting

Client Outcomes

Client Will (Specify Time Frame)

- Verbalize known fears
- State accurate information about the situation
- Identify, verbalize, and demonstrate those coping behaviors that reduce own fear
- Report and demonstrate reduced fear

• = Independent ▲ = Collaborative

Nursing Interventions

- Assess source of fear with the client.
- Assess for a history of anxiety.
- Have the client draw the object of his or her fear.
- Discuss the situation with the client and help distinguish between real and imagined threats to well-being.
- Encourage the client to explore underlying feelings that may be contributing to the fear.
- Stay with clients when they express fear; provide verbal and nonverbal (touch and hug with permission and if culturally acceptable) reassurances of safety if safety is within control.
- Explore coping skills previously used by the client to deal with fear; reinforce these skills and explore other outlets. Provide backrubs and massage for clients to decrease anxiety.
- ▲ Refer for cognitive behavior therapy.
- Encourage clients to express their fears in narrative form.

Pediatric

- Explore coping skills previously used by the client to deal with fear.
- Teach parents to use cognitive-behavioral strategies such as positive coping statements ("I am a brave girl [boy]. I can take care of myself in the dark.") And rewards of bravery tokens for appropriate behavior.
- Teach relaxation techniques to children to induce calmness.

Geriatric

- Establish a trusting relationship so that all fears can be identified. Monitor for dementia and use appropriate interventions.
- Provide a protective and safe environment, use consistent caregivers, and maintain the accustomed environmental structure.
- Observe for untoward changes if antianxiety drugs are taken.
- Assess for fear of falls in hospitalized clients with hip fractures to determine risk of poor health outcomes.
- Encourage exercises to improve physical skills and levels of mobility to decrease fear of falling.
- Assist the client in identifying and reducing risk factors for falls, including environmental hazards in and out of the home, the importance of good nutrition and activity, proper footwear, and how to stand up after a fall.

• = Independent   ▲ = Collaborative

F

Multicultural

- Assess for the presence of culture-bound anxiety and fear states.
- Assess for the influence of cultural beliefs, norms, and values on the client's perspective of a stressful situation.
- Identify what triggers fear response.
- Identify how the client expresses fear.
- Validate the client's feelings regarding fear.
- Assess for fears of racism in culturally diverse clients.

Home Care

- The previous interventions may be adapted for home care use.
- Assess to differentiate the presence of fear versus anxiety.
- Refer to care plan for **Anxiety.**
- During initial assessment, determine whether current or previous episodes of fear relate to the home environment (e.g., perception of danger in the home or neighborhood or of relationships that have a history in the home).
- Identify with the client what steps may be taken to make the home a "safe" place to be.
- ▲ Encourage the client to seek or continue appropriate counseling to reduce fear associated with stress or resolve alterations in irrational thought processes.
- ▲ Encourage the client to have a trusted companion, family member, or caregiver present in the home for periods when fear is most prominent. Pending other medical diagnoses, a referral to homemaker or home health aide services may meet this need.
- ▲ Offer to sit quietly with a terminally ill client as needed by the client or family, or provide hospice volunteers to do the same.

Client/Family Teaching and Discharge Planning

- Teach the client the difference between warranted and excessive fear.
- Teach clients to use guided imagery when they are fearful; have them use all senses to visualize a place that is "comfortable and safe" for them.
- Teach use of appropriate community resources in emergency situations (e.g., hotlines, emergency departments, law enforcement, judicial systems).
- Encourage use of appropriate community resources in nonemergency situations (e.g., family; friends; neighbors; self-help and support

groups; volunteer agencies; churches; recreation clubs and centers; seniors, youths, and others with similar interests).
- If fear is associated with bioterrorism, provide accurate information and ensure that health care personnel have appropriate training and preparation.

F

Ineffective infant Feeding pattern
NANDA-I Definition

Impaired ability of an infant to suck or coordinate the suck/swallow response, resulting in inadequate oral nutrition for metabolic needs

Defining Characteristics

Inability to coordinate sucking, swallowing, and breathing; inability to initiate an effective suck; inability to sustain an effective suck

Related Factors (r/t)

Neurological delay; neurological impairment (e.g., positive electroencephalogram, head trauma, seizure disorders); oral hypersensitivity; oropharyngeal defect; prematurity; prolonged nil per os (NPO) status

Client Outcomes

Infant Will (Specify Time Frame)

- Consume adequate calories that will result in appropriate weight gain and optimal growth and development
- Have opportunities for skin-to-skin (kangaroo care) experiences
- Have opportunities for "trophic" (i.e., small volume of breast milk/formula) enteral feedings prior to full oral feedings
- Progress to stable, neurobehavioral organization (i.e., motor, state, self-regulation, attention-interaction)
- Demonstrate presence of mature oral reflexes that are necessary for safe feeding
- Progress to safe, self-regulated oral feedings
- Coordinate the suck-swallow-breathe sequence while nippling
- Display clear behavioral cues related to hunger and satiety
- Display approach/engagement cues, with minimal avoidance/disengagement cues
- Have opportunities to pace own feeding, taking breaks as needed
- Display evidence of being in the "quiet-alert" state while nippling
- Progress to and engage in mutually positive parent/caregiver-infant/child interactions during feedings

• = Independent   ▲ = Collaborative

Parent/Family Will (Specify Time Frame)

* Recognize necessity of adequate calories for appropriate weight gain and optimal growth and development
* Learn to read and respond contingently to infant's behavioral cues (e.g., hunger, satiety, approach/engagement, stress/avoidance/disengagement)
* Learn strategies that promote organized infant behavior
* Learn appropriate positioning and handling techniques
* Learn effective ways to relieve stress behaviors during nippling
* Learn ways to help infant coordinate suck-swallow-breathe sequence (i.e., external pacing techniques)
* Engage in mutually positive interactions with infant during feeding
* Recognize ways to facilitate effective feedings: feed in quiet-alert state; keep length of feeding appropriate; burp; prepare/structure environment; recognize signs of sensory overload; encourage self-regulation; respect need for breaks and breathing pauses; avoid pulling and twisting nipple during pauses; allow infant to resume sucking when ready; provide oral support (cheek and/or jaw) as needed; use appropriate nipple hole size and flow rate

Nursing Interventions

* Refer to care plans for Disorganized **Infant** behavior, Risk for disorganized **Infant** behavior, Ineffective and Interrupted **Breastfeeding**, and Insufficient **Breast Milk** and assess as needed.
* Interventions follow a sequential pattern of implementation that can be adapted as appropriate.
* Assess coordination of infant's suck, swallow, and gag reflex.
▲ Provide developmentally supportive neonatal intensive care for preterm infants.
* Provide opportunities for kangaroo (i.e., skin-to-skin) care.
▲ Before the infant is ready for oral feedings, implement gavage feedings (or other alternative) as ordered, using breast milk whenever possible.
* Provide a naturalistic environment for tube feedings (naso-orogastric, gavage, or other) that approximates a pleasurable oral feeding experience: hold infant in semi-upright/flexed position; offer nonnutritive sucking; pace feedings; allow for semi-demand feedings contingent with infant cues; offer rest breaks; burp, as appropriate.

• = Independent   ▲ = Collaborative

- Foster direct breastfeeding as early as possible and enable the first oral feed to be at the breast in the neonatal intensive care unit (NICU).
- Allow parents to feed the infant when possible.
- Position infant in semi-upright position, with head, shoulders, and hips in straight line facing the mother with the infant's nose level with the mother's nipple.
- Feed infant in the quiet-alert state.
- Determine the appropriate shape, size, and hole of nipple to provide flow rate for preterm infants.
- Implement pacing for infants having difficulty coordinating breathing with sucking and swallowing.
- Provide infants with jaw and/or cheek support, as needed.
- Allow the stable newborn to breastfeed within the first half hour after birth.
- Allow appropriate time for nipple feeding to ensure infant's safety, limiting to 15 to 20 minutes for bottle feeding.
- Monitor length of breastfeeding so that it does not exceed 30 minutes. Breast milk transfer may last from as little as 5 to 20 minutes during breastfeeding depending on variations in milk supply during a 24-hour day (Flaherman et al, 2012).
- Encourage transitioning from scheduled to semi-demand feedings, contingent with infant behavior cues.
- ▲ Refer to a multidisciplinary team (e.g., neonatal/pediatric nutritionist, physical or occupational therapist, speech pathologist, lactation specialist) as needed.

Home Care

- The above appropriate interventions may be adapted for home care use.
- ▲ Infants with risk factors and clinical indicators of feeding problems present before hospital discharge should be referred to appropriate community early-intervention service providers (e.g., community health nurses, early learning programs [individualized per states], occupational therapy, speech pathologists, feeding specialists) to facilitate adequate weight gain for optimal growth and development.

Client/Family Teaching and Discharge Planning

- Provide anticipatory guidance for infant's expected feeding course.
- Teach various effective feeding methods and strategies to parents.

• = Independent   ▲ = Collaborative

- Teach parents how to read, interpret, and respond contingently to infant cues.
- Help parents identify support systems before hospital discharge.
- Provide anticipatory guidance for the infant's discharge.

F

Readiness for enhanced Fluid balance

NANDA-I Definition

A pattern of equilibrium between the fluid volume and chemical composition of body fluids, which can be strengthened

Defining Characteristics

Expresses desire to enhance fluid balance

Client Outcomes

Client Will (Specify Time Frame)

- Maintain light yellow urine output of at least 0.5 mL/kg/hr
- Maintain elastic skin turgor, moist tongue, and moist mucous membranes
- Explain measures that can be taken to improve fluid intake

Nursing Interventions

- Discuss normal fluid requirements.
- Recommend the client choose mainly water to meet fluid needs, although fruit juices and milk are also useful for hydration. The intake of beverages containing caffeine or alcohol is no longer thought to cause dehydration.
- Recommend the client choose and prepare foods with less salt, aiming for a maximum of 1500 mg per day, less than a teaspoon. The Centers for Disease Control and Prevention (2012) recommends that all salt-sensitive Americans, including everyone 40 years or older, should decrease daily sodium intake.
- Recommend the client avoid intake of soft drinks with sugar; instead, encourage the client to drink water.
- Recommend the client note the color of urine at intervals when voiding. Normal urine is straw-colored or amber.
- Recommend client monitor weight at intervals for alterations.

Geriatric

- Encourage older clients to develop a pattern of drinking water regularly.

• = Independent ▲ = Collaborative

- Ensure that when food intake is reduced or limited, it is compensated with an increase in water/fluid intake.
- Incorporate regular hydration into daily routines, such as providing an extra glass of fluid with medication or during social activities.

F

Deficient Fluid volume
NANDA-I Definition
Decreased intravascular, interstitial, and/or intracellular fluid. This refers to dehydration, water loss alone without change in sodium level

Defining Characteristics
Alteration in mental status; alteration in skin turgor; decrease in blood pressure; decrease in pulse pressure; decrease in pulse volume; decrease in tongue turgor; decrease in urine output; decreased venous filling; dry mucous membranes; dry skin; increase in body temperature; increase in heart rate; increase in hematocrit; increase in urine concentration; sudden weight loss; thirst; weakness

Client Outcomes
Client Will (Specify Time Frame)
- Maintain urine output of 0.5 mL/kg/hr or at least more than 1300 mL/day
- Maintain normal blood pressure, heart rate, and body temperature
- Maintain elastic skin turgor; moist tongue and mucous membranes; and orientation to person, place, and time
- Explain measures that can be taken to treat or prevent fluid volume loss
- Describe symptoms that indicate the need to consult with health care provider

Nursing Interventions
- Watch for early signs of hypovolemia, including thirst, restlessness, headaches, and inability to concentrate.
- Recognize symptoms of cyanosis; cold clammy skin, weak thready pulse, confusion, and oliguria as late signs of hypovolemia.
- Monitor pulse, respiration, and blood pressure of clients with deficient fluid volume every 15 minutes to 1 hour for the unstable client and every 4 hours for the stable client.
- Check orthostatic blood pressures with the client lying, sitting, and standing.

• = Independent ▲ = Collaborative

- Note skin turgor over bony prominences such as the hand or shin.
- Monitor for the existence of factors causing deficient fluid volume (e.g., hypovolemia from vomiting, diarrhea, difficulty maintaining oral intake, fever, uncontrolled type 2 diabetes, diuretic therapy).
- Observe for dry tongue and mucous membranes, and longitudinal tongue furrows.
- Recognize that checking capillary refill may not be helpful in identifying fluid volume deficit.
- Weigh client daily and watch for sudden decreases, especially in the presence of decreasing urine output or active fluid loss.
- Monitor total fluid intake and output every 4 hours (or every hour for the unstable client or the client who has urine output equal to or less than 0.5 mL/kg/hr). Recognize that urine output is an accurate indicator of fluid balance.
- Note the color of urine, urine osmolality, and specific gravity.
- Provide fresh water and oral fluids preferred by the client (distribute over 24 hours [e.g., 1200 mL on days, 800 mL on evenings, and 200 mL on nights]); provide prescribed diet; offer snacks (e.g., frequent drinks, fresh fruits, fruit juice); instruct significant other to assist the client with feedings as appropriate.
- ▲ Provide oral replacement therapy as ordered and tolerated with a hypotonic glucose-electrolyte solution when the client has acute diarrhea or nausea/vomiting. Provide small, frequent quantities of slightly chilled solutions.
- ▲ Administer antidiarrheals and antiemetics as ordered and appropriate.
- ▲ Hydrate the client with ordered isotonic IV solutions if prescribed.
- Assist with ambulation if the client has postural hypotension. Hypovolemia causes orthostatic hypotension, which can result in syncope when the client goes from a sitting to standing position (Wagner & Hardin-Pierce, 2014).

Critically Ill

- ▲ Monitor central venous pressure (CVP), pulmonary artery pressure, or stroke volume for decreasing trends for more accurate fluid volume status.
- ▲ Monitor serum and urine osmolality blood urea nitrogen (BUN)/creatinine ratio and hematocrit for elevations.

• = Independent   ▲ = Collaborative

▲ Insert an indwelling urinary catheter if ordered and measure urine output hourly. Notify health care provider if urine output is less than 0.5 mL/kg/hr.

▲ When ordered, initiate a fluid challenge of crystalloids (e.g., 0.9% normal saline or lactated Ringer's) for replacement of intravascular volume; monitor the client's response to prescribed fluid therapy and fluid challenge, especially noting vital signs, urine output, blood lactate concentrations, and lung sounds.

• Position the client flat with legs elevated when hypotensive, if not contraindicated.

▲ Monitor trends in serum lactic acid levels and base deficit obtained from blood gases as ordered.

▲ Consult provider if signs and symptoms of deficient fluid volume persist or worsen.

Pediatric

• Monitor the child for signs of deficient fluid volume, including sunken eyes, decreased tears, dry mucous membranes, poor skin turgor, and decreased urine output (Graves, 2013).

▲ Reinforce the health care provider recommendation for the parents to give the child oral rehydration fluids to drink in the amounts specified, especially during the first 4 to 6 hours to replace fluid losses. Consider using diluted oral rehydration fluids. Once the child is rehydrated, an orally administered maintenance solution should be used along with food.

• Recommend that the mother resume breastfeeding as soon as possible.

• Recommend that parents not give the child decarbonated soda, fruit juices, gelatin dessert, or instant fruit drink mix. Instead give the child oral rehydration fluids ordered and, when tolerated, food.

• Once the child has been rehydrated, begin feeding regular food, but avoid milk products (Guandalini et al, 2014).

Geriatric

• Monitor older clients for deficient fluid volume carefully, noting new onset of headache, weakness, dizziness, and postural hypotension.

• Evaluate the risk for dehydration using the Dehydration Risk Appraisal Checklist.

• Check skin turgor of older clients on the forehead and axilla; check for dry mucous membranes and sunken eyes.

• = Independent   ▲ = Collaborative

F

- Encourage fluid intake by offering fluids regularly to cognitively impaired clients.
- Incorporate regular hydration into daily routines (e.g., extra glass of fluid with medication or social activities) (Hooper et al, 2013).
- Because they have low water reserves, older adults should be encouraged to drink regularly even when not thirsty. Frequent and varied beverage offerings should be made available by hydration assistants to routinely offer increased beverages to clients in extended care.
- Flag the food tray of clients with chronic dehydration to indicate if the client is identified as having chronic dehydration and indicate that they should finish 75% to 100% of their food and fluids. Offering beverages in brightly colored cups may improve fluid intake.
- Recognize that lower blood pressure and a higher BUN/creatinine ratio can be significant signs of dehydration in older adults.
- Note the color of urine and compare against a urine color chart to monitor adequate fluid intake.
- Monitor older clients for excess fluid volume during the treatment of deficient fluid volume: auscultate lung sounds, assess for edema, and note vital signs.

Home Care

- Teach family members how to monitor output in the home (e.g., use of commode "hat" in the toilet, urinal, or bedpan, or use of catheter and closed drainage system). Instruct them to monitor both intake and output. Use common terms such as "cups" or "glasses of water a day" when providing education.
- When weighing the client, use same scale each day. Be sure scale is on a flat, not cushioned, surface. Do not weigh the client with scale placed on any type of rug.
- Teach family about complications of deficient fluid volume and when to call the health care provider.
- Teach the family the signs of hypovolemia, especially in older adults, and how to monitor for dizziness or unsteady gait.
- If the client is receiving IV fluids, there must be a responsible caregiver in the home. Teach caregiver about administration of fluids, complications of IV administration (e.g., fluid volume overload, speed of medication reactions), and when to call for assistance. Assist

• = Independent ▲ = Collaborative

caregiver with administration for as long as necessary to maintain client safety.
- Identify an emergency plan, including when to call 911.
- Deficient fluid volume may be a symptom of impending death in terminally ill clients. In palliative care situations, treatment of deficient fluid volume should be determined based on client/family goals. Information and support should be provided to assist the client/family in this decision. Support the family/client in a palliative care situation to decide if it is appropriate to intervene for deficient fluid volume or to allow the client to die without fluids.

F

Client/Family Teaching and Discharge Planning
- Instruct the client to avoid rapid position changes, especially from supine to sitting or standing.
- Teach the client and family about appropriate diet and fluid intake.
- Teach the client and family how to measure and record intake and output accurately.
- Teach the client and family about measures instituted to treat hypovolemia and to prevent or treat fluid volume loss.
- Instruct the client and family about signs of deficient fluid volume that indicate they should contact the health care provider.

Excess Fluid volume

NANDA-I Definition
Increased isotonic fluid retention

Defining Characteristics
Adventitious breath sounds; alteration in blood pressure; alteration in mental status; alteration in pulmonary artery pressure (PAP); alteration in respiratory pattern; alteration in urine specific gravity; anasarca; anxiety; azotemia; decrease in hematocrit; decrease in hemoglobin; dyspnea; edema; electrolyte imbalance; hepatomegaly; increased central venous pressure (CVP); intake exceeds output; jugular vein distention; oliguria; orthopnea; paroxysmal nocturnal dyspnea; pleural effusion; positive hepatojugular reflex; pulmonary congestion; restlessness; presence of S3 heart sound; weight gain over short period of time

Related Factors
Compromised regulatory mechanism; excessive fluid intake; excessive sodium intake

• = Independent   ▲ = Collaborative

F

Client Outcomes

Client Will (Specify Time Frame)

- Remain free of edema, effusion, anasarca
- Maintain body weight appropriate for the client
- Maintain clear lung sounds; no evidence of dyspnea or orthopnea
- Remain free of jugular vein distention, positive hepatojugular reflex, and S3 heart sound
- Maintain normal CVP, PAP, cardiac output, and vital signs
- Maintain urine output of 0.5 mL/kg/hr or more with normal urine osmolality and specific gravity
- Explain actions that are needed to treat or prevent excess fluid volume including fluid and dietary restrictions and medications
- Describe symptoms that indicate the need to consult with health care provider

Nursing Interventions

- Monitor location and extent of edema using the 1+ to 4+ scale to quantify edema; also measure the legs using a millimeter tape in the same area at the same time each day. Note differences in measurement between extremities.
- Monitor daily weight for sudden increases; use same scale and type of clothing at same time each day, preferably before breakfast.
- Monitor intake and output; note trends reflecting decreasing urine output in relation to fluid intake.
- Monitor vital signs; note decreasing blood pressure, tachycardia, and tachypnea. Monitor for S3 heart sounds. If signs of heart failure are present, see the care plan for Decreased **Cardiac** output.
- Auscultate lung sounds for crackles, monitor respiration effort, and determine the presence and severity of orthopnea.
- Monitor serum and urine osmolality, serum sodium, blood urea nitrogen (BUN)/creatinine ratio, and hematocrit for abnormalities.
- With head of bed elevated 30 to 45 degrees, monitor jugular veins for distention with the client in the upright position; assess for positive hepatojugular reflex.
- Monitor the client's behavior for restlessness, anxiety, or confusion; use safety precautions if symptoms are present.
- ▲ Monitor for the development of conditions that increase the client's risk for excess fluid volume, including heart failure, kidney failure,

and liver failure, all of which result in decreased glomerular filtration rate and fluid retention.

▲ Provide a restricted-sodium diet as appropriate if ordered.

▲ Monitor serum albumin level and provide protein intake as appropriate.

▲ Administer prescribed diuretics as appropriate; ensure adequate blood pressure before administration. If diuretic is administered intravenously, note and record the blood pressure and urine output following the dose.

• Monitor for side effects of diuretic therapy: orthostatic hypotension (especially if the client is also receiving angiotensin-converting enzyme [ACE] inhibitors), hypovolemia, and electrolyte imbalances (hypokalemia and hyponatremia).

▲ Implement fluid restriction as ordered, especially when serum sodium is low; include all routes of intake. Schedule limited intake of fluids around the clock, and include the type of fluids preferred by the client.

• Maintain the rate of all IV infusions, carefully using an IV pump.

• Turn clients with dependent edema at least every 2 hours.

▲ Provide ordered care for edematous extremities including compression, elevation, and muscle exercises.

• Promote a positive body image and good self-esteem. Refer to the care plan for Disturbed **Body Image.**

▲ Consult with the health care provider if signs and symptoms of excess fluid volume persist or worsen.

Critically Ill

• Insert an indwelling urinary catheter if ordered and measure urine output hourly. Notify health care provider if output is less than 0.5 mL/kg/hr.

▲ Monitor CVP, mean arterial pressure, PAP, and cardiac output/index; note and report trends of increasing or decreasing pressures over time.

▲ Monitor the effects of infusion of diuretic drips. Perform continuous renal replacement therapy (CRRT) as ordered if the client is critically ill and hemodynamically unstable and excessive fluid must be removed.

Geriatric

• Recognize that the presence of fluid volume excess is particularly serious in older adults.

• = Independent   ▲ = Collaborative

- Monitor electrolyte levels carefully, including sodium levels and potassium levels, with both increased and decreased levels possible.

Home Care

- Assess client and family knowledge of disease process causing excess fluid volume.
▲ Teach about disease process and complications of excess fluid volume, including when to contact the health care provider.
- Assess client and family knowledge and compliance with medical regimen, including medications, diet, rest, and exercise. Assist family with integrating restrictions into daily living.
▲ Teach and reinforce knowledge of medications. Instruct the client not to use over-the-counter (OTC) medications (e.g., diet medications) without first consulting the provider.
▲ Instruct the client to make the primary health care provider aware of medications ordered by other health care providers.
- Identify emergency plan for rapidly developing or critical levels of excess fluid volume when diuresing is not safe at home.
▲ Teach about signs and symptoms of both excess and deficient fluid volume, such as darker urine, and when to call the health care provider.

Client/Family Teaching and Discharge Planning

- Describe signs and symptoms of excess fluid volume and actions to take if they occur.
▲ Teach client on diuretics to weigh self daily in the morning and to notify the health care provider if there is a 2.2 pound (1 kg) or more weight gain (Wagner & Hardin-Pierce, 2014).
▲ Teach the importance of fluid and sodium restrictions. Help the client and family devise a schedule for intake of fluids throughout the entire day. Refer to a dietitian concerning implementation of a low-sodium diet.
- Teach clients how to measure and document intake and output with common household measurements, such as cups.
▲ Teach how to take diuretics correctly: take one dose in the morning and second dose (if taken) no later than 4 PM. Adjust potassium intake as appropriate for potassium-losing or potassium-sparing diuretics. Note the appearance of side effects such as weakness, muscle cramps, hypertension, palpitations, or irregular heartbeat (Wagner & Hardin-Pierce, 2014).

• = Independent   ▲ = Collaborative

• For the client undergoing hemodialysis, teach client the required restrictions in dietary electrolytes, protein, and fluid. Spend time with the client to detect any factors that may interfere with the client's compliance with the fluid restriction or restrictive diet.

Risk for Deficient Fluid volume

NANDA-I Definition

Vulnerable to experiencing decreased intravascular, interstitial, and/or intracellular fluid volumes, which may compromise health

Risk Factors

Active fluid volume loss; barrier to accessing fluid; compromised regulatory mechanism; deviations affecting fluid absorption; deviations affecting fluid intake; excessive fluid loss through normal route; extremes of age; extremes of weight; factors influencing fluid needs; fluid loss through abnormal route; insufficient knowledge about fluid needs; pharmaceutical agent

Client Outcomes, Nursing Interventions, and Client/Family Teaching and Discharge Planning

Refer to care plan for deficient **Fluid** volume.

Risk for imbalanced Fluid volume

NANDA-I Definition

Vulnerable to a decrease, increase, or rapid shift from one to the other of intravascular, interstitial, and/or intracellular fluid, which may compromise health; this refers to body fluid loss, gain, or both

Risk Factors

Apheresis; ascites; burns; intestinal obstruction; pancreatitis; sepsis; trauma; treatment regimen

Client Outcomes

• Lung sounds clear, respiratory rate 12 to 20 and free of dyspnea
• Urine output greater than 0.5 mL/kg/hr
• Blood pressure, pulse rate, temperature, and oxygen saturation within expected range
• Laboratory values within expected range, that is, normal serum sodium, hematocrit, and osmolarity
• Extremities and dependent areas free of edema
• Mental orientation appropriate based on previous condition

• = Independent   ▲ = Collaborative

Nursing Interventions
Surgical Clients

- Monitor the fluid balance. If there are symptoms of hypovolemia, refer to the interventions in the care plan for Deficient **Fluid** volume. If there are symptoms of hypervolemia, refer to the interventions in the care plan for Excess **Fluid** volume.

Preoperative

- Collect a thorough history and perform a preoperative assessment to identify clients with increased risk for hemorrhage or hypovolemia, that is, clients with recent traumatic injury, abnormal bleeding or altered clotting times, complicated kidney or liver disease, diabetes, cardiovascular disease, major organ transplant, history of aspirin and/or NSAID use, anticoagulant therapy, or history of hemophilia, von Willebrand's disease, or disseminated intravascular coagulation. Assess the client's use of over-the-counter agents to include herbal products.
- Recognize that NPO at midnight may or may not be appropriate for each surgical client. Guidelines from the American Society of Anesthesiologists (ASA) in 2011 recommend the following: healthy clients having elective surgery should be allowed to have clear liquids up to 2 hours before surgery.
- Determine length of time the client has been without normal intake, been NPO, or experienced fluid loss (e.g., vomiting, diarrhea, bleeding).
- Assess and document the client's mental status.
- Recognize that there is conflicting evidence regarding liberal intraoperative fluid management versus restrictive fluid management. Fluid administration during surgery is more restrictive to prevent pulmonary complications associated with excessive fluid administration (Assaad et al, 2013).
- Recognize that an individualized fluid management plan would be developed incorporating client-specific assessment parameters (e.g., existing comorbid diseases, age) and type of surgical procedure (Allison & George, 2014).
- Recognize the effects of general anesthetics, inhalational agents, and of regional anesthesia on perfusion in the body and decreasing the blood pressure.
- Monitor for signs of intraoperative hypovolemia: dry skin, dry mucous membranes, tachycardia, decreased urinary output, decreased

• = Independent   ▲ = Collaborative

central venous pressure, hypotension, increased pulse, and/or deep rapid respirations.

- Monitor for signs of intraoperative hypervolemia: dyspnea, coarse crackles, increased pulse and respirations, decreased oxygenation, and decreased urinary output, all of which could progress to pulmonary edema.
- In the critically ill surgical client, a pulmonary artery catheter or other minimally invasive cardiac output monitoring device may be used to determine fluid balance and guide fluid and vasoactive intravenous (IV) drip administration.
- Monitor the client for hyponatremia, that is, headache, anorexia, nausea and vomiting, diarrhea, tachycardia, general malaise, muscle cramps, weakness, lethargy, change in mental status, disorientation, seizures, and death.
- Monitor clients undergoing laparoscopic or hysteroscopic procedures for the development of hyponatremia, hypervolemia, and pulmonary edema when an irrigation fluid is used.
- Monitor clients undergoing transurethral resection of the prostate (TURP) procedures for development of hyponatremia and hypervolemia with symptoms of TURP syndrome: headache, visual changes, agitation, lethargy, vomiting, muscle twitching, bradycardia, diminished pupillary reflexes, hypertension, and respiratory distress.
- Measure the irrigation fluid used during urological and gynecological procedures accurately for volume deficit, that is, amount of irrigation used minus amount of irrigation recovered via suction.
- Monitor intraoperative intake and output including blood loss, urine output, and third-space losses, to provide an estimate of fluid volume.
- Observe the surgical client for hyperkalemia, that is, dysrhythmias, heart block, asystole, abdominal distention, and weakness.
- Maintain the client's core temperature at normal levels, using warming devices as needed.

Postoperative

- Continue to support restrictive fluid management postoperatively.
- Assess the client for development of tissue edema.
- Recognize that IV fluid replacement decisions incorporate multiple assessment parameters: hourly urine output, blood pressure, heart rate, respiratory rate, lung sounds, output from drains, and changes

in laboratory results (e.g., hemoglobin/hematocrit, serum electrolytes).

Geriatric

- Check skin turgor of older client on the forehead, subclavian area, or inner thigh; also look for the presence of longitudinal furrows on the tongue and dry mucous membranes.
- Closely monitor urine output, concentration of urine, and serum BUN/creatinine results.
- Monitor older clients for excess fluid volume during the treatment of deficient fluid volume: auscultate lung sounds, assess for edema, and trend vital signs.
- Assess the older client's cognitive status.

Pediatric

- Assess the pediatric client's weight, length of NPO status, underlying illness, and the surgical procedure to be performed.
- Recognize that newborns require very little fluid replacement when undergoing major surgical procedures during the first few days of life.
- Monitor pediatric surgical clients closely for signs of fluid loss.
- Administer fluids preoperatively until NPO status must be initiated so that fluid deficit is decreased.
- Perform an assessment for signs of fluid responsiveness in the pediatric client.

Frail Elderly syndrome

NANDA-I Definition

Dynamic state of unstable equilibrium that affects the older individual experiencing deterioration in one or more domains of health (physical, functional, psychological, or social) and leads to increased susceptibility to adverse health effects, particularly disability

Risk Factors

Activity intolerance; bathing self-care deficit; decreased cardiac output; dressing self-care deficit; fatigue; feeding self-care deficit; hopelessness; imbalanced nutrition: less than body requirements; impaired memory; impaired physical mobility; impaired walking; social isolation; toileting self-care deficit

Related Factors

Alteration in cognitive functioning; chronic illness; history of falls; living alone; malnutrition; prolonged hospitalization; psychiatric disorder; sarcopenia; sarcopenic obesity; sedentary lifestyle

Client Outcomes

Client Will (Specify Time Frame)

- Remain living as independently as possible in the home or care setting of his or her choice
- Maintain safety when engaging in activities of daily living and ambulation
- Increase exercise and/or daily physical activity in order to build muscle strength
- Maintain a healthy weight

Nursing Interventions

- Assess frailty with a tool such as the Edmonton Frail Scale.
- Recognize that balance and gait impairment are features of frailty and are risk factors for falls.
- Monitor physical frailty indicators such as slow gait speed and low physical activity.
- Assess falls using a falls risk assessment tool such as the Hendrich II Fall Risk Model.
- Evaluate the client's medications to determine whether medications increase the risk of frailty; if appropriate, consult with the client's health care provider regarding the client's medications.
- ▲ Refer to a dietitian for an individualized therapeutic diet.
- Refer to care plan for Readiness for enhanced **Nutrition** for additional interventions.
- Monitor weight loss.
- Encourage clients to engage in active lifestyles.
- Provide an exercise-training program.
- Promote the benefits of home-based exercise to older clients who are frail.
- Use a multidisciplinary and person-centered approach for supporting frail older adults.
- Develop a trusting and responsive relationship with frail clients.

Multicultural, Home Care, Client/Family Teaching and Discharge Planning

- The above interventions may be adapted for multicultural, home care, and client/family teaching and discharge planning.

• = Independent ▲ = Collaborative

Risk for Frail Elderly syndrome
NANDA-I Definition

Vulnerable to a dynamic state of unstable equilibrium that affects the older individual experiencing deterioration in one or more domains of health (physical, functional, or social) and leads to increased susceptibility to adverse health effects, in particular disability

Defining Characteristics

Activity intolerance; age >70 years; alteration in cognitive functioning; altered clotting process (e.g., factor VII, D-dimers); anorexia; anxiety; average daily physical activity is less than recommended for gender and age; chronic illness; constricted life space; decrease in energy; decrease in muscle strength; decrease in serum 25-hydroxyvitamin D concentration; depression; economically disadvantaged; endocrine regulatory dysfunction (e.g., glucose intolerance, increase in IGF-1, androgen, DHEA, and cortisol); ethnicity other than Caucasian; exhaustion; fear of falling; female gender; history of falls; immobility; impaired balance; impaired mobility; insufficient social support; living alone; low educational level; malnutrition; muscle weakness; obesity; prolonged hospitalization; sadness; sarcopenia; sarcopenic obesity; sedentary lifestyle; sensory deficit (e.g., visual, hearing); social isolation; social vulnerability (e.g., disempowerment, decreased life control); suppressed inflammatory response (e.g., IL-6, CRP); unintentional loss of 25% of body weight over 1 year; unintentional weight loss >10 pounds (>4.5 kg) in 1 year; walking 15 feet requires more than 6 seconds (4 m > 5 seconds)

Client Outcomes, Nursing Interventions, and Client/Family Teaching and Discharge Planning

Refer to care plan for **Frail Elderly** syndrome.

Impaired Gas exchange
NANDA-I Definition

Excess or deficit in oxygenation and/or carbon dioxide elimination at the alveolar-capillary membrane

Defining Characteristics

Abnormal arterial blood gases; abnormal arterial pH; abnormal breathing pattern (e.g., rate, rhythm, depth); abnormal skin color (e.g., pale, dusky, cyanosis); confusion; cyanosis; decrease in carbon dioxide (CO_2) levels; diaphoresis; dyspnea; headache upon awakening; hypercapnia; hypoxemia; hypoxia; irritability; nasal flaring; restlessness, somnolence; tachycardia; visual disturbances

• = Independent   ▲ = Collaborative

Related Factors (r/t)

Alveolar-capillary membrane changes; ventilation-perfusion imbalance

Client Outcomes

Client Will (Specify Time Frame)

- Demonstrate improved ventilation and adequate oxygenation as evidenced by blood gas levels within normal parameters for that client
- Maintain clear lung fields and remain free of signs of respiratory distress
- Verbalize understanding of oxygen supplementation and other therapeutic interventions

G

Nursing Interventions

- Monitor respiratory rate, depth, and ease of respiration. Watch for use of accessory muscles and nasal flaring.
- Auscultate breath sounds every 1 to 2 hours. The presence of crackles and wheezes may alert the nurse to airway obstruction, which may lead to or exacerbate existing hypoxia.
- Monitor the client's behavior and mental status for the onset of restlessness, agitation, confusion, and (in the late stages) extreme lethargy.
- ▲ Monitor oxygen saturation continuously using pulse oximetry. Note blood gas results as available.
- Observe for cyanosis of the skin; especially note color of the tongue and oral mucous membranes.
- Position the client in a semirecumbent position with the head of the bed at a 30- to 45-degree angle to decrease the aspiration of gastric, oral, and nasal secretions (Grap, 2009; Siela, 2010; Vollman & Sole, 2011). Historically, evidence shows that mechanically ventilated clients have a decreased incidence of aspiration pneumonia if the client is placed in a 30- to 45-degree semirecumbent position as opposed to a supine position.
- If the client has unilateral lung disease, position with head of bed at 30 to 45 degrees with "good lung down" for about 1 hour at a time (Burns, 2011).
- ▲ If the client is acutely dyspneic, consider having the client lean forward over a bedside table, resting elbows on the table if tolerated.
- Help the client deep breathe and perform controlled coughing. Have the client inhale deeply, hold the breath for several seconds, and cough two or three times with the mouth open while tightening the upper abdominal muscles as tolerated. If the client has excessive fluid

---

• = Independent   ▲ = Collaborative

in the respiratory system, see the interventions for ineffective **Airway** clearance.

▲ Monitor the effects of sedation and analgesics on the client's respiratory pattern; use judiciously.

• Schedule nursing care to provide rest and minimize fatigue.

▲ Administer humidified oxygen through an appropriate device (e.g., nasal cannula or Venturi mask per the health care provider's order); aim for an oxygen (O_2) saturation level of 90% or above. Watch for onset of hypoventilation as evidenced by increased somnolence.

• Once oxygen is started, arterial blood gases should be checked 30 to 60 minutes later to ensure satisfactory oxygenation without carbon dioxide retention or acidosis (GOLD, 2015).

• Assess nutritional status including serum albumin level and body mass index (BMI).

▲ Assist the client to eat small meals frequently and use dietary supplements as necessary. Engage dietitian in evaluating and creating an optimal nutrition plan. For some clients, drinking 30 mL of a supplement every hour while awake can be helpful.

• If the client is severely debilitated from chronic respiratory disease, consider the use of a wheeled walker to help in ambulation.

▲ Watch for signs of psychological distress including anxiety, agitation, and insomnia.

▲ Refer the COPD client to a pulmonary rehabilitation program.

Critical Care

▲ Assess and monitor oxygen indices such as the PF ratio (FIo_2:pO_2), venous oxygen saturation/oxygen consumption (SVO_2 or $ScVO_2$) (Headley & Guiliano, 2011; Burns, 2011).

▲ Turn the client every 2 hours. Monitor mixed venous oxygen saturation closely after turning. If it drops below 10% or fails to return to baseline promptly, turn the client back into the supine position and evaluate oxygen status. If the client does not tolerate turning, consider use of a kinetic bed that rotates the client from side to side in a turn of at least 40 degrees (Vollman and Powers, 2011).

▲ If the client has acute respiratory distress syndrome with difficulty maintaining oxygenation, consider positioning the client prone with the upper thorax and pelvis supported. Monitor oxygen saturation and turn the client back to supine position if desaturation occurs. NOTE: If the client becomes ventilator dependent, see the care plan for Impaired spontaneous **Ventilation.**

• = Independent   ▲ = Collaborative

▲ High levels of positive end-expiratory pressures likely improve oxygenation and gas exchange (Meade et al, 2008; Suzumura et al, 2014).

Geriatric

▲ Use central nervous system depressants and other sedating agents carefully to avoid decreasing respiration rate.

▲ Maintain low-flow oxygen therapy for clients with impaired gas exchange and hypoxemia (GOLD 2015; Burns, 2011).

G

Home Care

• Work with the client to determine what strategies are most helpful during times of dyspnea. Educate and empower the client to self-manage the disease associated with impaired gas exchange.

• Collaborate with health care providers regarding long-term oxygen administration for chronic respiratory failure clients with severe resting hypoxemia. Administer long-term oxygen therapy greater than 15 hours daily for pO_2 less than 55 or SaO_2 at or below 88% (GOLD, 2015).

• Assess the home environment for irritants that impair gas exchange. Help the client adjust the home environment as necessary (e.g., install an air filter to decrease the level of dust).

▲ Refer the client to occupational therapy as necessary to assist the client in adapting to the home and environment and in energy conservation (GOLD, 2015).

• Assist the client with identifying and avoiding situations that exacerbate impairment of gas exchange (e.g., stress-related situations, exposure to pollution of any kind, proximity to noxious gas fumes such as chlorine bleach).

• Refer to GOLD guidelines for management of home care and indications of hospital admission criteria (GOLD, 2015).

• Instruct the client to keep the home temperature above 68° F (20° C) and to avoid cold weather.

• Instruct the client to limit exposure to persons with respiratory infections.

• Instruct the family in the complications of the disease and the importance of maintaining the medical regimen, including when to call a health care provider.

▲ Refer the client for home health aide services as necessary for assistance with activities of daily living.

• = Independent   ▲ = Collaborative

- When respiratory procedures are being implemented, explain equipment and procedures to family members, and provide needed emotional support.
- When electrically based equipment for respiratory support is being implemented, evaluate home environment for electrical safety, proper grounding, and so on. Ensure that notification is sent to the local utility company, the emergency medical team, and police and fire departments.
- ▲ Assess family role changes and coping ability. Refer the client to medical social services as appropriate for assistance in adjusting to chronic illness.
- Support the family of the client with chronic illness.

Client/Family Teaching and Discharge Planning

- Teach the client how to perform pursed-lip breathing and inspiratory muscle training, and how to use the tripod position. Have the client watch the pulse oximeter to note improvement in oxygenation with these breathing techniques.
- Teach the client energy conservation techniques and the importance of alternating rest periods with activity. See nursing interventions for **Fatigue.**
- ▲ Teach the importance of not smoking. Refer to smoking cessation programs, and encourage clients who relapse to keep trying to quit. Ensure that clients receive appropriate medications to support smoking cessation from the primary health care provider.
- ▲ Instruct the family regarding home oxygen therapy if ordered (e.g., delivery system, liter flow, safety precautions).
- ▲ Teach the client the need to receive a yearly influenza vaccine.
- Teach the client relaxation techniques to help reduce stress responses and panic attacks resulting from dyspnea.
- Teach the client to use music, along with a rest period, to decrease dyspnea and anxiety (Loscalzo, 2013).

Dysfunctional Gastrointestinal motility

NANDA-I Definition

Increased, decreased, ineffective, or lack of peristaltic activity within the gastrointestinal system

• = Independent   ▲ = Collaborative

Defining Characteristics

Abdominal cramping; abdominal distention; abdominal pain; absence of flatus; acceleration of gastric emptying; bile-colored gastric residual; change in bowel sounds; diarrhea; difficulty with defecation; hard, formed stool; increase in gastric residual; nausea; regurgitation; vomiting

Related Factors (r/t)

Aging; anxiety; enteral feedings; food intolerance; immobility; ingestion of contaminated material (e.g., radioactive, food, water); malnutrition; prematurity; sedentary lifestyle; treatment regimen

G

Client Outcomes

Client Will (Specify Time Frame)

- Be free of abdominal distention and pain
- Have normal bowel sounds
- Pass flatus rectally at intervals
- Defecate formed, soft stool every day to every third day
- State has an appetite
- Be able to eat food without nausea and vomiting

Nursing Interventions

- Monitor for abdominal distention, and presence of abdominal pain, weight loss, nausea, vomiting, obstipation, or diarrhea.
- Inspect, auscultate for bowel sounds noting characteristics and frequency; palpate and percuss the abdomen.
- Review history noting any anorexia or nausea/vomiting. Other symptoms may include relation of symptoms to meals, especially if aggravated by food, satiety, postprandial fullness/bloating, and weight loss or weight loss with severe gastroparesis.
- Monitor for fluid deficits by checking skin turgor and moisture of tongue, daily weights, input and output, and electrolyte values. Refer to care plan for Deficient **Fluid** volume if relevant.
- ▲ Monitor for nutritional deficits by keeping close track of food intake. Review laboratory studies that affirm nutritional deficits, such as decreased albumin and serum protein levels, liver profile, glucose, and an electrolyte panel. Refer to care plans for Imbalanced **Nutrition:** less than body requirements or Risk for **Electrolyte** imbalance as appropriate.

Slowed Gastric Motility

- Monitor the client for signs and symptoms of decreased gastric motility, which may include nausea after meals, vomiting, feeling full

• = Independent   ▲ = Collaborative

quickly while eating, abdominal bloating, and abdominal pain (Bouras et al, 2013).

▲ Monitor daily laboratory studies and point of care testing blood glucose levels ensuring ordered glucose levels are performed and evaluated.

• Obtain a thorough gastrointestinal history if the client has diabetes, because he/she is at high risk for gastroparesis and gastric reflux.

▲ If client has nausea and vomiting, provide an antiemetic and intravenous fluids as ordered. Refer to the care plan for **Nausea.**

▲ Evaluate medications that the client is taking. Recognize that vasopressors, opioids, or anticholinergic medications can cause gastric slowing (Aderinto-Adike & Quigley, 2014).

▲ Review laboratory and other diagnostic tools, including complete blood count, amylase, and thyroid-stimulating hormone level, glucose with other metabolic studies, upper endoscopy, and gastric-emptying scintigraphy.

▲ Obtain a nutritional consult, considering a small particle size diet or diets lower or higher in liquids or solids, depending on gastric motility.

▲ If client is unable to eat or retain food, consult with the registered dietitian and health care provider, considering further nutritional support in the form of enteral or parenteral feedings for the client with gastroparesis.

▲ If client is receiving gastric enteral nutrition, see the care plan for risk for **Aspiration.**

▲ Administer medications that increase gastrointestinal motility as ordered (Chang et al, 2011).

Postoperative Ileus

• Observe for complications of delayed intestinal motility. Symptoms include vague abdominal pain and distention, nausea, vomiting, anorexia, sometimes bloating, and tympany to percussion. Clients may or may not pass flatus and some stool (Cagir, 2013).

▲ Recommend chewing gum for the abdominal surgery client who is experiencing an ileus, is not at risk for aspiration, and has normal dentition.

• Help the client out of bed to walk at least two times per day. Assist client to sit in a rocking chair to rock back and forth.

▲ If postoperative ileus is associated with opioid pain medication, ensure opioids are decreased or ideally discontinued. Use

• = Independent   ▲ = Collaborative

nonsteroidal anti-inflammatory drugs for pain as feasible and if not contraindicated (Cagir, 2013).

▲ Note serum electrolyte levels, especially potassium and magnesium.

Increased Gastrointestinal Motility

▲ Observe for complications of gastric surgeries such as dumping syndrome.

· Watch for nausea, vomiting, bloating, cramping, diarrhea, dizziness, and fatigue.

· Monitor for low blood sugar, weakness, sweating, and dizziness 1 to 3 hours after eating as this is when late rapid gastric emptying may occur. Late rapid gastric emptying is associated with low blood sugar (Bosnic, 2014).

▲ Order a nutritional consult to discuss diet changes. The diet may vary depending on the kind of surgery causing dumping syndrome.

▲ Give intravenous fluids as ordered for the client complaining of diarrhea with weakness and dizziness. Monitor electrolyte panel.

· Offer bathroom, commode, or bedpan assistance, depending on frequency, amount of diarrhea, and condition of client.

· Monitor rectal area for decreased skin integrity, apply barrier creams as needed to protect and treat skin.

· Refer to the care plans for Deficient **Fluid** volume, **Nausea,** Impaired **Skin** integrity, and **Diarrhea** as relevant.

Pediatric

· Assess infants and children with suspected delayed gastric emptying for fullness and vomiting.

▲ Observe for nutritional and fluid deficits with assessment of skin turgor, mucous membranes, fontanels, furrows of the tongue, electrolyte panel, fluid status, input and output, and daily weights (Saliakellis & Fotoulaki, 2013).

▲ Recommend gentle massage for preterm infants as appropriate.

Geriatric

· Closely monitor diet and medication use/side effects as they affect the gastrointestinal system. Watch for constipation.

▲ Watch for symptoms of dysphagia, gastroesophageal reflux disease, dyspepsia, irritable bowel syndrome, maldigestion, and reduced absorption of nutrients.

Client/Family Teaching and Discharge Planning

· Teach the client and caregivers about medications, reinforcing side effects as they relate to gastrointestinal function.

- Teach client and caregivers to report signs and symptoms that may indicate further complications including increased abdominal girth, projectile vomiting, and unrelieved acute cramping pain (bowel obstruction).
- Review signs and symptoms of dehydration with client and caregivers.

G

Risk for dysfunctional Gastrointestinal motility

NANDA-I Definition

Vulnerable to a decrease in normal frequency of defecation accompanied by difficult or incomplete passage of stool, which may compromise health

Risk Factors

Aging; anxiety; change in water source; decrease in gastrointestinal circulation; diabetes mellitus; eating habit change (e.g., foods, eating times); food intolerance; gastroesophageal reflux disease; immobility; infection; pharmaceutical agent; prematurity; sedentary lifestyle; stressors; unsanitary food preparation

Client Outcomes, Nursing Interventions, and Client/Family Teaching and Discharge Planning

Refer to care plan for Dysfunctional **Gastrointestinal** motility.

Risk for ineffective Gastrointestinal perfusion

NANDA-I Definition

Vulnerable to decrease in gastrointestinal circulation, which may compromise health

Risk Factors

Abdominal aortic aneurysm; abdominal compartment syndrome; abnormal partial thromboplastin time (PTT); abnormal prothrombin time (PT); acute gastrointestinal hemorrhage; age >60 years; anemia; cerebral vascular accident; coagulopathy (e.g., sickle cell anemia); decrease in left ventricular performance; diabetes mellitus; disseminated intravascular coagulopathy; female gender; gastroesophageal varices; gastrointestinal condition (e.g., ulcer, ischemic colitis, ischemic pancreatitis); myocardial infarction; renal disease (e.g., polycystic kidney, renal artery stenosis, failure); smoking; trauma; treatment regimen; vascular disease

• = Independent   ▲ = Collaborative

Client Outcomes

Client Will (Specify Time Frame)

- Maintain blood pressure within normal limits
- Remain free from abdominal distention
- Tolerate feedings without nausea, vomiting, or abdominal discomfort
- Pass stools of normal color, consistency, frequency, and amount
- Describe prescribed diet regimen
- Describe prescribed medication regimen including medication actions and possible side effects
- Verbalize understanding of treatment regimen including monitoring for signs and symptoms that may indicate problems with gastrointestinal tissue perfusion, the importance of diet and exercise to gastrointestinal health

Nursing Interventions

Critical Care

▲ Complete a pain assessment. Assess and document the onset, intensity, character, location, duration, aggravating factors, and relieving factors. Determine whether the pain is exacerbated by eating. Notify the provider for any significant increase in pain.

- Perform a physical abdominal examination including inspection, auscultation, percussion, and palpation. Complete the assessment in the described order.
- Monitor vital signs frequently as needed, watching for hypotension and tachycardia.
- Monitor frequency, consistency, color, and amount of stools.
- Assess for abdominal distention. Measure abdominal girth and compare to client's accustomed waist or belt size.
- Review the client's medical and surgical history. Certain conditions place clients at higher risk for ineffective tissue perfusion (see risk factors above). In addition to medical or surgical conditions, lifestyle choices such as smoking or cocaine and amphetamine use affect tissue perfusion (Hauser, 2011).
- Recognize that any client who has been in a shock state has decreased gastrointestinal perfusion due to compensatory mechanisms, and watch for symptoms as identified. See care plan for Risk for **Shock.**

▲ Monitor intake and output to evaluate fluid and electrolyte balance, and review laboratory data as ordered.

• = Independent   ▲ = Collaborative

▲ Prepare client for diagnostic or surgical procedures. Diagnostic studies may include abdominal x-ray study to rapidly rule out intestinal obstruction, computed tomography, angiography, and abdominal ultrasound. Surgical procedures include exploratory laparotomy, thrombectomy, surgical revascularization, and/or stent placement (Dang & Su, 2014).

Pediatric

• Monitor vital signs frequently. Notify health care provider if there is significant deviation from baseline or findings are significantly abnormal.

• Monitor oxygen saturation and provide oxygen therapy as ordered. Take steps to prevent hypovolemia and hypotensive episodes.

• Monitor tolerance of enteral feedings. Measure gastric residual and note color and consistency.

Geriatric

▲ Monitor for gastrointestinal side effects from medications, especially nonsteroidal antiinflammatory drugs (NSAIDs).

▲ Recognize that decreased gastrointestinal perfusion, either acute or chronic, is much more common in older adults.

▲ Be aware that gastrointestinal bleeding that is difficult to control in older adults may be associated with decreased gastrointestinal perfusion (Hauser, 2011).

Risk for unstable blood Glucose level

NANDA-I Definition

Vulnerable to variation in blood glucose/sugar levels from the normal range, which may compromise health

Risk Factors

Alteration in mental status; average daily physical activity is less than recommended for gender and age; compromised physical health status; delay in cognitive development; does not accept diagnosis; excessive stress; excessive weight gain; excessive weight loss; inadequate blood glucose monitoring; ineffective medication management; insufficient diabetes management; insufficient dietary intake; insufficient knowledge of disease management; nonadherence to diabetes management plan; pregnancy; rapid growth period

• = Independent   ▲ = Collaborative

Client Outcomes

Client Will (Specify Time Frame)

- Maintain A_{1C} less than 7% (normal level 4% to 6%) (American Diabetes Association [ADA], 2014a)
- Maintain outpatient preprandial blood glucose in adults between 70 and 130 mg/dL (ADA, 2014a); consult primary care provider for client-specific goals
- Maintain preprandial blood glucose for preschoolers (0 to 6 years) between 100 and 180 mg/dL; school age (6 to 12 years) between 90 and 180 mg/dL; adolescents and young adults (13 to 19 years) between 90 and 130 mg/dL (ADA, 2014a)
- Maintain outpatient peak postprandial (1 to 2 hours after beginning of meal) glucose below 180 mg/dL (ADA, 2014a)
- Maintain preprandial blood glucose for gestational diabetes ≤95 mg/dL, 1-hour pc level at or below 140 mg/dL, and 2-hour pc level at or below 120 mg/dL (ADA, 2014a)
- Maintain premeal, bedtime, and overnight blood glucose for a pregnant mother with preexisting type 1 or 2 diabetes at 60 to 99 mg/dL, peak postprandial glucose at 100 to 129 mg/dL, and A_{1C} <6% (ADA, 2014a)
- Maintain blood glucose in critically ill hospitalized clients between 140 and 180 mg/dL (ADA, 2014a)
- Maintain premeal blood glucose values in non-critically ill hospitalized clients below 140 mg/dL and random blood glucose values below 180 mg/dL (ADA, 2014a)
- Demonstrate how to accurately test blood glucose
- Identify self-care actions to take to maintain target glucose levels
- Identify self-care actions to take if blood glucose level is too low or too high
- Demonstrate correct administration of prescribed medications
- Demonstrate knowledge of appropriate diet and carbohydrate intake

Nursing Interventions

▲ Obtain blood glucose before meals and snacks. Obtain blood glucose every 4 to 6 hours in the client not receiving nutrition.

▲ Evaluate blood glucose levels in hospitalized clients before administering oral hypoglycemic agents or insulin. Adjust timing of medication appropriately with meal times.

• = Independent   ▲ = Collaborative

▲ Recognize that SMBG may not be beneficial in clients who have had type 2 diabetes for more than 1 year and who are not taking insulin.

▲ Monitor blood glucose every 30 minutes to 2 hours for clients on continuous insulin drips.

• Consider continuous glucose monitoring (CGM) in clients with type 1 diabetes on intensive insulin regimens.

G

▲ Evaluate A_{1C} level for glucose control over previous 2 to 3 months.

• Consider monitoring 1 to 2 hours after meals in individuals who have premeal glucose values within target but have A_{1C} values above target.

• Monitor for signs and symptoms of hypoglycemia, such as shakiness, dizziness, sweating, hunger, headache, pallor, behavior changes, confusion, or seizures.

▲ Be alert for hypoglycemia in clients receiving 0.6 unit/kg insulin or more daily, and in clients receiving NPH insulin.

▲ If client is experiencing signs and symptoms of hypoglycemia, test glucose; if result is below 70 mg/dL, administer 15 to 20 g glucose. Pure glucose is the preferred treatment, but any form of carbohydrate that contains glucose will suffice (½ cup fruit juice or regular [not diet] soda, 1 cup milk, 1 small piece of fruit, or 3 to 4 glucose tablets). Avoid treating with foods that contain fat. Repeat test in 15 minutes and repeat treatment if indicated. Once blood glucose returns to normal, the individual should consume a meal or snack to prevent recurrence of hypoglycemia.

▲ If the client is unable to swallow, parenteral glucagon may be given by a trained family member or by medical personnel. In unresponsive clients, intravenous glucose should be given.

▲ Clients who do not experience symptoms of hypoglycemia should raise their glucose targets to avoid hypoglycemia for several weeks.

▲ In clients with type 2 diabetes who become hypoglycemic and have been treated with an alpha-glucosidase inhibitor (e.g., acarbose [Precose] or miglitol [Glyset]) in addition to insulin or an insulin release stimulator, oral glucose rather than more complex carbohydrates must be given.

• Monitor for signs and symptoms of hyperglycemia, such as increased thirst or urination, or high blood or urine glucose levels.

▲ Ensure an acutely ill client is receiving adequate fluids and nutrition. Adjustment in oral hypoglycemic or insulin therapy may be required.

• = Independent   ▲ = Collaborative

▲ Test urine or blood for ketones in ketosis-prone clients during acute illness, trauma, surgery, or stress.

▲ Prime intravenous (IV) tubing with 20 mL of diluted insulin solution before initiating insulin drip.

▲ Evaluate client's medication regimen for medications that can alter blood glucose.

▲ Refer client to dietitian for carbohydrate counting instruction.

▲ Refer overweight clients to dietitian for weight loss counseling.

• For interventions regarding foot care, refer to the care plan for Ineffective peripheral **Tissue Perfusion.**

G

Geriatric

• Watch for age-related cognitive changes that can impair self-management of diabetes.

• Monitor for vision and dexterity impairments that may affect the older client's ability to accurately measure insulin doses.

▲ Consider relaxing glucose targets for older adults with advanced diabetes complications, life-limiting comorbid illness, or substantial cognitive or functional impairment.

• Teach older clients the importance of verifying symptoms with a glucometer reading.

Pediatric

• Be aware that young children (<7 years) may not be aware of symptoms of hypoglycemia.

• Teach children and adolescents (and their parents) with type 1 diabetes or on intensive insulin regimens (MDI or insulin pump therapy) to perform SMBG before meals and snacks, occasionally postprandially, at bedtime, before exercise, when they suspect low blood glucose, after treating low blood glucose until they are normoglycemic, and before critical tasks such as driving.

• Teach self-efficacy measures to adolescents with type 1 diabetes who are involved in family conflict.

Home Care

▲ Teach family and others having close contact with the person with diabetes how to use an emergency glucagon kit (if prescribed).

Multicultural

• Provide culturally appropriate diabetes health education.

• Involve Hispanic community workers (promotoras) when working with Hispanic clients with diabetes.

• = Independent   ▲ = Collaborative

- Provide culturally adapted diabetes self-management education for African American clients with diabetes.
- Encourage involvement of African American client's family and friends in diabetes education activities.

Client/Family Teaching and Discharge Planning

- Provide "survival skills" education or review for hospitalized clients, including information about (1) identification of the health care provider who will provide diabetes care after discharge, (2) diagnosis of diabetes, SMBG, and explanation of home blood glucose goals, (3) information on consistent eating patterns, (4) when and how to take medications including insulin administration, (5) proper use and disposal of needles and syringes if applicable, (6) definition, recognition, treatment, and prevention of hyperglycemia and hypoglycemia, and (7) sick-day management.
- Evaluate client's monitoring technique initially and at regular intervals.
- Teach client how to match prandial insulin dose to carbohydrate intake, premeal blood glucose, and anticipated activity.
- ▲ Refer client for Blood Glucose Awareness Training (BGAT) or Web-based training available at http://www.BGAThome.com for instruction in detection, anticipation, avoidance, and treatment of extremes in blood glucose levels.
- Teach client to maintain a blood glucose log. A results log can help clients track their response to treatment. Many logs are available online (ADA, 2014b).
- Provide group-based training programs for instruction.
- Teach client the importance of at least 150 minutes/week of moderate-intensity aerobic physical activity (50% to 70% of maximum heart rate), spread over at least 3 days per week.
- Discuss recommending resistance training with client's provider.
- Teach client with type 1 diabetes to avoid vigorous activity if ketones are present in urine or blood. Exercise can worsen hyperglycemia and ketosis in people deprived of insulin for 12 to 48 hours (ADA, 2014a).
- Teach clients who are treated with insulin or insulin-stimulating oral agents to eat added carbohydrates before exercise if glucose levels are below 100 mg/dL. Physical activity can cause hypoglycemia if medication dose or carbohydrate consumption is not altered (ADA, 2014a).

• = Independent ▲ = Collaborative

▲ Teach clients on multiple-dose insulin or insulin pump therapy to perform SMBG before critical tasks such as driving.
▲ Teach clients to use alcohol with caution.

Grieving
NANDA-I Definition

A normal complex process that includes emotional, physical, spiritual, social, and intellectual responses and behaviors by which individuals, families, and communities incorporate an actual, anticipated, or perceived loss into their daily lives

Defining Characteristics

Alteration in activity level; alteration in dream pattern; alteration in immune functioning; alteration in neuroendocrine functioning; alteration in sleep pattern; anger; blaming; despair; detachment; disorganization; finding meaning in a loss; guilt about feeling relieved; maintaining a connection to the deceased; pain; panic behavior; personal growth; psychological distress; suffering

Related Factors (r/t)

Anticipatory loss of significant object (e.g., possession, job status); anticipatory loss of significant other; death of significant other; loss of significant object (e.g., possession, job, status, home, body part)

Client/Family Outcomes
Client/Family Will (Specify Time Frame)

• Discuss meaning of the loss to his/her life and the functioning of the family
• Identify ways to support family members and articulate methods of support he/she requires from family and friends
• Accept assistance in meeting the needs of the family from friends/extended family

Nursing Interventions
Anticipatory Grieving Interventions

• Grieving of a critically ill or dying client and client's family/relatives for the losses experienced during the deteriorating illness, and the future that will be filled with loss.
• Develop a trusting relationship both with the client and with the family by using presence and therapeutic communication techniques.

• = Independent   ▲ = Collaborative

- Keep the family apprised of the client's ongoing condition as much as possible. Consult with the family for decision-making as appropriate.
- Keep the family informed of client's needs for physical care and support in symptom control, and inform them about health care options at the end of life, including palliative care, hospice care, and home care.

G

- Discuss preferred place of death (PPD) with client.
- Ask family members if they are receiving sufficient sleep. If a family member desires to be in the room for sleep, provide a reclining chair or portable bed, if possible, and bedding to keep the family member comfortable. If needed, find housing for family member from out of town with support of case manager or social worker.
- Ask family member about having adequate resources to care for themselves and the critically ill family member.
- Listen to the family member's story.
- Encourage family members to show their caring feelings and talk to the client.
- Recognize and respect different feelings and wishes from both the family members and the client.
- If necessary, refer a family member for counseling or to a minister/priest to help him/her cope with the existential questions and current overwhelming reality.
- Recognize that one family member may be in a state of caregiver role strain from a long caregiving situation.
- Promote the family roles as appropriate.
- Promote mutual goal setting where decisions are made together that affect the family.

Grieving Interventions When Death of a Loved One Occurs

- Use the following activities when interacting with the bereaved person:
  - Be present and attentive, use active empathetic listening.
  - Validate the client's feelings of grief and feeling hurt, stressful, anxious, out of control, and further symptoms of grieving.
  - Provide time and space for the person to tell their story of loss.
  - Offer condolences: "I am sorry that you lost your husband."
  - Explain that feelings will oscillate as the person does grief work, from coping to accept the loss to coping to build a new life without the loved one.

• = Independent ▲ = Collaborative

- ○ Intentionally schedule meetings with family members to provide support during grieving.
- Refer to mental health providers as needed.
- Help the client use a method to give voice to his unique story of loss. Methods include keeping a personal journal to record feelings and insights, retelling of the loss narrative to a caring person, music therapy techniques with a trained therapist or listening to music that has significance to the relationship, use of the "virtual dream," which is a dreamlike short story written by the grieving person to tell the narrative of the loss.
- Discuss coping methods with the grieving person. Common coping techniques include exercise, telling the story of grief to a caring person, journaling, pets, and developing a legacy for the deceased.
- Encourage the family to create a quiet and comfortable healing environment, and follow comforting grief rituals such as prayer, interacting with nature, or lighting votive candles.
- Refer the family members for spiritual counseling if desired.
- Help the family determine the best way and place to find social support. Encourage family members to continue to use supports as needed for years.
- Identify available community resources, including bereavement groups at local hospitals and hospice centers. Volunteers who provide bereavement support can also be effective.
- Refer to Complicated **Grieving** if grieving fails to follow normative (or cultural) expectations and manifests in functional impairment.

Pediatric/Parent

- Treat the child/parents with respect, give him/her opportunity to talk about concerns and answer questions honestly.
- Listen to the child's expression of grief.
- Help parents recognize that the grieving child does not have to be "fixed"; instead they need support going through an experience of grieving just as adults do.
- Consider the use of art for children in hospice care who are dying or dealing with the death of a parent, sibling, or other family member.
- ▲ Refer grieving children and parents to a program to help facilitate grieving if desired, especially if the death was traumatic.

• = Independent   ▲ = Collaborative

- Help the adolescent determine sources of support and how to use them effectively.
- Encourage grieving parents to take good care of their own health.
▲ Encourage grieving parents to seek mental health services as needed. The death of a child is regarded as among the most traumatic, incomprehensible, and devastating of losses, with the potential to precipitate a crisis of meaning for the bereaved parent.
- Recognize that men and women often grieve differently, and explain this to parents if it becomes an issue.
- Recognize that mothers who have a miscarriage/stillbirth grieve and experience sorrow because of loss of the child.

Geriatric
- Monitor an older adult who has been treated for bereavement-related depression for relapse or recurrence.
- Provide support for the family when the loss is associated with dementia of the family member.
- Determine the social supports of older adults.

Multicultural
- See interventions for Complicated **Grieving** and Chronic **Sorrow**.

Home Care
- The interventions previously described may be adapted for home care use.
- Assessment of activities of daily living (ADLs) and instrumental ADLs is essential as part of comprehensive care after a home care client has suffered the loss of a loved one.
- Actively listen as the client grieves for his or her own death or for real or perceived loss. Normalize the client's expressions of grief for self. Demonstrate a caring and hopeful approach.
▲ Refer the client to social services as necessary for losses not related to death. Support is helpful to grief work for all types of losses. Social workers can help the client plan for financial changes as a result of job losses and help with community referrals as appropriate.
▲ Refer the bereaved to hospice bereavement programs or an Internet self-help group. Relief of the suffering of clients and families (physical, emotional, and spiritual) is the goal of hospice care.

• = Independent   ▲ = Collaborative

Complicated Grieving

NANDA-I Definition

A disorder that occurs after the death of a significant other in which the experience of distress accompanying bereavement fails to follow normative expectations and manifests in functional impairment

Defining Characteristics

Anger; anxiety; avoidance of grieving; decrease in functioning in life roles; depression; disbelief; distress about the deceased person; excessive stress; experiencing symptoms the deceased experienced; fatigue; feeling dazed; feeling of detachment from others; feeling of shock; feeling stunned; feelings of emptiness; insufficient same of well-being; longing for the deceased person; low levels of intimacy; mistrust; non-acceptance of a death; persistent painful memories; preoccupation with thoughts about a deceased person; rumination; searching for a deceased person; self-blame; separation distress; traumatic distress; yearning for deceased person

Related Factors (r/t)

Death of a significant other; emotional disturbance; insufficient social support (adapted from the work of NANDA-I)

Client Outcomes

Client Will (Specify Time Frame)

- Express appropriate feelings of guilt, fear, anger, or sadness
- Identify somatic distress associated with grief (e.g., anxiety, changes in appetite, insomnia, nightmares, loss of libido, decreased energy, altered activity levels)
- Seek support in dealing with grief-associated issues
- Identify personal strengths and effective coping strategies
- Function at a normal developmental level and begin to successfully and increasingly perform activities of daily living

Nursing Interventions

- Assess for signs of complicated grieving that include symptoms that persist at least 6 months after the death and are experienced at least daily or to a disabling degree. Symptoms include feeling emotionally numb, stunned, shocked, and that life is meaningless; dysfunctional thoughts and maladaptive behaviors; experiencing mistrust and estrangement from others; anger and bitterness over the loss; identity confusion; avoidance of the reality of the loss, or excessive proximity seeking to try to feel closer to the deceased, sometimes focused on wishes to die or suicidal statements and behavior; or difficulty moving on with life.

• = Independent   ▲ = Collaborative

▲ Determine the client's state of grieving. Use a tool such as the Prolonged Grief Disorder (PGD) scale (Jordan & Litz, 2014), the Grief Support in Health Care Scale (Anderson et al, 2010), the Hogan Grief Reaction Checklist (Hogan et al, 2004), and the Beck Depression Inventory.

▲ Determine whether the client is experiencing depression, suicidal tendencies, or other emotional disorders. Refer the client for counseling or therapy as appropriate.

• Educate the client and his or her support systems that grief resolution is not a sequential process and that the positive outcome of grief resolution is the integration of the deceased into the ongoing life of the griever.

▲ Assess caregivers, particularly younger caregivers, for pessimistic thinking and additional stressful life events. Refer for appropriate support.

• See the interventions for **Grieving** and Chronic **Sorrow**.

Pediatric/Parent

▲ Refer grieving children and parents to a program to help facilitate grieving if desired, especially if the death was traumatic.

• Encourage grieving parents to take part in activities that are supportive, such as faith-based activities.

• Encourage grieving parents to seek mental health services as needed.

• Help the adolescent determine sources of support and how to use them effectively. If client is an adolescent exposed to a peer's suicide, watch for symptoms of traumatic grief as well as post-traumatic stress disorder, which include numbness, preoccupation with the deceased, functional impairment, and poor adjustment to the loss.

Geriatric

• Assess for deterioration in bereaved older adult self-care.

• Those who have lived with older adults with dementia and experienced significant feelings of loss before the loved one's death may be at risk for more intense feelings of grief after the death of the client with dementia.

• Monitor the older client for complicated grieving manifesting in physical and mental health problems.

Multicultural

• Assess for the influence of cultural beliefs, norms, and values on the client's grief and mourning practices.

• = Independent   ▲ = Collaborative

- Encourage discussion of the grief process.
- Identify whether the client had been notified of the health status of the deceased and was able to be present during illness and death.

Home Care
- Consider providing support via the Internet.

Risk for complicated Grieving

G

NANDA-I Definition

Vulnerable to a disorder that occurs after death of a significant other in which the experience of distress accompanying bereavement fails to follow normative expectations and manifests in functional impairment, which may compromise health

Risk Factors

Death of a significant other; insufficient social support; emotional disturbance

Client Outcomes, Nursing Interventions, and Client/Family Teaching and Discharge Planning

Refer to care plan for Complicated **Grieving.**

Risk for disproportionate Growth

NANDA-I Definition

Vulnerable to growth above the 97th percentile or below the 3rd percentile for age, crossing two percentile channels, which may compromise health

Risk Factors

Caregiver

Alteration in cognitive functioning; learning disability; mental health issue (e.g., depression, psychosis, personality disorder, substance abuse); presence of abuse (e.g., physical, psychological, sexual)

Environmental

Deprivation; economically disadvantaged; exposure to teratogen; exposure to violence; lead poisoning; natural disaster

Individual

Anorexia; chronic illness; infection; insatiable appetite; maladaptive feeding behavior by caregiver; maladaptive self-feeding behavior; malnutrition; prematurity; substance abuse

• = Independent ▲ = Collaborative

Prenatal

Congenital disorder; exposure to teratogen; genetic disorder; inadequate maternal nutrition; maternal infection; multiple gestation; substance abuse

Client Outcomes

Client/Parents/Primary Caregiver Will (Specify Time Frame)

- State information related to possible teratogenic agents
- Identify components of healthy nutrition that will promote growth
- Maintain or improve weight to be within a healthy range for age and sex

Nursing Interventions

Preconception/Pregnancy

- Counsel women who smoke to quit smoking prior to conception if possible and to avoid smoking and secondhand smoke while pregnant.
- Assess alcohol consumption of pregnant women and advise those who drink alcohol to discontinue all use of alcohol through the pregnancy.
- Assess and limit exposure to all drugs (prescription, "recreational," and over the counter) and give the mother information on known teratogenic agents.
- All women of childbearing age who are capable of becoming pregnant should take 400 mcg of folic acid daily.
- ▲ Promote a team approach toward preconception and pregnancy glucose control for women with diabetes.
- ▲ Advise women with mental health disorders to seek appropriate counseling before pregnancy.

Pediatric

- Consider regular breast milk and protein-fortified breast milk for low-birth-weight infants in the neonatal intensive care unit.
- Provide tube feedings per health care provider's orders when appropriate for clients with neuromuscular impairment.
- Provide for adequate nutrition and nutritional monitoring in clients with medical disorders requiring long-term medication and those with developmental delay.
- Adequate intake of vitamin D is set at 400 IU/day by the National Academy of Sciences. Because adequate sunlight exposure is difficult to determine, a supplement of 400 IU/day is recommended for the

• = Independent   ▲ = Collaborative

following groups to prevent rickets and vitamin D deficiency in
healthy infants and children:

- ○ All breastfed infants unless they are weaned to at least
  500 mL/day of vitamin D–fortified formula or milk
- ○ All non-breastfed infants who are ingesting less than
  500 mL/day of vitamin D–fortified formula or milk
- ○ Children and adolescents who do not receive regular sunlight
  exposure, do not ingest at least 500 mL/day of vitamin
  D–fortified milk, or do not take a daily multivitamin supplement
  containing at least 400 IU of vitamin D

G

- Provide adequate nutrition to clients with active intestinal
  inflammation.
- Encourage limiting "screen time" (television, video games,
  Internet, smartphones, and tablets) to less than 2 hours/day for
  children.

Multicultural

- Assess the influence of cultural beliefs, norms, values, and
  expectations on parents' perceptions of normal growth and
  development.
- Focus nutritional education on promoting good nutrition and
  physically active lifestyles for healthy child development as opposed
  to only for prevention or reduction of overweight.
- Assess for the influence of acculturation.
- Assess parents' understanding of appropriate nutrition for infants.
- Assess the influence of family/parents on patterns of nutritional
  intake.
- Negotiate with clients regarding which aspects of healthy nutrition
  can be modified while still honoring cultural beliefs.
- Encourage parental efforts at increasing physical activity and
  decreasing dietary fat for their children.

Home Care

- The interventions previously described may be adapted for home care
  use.
- Assess parental perception of their child's weight.
- Assess family meal planning and family participation in mealtime
  activities such as eating together at a scheduled time.
- Educate families and children about providing healthy meals and
  healthy eating to improve learning ability.

• = Independent   ▲ = Collaborative

Deficient community Health
NANDA-I Definition

Presence of one or more health problems or factors that deter wellness or increase the risk of health problems experienced by an aggregate

Defining Characteristics

Health problem experienced by aggregates or populations; program unavailable to eliminate health problems of an aggregate or population; program unavailable to enhance wellness of an aggregate or population; program unavailable to prevent health problems of an aggregate or population; program unavailable to reduce health problems of an aggregate or population; risk of hospitalization experienced by aggregates or population; risk of physiological states experienced by aggregates or populations; risk of psychological states experienced by aggregates or population

Related Factors

Inadequate consumer satisfaction with program; inadequate program budget; inadequate program evaluation plan; inadequate program outcome data; inadequate social support for program; insufficient access to healthcare provider; insufficient community experts; insufficient resources (e.g., financial, social, knowledge); program incompletely addresses health problem

Client Outcomes

Community/Adolescents/Minority Clients Will (Specify Time Frame)

- Provide programs for healthy behaviors
- Demonstrate goal setting
- Describe and comply with healthy behaviors
- Describe and demonstrate compliance with HBV education and testing

Nursing Interventions

Refer to care plans: Readiness for enhanced community **Coping,** Ineffective community **Coping,** Ineffective **Health** maintenance, Impaired **Home** maintenance, Risk for other-directed **Violence.**

- Assess for the presence of demographic variables that predict community mortality.
- Assess for needs related to the community's priority health concerns.
- Encourage healthy nutrition and exercise among community members using the resources available to the community.
- Facilitate goal setting in the community for behavior change related to diet and exercise for overweight and obese adults.

• = Independent ▲ = Collaborative

- Utilize a community forum approach to increase community knowledge and awareness of community health issues.

Pediatric

▲ Consider a community-based program for young people that encourages health-related behavior changes, increasing fruit and vegetable intake, and engaging in activity.

▲ Support religious affiliation and positive school climates for adolescents, particularly for lesbian, gay, and bisexual youths in the community.

Geriatric

▲ Assess homeless older veterans in the community for post-traumatic stress disorder and/or suicidal behavior and make appropriate referrals.

▲ Provide community-dwelling older women with psychoeducation about aging skills and behaviors and cognitive function using group discussion.

Multicultural

- Provide information and venues for testing about the pervasiveness and deadly consequence of hepatitis B virus (HBV) for Asians in the United States.

- Provide culturally and linguistically appropriate risk reduction programs to individuals living in rural and border regions of the country.

Home Care, Client/Family Teaching, and Discharge Planning

- The above interventions may be adapted for home care and client/family teaching.

- Provide support for establishment of a community garden.

Risk-prone Health behavior

NANDA-I Definition

Impaired ability to modify lifestyle/behaviors in a manner that improves health status

Defining Characteristics

Failure to achieve optimal sense of control; failure to take action that prevents health problem; minimizes health status change; nonacceptance of health status change

• = Independent   ▲ = Collaborative

Related Factors (r/t)

Economically disadvantaged; inadequate comprehension; insufficient social support; low self-efficacy; negative attitude toward health care; smoking; stressors; substance abuse

Client Outcomes

Client Will (Specify Time Frame)

- State acceptance of change in health status
- Request assistance in altering behaviors to adapt to change
- State personal goals for dealing with change in health status and means to prevent further health problems
- State experience of a period of grief that is proportional to the actual or perceived effect of the loss
- Report and/or demonstrate behavior changes mutually agreed upon with nurse as evidence of positive adaptation

Nursing Interventions

- Assess the client's definitions of health and wellness and major barriers to health and wellness.
- Use motivational interviewing to help the client identify and change unhealthy behaviors.
- Encourage mindfulness and meditation to help the client cope with changes in health status.
- Allow the client adequate time to express feelings about the change in health status.
- Use open-ended questions to allow the client free expression (e.g., "Tell me about your last hospitalization" or "How does this time compare?").
- Help the client work through the stages of grief that occur as part of a psychological adaptation to illness or life change. Assess for signs of nonacceptance to illness or change.
- Assess the client for depression and refer to for counseling or medical follow-up, as appropriate.
- Discuss the client's current goals and assist in modification, if appropriate. Have the client list goals so that they can be referred to and steps can be taken to accomplish them. Support hope that the goals will be accomplished.
- ▲ Encourage participation in appropriate wellness programs associated with health changes.
- Provide assistance with activities as needed.

• = Independent   ▲ = Collaborative

- Give the client positive feedback for accomplishments, no matter how small. Support the client and family and promote their strengths and coping skills.
- Manipulate the environment to decrease stress; allow the client to display personal items that have meaning.
- Maintain consistency and continuity in daily schedule. When possible, provide the same caregiver.
▲ Promote use of positive spiritual influences, as appropriate.
▲ Refer to community resources. Provide general and contact information for ease of use.

H

Pediatric
- Include social history in client assessment to help identify past abuse and traumatic experiences.
- Encourage visitation of children when family members are in intensive care.
- Encourage parents to process and express grief, uncertainty, and discouragement after learning about their child's diagnosis, prognosis, and treatments. Provide parents with resources and tools to help further their understanding of the illness.
▲ Refer parents of critically ill children to an intervention program such as COPE, a theory-based intervention program.
- Use visualization and distraction with children undergoing procedures or treatment with unpleasant side effects.
- Discuss with parents and children possible adverse or unpleasant side effects associated with a treatment and assist with developing a plan to cope with these effects.

Geriatric
▲ Assess for signs of depression resulting from illness-associated changes and make appropriate referrals.
- Use open-ended questions in screening for depression in older adults (Magnil et al, 2011).
- Support activities that promote usefulness of older adults.
▲ Encourage social support.

Multicultural
- Assess for the influence of cultural beliefs, norms, and values on the client's ability to modify health behavior.
- Assess the role of fatalism on the client's ability to modify health behavior.
- Encourage spirituality as a source of support for coping.

• = Independent   ▲ = Collaborative

- Negotiate with the client regarding the aspects of health behavior that will need to be modified.
- Acknowledge client's identified gender and sexual orientation and refer client and family members to support networks that have experience with lesbian, gay, bisexual, or transgender (LGBT) issues, as appropriate.

Home Care
- The above interventions may be adapted for home care use.
- Take the client's perspective into consideration and use a holistic approach in assessing and responding to client planning for the future.
- Assist the client to adapt to his/her diagnosis and to live with their disease.
- Ensure that evaluations of the client's ability to perform activities of daily living are age appropriate and consider existing, as well as new, diagnoses.
- ▲ Refer the client to a counselor or therapist for follow-up care. Initiate community referrals as needed (e.g., grief counseling, self-help groups).
- Refer to care plan for **Powerlessness.**

Client/Family Teaching and Discharge Planning
- Assess family/caregivers for coping and teaching/learning styles.
- Foster communication between the client/family and medical staff.
- Educate and prepare families regarding the appearance of the client and the environment before initial exposure.
- Help the client to enjoy a sense of "wellness." Provide support for progress and support enjoyment of the physical, emotional, spiritual, and social aspects of life.
- Teach a client and his/her family relaxation techniques (controlled breathing, guided imagery) and help them practice.
- Allow the client to proceed at own pace in learning; provide time for return demonstrations (e.g., self-injection of insulin). Tailor teaching and learning materials as appropriate for client and caregiver literacy level.
- If long-term deficits are expected, inform the family as soon as possible.
- Provide clients with information on how to access and evaluate available health information via the Internet.

• = Independent   ▲ = Collaborative

Ineffective Health management

NANDA-I Definition

Pattern of regulating and integrating into daily living a therapeutic regimen for the treatment of illness and its sequelae that is unsatisfactory for meeting specific health goals

Defining Characteristics

Difficulty with prescribed regimen; failure to include treatment regimen in daily living; failure to take action to reduce risk factors; ineffective choices in daily living for meeting health goals

Related Factors (r/t)

Complex treatment regimen; complexity of health care system; decisional conflict; economically disadvantaged; excessive demands; family conflict; family pattern of health care; inadequate number of cues to action; insufficient knowledge of therapeutic regimen; insufficient social support; perceived barrier; perceived benefit; perceived seriousness of condition; perceived susceptibility; powerlessness

Client Outcomes

Client Will (Specify Time Frame)

- Describe daily food and fluid intake that meets therapeutic goals
- Describe activity/exercise patterns that meet therapeutic goals
- Describe scheduling of medications that meets therapeutic goals
- Verbalize ability to manage therapeutic regimens
- Collaborate with health professionals to decide on a therapeutic regimen that is congruent with health goals and lifestyle

Nursing Interventions

NOTE: This diagnosis does not have the same meaning as the diagnosis **Noncompliance.** This diagnosis is made with the client, so if the client does not agree with the diagnosis, it should not be made. The emphasis is on helping the client direct his or her own life and health, not on the client's compliance with the provider's instructions.

- Establish a collaborative partnership with the client for purposes of meeting health-related goals.
- Explore the client's perception of their illness experience and identify uncertainties and needs through open-ended questions.
- Assist the client to enhance self-efficacy or confidence in his or her own ability to manage the illness.
- Involve family members in knowledge development, planning for self-management, and shared decision-making.

• = Independent ▲ = Collaborative

- Review factors of the health belief model (HBM) (individual perceptions of seriousness and susceptibility, demographic and other modifying factors, and perceived benefits and barriers) with the client.
- Use various formats to provide information about the therapeutic regimen, including group education, brochures, videotapes, written instructions, computer-based programs, and telephone contact.
- Help the client identify and modify barriers to effective self-management.
- Help the client self-manage his or her own health through education about strategies for changing habits such as overeating, sedentary lifestyle, and smoking.
- Develop a contract with the client to maintain motivation for changes in behavior.
- Use focus groups to evaluate the implementation of self-management programs.
- Refer to the care plan for Ineffective Family **Health** management.

Geriatric
- Identify the reasons for behaviors that are not therapeutic and discuss alternatives.

Multicultural
- Assess the influence of cultural beliefs, norms, and values on the individual's perceptions of the therapeutic regimen.
- Discuss all strategies with the client in the context of the client's culture.
- Provide health information that is consistent with the health literacy of clients.
- Assess for barriers that may interfere with client follow-up of treatment recommendations.
- Use electronic monitoring and dosing to improve management of medications.
- Validate the client's feelings regarding the ability to manage his/her own care and the impact on lifestyle.

Home Care
- Prepare and instruct clients and family members in the use of a medication box. Set up an appropriate schedule for filling of the medication box, and post medication times and doses in an accessible area (e.g., attached by a magnet to the refrigerator).

• = Independent   ▲ = Collaborative

- Monitor self-management of the medical regimen.
- Refer to health care professionals for questions and self-care management.

Client/Family Teaching and Discharge Planning

- Identify the client's and/or family's current knowledge and adjust teaching accordingly. Teach the client and family about all aspects of the therapeutic regimen, providing as much knowledge as the client and family will accept, in a culturally congruent manner.
- Teach ways to adjust activities of daily living (ADLs) for inclusion in therapeutic regimens.
- Teach safety in taking medications.
- Teach the client to act as a self-advocate with health providers who prescribe therapeutic regimens.

Ineffective Family Health management

NANDA-I Definition

A pattern of regulating and integrating, into family processes, a program for the treatment of illness and its sequelae that is unsatisfactory for meeting specific health goals

Defining Characteristics

Acceleration of illness symptoms of a family member; decrease in attention to illness; difficulty with prescribed regimen; failure to take action to reduce risk factors; inappropriate family activities for meeting health goals

Related Factors (r/t)

Complex treatment regimen; complexity of health care system; decisional conflict; economically disadvantaged; family conflict

Client Outcomes

Client Will (Specify Time Frame)

- Make adjustments in usual activities (e.g., diet, activity, stress management) to incorporate therapeutic regimens of its members
- Reduce illness symptoms of family members
- Desire to manage therapeutic regimens of its members
- Describe a decrease in the difficulties of managing therapeutic regimens
- Describe actions to reduce risk factors

• = Independent   ▲ = Collaborative

Nursing Interventions

- Base family interventions on knowledge of the family, family context, family dynamics, family structure, and family function.
- Use a family approach when helping an individual with a health problem that requires therapeutic management.
- Review with family members the congruence and incongruence of family behaviors and health-related goals.
- Acknowledge the challenge of integrating therapeutic regimens with family behaviors.
- Review the symptoms of specific illnesses and work with the family toward development of greater self-efficacy in relation to these symptoms.
- Support family decisions to adjust therapeutic regimens as indicated.
- Advocate for the family in negotiating therapeutic regimens with health providers.
- Help the family mobilize social supports.
- Help family members modify perceptions as indicated.
- Use one or more theories of family dynamics to describe, explain, or predict family behaviors (e.g., theories of Bowen, Satir, and Minuchin).
- ▲ Collaborate with expert nurses or other consultants regarding strategies for working with families.
- Coaching methods can be used to help families improve their health.

Pediatric

- Support kangaroo care for infants at risk at birth. Keep infants in an upright position in skin-to-skin contact until they no longer tolerate it.

Geriatric

- Recommend that clients use the "Ask Me 3" program when communicating with their pharmacist (What is my main problem? What do I need to do? Why is it important for me to do this?).

Multicultural

- Acknowledge racial and ethnic differences at the onset of care.
- Ensure that all strategies for working with the family are congruent with the culture of the family.
- Use a family-centered approach when working with Latino, Asian, African American, and Native American clients. Facilitate modeling and role playing for the family regarding healthy ways to communicate and interact.

• = Independent   ▲ = Collaborative

- Use the nursing intervention of cultural brokerage to help families deal with the health care system.

Client/Family Teaching and Discharge Planning

- Teach about all aspects of therapeutic regimens. Provide as much knowledge as family members will accept, adjust instruction to account for what the family already knows, and provide information in a culturally congruent manner.
- Teach ways to adjust family behaviors to include therapeutic regimens, such as safety in taking medications and teaching family members to act as self-advocates with health providers who prescribe therapeutic regimens.

H

Readiness for Enhanced Health management

NANDA-I Definition

A pattern of regulating and integrating into daily living a therapeutic regimen for treatment of illness and its sequelae, which can be strengthened

Defining Characteristics

Expresses desire to enhance choices of daily living for meeting goals; expresses desire to enhance management of illness; expresses desire to enhance management of prescribed regimens; expresses desire to enhance management of risk factors; expresses desire to enhance management of symptoms; expresses desire to enhance immunization/vaccination status

Client Outcomes

Client Will (Specify Time Frame)

- Describe integration of therapeutic regimen into daily living
- Demonstrate continued commitment to integration of therapeutic regimen into daily living routines

Nursing Interventions

- Acknowledge the expertise that the client and family bring to health management.
- Review factors that contribute to the likelihood of health promotion and health protection. Use Pender's Health Promotion Model and Becker's Health Belief Model to identify contributing factors (Pender et al, 2015).

• = Independent   ▲ = Collaborative

- Further develop and reinforce contributing factors that might change with ongoing management of the therapeutic regimen (e.g., knowledge, self-efficacy, self-esteem, and perceived benefits).
- Support all efforts to manage therapeutic regimens.
- Review the client's strengths in the management of the therapeutic regimen.
- Collaborate with the client to identify strategies to maintain strengths and develop additional strengths as indicated.

H

- Identify contributing factors that may need to be improved now or in the future.
- Provide knowledge as needed related to the pathophysiology of the disease or illness, prescribed activities, prescribed medications, and nutrition.
- Support positive health promotion and health protection behaviors.
- Help the client maintain existing support and seek additional supports as needed.

Geriatric

- Facilitate the client and family to obtain health insurance and drug payment plans whenever needed and possible.

Multicultural

- Assess client's cultural perspectives on health management.
- Assess health literacy in clients of diverse backgrounds.
- Validate the client's feelings regarding the ability to manage his/her own care and the impact on current lifestyle.
- Facilitate the client and family to obtain financial assistance in the form of health insurance and drug payment plans whenever needed and possible.
- Use electronic monitoring to improve medication adherence.
- Discuss with clients their beliefs about medication and treatment to enhance medication and treatment adherence.

Community Teaching

- Review therapeutic regimens and their optimal integration with daily living routines.
- Teach disease processes and therapeutic regimens to clients and peer supporters for management of disease processes.

• = Independent   ▲ = Collaborative

Ineffective Health maintenance

NANDA-I Definition

Inability to identify, manage, and/or seek out help to maintain health

Defining Characteristics

Absence of adaptive behaviors to environmental changes; absence of interest in improving health behaviors; inability to take responsibility for meeting basic health practices; insufficient knowledge about basic health practices; insufficient social support; pattern of lack of health-seeking behavior

Related Factors (r/t)

Alteration in cognitive functioning; complicated grieving; decrease in fine motor skills; decrease in gross motor skills; impaired decision-making; ineffective communication skills; ineffective coping strategies; insufficient resources (e.g., financial, social knowledge); perceptual impairment; spiritual distress; unachieved developmental tasks

Client Outcomes

Client Will (Specify Time Frame)

- Discuss fear of or blocks to implementing health regimen
- Follow mutually agreed on health care maintenance plan
- Meet goals for health care maintenance

Nursing Interventions

- Assess the client's feelings, values, and reasons for not following the prescribed plan of care. See Related Factors.
- Assess for family patterns, economic issues, spiritual, and cultural patterns that influence compliance with a given medical regimen.
- Involve the client in shared decision-making regarding health maintenance.
- Show genuine interest in client's individual needs.
- Assist the client in finding methods to reduce stress.
- Help the client determine how to manage complex medication schedules (e.g., HIV/AIDS regimens or polypharmacy).
- Identify complementary healing modalities, such as herbal remedies, acupuncture, healing touch, yoga, or cultural shamans that the client can use in addition to or instead of the prescribed allopathic regimen along with the client's perception of the complementary healing modalities.
- ▲ Refer the client to appropriate medical and social services as needed, providing adequate information on details about the service, including scheduling.

• = Independent   ▲ = Collaborative

- Identify support groups related to the disease process.
- Use social media such as text messaging to remind clients of scheduled appointments.
- Use telehealth interventions to facilitate self-care.

Geriatric

- Assess the client's perception of health and health maintenance.
- Assist client to identify both life- and health-related goals.
- Provide information that supports informed decision-making.
- Discuss realistic goal setting for changes in health maintenance with the client and support person.
- Educate the client about the symptoms of life-threatening illness, such as myocardial infarction (MI), and the need for timeliness in seeking care.

Multicultural

- Assess influence of cultural beliefs, norms, and values on the client's ability to modify health behavior.
- Assess the effect of fatalism on the client's ability to modify health behavior.
- Clarify culturally related health beliefs and practices.
- Provide culturally appropriate education and health care services.

Home Care

- The interventions described previously may be adapted for home care use.
- ▲ Provide nurse-led case management.
- Provide a health promotion focus for the client with disabilities, with the goals of reducing secondary conditions (e.g., obesity, hypertension, pressure sores), maintaining functional independence, providing opportunities for leisure and enjoyment, and enhancing overall quality of life.
- Provide support and individual training for caregivers before the client is discharged from the hospital.
- Assist client to develop confidence in ability to manage the health condition.

Client/Family Teaching and Discharge Planning

- Provide the family with credible sources where information can be obtained from social media. (Most libraries have Internet access with printing capabilities.)
- ▲ Develop collaborative multidisciplinary partnerships.

• = Independent   ▲ = Collaborative

- Tailor both the information provided and the method of delivery of information to the specific client and/or family.
- Explain nonthreatening qualities before introducing more anxiety-producing information regarding possible side effects of the disease or medical regimen.

Impaired Home maintenance

H

NANDA-I Definition

Inability to independently maintain a safe, growth-promoting immediate environment

Defining Characteristics

Difficulty maintaining a comfortable environment; excessive family responsibilities; financial crisis (e.g., debt, insufficient finances); insufficient clothing; insufficient cooking equipment; insufficient equipment for maintaining home; insufficient linen; pattern of disease caused by unhygienic conditions; pattern of infection caused by unhygienic conditions; request for assistance with home maintenance; unsanitary environment

Related Factors (r/t)

Alteration in cognitive functioning; condition impacting ability to maintain home (e.g., disease, illness, injury); illness impacting ability to maintain home; injury impacting ability to maintain home; insufficient family organization; insufficient family planning; insufficient knowledge of home maintenance; insufficient knowledge of neighborhood resources; insufficient role model; insufficient support system

Client Outcomes

Client Will (Specify Time Frame)

- Maintain a healthy home environment
- Use community resources to assist with home care needs
- Maintain a safe home environment

Nursing Interventions

- Assess the concerns of family members, especially the primary caregiver, about home care for a long time.
- Provide home safety education and safety equipment when possible.
- ▲ Consider a predischarge home assessment referral to determine the need for accessibility and safety-related environmental changes.
- Use an assessment tool to identify environmental safety hazards in the home.

• = Independent   ▲ = Collaborative

- Establish an individualized plan of care for improved home maintenance with the client and family based on the client's needs and the caregiver's capabilities.
- Set up a system of relief for the main caregiver in the home and a plan for sharing of household duties and/or outside assistance.
▲ Provide a multidisciplinary approach to target the home environment and the client's ability to function in the home.
- Assess the quality of relationships among family members.

H Geriatric

- All of the previously mentioned interventions are applicable for the geriatric population.
- Assess injury prevention knowledge and practices of the client and caregivers and provide information as appropriate.
- Assess functional ability to manage safely after hospital discharge.
- Explore community resources to assist with home maintenance (e.g., senior centers, Department of Aging, hospital case managers, friends and relatives, the Internet, or church parish nurse).
- Support "aging in place" by providing assistive technology devices: home modification, daily living aids, mobility aids, seating and positioning devices, and sensory aids.
- Focus on the interaction between the older client and the technology, assisting the client to be an active participant in choices of and uses for technology.
- See the care plans for Risk for **Injury** and Risk for **Falls.**

Multicultural

- Acknowledge the stresses unique to racial/ethnic communities.

Home Care

- The previously mentioned interventions incorporate these resources.
- See care plans for **Contamination** and Risk for **Contamination.**

Client/Family Teaching and Discharge Planning

- Identify support groups within the community to assist families in the caregiver role.
- Provide counseling and support for clients and for caregivers of clients.
- Focus teaching on environmental hazards identified in the nursing assessment. Areas may include, but are not limited to:
  ○ **Home Safety.** Identify the need for and use of common safety devices in the home.

• = Independent   ▲ = Collaborative

- ○ **Food Safety.** Instruct client to avoid microbial food-borne illness by storing and cooking food at the proper temperature; regularly washing hands, food contact surfaces, and fruits and vegetables; and monitoring expiration dates.
- Teach clients to assess their homes for potential environmental health hazards in the home, including risks related to structure, moisture/mold, fire, pets, electrical, ventilation, pests, and lifestyle.
- See care plans for **Contamination,** Risk for **Contamination,** Risk for **Falls,** Risk for **Infection,** and Risk for **Injury.**

H

Readiness for enhanced Hope

NANDA-I Definition

A pattern of expectations and desires for mobilizing energy on one's own behalf, which can be strengthened

Defining Characteristics

Expresses desire to enhance ability to set achievable goals; expresses desire to enhance belief in possibilities; expresses desire to enhance congruency of expectations with goals; expresses desire to enhance connectedness with others; expresses desire to enhance hope; expresses desire to enhance problem solving to meet goals; expresses desire to enhance sense of meaning in life; expresses desire to enhance spirituality

Client Outcomes

Client Will (Specify Time Frame)

- Describe values, expectations, and meanings
- Set achievable goals that are consistent with values
- Design strategies to achieve goals
- Express belief in possibilities

Nursing Interventions

- Develop an open, caring, and empathetic relationship that enables the client to discuss hope.
- Assist clients to identify sources of gratitude in their lives using a future-oriented focus.
- Assist families to identify sources of gratitude in their lives.
- Screen the client for hope using a valid and reliable instrument as indicated.
- Focus on the positive aspects of hope, rather than the prevention of hopelessness.

• = Independent   ▲ = Collaborative

H

- Assist the client to expect positive outcomes and recognize the pathways to achieve the positive outcomes.
- Assist clients in developing realistic goals for their recovery.
- Assist clients to set a goal, write down what steps are needed to achieve the goal, and visualize themselves reaching the goal.
- Teach individuals how to become aware of attention that is focused on unwanted aspects of life and how to redirect attention toward things that feel more wanted or desired by using a future-directed approach.
- Engage the client in a therapeutic relationship to enhance social connectedness and social support networks.
- Provide emotional support and encourage hope.
- Help the client identify his or her desires and expectations.
- Use a family-oriented approach when discussing hope.
- Review internal and external resources to enhance hope.
- Identify spiritual beliefs and practices.
- Assist the client to consider possible adaptations to changes.

Home Care

- The above interventions may be adapted for home care use.

Client/Family Teaching and Discharge Planning

- Assess client and family hope before teaching.
- Incorporate client and family goal setting within teaching content.
- Teach alternative coping strategies such as physical activity.
- Provide information to the client and family regarding all aspects of the client's health condition.
- Offer emotional support, active listening, and coping assistance to client's family.

Hopelessness
NANDA-I Definition

Subjective state in which an individual sees limited or no alternatives or personal choices available and is unable to mobilize energy on own behalf

Defining Characteristics

Alteration in sleep pattern; decrease in affect; decrease in appetite; decrease in initiative; decrease in response to stimuli; decrease in verbalization; despondent verbal cues (e.g., "I can't," sighing); inadequate involvement in care; passivity; poor eye contact; shrugging in response to speaker; turning away from speaker

• = Independent   ▲ = Collaborative

Related Factors (r/t)

Chronic stress; deterioration in physiological condition; history of abandonment; loss of belief in spiritual power; loss of belief in transcendent values; prolonged activity restriction; social isolation

Client Outcomes

Client Will (Specify Time Frame)

- Verbalize feelings
- Participate in care
- Make positive statements (e.g., "I can" or "I will try")
- Set goals
- Make eye contact; focus on speaker
- Maintain appropriate appetite for age and physical health
- Sleep appropriate length of time for age and physical health
- Express concern for another
- Initiate activity

Nursing Interventions

▲ Assess for, monitor, and document the potential for suicide. (Refer the client for appropriate treatment if a potential for suicide is identified.) Refer to the care plan for Risk for **Suicide** for specific interventions.

▲ Assess and monitor potential for depression. (Refer the client for appropriate treatment if depression is identified.)

▲ Assess for hopelessness with the modified Beck Hopelessness Scale.

- Engage the client in a therapeutic relationship to enhance social connectedness and social support networks.
- Assess and monitor family caregivers for symptoms of hopelessness.
- Determine appropriate approaches based on the underlying condition or situation that is contributing to feelings of hopelessness.
- Assess for pain and respond with appropriate measures for pain relief.
- Facilitate access to resources to support spiritual well-being.
- Facilitate sources of the client's resilience.
- Assist the client to expect positive outcomes and recognize the pathways to achieve the positive outcomes.
- Assist the client in looking at alternatives and setting long- and short-term goals that are important to him/her.
- Encourage clients to discuss hope, because discussion may be helpful in increasing hope.
- Assist clients in developing realistic goals for their recovery.

• = Independent   ▲ = Collaborative

- Assist clients to set a goal, write down what steps are needed to achieve the goal, and visualize themselves reaching the goal.
- Provide accurate information.
- Encourage decision-making and problem solving.
- Spend one-on-one time with the client. Use empathy; try to understand what the client is saying and communicate this understanding to the client to create a nonjudgmental trusting environment in order to develop therapeutic relationships with the client.
- Teach alternative coping strategies such as physical activity.
- Use a future-directed approach that teaches individuals how to become aware of attention that is focused on unwanted aspects of life and how to redirect attention toward things that feel more wanted or desired.
- Review the client's strengths and resources in conjunction with the client.
- Encourage the client to adopt active coping strategies.
- Involve family and significant others in the plan of care.
- Offer emotional support, active listening, and coping assistance to client's family.
- For additional interventions, see the care plans for Readiness for enhanced **Hope, Spiritual** distress, Readiness for enhanced **Spiritual** well-being, and Disturbed **Sleep** pattern.

Geriatric
- Previous interventions may be adapted for geriatric clients.
- ▲ If depression is suspected, confer with the primary health care provider regarding referral for mental health services.
- Take threats of self-harm or suicide seriously and intervene as needed.
- Use reminiscence and life-review therapies to identify past coping skills.
- Encourage visits from children and family members.
- Consider videoconferencing for older adults in nursing homes with relatives as alternatives to "live visits."
- Position the client by a window, take the client outside, or encourage such activities as gardening (if ability allows).
- Provide esthetic forms of expression, such as dance, music, literature, and pictures
- Consider "biblio and telephone therapy" (BTT).

• = Independent   ▲ = Collaborative

Multicultural

- Assess for the influence of cultural beliefs, norms, and values on the client's feelings of hopelessness.
- Assess the effect of fatalism on the client's expression of hopelessness.
▲ Assess for depression and refer to appropriate services.
- Encourage spirituality as a source of support for hopelessness.

Home Care

- Previously mentioned interventions may be adapted for home care use.
▲ Assess for isolation within the family unit. Encourage the client to participate in family activities. If the client cannot participate, encourage him/her to be in the same area and watch family activities. Refer for telephone support.
- Reminisce with the client about his/her life.
- Identify areas in which the client can have control.
- If illness precipitated the hopelessness, discuss knowledge of and previous experience with the disease.
▲ Provide plant or pet therapy if possible.

Client/Family Teaching and Discharge Planning

- Provide information regarding the client's condition, treatment plan, and progress.
- Teach family caregivers skills to provide care in the home.
- Provide positive reinforcement, praise, and acknowledgment of the challenges of caregiving to family members.
▲ Refer the client to self-help groups, such as "I Can Cope" and "Make Today Count."
▲ Consider an Internet-based behavior change intervention when depression is identified by primary care provider in adolescents.

Risk for compromised Human Dignity

NANDA-I Definition

Vulnerable for perceived loss of respect and honor, which may compromise health

Risk Factors

Cultural incongruence; dehumanizing treatment; disclosure of confidential information; exposure of the body; humiliation; insufficient

• = Independent   ▲ = Collaborative

comprehension of health information; intrusion by clinician; invasion of privacy; limited decision-making experience; loss of control over body function; stigmatization

Client-Based Outcome

Client/Caregiver Will (Specify Time Frame)

- Perceive that dignity is maintained throughout hospitalization/encounter
- Consistently call client by name of choice
- Maintain client's privacy

Nursing Interventions

- Be authentically present when with the client, try to limit extraneous thoughts of self or others, and concentrate on the well-being of the client.
- Enter into and stay within the other's frame of reference. Connect with the inner life world of meaning and spirit of the other. Join in a mutual search for meaning and wholeness of being and becoming to potentiate comfort measures, pain control, a sense of well-being, wholeness, or even spiritual transcendence of suffering.
- Determine the client's perspective about his/her health. Example questions include "Tell me about your health." "What is it like to be in your situation?" "Tell me how you perceive yourself in this situation." "What meaning are you giving to this situation?" "Tell me about your health priorities." "Tell me about the harmony you wish to reach."
- Determine the client's preferences for when and how nursing care is needed and follow the client's guidelines if possible.
- Include the client in all decision-making; if the client does not choose to be part of the decision or is no longer capable of making a decision, use the named surrogate decision maker.
- Maintain client's privacy at all times.
- Actively listen to what the client is saying both verbally and nonverbally.
- Encourage the client to share thoughts about spirituality as desired.
- Use interventions to instill increased hope; see the care plan for Readiness for enhanced **Hope.**
- For further interventions on spirituality, see the care plan for Readiness for enhanced **Spiritual** well-being.

• = Independent   ▲ = Collaborative

Geriatric

- Always ask the client how he/she would like to be addressed. Avoid calling older clients "sweetie," "honey," "Gramps," or other terms that can be demeaning unless this is acceptable in the client's culture or requested by the client.
- Treat the older client with the utmost respect, even if delirium or dementia is present with confusion.

Multicultural

- Assess for the influence of cultural beliefs, norms, and values on the client's way of communicating, and follow the client's lead in communicating in matters of eye contact, amount of personal space, voice tones, and amount of touching. If in doubt, ask the client.

Home Care

- Most of the interventions described previously may be adapted for home care use.
- Recognize that the client with the caregiver has complete autonomy in the home.

Client/Family Teaching and Discharge Planning

- Teach family and caregivers the need for the dignity of the client to be maintained at all times. How an individual cognitively perceives and emotionally deals with the illness can depend on the person's family and social relationships and ultimately can affect the ability to heal. NOTE: Caring is integral to maintaining dignity.

Hyperthermia

NANDA-I Definition

Core body temperature above the normal diurnal range due to failure of thermoregulation

Defining Characteristics

Abnormal posturing; apnea; coma; convulsions; flushed skin; hypotension; infant does not maintain suck; irritability; lethargy; seizure; skin warm to touch; stupor; tachycardia; tachypnea; vasodilation

Related Factors (r/t)

Decreased sweat response; dehydration; high environmental temperature; illness; inappropriate clothing; increase in metabolic rate; ischemia; pharmaceutical agent; sepsis; trauma; vigorous activity

Client Outcomes

Client Will (Specify Time Frame)

- Maintain core body temperature within adaptive levels (less than 104°F, 40°C)
- Remain free of complications of malignant hyperthermia
- Remain free of complications of neuroleptic malignant syndrome
- Remain free of dehydration
- Remain free from infection
- Verbalize signs and symptoms of heat stroke and actions to prevent heat stroke
- Verbalize personal risks for malignant hyperthermia and neuroleptic malignant syndrome to be reported during health history reviews to all health care professionals, including pharmacists

Nursing Interventions

Temperature Measurement

- Recognize that hyperthermia is a rise in body temperature above 40°C (104°F) that is not regulated by the hypothalamus, resulting in an uncontrolled increase in body temperature exceeding the body's ability to lose heat, and is a medical emergency (Dinarello & Porat, 2011; Saltzberg, 2013).
- Measure and record a client's temperature every hour and more frequently as clinically indicated. Two modes of temperature monitoring may be indicated. Continuous temperature monitoring using an indwelling method of temperature measurement is usually indicated to monitor effectiveness of interventions in lowering the body temperature.
- Use the same site and method (device) for temperature measurement for a given client so that temperature trends are assessed accurately; record site of temperature measurement.
- ▲ Work with the health care provider to help determine the cause of the temperature increase, hyperthermia, which will often help direct appropriate treatment.
- Refer to care plan for Ineffective **Thermoregulation** for interventions to manage fever (pyrexia).

Heat Stroke

- Recognize that heat stroke may be separated into two categories: classic and exertional.

• = Independent ▲ = Collaborative

- Watch for risk factors for classic heat stroke, which include (Leon & Helwig, 2010):
  - ○ Medications, especially diuretic agents, anticholinergic agents, anti-Parkinson medications
  - ○ Alcoholism
  - ○ Mental illness
- Risk factors of exertional heat stroke include (Kerr et al, 2014):
  - ○ Preexisting illness
  - ○ Drug use (e.g., alcohol, amphetamines, ecstasy)
  - ○ Wearing protective clothing (uniforms and athletic gear) that limits heat dissipation
- Recognize signs and symptoms of hyperthermia: core body temperature greater than 40°C (104°F), exercise-associated muscle cramps, tachycardia, tachypnea, orthostatic dizziness, weakness, vomiting, headache, confusion, delirium, seizures, coma, acute kidney injury (rhabdomyolysis), hot dry skin (classic heat stroke) (Pryor et al, 2013; Brege, 2009; Dinarello & Porat, 2011; Leon & Helwig, 2010).
- Recognize that antipyretic agents are of little use in treatment of hyperthermia.
- ▲ Assess fluid loss and facilitate oral intake or administer intravenous fluids as ordered to accomplish fluid replacement and support the cardiovascular system.
- Use external cooling measures carefully: loosen or remove excessive clothing, give a tepid water bath, provide cool liquids if the client is alert enough to swallow, fan the client's face.
- Recognize that cooling with ice packs, cooled intravenous solution, or a hypothermia blanket may be required to lower the body temperature quickly (Dinarello & Porat, 2011; Leon & Helwig, 2010). When using a cooling blanket, choose a circulating water cooling device if available and set the temperature regulator to 0.5°C to 1°C (1°F to 2°F) below the client's current temperature to prevent shivering.
- ▲ Continually assess the client's neurological and other organ function, especially kidney function (i.e., signs of rhabdomyolysis), for signs of injury from hyperthermia.

Malignant Hyperthermia

- ▲ If the client has just received general anesthesia, especially sevoflurane, desflurane, enflurane, isoflurane, or succinylcholine, recognize that the hyperthermia may be caused by malignant hyperthermia and requires immediate treatment to prevent death.

- Recognize that signs and symptoms of malignant hyperthermia typically occur suddenly after exposure to the anesthetic agent and include rapid rise in core body temperature, hypercarbia (increase in end tidal carbon dioxide), muscle rigidity, arrhythmias, tachycardia, tachypnea, rhabdomyolysis, and acute kidney injury, and elevated serum calcium and potassium, progressing to disseminated intravascular coagulation and cardiac arrest (Seifert et al, 2014; Stewart, 2014; Hopkins, 2011).
▲ If the client has malignant hyperthermia, begin treatment as ordered, including cessation of the anesthetic agent and intravenous administration of dantrolene sodium, stat, along with antiarrhythmics, and continued support of the cardiovascular system.
- Provide client and family education when malignant hyperthermia occurs, as it is an inherited muscle disorder.

Neuroleptic Malignant Syndrome

▲ Recognize that neuroleptic malignant syndrome is a rare condition associated with clients who are taking typical and atypical antipsychotic agents (Takanobu et al, 2015; Paden et al, 2013; Gillman, 2010; Trollor et al, 2009).
- Watch for signs and symptoms that can range from mild to severe and include a sudden change in mental status, rapid rise in body temperature, muscle rigidity, tachycardia, tachypnea, elevated or labile blood pressure, diaphoresis, rhabdomyolysis, and acute kidney injury (Paden et al, 2013).
▲ Begin treatment when diagnosed, including cessation of the neuroleptic or dopamine antagonist agent; order administration of dantrolene and continued support of the cardiovascular, pulmonary, and renal systems (Dinarello & Porat, 2011).
- A client health history that reports extrapyramidal reaction to any medication should be further explored for risk of neuroleptic malignant syndrome, because this syndrome can occur at any time during a client's treatment with typical and atypical antipsychotic agents (Takanobu et al, 2015; Paden et al, 2013; Trollor et al, 2009).
- Recognize that clients receiving rapid dose escalation of antipsychotic agents (e.g., haloperidol) intramuscularly for acute

• = Independent   ▲ = Collaborative

treatment of delirium may be at increased risk for neuroleptic malignant syndrome (Takanobu et al, 2015; Paden et al, 2013).

Pediatric

- Assess risk factors of malignant hyperthermia as this has an increased prevalence in the pediatric population.
▲ Administer dantrolene, provide oxygen and assist with ventilation, monitor heart rate and rhythm, and treat electrolyte and acid-base disorders (i.e., metabolic acidosis) as ordered if malignant hyperthermia is present.

Geriatric

- Help the client seek medical attention immediately if elevated core temperature is present. To diagnose the hyperthermia, assess for possible precipitating factors, including changes in medication, environmental changes, and recent medical interventions or infectious exposures.
- In hot weather, encourage the client to wear lightweight cotton clothing (Sadler, 2011).
- Provide education on the importance of drinking eight glasses of fluid per day (within their cardiac and renal reserves) regardless of whether they are thirsty. Assess for the need for and presence of fans or air conditioning, and also appropriate clothing.
▲ In hot weather, monitor the older client for signs of heat stroke: rising temperature, orthostatic blood pressure drop, weakness, restlessness, mental status changes, faintness, thirst, nausea, and vomiting. If signs are present, move the client to a cool place, have the client lie down, give sips of water, check orthostatic blood pressure, spray with lukewarm water, cool with a fan, and seek medical assistance immediately.
- During warm weather, help the client obtain a fan or an air conditioner to increase evaporation, as needed. Help the older client locate a cool environment to which they can go for safety in hot weather.
- Take the temperature of the older client in hot weather.

Home Care

- Some of the interventions described previously may be adapted for home care use.
- Determine whether the client or family has a functioning thermometer and know how to use it. Refer to the interventions above on taking a temperature.

• = Independent ▲ = Collaborative

- Help the client and caregivers prevent and monitor for heat stroke/ hyperthermia during times of high outdoor temperatures.
- To prevent heat-related injury in athletes, laborers, and military personnel, instruct them to acclimate gradually to the higher temperatures, increase fluid intake, wear vapor-permeable clothing, and take frequent rests (Kerr et al, 2014; CDC, 2013).
- In the event of temperature elevation above the adaptive range, institute measures to decrease temperature (e.g., get the client out of the sun and into a cool place, remove excess clothing, have the client drink fluids, spray the client with lukewarm water, and fan with cool air). Initiate emergency transport.

H

Client/Family Teaching and Discharge Planning

▲ Instruct to increase fluids to prevent heat-induced hyperthermia and dehydration in the presence of fever.
- Teach the client to stay in a cooler environment during periods of excessive outdoor heat or humidity. If the client does go out, instruct him/her to avoid vigorous physical activity; wear lightweight, loose-fitting clothing; and wear a hat to minimize sun exposure.

Hypothermia
NANDA-I Definition

Core body temperature below normal diurnal range due to failure of thermoregulation

Defining Characteristics

Acrocyanosis; bradycardia; cyanotic nail beds; decrease in blood glucose level; decrease in ventilation; hypertension; hypoglycemia; hypoxia; increase in metabolic rate; increase in oxygen consumption; peripheral vasoconstriction; piloerection; shivering; skin cool to touch; slow capillary refill; tachycardia

Accidental Low Body Temperature in Children and Adults

Mild hypothermia, core temperature approaching 32°C to 35°C; moderate hypothermia, core temperature approaching 30°C to 32°C; severe hypothermia, core temperature <30°C

Injured Adults and Children

Hypothermia, core temperature <35°C; severe hypothermia, core temperature <32°C

• = Independent   ▲ = Collaborative

Neonates

Grade 1 hypothermia, core temperature 36°C to 36.5°C; grade 2 hypothermia, core temperature 35°C to 35.9°C; grade 3 hypothermia, core temperature 34°C to 34.9°C; grade 4 hypothermia, core temperature <34°C; infant with insufficient energy to maintain sucking; infant with insufficient weight gain (<30 g/d); irritability; jaundice; metabolic acidosis; pallor; respiratory distress

Related Factors (r/t)

Alcohol consumption; damage to hypothalamus; decrease in metabolic rate; economically disadvantaged; extremes of age; extremes of weight; heat transfer (e.g., conduction, convection, evaporation, radiation); inactivity; insufficient caregiver knowledge of hypothermia prevention; insufficient clothing; insufficient supply of subcutaneous fat; low environmental temperature; malnutrition; pharmaceutical agent; radiation; trauma

Neonates

Delay in breastfeeding; early bathing of newborn; high-risk out-of-hospital birth; immature stratum corneum; increased body surface area to weight ratio; increase in oxygen demand; increase in pulmonary vascular resistance; ineffective vascular control; inefficient nonshivering thermogenesis; unplanned out-of-hospital birth

Client Outcomes

Client Will (Specify Time Frame)

- Maintain body temperature within normal range
- Identify risk factors of hypothermia
- State measures to prevent hypothermia
- Identify symptoms of hypothermia and actions to take when hypothermia is present
- If hypothermia is medically induced, client/family will state goals for hypothermia treatment

Nursing Interventions

Temperature Measurement

- Recognize hypothermia as a drop in core body temperature below 35°C (95°F) (Danzl et al, 2011; Turk, 2010).
- Measure the client's temperature at least hourly and with changes in client condition (e.g., chills, change in mental status); if more than mild hypothermia is present (temperature lower than 35°C [95°F]), use a continuous temperature-monitoring device. Two modes of temperature monitoring may be indicated. Continuous temperature monitoring using an indwelling method of temperature measurement

is usually indicated to monitor effectiveness of treating body alterations in core body temperature.

- Use the same site and method (device) for temperature measurement for a given client so that temperature trends are assessed accurately and record site of temperature measurement.
- Bladder temperature may be used as an indwelling urinary catheter and is often inserted in the management of hypothermia to monitor diuresis.
- See the care plan for Ineffective **Thermoregulation** as appropriate.

Accidental Hypothermia

- Recognize that there are three types of accidental hypothermia (environmental causes):
  - ○ Acute hypothermia, also called immersion hypothermia, often from sudden exposure to cold through immersion in cold water or snow
  - ○ Exhaustion hypothermia, caused by exposure to cold in association with lack of food and exhaustion
  - ○ Chronic hypothermia that occurs over days or weeks and primarily affects older adults (Guly, 2011; Petrone, 2014)
- Remove the client from the cause of the hypothermic episode (e.g., cold environment, cold or wet clothing) and bring into a warm environment. Cover the client with warm blankets and apply a covering to the head and neck to conserve body heat.
- Watch the client for signs of hypothermia: shivering, slurred speech, confusion, clumsy movements, fatigue, and dehydration. As hypothermia progresses, the skin becomes pale, muscles are tense, fatigue and weakness progress, breathing is decreased, and pulmonary congestion is present, compromising oxygenation; pulses are decreased and blood pressure and heart rate decrease, progressing to lethal arrhythmias (e.g., ventricular fibrillation).
- ▲ Administer oxygen as ordered.
- Monitor the client's vital signs every hour and as appropriate. Note changes associated with hypothermia, such as initially increased pulse rate, respiratory rate, and blood pressure as well as diuresis with mild hypothermia, and then decreased pulse rate, respiratory rate, and blood pressure as well as oliguria with moderate to severe hypothermia.
- ▲ Attach electrodes and a cardiac monitor. Watch for dysrhythmias.

• = Independent   ▲ = Collaborative

▲ Monitor for signs of coagulopathy (e.g., oozing of blood from any open areas or from intravascular catheter sites or mucous membranes). Also note results of clotting studies as available.

• For mild hypothermia (core temperature of 32.2°C to 35°C [90°F to 95°F]), rewarm client passively:
  ○ Set room temperature to 21°C to 24°C (70°F to 75°F)
  ○ Keep the client dry; remove any damp or wet clothing
  ○ Layer clothing and blankets and cover the client's head; use insulated metallic blankets
  ○ Offer warm fluids; avoid alcohol or caffeine

▲ For moderate hypothermia (core temperature 28°C to 32.1°C [82.4°F to 90°F]), use active external rewarming methods. The rewarming rate should not exceed 0.5°C to 1°C (1.8°F) per hour. Methods include the following (Danzl et al, 2011; Galvao et al, 2010):
  ○ Forced-air warming blankets
  ○ Circulation of water through external heat exchange pads
  ○ Radiant heat sources

▲ For severe hypothermia (core temperature below 28°C [82.4°F]), use active core rewarming techniques as ordered (Danzl et al, 2011; Petrone, 2014; Soreide, 2014):
  ○ Recognize that extracorporeal blood rewarming methods, such as coronary artery bypass, are most effective
  ○ Use intravascular countercurrent in-line heat exchange to deliver warmed fluid or blood (Danzl et al, 2011)
  ○ Use heated and humidified oxygen through the ventilator as ordered
  ○ Administer heated intravenous (IV) fluids at prescribed temperature
  ○ Use heated irrigation of the gastrointestinal tract (nasogastric lavage) or bladder irrigations as ordered

• Rewarm clients slowly, generally at a rate of 0.5°C to 1°C every hour.

• Check blood pressure frequently when rewarming; watch for hypotension.

▲ Administer IV fluids, using a rapid infuser IV fluid warmer as ordered.

• Determine the factors leading to the hypothermic episode; see Related Factors.

• = Independent   ▲ = Collaborative

▲ Request a social service referral to help the client obtain the heat, shelter, and food needed to maintain body temperature.

▲ Encourage proper nutrition and hydration.

Targeted Temperature Hypothermia

• Recognize that targeted temperature management, also called therapeutic hypothermia, is the active lowering of the client's body temperature, in a controlled manner, to preserve neurological function after an acute myocardial injury or cardiac arrest.

H

• Recognize that controlled cooling of clients should be considered for all unconscious survivors of out-of-hospital ventricular tachycardia arrest as well as clients experiencing in-hospital arrests (Neumer et al, 2011; Scirica, 2013; Kim et al, 2015). The optimal targeted temperature for therapy is between 34°C and 36°C for up to 48 hours (Azmoon et al, 2011; Neumer et al, 2011; Scirica, 2013; Bravo & Kim, 2014).

• Monitor core or near core temperatures continuously using two methods of temperature monitoring.

• Recognize that cooling may be achieved noninvasively, using fluid-filled cooling devices that are placed next to the client's skin, or invasively, infusing iced solution.

• Obtain vital signs hourly (or via continuous monitoring) to include continuous electrocardiogram monitoring. Observe for signs of hypotension, bradycardia, and arrhythmias. Mechanical ventilation is required to protect the client's airway and breathing during treatment.

▲ Observe for shivering and administer sedation agents as prescribed.

▲ Closely inspect the skin before and throughout the cooling intervention to prevent skin breakdown associated with the treatment. Implement frequent turning and other pressure reduction interventions as indicated.

▲ Monitor and treat serum electrolytes (e.g., potassium, magnesium, calcium, and phosphorus) and serum glucose closely during targeted hypothermia and during rewarming of the client. Electrolytes will fluctuate as the client is rewarmed.

▲ Observe for signs and symptoms of coagulopathy during targeted hypothermia treatment. Hemoconcentration may be noticed as fluids shift during treatment.

• = Independent   ▲ = Collaborative

- Rewarming should occur in a controlled manner with a rise in body temperature of 0.5°C to 1°C per hour and with a targeted goal of normothermia, 37°C.
▲ Neurological and cognitive function should be assessed during targeted temperature treatment and after rewarming.

Pediatric

- Recognize that pediatric clients have a decreased ability to adapt to temperature extremes. Take the following actions to maintain body temperature in the infant/child:
  ○ Keep the head covered
  ○ Use blankets to keep the client warm
  ○ Keep the client covered during procedures, transport, and diagnostic testing
  ○ Keep the room temperature at 22.2°C (72°F)
▲ For the preterm or low-birth-weight newborn, use specially designed bags, skin-to-skin care, transwarmer mattresses, and radiant warmers to keep the infant warm.
▲ Targeted hypothermia may be implemented in the treatment of neonates with hypoxic-ischemic encephalopathy.

Geriatric

- Normal aging often includes changes in touch-related sensations, making it harder to differentiate cool and cold.
- Recognize that older adults can develop indoor hypothermia from air conditioning or ice baths.
- Assess neurological signs frequently, watching for confusion and decreased level of consciousness.
- Recognize that older adults often wear socks and sweaters to protect themselves from feeling cold, even in warmer weather (Sadler, 2011).

Home Care

Hypothermia is not a symptom that appears in the normal course of home care. When it occurs, it is a clinical emergency, and the client/family should access emergency medical services immediately.

- Some of the interventions described earlier may be adapted for home care use.
- Before a medical crisis occurs, confirm that the client or family has a thermometer and can read it. Instruct as needed. Verify that the thermometer registers accurately.
- Instruct the client or family to take the temperature when the client displays cyanosis, pallor, or shivering.

• = Independent   ▲ = Collaborative

▲ Monitor temperature every hour, as noted previously. If the temperature of the client begins dropping below the normal range, apply layers of clothing or blankets, or adjust environmental heat to the comfort level. Do not overheat. Contact a health care provider.

▲ If temperature continues to drop, activate the emergency system and notify a health care provider.

▲ If the client is in hospice care or is terminally ill, follow advance directives, client wishes, and the health care provider's orders. Keep the client free of pain.

H

Client/Family Teaching and Discharge Planning

• Teach the client and family signs of hypothermia and the method of taking the temperature (age appropriate).

• Teach the client methods to prevent hypothermia: wearing adequate clothing, including a hat and mittens; heating the environment to a minimum of 20°C (68°F); and ingesting adequate food and fluid.

▲ Teach the client and family about medications such as sedatives, opioids, and anxiolytics that predispose the client to hypothermia (as appropriate).

Risk for Hypothermia
NANDA-I Definition

Vulnerable to a failure of thermoregulation that may result in a core body temperature below the normal diurnal range, which may compromise health

Risk Factors

Alcohol consumption; damage to hypothalamus; economically disadvantaged; extremes of age; extremes of weight; heat transfer (e.g., conduction, convection, evaporation, radiation); inactivity; insufficient caregiver knowledge of hypothermia prevention; insufficient clothing; insufficient supply of subcutaneous fat; low environmental temperature; malnutrition; pharmaceutical agent; radiation; trauma

Children and Adults: Accidental

Mild hypothermia, core temperature approaching 35°C; moderate hypothermia, core temperature approaching 32°C; severe hypothermia, core temperature approaching 30°C

Neonates

Decrease in metabolic rate; delay in breastfeeding; early bathing of newborn; grade 1 hypothermia, core temperature approaching 36.5°C; grade 2 hypothermia, core temperature approaching 36°C; grade 3 hypothermia, core temperature approaching 35°C; grade 4 hypothermia, core temperature approaching 34°C; high-risk out-of-hospital birth; immature stratum corneum; increased body surface area to weight ratio; increase in oxygen demand; increase in pulmonary vascular resistance; ineffective vascular control; inefficient nonshivering thermogenesis; unplanned out-of-hospital birth

Client Outcomes, Nursing Interventions, and Client/Family Teaching and Discharge Planning

Refer to care plan for **Hypothermia.**

Risk for Perioperative Hypothermia

NANDA-I Definition

Vulnerable to an inadvertent drop in core body temperature below 36°C (96.8°F) occurring 1 hour before to 24 hours after surgery, which may compromise health

Risk Factors

American Society of Anesthesiologist (ASA) Physical Status classification score >1; cardiovascular complications; combined regional and general anesthesia; diabetic neuropathy; heat transfer (e.g., high volume of unwarmed infusion, unwarmed irrigation >20 L); low body weight; low environmental temperature; low preoperative temperature (<36°C [96.8°F]); surgical procedure

Client Outcomes

Client Will (Specify Time Frame)

- Maintain body temperature within normal range
- Identify risk factors of hypothermia
- State measures to prevent hypothermia
- Identify symptoms of hypothermia and actions to take when hypothermia is present
- Be free of surgical site infection

Nursing Interventions

Temperature Measurement

- Recognize perioperative hypothermia as a drop in core body temperature below 36°C (96.8°F) (Campbell et al, 2015; CDC, 2015).

• = Independent ▲ = Collaborative

- Measure the client's temperature frequently, and with changes in client condition (e.g., chills, change in mental status); if more than mild hypothermia is present (temperature lower than 36°C [96.85°F], use a continuous temperature-monitoring device. Two modes of temperature monitoring may be indicated. Continuous temperature monitoring using an indwelling method of temperature measurement is usually indicated to monitor effectiveness of treating body alterations in core body temperature.

H
- Use the same site and method (device) for temperature measurement for a given client so that temperature trends are assessed accurately, and record site of temperature measurement.
- Bladder temperature may be used as an indwelling urinary catheter and is often inserted in the management of hypothermia to monitor diuresis.

Unintentional Perioperative Hypothermia

- Keep the client warm throughout the perioperative period (preoperatively, intraoperatively, and postoperatively) to prevent unintentional perioperative hypothermia.
- Closely monitoring and preventing unintentional perioperative hypothermia are necessary to prevent adverse patient outcomes.
- Several interventions should be implemented to prevent unintentional perioperative hypothermia:
  - Use warming and booties perioperatively
  - Use warming blankets over and under the client perioperatively
  - Use warming blankets under the client on the operating table
  - Adjust environmental room controls to prevent cool ambient room temperature in the perioperative and operative rooms
  - Use warmed forced-air blankets preoperatively, during surgery, and in the postanesthesia care unit
  - Use warmed IV fluids and irrigation solutions
  - Designate responsibility and accountability for thermoregulation
- Using warmed IV fluids and irrigation solutions during the operative period may assist with reducing the client's risk of unintentional perioperative hypothermia.
- Active warming interventions include the use of warm blankets and forced-air warming devices.

• = Independent   ▲ = Collaborative

- Watch the client for signs of hypothermia: shivering, slurred speech, confusion, clumsy movements, fatigue, dehydration. As hypothermia progresses, the skin becomes pale, muscles are tense, fatigue and weakness progress, breathing is decreased, and pulmonary congestion is present, compromising oxygenation; pulses are decreased and blood pressure and heart rate decrease, progressing to lethal arrhythmias (e.g., ventricular fibrillation) (Danzl, 2011; Petrone, 2014).
▲ Administer oxygen as ordered.
▲ Attach electrodes and a cardiac monitor. Watch for dysrhythmias.
▲ Monitor for signs of coagulopathy (e.g., oozing of blood from any open areas or from intravascular catheter sites or mucous membranes). Also note results of clotting studies as available.
▲ Monitor for signs of surgical site infection (e.g., increased incisional pain, drainage, poor healing, poor incision approximation).
- See care plans for Ineffective **Thermoregulation** and **Hypothermia** as appropriate.

Pediatric
- Interventions implemented in the care of adult clients are similar when providing care to pediatric clients to prevent hypothermia.

Home Care
▲ Hypothermia is not a symptom that appears in the normal course of postoperative home care. If the client continues to complain of chills or feeling cold after discharge home from a surgical procedure, provide the client with warm blankets. If the client is allowed to drink, provide warm fluids by mouth.
▲ Monitor temperature every hour, as noted previously. If the temperature of the client begins dropping below the normal range, apply layers of clothing or blankets, or adjust environmental heat to the comfort level. Do not overheat. Contact a health care provider.
▲ If temperature continues to drop, activate the emergency system and notify a health care provider.

Client/Family Teaching and Discharge Planning
- Teach the client/family signs of hypothermia and the method of taking the temperature (age appropriate).
▲ Teach the client and family about medications such as sedatives, opioids, and anxiolytics that predispose the client to hypothermia (as appropriate).

• = Independent   ▲ = Collaborative

Disturbed personal Identity

NANDA-I Definition

Inability to maintain an integrated and complete perception of self

Defining Characteristics

Alteration in body image; confusion about cultural values; confusion about goals; confusion about ideological values; delusional description of self; feeling of emptiness; feeling of strangeness; fluctuating feelings about self; gender confusion; inability to distinguish between internal and external stimuli; inconsistent behavior; ineffective coping strategies; ineffective relationships; ineffective role performance

Related Factors

Alteration in social role; cult indoctrination; cultural incongruence; developmental transition; discrimination; dissociative identity disorder; dysfunctional family processes; exposure to toxic chemical; low self-esteem; manic states; organic brain disorder; perceived prejudice; pharmaceutical agent; psychiatric disorder; situational crisis; stages of growth

Client Outcomes

Client Will (Specify Time Frame)

- Demonstrate new purposes for life
- Show interests in surroundings
- Perform self-care and self-control activities appropriate for age
- Acknowledge personal strengths
- Engage in interpersonal relationships

Nursing Interventions

- Assess and support family strengths of commitment, appreciation, and affection toward each other, positive communication, time together, a sense of spiritual well-being, and the ability to cope with stress and crisis.
- ▲ Assess for suicidal ideation and make appropriate referral for clients dealing with diversity or mental or chronic somatic illness.
- ▲ Assess clients with mood disorders and make appropriate referrals for treatment.
- ▲ Assess and make appropriate referrals for clients with physical or mental disabilities.
- ▲ Assess clients for substance abuse and make appropriate referral.
- Use empathetic communication and encourage the client and family to verbalize fears, express emotions, and set goals.
- Be present for clients physically or by telephone.

• = Independent   ▲ = Collaborative

- Empower the client to set realistic goals and engage in problem solving.
- Encourage expression of positive thoughts and emotions.
- Encourage the client to use coping mechanisms.
- Help clients with serious and chronic conditions to maintain social support networks or assist in building new ones.
▲ Refer women facing diagnostic and curative breast cancer surgery for psychosocial support.
- Refer for cognitive behavioral therapy (CBT).
▲ Refer clients with borderline personality disorder (BPD) and dual-diagnosed BPD and substance-dependent female clients for dialectical behavior therapy (DBT) and psychoanalytical-orientated day-hospital therapy.
▲ Refer to the care plans for Readiness for enhanced **Communication** and Readiness for enhanced **Spiritual** well-being.

Pediatric
- Encourage adolescents to promote positive self-esteem, to enhance coping, and to prevent behavioral and psychological problems.
- Evaluate and refer children and adolescents for eating disorder prevention programs to include medical care, nutritional intervention, and mental health treatment and care coordination.
- Provide children with low self-esteem with appropriate support.
- Use computer-mediated support groups to enhance identity formation.

Geriatric
- Evaluate the effectiveness of nursing interventions used to promote positive self-identity in older adults.
- Consider the use of telephone/interview/group/computer support for caregivers of family members with dementia.
- Encourage clients to discuss "life history." Life history-based interventions and self-esteem and life-satisfaction questionnaires may be used to reinforce personal identity and foster hope.
▲ Refer the older client to self-help support groups.
▲ Refer the client with Alzheimer's disease who is terminally ill to hospice.

Multicultural
- Assess an individual's sociocultural background in teaching self-management and self-regulation as a means of supporting hope and coping.

• = Independent   ▲ = Collaborative

- Decrease discrimination to promote positive ethnic identity.
- Refer to care plan for Ineffective **Coping.**

Home Care

- The interventions described previously may be adapted for home care use.
- Provide an Internet-based health coach to encourage self-management for clients with chronic conditions such as depression, impaired mobility, and chronic pain. Use computer-mediated support groups to enhance identity formation.
- ▲ Refer the client to mutual health support groups. Participating in mutual health support groups led to enhanced coping by improving psychological and social functioning.
- ▲ Refer cancer clients and their spouses to family programs that include family-based interventions for communication, hope, coping, uncertainty, and symptom management.
- Refer combat veterans and service members directly involved in combat, as well as those providing support to combatants, including nurses, for mental health services.

Client/Family Teaching and Discharge Planning

- Teach the client about available community resources (e.g., therapists, ministers, counselors, self-help groups, family education groups).
- Teach coping skills to family caregivers of cancer clients.
- Teach caregivers the COPE intervention (creativity, optimism, planning, expert information) to assist with symptom management.

Risk for disturbed personal Identity

NANDA-I Definition

Vulnerable to the inability to maintain an integrated and complete perception of self, which may compromise health

Risk Factors

Alteration in social role; cult indoctrination; cultural incongruence; developmental transition; discrimination; dissociative identity disorder; dysfunctional family processes; exposure to toxic chemical; low self-esteem; manic states; organic brain disorder; perceived prejudice; pharmaceutical agent; psychiatric disorder; situational crisis; stages of growth

• = Independent   ▲ = Collaborative

Client Outcomes, Nursing Interventions, and Client/Family Teaching and Discharge Planning

Refer to care plan for Disturbed personal **Identity.**

Ineffective Impulse control
NANDA-I Definition

A pattern of performing rapid, unplanned reactions to internal or external stimuli without regard for the negative consequences of these reactions to the impulsive individual or to others

Defining Characteristics

Acting without thinking; asking personal questions despite the discomfort of others; gambling addiction; inability to save money or regulate finances; inappropriate sharing of personal details; irritability; overly familiar with strangers; sensation seeking; sexual promiscuity; temper outbursts; violent behavior

Related Factors

Alteration in cognitive functioning; alteration in development; hopelessness; mood disorder; organic brain disorder; personality disorder; smoking; substance abuse

Client Outcomes

Client Will (Specify Time Frame)

- Be free from harm
- Cooperate with behavioral modification plan
- Verbalize adaptive ways to cope with stress by means other than impulsive behaviors
- Delay gratification and use adaptive coping strategies in response to stress
- Verbalize understanding that behavior is unacceptable
- Accept responsibility for own behavior

Nursing Interventions

- Refer to mental health treatment for cognitive behavioral therapy (CBT).
- Assess the circumstances that led the client to seek help for their impulse control disorder.
- Implement motivational interviewing for clients with impulse control disorders.
- Teach client mindfulness meditation techniques. Mindfulness meditation includes observing experiences in the present moment,

• = Independent   ▲ = Collaborative

describing those experiences without judgments or evaluations, and participating fully in one's current context.

- Refer to self-help groups such as Gambler's Anonymous or Overeaters Anonymous as needed.
- Remove positive reinforcements associated with excessive behavior.
- Assist the client to recognize patterns and cues of impulsive behavior.
- Teach clients to use urge surfing techniques when impulses are triggered. A core skill associated with urge surfing is the ability to observe within oneself the rise and fall of urges and to "surf" or stay with these urges without acting on them.
- Implement cue elimination procedures as a stimulus control technique.
- Implement strategies to engage a high level construal mind-set by asking "why" abstaining from the targeted behavior will benefit the client.

Pediatric

- Assess children who have been exposed to violence in their environment for impulsive behavior.
- Implement in situ training to address impulsive behavior followed by role-play, differential reinforcement, corrective feedback, and rehearsal in young children and adolescents.
- Refer to mental health treatment for CBT.

Geriatric

- Assess for impulsive symptoms and maintain increased surveillance of the client whenever use of dopamine agonists has been initiated.
- Implement fall risk screening and precautions for geriatric clients with inattention and impulse control symptoms.
- Monitor caregivers for evidence of caregiver burden.

Client/Family Teaching and Discharge Planning

- Provide families with information about services such as addiction or marriage counseling.
- Families should be encouraged to employ practical measures to manage behavior such as limiting access to credit cards and restricting Internet access to gambling and casino websites and other addictive social media.

• = Independent   ▲ = Collaborative

Bowel Incontinence

NANDA-I Definition

Change in normal bowel elimination habits characterized by involuntary passage of stool

Defining Characteristics

Bowel urgency; constant passage of soft stool; does not recognize urge to defecate; fecal odor; fecal staining of bedding; fecal staining of clothing; inability to delay defecation; inability to expel formed stool despite recognition of rectal fullness; inability to recognize rectal fullness; inattentive to urge to defecate; reddened perianal skin

Related Factors

Increase in abdominal pressure; abnormal increase in intestinal pressure; alteration in cognitive functioning; chronic diarrhea; colorectal lesion; deficient dietary habits; difficulty with toileting self-care; dysfunctional rectal sphincter; environmental factor (e.g., inaccessible bathroom); generalized decline in muscle tone; immobility; impaction; impaired reservoir capacity; incomplete emptying of bowel; laxative abuse; lower motor nerve damage; pharmaceutical agent; rectal sphincter abnormality; stressors; upper motor nerve damage

Client Outcomes

Client Will (Specify Time Frame)

- Have regular, complete evacuation of fecal contents from the rectal vault (pattern may vary from every day to every 3 days)
- Have regulation of stool consistency (soft, formed stools)
- Reduce or eliminate frequency of incontinent episodes
- Exhibit intact skin in the perianal/perineal area
- Demonstrate the ability to isolate, contract, and relax pelvic muscles (when incontinence is related to sphincter incompetence or high-tone pelvic floor dysfunction)
- Increase pelvic muscle strength (when incontinence is related to sphincter incompetence)
- Identify triggers that precipitate change in bowel continence

Nursing Interventions

- In a private setting, directly question client about the presence of fecal incontinence. If the client reports altered bowel elimination patterns, problems with bowel control, or "uncontrollable diarrhea," complete a focused nursing history including previous and present bowel elimination routines, dietary history, frequency and volume of uncontrolled stool loss, and aggravating and alleviating factors.

• = Independent   ▲ = Collaborative

- Recognize that risk factors for fecal incontinence include older individuals, female sex, impaired mobility, cognitive impairment, and structural or functional impairment of bowel function (Aitola et al, 2010; Langemo et al, 2011; Willson et al, 2014).
- Recognize that additional risk factors for bowel incontinence in hospitalized clients include antibiotic therapy, medications, enteral feeding, immobility, inability to communicate elimination needs, acute disease processes and procedures (e.g., cancer, abdominal surgery), sedation, and mechanical ventilation (Hurnauth, 2011; Makic et al, 2011; Chang & Huang, 2013).
▲ Conduct a health history assessment that includes a review of current bowel patterns/habits to include constipation and use of laxatives; pelvic floor injury with childbirth; acute trauma to organs, muscles, or nerves involved in defecation; gastrointestinal inflammatory disorders; functional disability; and medications (Nurko & Scott, 2011; Kaiser et al, 2014).
▲ Closely inspect the perineal skin and skin folds for evidence of skin breakdown in clients with incontinence.
▲ Use a validated tool that focuses on bowel elimination patterns to help provide a more clear understanding of the client's individual challenges with fecal incontinence (Gillibrand, 2012; Langemo et al, 2011).
▲ Complete a focused physical assessment, including inspection of perineal skin, pelvic muscle strength assessment, digital examination of the rectum for presence of impaction and anal sphincter strength, and evaluation of functional status (mobility, dexterity, visual acuity).
- Complete an assessment of cognitive function; explore for a history of dementia, delirium, or acute confusion (Bliss et al, 2011; Drennan et al, 2014).
- Document patterns of stool elimination and incontinent episodes through a bowel record, including frequency of bowel movements, stool consistency, frequency and severity of incontinent episodes, precipitating factors, and dietary and fluid intake.
- Assess stool consistency and its influence on risk for stool loss.
- Identify conditions contributing to or causing fecal incontinence.
- Improve access to toileting:
  ○ Identify usual toileting patterns and plan opportunities for toileting accordingly.

• = Independent ▲ = Collaborative

- ○ Provide assistance with toileting for clients with limited access or impaired functional status (mobility, dexterity, access).
- ○ Institute a prompted toileting program for persons with impaired cognitive status.
- ○ Provide adequate privacy for toileting.
- ○ Respond promptly to requests for assistance with toileting.
- Review the client's nutritional history and evaluate methods to normalize stool consistency with dietary adjustments (e.g., avoiding high-fat content foods) and use of fiber (Nurko & Scott, 2011; Willson et al, 2014; International Foundation for Functional Gastrointestinal Disorders [IFFGD], 2014).
- Encourage the client to keep a nutrition log to track foods that irritate the bowel (Nurko & Scott, 2011).
- For hospitalized clients with tube feeding–associated fecal incontinence, involve the nutrition specialist to evaluate the formula composition, osmolality, and fiber content.
- For the client with intermittent episodes of fecal incontinence related to acute changes in stool consistency, begin a bowel reeducation program consisting of:
  - ○ Cleansing the bowel of impacted stool if indicated
  - ○ Normalizing stool consistency by adequate intake of fluids (30 mL/kg of body weight/day) and dietary or supplemental fiber
  - ○ Establishing a regular routine of fecal elimination based on established patterns of bowel elimination (patterns established before onset of incontinence)
- ▲ Implement a scheduled stimulation defecation program for persons with neurological conditions causing fecal incontinence:
  - ○ Cleanse the bowel of impacted fecal material before beginning the program.
  - ○ Implement strategies to normalize stool consistency, including adequate intake of fluid and fiber and avoidance of foods associated with diarrhea.
  - ○ Determine a regular schedule for bowel elimination (typically every day or every other day) based on prior patterns of bowel elimination.
  - ○ Provide a stimulus before assisting the client to a position on the toilet; digital stimulation, a stimulating suppository, "mini-enema," or pulsed evacuation enema may be used for stimulation.

• = Independent   ▲ = Collaborative

▲ Begin a reeducation or pelvic floor muscle exercise program for the person with sphincter incompetence or high-tone pelvic floor muscle dysfunction of the pelvic muscles, or refer persons with fecal incontinence related to sphincter dysfunction to a nurse specialist or other therapist with clinical expertise in these techniques of care.

▲ Consider a sacral nerve stimulation program in clients with urgency to defecate and fecal incontinence related to weakened sphincter muscles or sphincter defect.

• Institute a structured skin care regimen that incorporates three essential steps: cleanse, moisturize, and protect:

  ○ Select a cleanser with a pH range comparable to that of normal skin (usually labeled "pH balanced").

  ○ Moisturize with an emollient to replace lipids removed with cleansing and protect with a skin. Products containing petrolatum, dimethicone, or zinc oxide base or a no-sting skin barrier should be used.

  ○ Routine incontinence care should include daily perineal skin cleansing and following each episode of incontinence.

  ○ When feasible, select a product that combines two or all three of these processes into a single step. Ensure that products are available at the bedside when caring for a client with total incontinence in an inpatient facility.

▲ Use of absorptive pads or adult containment briefs that are applied next to the client's skin increases the risk of incontinence-associated dermatitis. Absorbent underpads that wick moisture away from skin may be used with immobile clients.

▲ Consult the provider if a fungal infection is suspected. An antifungal cream or powder beneath a protective ointment may be indicated (Black et al, 2011; Langemo et al, 2011; Makic et al, 2011; Willson et al, 2014).

• Assist the client to select and apply a containment device for occasional episodes of fecal incontinence. A fecal containment device will prevent soiling of clothing and reduce odors in the client with uncontrolled stool loss.

• In the client with frequent episodes of fecal incontinence and limited mobility, monitor the sacrum and perineal area for pressure ulcerations.

• = Independent   ▲ = Collaborative

- With acutely ill clients, anticipate and evaluate the cause of acute diarrhea. Anticipate diarrhea associated with treatment or specific interventions (e.g., medications, initiation of tube feedings).
▲ Consult a provider about insertion of a bowel management system in the critically ill client when conservative measures have failed and fecal incontinence is excessive and/or produces perianal skin injury or incontinence-associated dermatitis.

Geriatric

- Evaluate all older clients for established or acute fecal incontinence when the older client enters the acute or long-term care facility and intervene as indicated.
- Determine the client's cognitive level using a screening tool such as the Mini-Mental State Exam (MMSE), the CAM, or Mini-Cog.
  ○ Teach nursing colleagues, nonprofessional care providers, family, and clients the importance of providing toileting opportunities and adequate privacy for the client in an acute or long-term care facility.

Home Care

- The preceding interventions may be adapted for home care use.
- Assess and teach a bowel management program to support continence. Address timing, diet, fluids, and actions taken independently to deal with bowel incontinence.
- Instruct caregiver to provide clothing that is nonrestrictive, can be manipulated easily for toileting, and can be changed with ease.
- Evaluate self-care strategies of community-dwelling older adults, strengthen adaptive behaviors, and counsel older adults about altering strategies that compromise general health.
- Assist the family in arranging care in a way that allows the client to participate in family or favorite activities without embarrassment.
▲ If the client is limited to bed (or bed and chair), provide a commode or bedpan that can be easily accessed. Involve occupational and physical therapy services as indicated to promote safe transfers.
▲ If the client is frequently incontinent, refer for home health aide services to assist with hygiene and skin care.
▲ Refer the family to support services to assist with in-home management of fecal incontinence as indicated.

NOTE: Refer to care plans for **Diarrhea** and **Constipation** for detailed management of these related conditions.

• = Independent   ▲ = Collaborative

Functional urinary Incontinence

NANDA-I Definition

Inability of usually continent person to reach toilet in time to avoid unintentional loss of urine

Defining Characteristics

Completely empties bladder; early morning urinary incontinence; sensation of need to void; time between sensation of urge and ability to reach toilet is too short; voiding prior to reaching toilet

Related Factors (r/t)

Alteration in cognitive functioning; alteration in environmental factor; impaired vision; neuromuscular impairment; psychological disorder; weakened supporting pelvic structure

Client Outcomes

Client Will (Specify Time Frame)

- Eliminate or reduce incontinent episodes
- Eliminate or overcome environmental barriers to toileting
- Use adaptive equipment to reduce or eliminate incontinence related to impaired mobility or dexterity
- Use portable urinary collection devices or urine containment devices when access to the toilet is not feasible

Nursing Interventions

- Introduce yourself to the client and anyone accompanying him or her and inform them of your role.
- Gain consent to carry out care before proceeding further with the assessment. In clients unable to give consent, liaise with relevant health care professionals and/or family members.
- Wash hands using a recognized technique.
- Assess usual pattern of bladder management and establish the extent of the problem to include the following: A detailed and accurate assessment of the client enables the nurse to plan interventions, monitor outcomes, and evaluate care, ensuring no unnecessary treatment is carried out (Matthews, 2011).
- Bladder Habits
  - ○ Episodes of incontinence during the day and night
  - ○ Alleviating and aggravating factors
  - ○ Current management strategies to include containing/collection devices, restriction of fluid intake, and avoidance of fluid/food groups that cause bladder irritation

• = Independent   ▲ = Collaborative

- Lifestyle and Risk Assessment: Toilet facility access and ability to use including:
  - ○ Distance of the toilet from the bed, chair, and living quarters
  - ○ Characteristics of the bed, including presence of side rails and distance of the bed from the floor
  - ○ Characteristics of the pathway to the toilet, including barriers such as stairs, loose rugs on the floor, and inadequate lighting
  - ○ Characteristics of the bathroom, including patterns of use, lighting, height of the toilet from the floor, presence of handrails to assist transfers to the toilet, and breadth of the door and its accessibility for a wheelchair, walker, or other assistive device
- Physical and Mental Abilities
  - ○ Ability to rise from chair and bed, transfer to the toilet, and ambulate, and the need for physical assistive devices such as a cane, walker, or wheelchair.
  - ○ Ability to manipulate buttons, hooks, snaps, loop and pile closures, and zippers as needed to remove clothing.
  - ○ Functional and cognitive status assessment using a tool such as the Mini Mental Status Examination for the older client with functional incontinence.
  - ○ Daily fluid intake included amount of types of fluids drank
  - ○ Risk of falls due to dizziness, impaired vision, and hearing
  - ○ Functional ability decline secondary to comorbidities (cerebral vascular incidents, amputation—see Past Medical History)
  - ○ Discuss quality-of-life issues relating to socialization and family events
- Past Medical History
  - ○ Obstetrical/gynecological/urological history and surgeries
  - ○ Relevant comorbidities—cardiac, respiratory, renal, or neurological
  - ○ Recurrent urinary tract infections
- Teach the client, the client's care providers, or the family to complete a bladder diary; each 24-hour period is subdivided into 1- to 2-hour periods and includes number of urinations occurring in the toilet, actual episodes of incontinence and amount of urine leaked, reasons for episode of incontinence, type and amount of liquid intake, number of bowel movements, and incontinence pads or other products used.

• = Independent   ▲ = Collaborative

- Consult with the health care provider and carry out a medication review relating to side effects and contraindications. Antimuscarinic medications in clients receiving cholinesterase reuptake inhibitors for Alzheimer's-type dementia may experience adverse drug interactions.
- Provide an appropriate, safe urinary receptacle such as a three-in-one commode, female or male hand-held urinal, no-spill urinal, or containment device when toileting access is limited by immobility or environmental barriers and while other interventions are being put in place.
- Refer to occupational therapy for help in obtaining assistive devices and adapting the home for optimal toilet accessibility.
- Provide advice to clients relating to loose-fitting clothing with stretch waistbands rather than buttoned or zippered waist; minimize buttons, snaps, and multilayered clothing; and substitute a loop-and-pile closure or other easily loosened systems such as Velcro for buttons, hooks, and zippers in existing clothing.
- Work with client on retraining the bladder by regular timed toileting regimens (every 2 hours). For the older client in the home or a long-term care facility who has functional incontinence and dementia:
  - ○ Determine the frequency of current urination using an alarm system or check-and-change device.
  - ○ Record urinary elimination and incontinent patterns in a bladder log to use as a baseline for assessment and evaluation of treatment efficacy.
  - ○ Begin a prompted toileting program based on the results of this program; toileting frequency may vary from every 1.5 to 2 hours to every 4 hours.
  - ○ Provide positive reinforcement.
- Monitor older clients in a long-term care facility, acute care facility, or home for dehydration.
- Inspect the perineal and perianal skin for evidence of incontinence-associated dermatitis, including inflammation, vesicles in skin exposed to urinary leakage, and especially skin folds or denudation of the skin, particularly when incontinence is managed by absorptive pads or containment briefs.

• = Independent   ▲ = Collaborative

- Begin a preventive skin care regimen for all clients with urinary incontinence and treat clients with incontinence-associated dermatitis or related skin damage.
- Advise the client about the advantages of using disposable or reusable insert pads, pad-pant systems, or replacement briefs specifically designed for urinary incontinence as indicated for short-term/long-term use, including social events.
- Consider the use of an indwelling catheter for continuous drainage in the client who is both homebound and bed-bound and is receiving palliative or end-of-life care (requires a health care provider's order).
- When an indwelling urinary catheter is in place, follow prescribed maintenance protocols for managing the catheter, taping and replacing the catheter, drainage bag, and care of perineal skin and urethral meatus. Teach infection control measures adapted to the home care setting.
- Assist the client in adapting to the catheter. Encourage discussion of the client's response to the catheter.
- Provide client with comprehensive written information about bladder care.
- Document all care and advice given in a factual and comprehensive manner.

Overflow urinary Incontinence

NANDA-I Definition

Involuntary loss of urine associated with overdistention of the bladder

Defining Characteristics

Bladder distention; high postvoid residual volume; involuntary leakage of small volume of urine; nocturia

Related Factors

Bladder outlet obstruction; detrusor external sphincter dyssynergia; detrusor hypocontractility; fecal impaction; severe pelvic prolapse; treatment regimen; urethral obstruction

Client Outcomes, Nursing Interventions, and Client/Family Teaching and Discharge Planning

Refer to care plan for **Urinary Retention.**

• = Independent   ▲ = Collaborative

Reflex urinary Incontinence

NANDA-I Definition

Involuntary loss of urine at somewhat predictable intervals when a specific bladder volume is reached

Defining Characteristics

Absence of sensation of bladder fullness; absence of urge to void; absence of voiding sensation; inability to voluntarily inhibit voiding; inability to voluntarily initiate voiding; incomplete emptying of bladder with lesion above pontine micturition center; predictable pattern of voiding; sensation of bladder fullness; sensation of urgency to void without voluntary inhibition of bladder contraction

NOTE: Reflex urinary incontinence may be associated with sweating and acute elevation in blood pressure and pulse rate in clients with spinal cord injury. Refer to the care plan for **Autonomic Dysreflexia.**

Related Factors (r/t)

Neurological impairment above level of pontine micturition center; neurological impairment above level of sacral micturition center; tissue damage

Client Outcomes

Client Will (Specify Time Frame)

- Follow prescribed schedule for bladder emptying
- Have intact perineal skin
- Remain clear of symptomatic urinary tract infection
- Demonstrate how to apply containment device or insert intermittent catheter or be able to provide caregiver with instructions for performing these procedures

Nursing Interventions

- Introduce yourself to the client and anyone accompanying him/her and inform them of your role.
- Gain consent to carry out care before proceeding further with the assessment.
- Wash hands using a recognized technique.
- Assess usual pattern of bladder management and establish the extent of the problem (refer to Functional urinary **Incontinence** care plan).
- Ask the client to complete a bladder diary/log to determine the pattern of urine elimination, any incontinence episodes, and current bladder management program. An electronic voiding diary may be kept whenever feasible.

• = Independent   ▲ = Collaborative

- Consult with the health care provider concerning current bladder function and the potential of the bladder to produce hydronephrosis, vesicoureteral reflux, febrile urinary tract infection, or compromised renal function.
- Consult with the health care provider and physical therapist concerning the neuromuscular ability to perform bladder management. The type of neurological disorder, as well as the level of neurological impairment and the ability to use the hands effectively, determines the method of urine management in reflex incontinence.
- Inspect the perineal and perigenital skin for signs of incontinence-associated dermatitis and pressure ulcers.
- In consultation with the rehabilitation team, counsel the client and family concerning the merits and potential risks associated with each possible bladder management program, including spontaneous voiding, intermittent self-catheterization, and reflex voiding with condom catheter containment and, in some cases, indwelling suprapubic catheterization.

Intermittent Self-Catheterization (ISC)

- Begin intermittent catheterization as ordered using sterile technique; the client may be taught to use clean technique in the home situation.
- Schedule the frequency of intermittent catheterization based on the frequency/volume records of previous catheterizations, functional bladder capacity, and the impact of catheterization on the quality of the client's life.
- Teach the client to recognize signs of symptomatic urinary tract infection and to seek care promptly when these signs occur. The signs of symptomatic infection are the following:
  - ○ Discomfort over the bladder or during urination
  - ○ Acute onset of urinary incontinence
  - ○ Fever
  - ○ Markedly increased spasticity of muscles below the level of the spinal lesion
  - ○ Malaise, lethargy
  - ○ Hematuria
  - ○ Autonomic dysreflexia (hyperreflexia) symptoms
- Recognize that intermittent catheterization is typically associated with asymptomatic bacteriuria, and the indwelling catheter is routinely associated with asymptomatic colonization.

• = Independent   ▲ = Collaborative

- Teach intermittent catheterization as the client approaches discharge as per operational guidelines and best practice. Instruct the client and at least one family member in the performance of catheterization. Teach the client with quadriplegia how to instruct others to perform this procedure.
- Teach the client managed by intermittent catheterization to self-administer antispasmodic (parasympatholytic) medications as prescribed by consulting health care provider and to recognize and manage potential side effects as needed.

Condom Catheter/Sheath System

- For a male client with reflex incontinence who does not have urinary retention and cannot manage the condition effectively with spontaneous voiding, does not choose to perform intermittent catheterization, or cannot perform catheterization, teach the client and his family to obtain, select, and apply an external collective device and urinary drainage system. Assist the client and family to choose a product that adheres to the glans penis or penile shaft without allowing seepage of urine onto surrounding skin or clothing, that avoids provoking hypersensitivity reactions on the skin, and that includes a urinary drainage reservoir that is easily concealed under the clothing and does not cause irritation to the skin of the thigh.
- Teach the client whose incontinence is managed by a condom catheter to routinely inspect the skin with each catheter change for evidence of lesions caused by pressure from the containment device or by exposure to urine, to cleanse the penis thoroughly, and to reapply a new device daily or every other day.
- Ensure the client is aware of when and how to report any problems and/or complications of reflex incontinence care when at home.
- Encourage a mindset and program of self-care management.
- Assist the family with arranging care in a way that allows the client to participate in family or favorite activities without embarrassment. Elicit discussion of the client's concerns about the social or emotional burden of incontinence.
- Teach the client to ensure good hydration. Total daily fluid intake should be approximately 2.7 L per day for women and 3.7 L per day for men.
- Teach the client with a spinal injury the signs of autonomic dysreflexia, its relationship to bladder fullness, and management of the condition. Refer to the care plan for **Autonomic Dysreflexia.**

• = Independent   ▲ = Collaborative

- Provide client with comprehensive written information about bladder care.
- Document all care and advice given in a factual and comprehensive manner.

Risk for Urge Urinary Incontinence

NANDA-I Definition

Vulnerable to involuntary passage of urine occurring soon after a strong sensation or urgency to void, which may compromise health

Risk Factors

Alcohol consumption; atrophic urethritis; atrophic vaginitis; detrusor hyperactivity with impaired bladder contractility; ineffective toileting habits; involuntary sphincter relaxation; small bladder capacity; treatment regimen

Client Outcomes, Nursing Interventions, and Client/Family Teaching and Discharge Planning

Refer to care plan for Urge urinary **Incontinence.**

Stress Urinary Incontinence

NANDA-I Definition

Sudden leakage of urine with activities that increase intra-abdominal pressure

Defining Characteristics

Involuntary leakage of small volume of urine (e.g., with coughing, laughing, sneezing, on exertion); involuntary leakage of small volume of urine in the absence of detrusor contraction; involuntary leakage of small volume of urine in the absence of overdistended bladder

Related Factors (r/t)

Degenerative changes in pelvic muscles; increase in intra-abdominal pressure; intrinsic urethral sphincter deficiency; weak pelvic muscles

Client Outcomes

Client Will (Specify Time Frame)

- Report fewer stress incontinence episodes and/or a decrease in the severity of urine loss
- Experience reduction in frequency of urinary incontinence episodes as recorded on voiding diary (bladder log)
- Identify containment devices that assist in management of stress incontinence

• = Independent   ▲ = Collaborative

Nursing Interventions

- Introduce yourself to the client and anyone accompanying him/her and inform them of your role.
- Gain consent to carry out care before proceeding further with the assessment. In clients unable to give consent, liaise with relevant health care professionals and/or family members.
- Wash hands using a recognized technique.
- Assess usual pattern of bladder management and establish pattern of bladder management and extent of the problem to include: (refer to Functional urinary **Incontinence** care plan).
- Past Medical History (risk factors for stress incontinence): pregnancy, parity, large babies, forceps or breech deliveries, obesity, chronic cough, physical activity, previous urinary tract or gynecological surgery.
- Medication Review (diuretics, lithium, adrenergic blockers, diabetes, and smoking).
- Bladder Habits
  - ○ Onset and duration of urinary leakage
  - ○ Related lower urinary tract symptoms, including voiding frequency (day/night), urgency, severity (small, moderate, large amounts) of urinary leakage
  - ○ Factors provoking urine loss (diuretics, bladder irritants, alcohol), focusing on the differential diagnosis of stress, urge or mixed stress, and urge urinary symptoms. Consider using a symptom questionnaire that elicits relevant lower urinary tract symptoms and provides differentiation between stress and urge incontinence symptoms.
- Assess for mixed urinary incontinence (a combination of stress and urge incontinence):
  - ○ Can you delay urination for a 2-hour movie or car ride?
  - ○ How often do you arise at night to urinate?
  - ○ When you have the urge to urinate, can you reach the toilet without leaking?
- Lifestyle Assessment: impact on the individual's lifestyle. Inquire about incontinence pad use and change in daily, social, or recreational activities, as well as emotional impact.
- Inspect the perineal skin for evidence of incontinence-associated dermatitis, including inflammation, vesicles in skin exposed to urinary leakage, and especially skin folds or denudation of the skin,

• = Independent   ▲ = Collaborative

particularly when incontinence is managed by absorptive pads or containment briefs.

- Refer client for specific testing to further confirm diagnosis. If trained to do so, carry out cough stress test, request 24-hour pad test (if appropriate) and urodynamic studies (to include urine speed and flow, post-void residual measurement, leak point pressure, and pressure flow study).
- Establish with client his/her current use of containment devices; evaluate the devices for their ability to adequately contain urine loss, protect clothing, and control odor. Assist the client in identifying containment devices specifically designed to contain urinary leakage.
- Teach the client to complete a bladder diary by recording voiding frequency, the frequency and degree of urinary incontinence episodes, their association with urgency (a sudden and strong desire to urinate that is difficult to defer), fluid intake, and pad usage over a 3- to 7-day period. An electronic voiding diary may be kept whenever feasible.
- With the client and in close consultation with the health care provider, review treatment options, including behavioral management; drug therapy; use of a pessary, vaginal device, or urethral insert; and surgery. Outline their potential benefits, efficacy, and side effects.

Pelvic Floor Training Program

- Teach the client undergoing pelvic floor muscle training to identify, contract, and relax the pelvic floor muscles without contracting distal muscle groups (e.g., abdominal muscles or gluteus muscles) using verbal feedback based on vaginal or anal palpation, biofeedback, or electrical stimulation, utilizing the assistance of an incontinence specialist or health care provider as necessary.
- Incorporate principles of exercise physiology into a pelvic muscle training program using the following strategies:
  - Begin a graded exercise program, usually starting with 5 to 10 repetitions and advancing gradually to no more than 35 to 50 repetitions every day or every other day based on baseline and ongoing evaluation of maximal strength and endurance.
  - Continue exercise sessions over a period of 3 to 6 months.
  - Integrate muscle training into activities of daily living.
  - Assess progress every 2 weeks during the first month and every 4 to 6 weeks thereafter.

Bladder Training Program

- Assist the client in completing a bladder diary over a period of a minimum of 3 days or up to 7 days.
  - ○ Review the results with the client, determining typical voiding frequency and establishing goals for voiding frequency.
  - ○ Using baseline voiding frequency, as determined by the diary, teach the client to urinate by the clock when awake, typically every 30 to 120 minutes.
  - ○ Encourage adherence to the program with timing devices, as well as verbal encouragement and support, and address individual reasons for schedule interruption.
  - ○ Gradually increase the time between urinations to the negotiated goal. Time intervals between voiding are typically increased in increments of 15 to 30 minutes for clients with a baseline frequency of less than every 60 minutes and increments of 25 to 30 minutes for clients with a baseline frequency of more than every 60 minutes.
- Teach the client to self-administer duloxetine and imipramine as ordered by consulting health care provider, and to monitor for adverse side effects.
- Teach the client to self-administer topical (vaginal) estrogens as directed, and to monitor for adverse side effects.
- Refer the female client with stress urinary incontinence and pelvic organ prolapse who wishes to employ a pessary to manage stress incontinence to a nurse specialist or gynecologist with expertise in the placement and maintenance of these devices.
- Discuss potentially reversible or controllable risk factors, such as weight loss, with the client with stress incontinence and assist the client to formulate a strategy to eliminate these conditions.
- Provide information about support resources such as the National Association for Continence, the Simon Foundation for Continence, and the Total Control Program.
- Refer the client with persistent stress incontinence to a continence service, health care provider, or nurse who specializes in the management of this condition.
- Teach the client to ensure good hydration. Total daily fluid intake should be approximately 2.7 L per day for women and 3.7 L per day for men.

• = Independent ▲ = Collaborative

- Provide client with comprehensive written information about bladder care.
- Encourage a mindset and program of self-care management.
- Assist the family with arranging care in a way that allows the client to participate in family or favorite activities without embarrassment. Elicit discussion of the client's concerns about the social or emotional burden of incontinence.
- Document all care and advice given in a factual and comprehensive manner.

Urge urinary Incontinence

NANDA-I Definition

Involuntary passage of urine occurring soon after a strong sense of urgency to void

Defining Characteristics

Inability to reach toilet in time to avoid urine loss; involuntary loss of urine with bladder contractions; involuntary loss of urine with bladder spasms; urinary urgency

Related Factors (r/t)

Alcohol consumption; atrophic urethritis; atrophic vaginitis; bladder infection; caffeine intake; decrease in bladder capacity; detrusor hyperactivity with impaired bladder contractility; fecal impaction; treatment regimen

Client Outcomes

Client Will (Specify Time Frame)

- Report relief from urge urinary incontinence or a decrease in the frequency of incontinent episodes
- Identify containment devices that assist in the management of urge urinary incontinence

Nursing Interventions

- Introduce yourself to the client and anyone accompanying him/her and inform them of your role.
- Gain consent to carry out care before proceeding further with the assessment.
- Wash hands using a recognized technique.
- Assess usual pattern of bladder management and establish pattern of bladder management and extent of the problem. Refer to Functional urinary **Incontinence** care plan.

• = Independent   ▲ = Collaborative

- Bladder Habits and Quality-of-Life Issues:
  - ○ Diurnal frequency (voiding more than once every 2 hours while awake)
  - ○ Urgency, daytime frequency, and nocturia
  - ○ Involuntary leakage and leakage accompanied by or preceded by urgency
  - ○ Amount of urine loss—moderate or large volume
  - ○ Severity of symptoms
  - ○ Alleviating and aggravating factors
  - ○ Effect on quality of life
- Ask specific questions relating to urge presentation:
  - ○ Can you delay urination for a 2-hour movie or car ride?
  - ○ How often do you wake at night to urinate?
  - ○ When you have the urge to urinate, can you reach the toilet without leaking?
- In close consultation with a health care practitioner or advanced practice nurse, consider administering a symptom questionnaire that elicits relevant lower urinary tract symptoms and differentiates stress and urge incontinence symptoms.
- Assess the severity of incontinence as well as the impact on the individual's lifestyle; inquire about incontinence pad use and change in daily, social, or recreational activities, as well as emotional impact.
- Perform a focused physical assessment, if competent to do so, alternatively in close consultation with a health care practitioner or advanced practice nurse including:
  - ○ Bladder palpation after voiding to check for retention
  - ○ Bladder scanning for post-void residual
  - ○ Inspection of the perineal skin
  - ○ Vaginal examination to determine hypoestrogenic changes in the mucosa (may contribute to urge incontinence)
  - ○ Pelvic examination to determine the presence, location, and severity of vaginal wall prolapse, and reproduction of stress urinary incontinence with the cough test
  - ○ Anal tone and constipation should be assessed.
- Inspect the perineal and perianal skin for evidence of incontinence-associated dermatitis, including inflammation, vesicles in skin exposed to urinary leakage, and especially skin folds or denudation of the skin, particularly when incontinence is managed by absorptive pads or containment briefs.

• = Independent ▲ = Collaborative

- Teach the client to complete a bladder diary by recording voiding frequency, the frequency and degree of urinary incontinence episodes, their association with urgency (a sudden and strong desire to urinate that is difficult to defer), fluid intake, and pad usage over a 3- to 7-day period. An electronic voiding diary may be kept whenever feasible. In addition to these parameters, the client may be asked to record voided volume and fluid intake.
- Review all medications the client is receiving, paying particular attention to sedatives, opioid analgesics, diuretics, antidepressants, psychotropic drugs, and cholinergics. Consult the health care practitioner or nurse practitioner about altering or eliminating these medications if they are suspected of affecting incontinence.
- Assess the client for urinary retention (see the care plan for **Urinary Retention**).
- Assess the client for functional limitations (environmental barriers, limited mobility or dexterity, impaired cognitive function).
- Consult the health care practitioner concerning diabetic management or pharmacotherapy for urinary tract infection when indicated. In specific cases, urgency and an increased risk of urge incontinence may be related to bacteriuria or urinary tract infection (Rodhe et al, 2008).
- Assess for signs and symptoms of atrophic vaginal changes in the perimenopausal or postmenopausal woman, including vaginal dryness, tenderness to touch, mucosal dryness, friability, and discomfort with gentle palpation. Specifically query the woman with atrophic vaginitis concerning associated lower urinary tract symptoms (usually voiding frequency, urgency, and dysuria). Refer the woman with atrophic vaginal changes and bothersome lower urinary tract symptoms to a gynecologist, urologist, or women's health nurse practitioner for further evaluation and management.

Pelvic Floor Training Program

- Teach the client undergoing pelvic floor muscle training to identify, contract, and relax the pelvic floor muscles without contracting distal muscle groups (e.g., abdominal muscles or gluteus muscles) using verbal feedback based on vaginal or anal palpation, biofeedback, or electrical stimulation, utilizing the assistance of an incontinence specialist or health care practitioner as necessary.

• = Independent   ▲ = Collaborative

- Incorporate principles of exercise physiology into a pelvic muscle training program using the following strategies:
  - ○ Begin a graded exercise program, usually starting with 5 to 10 repetitions and advancing gradually to no more than 35 to 50 repetitions every day or every other day based on baseline and ongoing evaluation of maximal strength and endurance.
  - ○ Continue exercise sessions over a period of 3 to 6 months.
  - ○ Integrate muscle training into activities of daily living.
  - ○ Assess progress every 2 weeks during the first month and every 4 to 6 weeks thereafter.

Bladder Training Program

- Assist the client in completing a voiding diary over a period of a minimum of 3 days or up to 7 days.
- Review the results with the client, determining typical voiding frequency and establishing goals for voiding frequency based on the longest time interval between voids that is comfortable for the client.
- Using baseline voiding frequency, as determined by the diary, teach the client to void first thing in the morning, every time the predetermined voiding interval passes, and before going to bed at night.
- Encourage adherence to the program with timing devices and verbal encouragement and support, and address individual reasons for schedule interruption.
- Teach distraction and urge suppression techniques (see later discussion) to control urgency while the client postpones urination.
- Gradually increase the time between urinations to the negotiated goal. Time intervals between voiding are typically increased in increments of 15 to 30 minutes for clients with a baseline frequency of less than every 60 minutes and increments of 25 to 30 minutes for clients with a baseline frequency of more than every 60 minutes. The voiding interval should be increased by 15 to 30 minutes each week (based on the client's tolerance) until a voiding interval of 3 to 4 hours is achieved. Utilize a bladder diary to monitor progress.
- Review with the client the types of beverages consumed, focusing on the intake of caffeine, which is associated with a transient effect on lower urinary tract symptoms. Advise all clients to reduce or eliminate intake of caffeinated beverages and over-the-counter

• = Independent ▲ = Collaborative

medications or dietary aids containing caffeine. Identify and counsel the client to eliminate other bladder irritants that may exacerbate incontinence, such as smoking, carbonated beverages, citrus, sugar substitutes, and tomato products.

- Review with the client the volume of fluids consumed; fluids may be reduced with caution, particularly in clients who do not drink more than 1500 mL during the day, to alleviate urinary frequency, especially in the evening after 6 PM or 3 to 4 hours before bedtime to reduce nocturia.

- Teach the client methods to avoid constipation (refer to **Constipation** care plans) such as increasing dietary fiber, moderately increasing fluid intake, exercising, and establishing a routine defecation schedule.

Urge Suppression

- Teach the client the following techniques:
  - ○ When a strong or precipitous urge to urinate is perceived, teach the client to avoid running to the toilet.
  - ○ Pause, sit down, and relax the entire body.
  - ○ Perform repeated, rapid pelvic muscle contractions until the urge is relieved.
  - ○ Use distraction: count backward from 100 by sevens, recite a poem, write a letter, balance a checkbook, do handwork such as knitting, take five deep breaths, focusing on breathing.
  - ○ Relief is followed by micturition within 5 to 15 minutes, using nonhurried movements when locating a toilet and voiding.
  - ○ Use urge suppression strategies on waking during the night. If the urge subsides, the client should be encouraged to go back to sleep. If after a minute or two it does not, clients should be instructed to get up to void to avoid sleep interruption.

- Teach the client to self-administer antimuscarinic (anticholinergic) drugs as directed. Teach dosage side effects and administration of the medication and the importance of combining pharmacotherapy with scheduled voiding, adequate fluid intake, restriction of bladder irritants, and urge suppression techniques.

- Assist the client in selecting, obtaining, and applying a containment device for urine loss as indicated.

- Provide the client with information about incontinence support groups such as the National Association for Continence and the Simon Foundation for Continence. A helpful website titled Total

Control (http://www.totalcontrolprogram.com/Pelvic+Health/
Bladder+Health) can be accessed to give support and information to
women with incontinence.
- Assess the functional and cognitive status of all clients with urge
  incontinence; use interventions to improve mobility.
- Refer client for occupational therapy for help in obtaining assistive
  devices and adapting the home for optimal toilet accessibility.
- Encourage the client to develop an action plan for self-care
  management of incontinence.
- Provide client with comprehensive written information about
  bladder care.
- Document all care and advice given in a factual and comprehensive
  manner.

Disorganized Infant behavior
NANDA-I Definition
Disintegrated physiological and neurobehavioral responses of infant to the
environment
Defining Characteristics
Attention-Interaction System
Impaired response to sensory stimuli (e.g., difficult to soothe, unable to
sustain alertness)
Motor System
Alteration in primitive reflexes; exaggerated startle response; finger splay-
ing; fisting; hands to face; hyperextension of extremities; impaired motor
tone; jitteriness; tremor; twitching; uncoordinated movement
Physiological
Abnormal skin color (e.g., pale, dusky, cyanosis); arrhythmia; bradycardia;
desaturation; feeding intolerance; tachycardia; time-out signals (e.g., gaze,
hiccough, sneeze, slack jaw, open mouth, tongue thrust)
Regulatory Problems
Inability to inhibit startle reflex; irritability
State-Organization System
Active-awake (e.g., fussy, worried gaze); diffuse alpha EEG activity with
eyes closed; irritable crying; quiet-awake (e.g., staring, gaze aversion); state
oscillation

• = Independent   ▲ = Collaborative

Related Factors

Caregiver

Cue misreading; environmental overstimulation; insufficient knowledge of behavioral cues

Environmental

Inadequate physical environment; insufficient containment within environment; insufficient sensory stimulation; sensory deprivation; sensory overstimulation

Individual

Illness; immature neurological functioning; low postconceptual age; prematurity

Postnatal

Feeding intolerance; impaired motor functioning; invasive procedure; malnutrition; oral impairment; pain

Prenatal

Congenital disorder; exposure to teratogen; genetic disorder

Client Outcomes

Client Will (Specify Time Frame)

Infant/Child

- Display physiological/autonomic stability: cardiopulmonary, digestive functioning
- Display signs of organized motor system (Wyngarden et al, 1999)
- Display signs of organized state system: ability to achieve and maintain a state, and transition smoothly between states (Wyngarden et al, 1999)
- Demonstrate progress toward effective self-regulation (Wyngarden et al, 1999)
- Demonstrate progress toward or ability to maintain calm attention
- Demonstrate progress or ability to engage in positive interactions
- Demonstrate ability to respond to sensory information (visual, auditory, tactile) in an adaptive way

Parent/Significant Other

- Recognize infant/child behaviors as complex communication system that express specific needs and wants (e.g., hunger, pain, stress, desire to engage or disengage)
- Educate parents/caregivers to recognize infant's avenues of neurobehavioral communication: autonomic/physiological, motor, state, attention/interaction
- Recognize how infants respond to environmental sensory input through stress/avoidance and approach/engagement behaviors

• = Independent   ▲ = Collaborative

- Recognize and support infant's self-regulatory, coping behaviors used to regain or maintain homeostasis
- Teach parents to "tune in" to their own interactive style and how that affects their infant's behavior
- Teach parents ways to adapt their interactive style in response to infant's style of communication
- Identify appropriate positioning and handling techniques that will enhance normal motor development (Wyngarden et al, 1999)
- Promote infant/child's attention capabilities that support visual and auditory development (Wyngarden et al, 1999)
- Engage in pleasurable parent-infant interactions that encourage bonding and attachment (Wyngarden et al, 1999)
- Structure and modify the environment in response to infant/child's behavior and personal needs (Wyngarden et al, 1999)
- Identify available community resources that provide early intervention services, emotional support, community health nursing, and parenting classes (Wyngarden et al, 1999)

Nursing Interventions

- Recognize the neurobehavior systems through which infants communicate organization and/or disorganization/stress (i.e., physiological/autonomic, motor, states, attention/interactional, self-regulatory).
- Recognize behavior used to communicate stress/avoidance and approach/engagement.
- Provide high-quality individualized developmental care for low-birth-weight preterm infants, which is shown to positively influence neurodevelopmental outcomes.
- Identify and manage pain using appropriate pain management techniques during invasive procedures (e.g., tube insertion, heel sticks, intravenous lines).
- Provide developmentally appropriate positioning to optimize musculoskeletal development and neurological development, and minimize complications; alternate positions over 24-hour period between prone, supine, and lateral side lying to support body alignment, flexion, midline orientation, and hand to mouth and to avoid head and neck hyperextension.
- Provide care that supports development of state organization: ability to achieve and maintain quiet sleep and quiet awake states and to transition smoothly between sleep and awake states.

• = Independent   ▲ = Collaborative

- Monitor level of noise in NICU environment; guidelines recommend 49 dB (1 ± 1.4).
- Recognize and expand infant's ability to focus attention on voices and faces.
- Provide infants with several opportunities for nonnutritive sucking.
- Provide parents opportunities to experience physical closeness through loving touch, massage, cuddling, skin-to-skin (kangaroo care), which enhances parent-infant attachment.
- Educate parents in ways to support infant's self-regulating behaviors.
- Encourage parents to be active collaborators in their infant's care.
- Provide infants with positive sensory experiences (i.e., visual, auditory, tactile, olfactory, vestibular, proprioceptive) to enhance development of sensory pathways.

Multicultural
- Identify cultural beliefs, norms, and values of family's perceptions of infant/child behavior.
- Recognize and support positive mother-infant interactive behaviors and be sensitive to cultural differences and ethnic backgrounds.

Client/Family Teaching and Discharge Planning
- ▲ Provide information or refer to community-based follow-up programs for preterm/at-risk infants and their families.
- Educate parents on safe "Back-to-Sleep" practice before NICU discharge.
- Encourage parents during infant awake periods to use a variety of development positions and handling that encourage body movement, hand-to-mouth, eye-hand coordination, and visual scanning; avoid overuse of infant carriers.
- Nurture parents so that they in turn can nurture their infant/child.

Home Care
- The preceding interventions may be adapted for home care use.
- Educate families in ways of preparing the home environment.
- Prepare families for realistic challenges occurring the first weeks and/or months of transition from NICU to home.
- Encourage families to teach extended family and support persons to recognize and respond appropriately to infant's behavioral cues; supportive help may be most appreciated doing physical tasks.

• = Independent   ▲ = Collaborative

• Provide families information about community resources, developmental follow-up services, parent-to-parent support programs, and the like; request parents ask primary health care provider to correct age for preterm birth until child is at minimal of 2 years of age, and to monitor developmental milestones to identify adverse neurological development.

Readiness for enhanced organized Infant behavior

NANDA-I Definition

A pattern of modulation of the physiological and behavioral systems of functioning (i.e., autonomic, motor, state organization, self-regulatory, and attentional-interactional systems) in an infant, which can be strengthened

Defining Characteristics

Parent expresses desire to enhance cue recognition; parent expresses desire to enhance recognition of infant's self-regulatory behaviors

Client Outcomes, Nursing Interventions, and Client/Family Teaching and Discharge Planning

Refer to care plans for Disorganized **Infant** behavior and Risk for disorganized **Infant** behavior.

Risk for disorganized Infant behavior

NANDA-I Definition

Vulnerable to alteration in integration and modulation of the physiological and behavioral systems of functioning (i.e., autonomic, motor, state organization, self-regulatory, and attentional-interactional systems), which may compromise health

Risk Factors

Impaired motor functioning; insufficient containment within environment; invasive procedure; oral impairment; pain; parent expresses desire to enhance environmental conditions; prematurity; procedure

Client Outcomes, Nursing Interventions, and Client/Family Teaching and Discharge Planning

Refer to Disorganized **Infant** behavior.

• = Independent   ▲ = Collaborative

Risk for Infection

NANDA-I Definition

Vulnerable to invasion and multiplication of pathogenic organisms, which may compromise health

Risk Factors

Chronic illness (e.g., diabetes mellitus); inadequate vaccination; insufficient knowledge to avoid exposure to pathogens; invasive procedure; malnutrition; obesity

Inadequate Primary Defenses

Alteration in peristalsis; alteration in pH of secretions; alteration in skin integrity; decrease in ciliary action; premature rupture of amniotic membrane; prolonged rupture of amniotic membrane; smoking; stasis of body fluids

Inadequate Secondary Defenses

Decrease in hemoglobin; immunosuppression; leukopenia; suppressed inflammatory response (e.g., IL-6, C-reactive protein [CRP]); inadequate vaccination

Increased Environmental Exposure to Pathogens

Exposure to disease outbreak

Client Outcomes

Client Will (Specify Time Frame)

- Remain free from symptoms of infection during contact with health care providers
- State symptoms of infection before initiating a health care–related procedure
- Demonstrate appropriate care of infection-prone sites within 48 hours of instruction
- Maintain white blood cell count and differential within normal limits within 48 hours of treatment initiation
- Demonstrate appropriate hygienic measures such as handwashing, oral care, and perineal care within 24 hours of instruction

Nursing Interventions

- Implement targeted surveillance for methicillin-resistant *Staphylococcus aureus* (MRSA) (screen clients at risk for MRSA on admission) and other multidrug-resistant organisms.
- Obtain a travel history from clients presenting to health care site (e.g., emergency department, clinic).

• = Independent ▲ = Collaborative

- Observe and report signs of infection such as redness, warmth, discharge, and increased body temperature.
- Assess temperature of neutropenic clients; report a single temperature of greater than 100.5° F.
- Oral, rectal, tympanic, temporal artery, or axillary thermometers may be used to assess temperature in adults and infants.
▲ Note and report laboratory values (e.g., white blood cell count and differential, serum protein, serum albumin, and cultures).
- Assess skin for color, moisture, texture, and turgor (elasticity). Keep accurate, ongoing documentation of changes.
- Carefully wash and pat dry skin, including skinfold areas. Use hydration and moisturization on all at-risk surfaces.

Refer to care plan for Risk for impaired **Skin** integrity.
▲ Monitor client's vitamin D level.

Refer to care plan for Readiness for enhanced **Nutrition** for additional interventions.

- Use strategies to prevent health care–acquired pneumonia (IHI, 2011); assess lung sounds and sputum color and characteristics; provide daily oral care with chlorhexidine; use sterile technique when suctioning; suction secretions above tracheal tube before suctioning; drain accumulated condensation in ventilator tubing into a fluid trap or other collection device before repositioning the client; assess patency and placement of nasogastric tubes; elevate the client's head to 30 degrees or higher to prevent gastric reflux of organisms in the lung (Peyrani, 2014).
- Encourage fluid intake.
- Use appropriate hand hygiene (i.e., handwashing or use of alcohol-based hand rubs).
- When using an alcohol-based hand rub, apply ample amount of product to palm of one hand and rub hands together, covering all surfaces of hands and fingers, until hands are dry. Note that the volume needed to reduce the number of bacteria on hands varies by product.
- Follow standard precautions and wear gloves during any contact with blood, mucous membranes, nonintact skin, or any body substance except sweat. Use goggles and gowns when appropriate. Standard precautions apply to all clients. You must assume all clients are carrying blood-borne pathogens (CDC, 2007).
- Implement respiratory hygiene/cough etiquette.

• = Independent   ▲ = Collaborative

- Follow transmission-based precautions for airborne-, droplet-, and contact-transmitted microorganisms:
  - **Airborne:** Isolate the client in a room with monitored negative air pressure, with the room door closed and the client remaining in the room. Always wear appropriate respiratory protection when you enter the room. Limit the movement and transport of the client from the room to essential purposes only. Have the client wear a surgical mask during transport.
  - **Droplet:** Keep the client in a private room, if possible. If not possible, maintain a spatial separation of 3 feet from other beds or visitors. The door may remain open. Wear a surgical mask when you must come within 3 feet of the client. Some hospitals may choose to implement a mask requirement for droplet precautions for anyone entering the room. Limit transport to essential purposes and have the client wear a mask, if possible.
  - **Contact:** Place the client in a private room, if possible, or with someone (cohorting) who has an active infection from the same microorganism. Wear clean, nonsterile gloves when entering the room. When providing care, change gloves after contact with any infective material such as wound drainage. Remove the gloves and clean your hands before leaving the room and take care not to touch any potentially infectious items or surfaces on the way out. Wear a gown if you anticipate your clothing may have substantial contact with the client or other potentially infectious items. Remove the gown before leaving the room. Limit transport of the client to essential purposes and take care that the client does not contact other environmental surfaces along the way. Dedicate the use of noncritical client care equipment to a single client. If use of common equipment is unavoidable, adequately clean and disinfect equipment before use with other clients.
- ▲ Use alternatives to indwelling catheters whenever possible (external catheters, incontinence pads, bladder control techniques).
- If a urinary catheter is necessary, follow catheter management practices: All indwelling catheters should be connected to a sterile, closed drainage system (i.e., not broken), except for good clinical reasons. Cleanse the perineum and meatus twice daily using soap and water.

• = Independent   ▲ = Collaborative

- Use evidence-based practices and educate personnel in care of peripheral catheters: use aseptic technique for insertion and care, label insertion sites and all tubing with date and time of insertion, inspect every 8 hours for signs of infection, record, and report.
- Use sterile technique wherever there is a loss of skin integrity.
- Ensure the client's appropriate hygienic care with handwashing, bathing, oral care, and hair, nail, and perineal care performed by either the nurse or the client.
- Recommend responsible use of antibiotics; use antibiotics sparingly.

Pediatric

NOTE: Many of the preceding interventions are appropriate for the pediatric client.

- Follow meticulous hand hygiene when working with children.
- Cluster nursing procedures to decrease number of contacts with infants, allowing time for appropriate hand hygiene.
- Avoid the prophylactic use of topical cream in premature infants.
- Encourage early enteral feeding with human milk.
- ▲ Monitor recurrent antibiotic use in children.
- Instruct parents on appropriate indicators for medical visits and the risks associated with overuse of antibiotics.

Geriatric

- ▲ Suspect pneumonia when the client has symptoms of lethargy or confusion. Assess response to treatment, especially antibiotic therapy.
- Most clients develop health care-associated pneumonia (HCAP) by either aspirating contaminated substances or inhaling airborne particles. Refer to care plan for Risk for **Aspiration.**
- ▲ Carefully screen older women with incontinence for urinary tract infections.
- Observe and report if the client has a low-grade fever or new onset of confusion.
- Recommend that the geriatric client receive an annual influenza immunization and one-time pneumococcal vaccine.
- Recognize that chronically ill geriatric clients have an increased susceptibility to *Clostridium difficile* infection; practice meticulous hand hygiene; monitor antibiotic response to antibiotics.

Home Care

- Adapt the above interventions for home care as needed.
- Assess and treat wounds in the home.
- Review standards for surveillance of infections in home care.

• = Independent   ▲ = Collaborative

- Maintain infection-prevention policies.
- Refer for nutritional evaluation; implement dietary changes to support recovery and maintain health.

Client/Family Teaching and Discharge Planning

- Teach the client risk factors contributing to surgical wound infection.
- Teach the client and family the importance of hand hygiene in preventing postoperative infections.
- ▲ Encourage high-risk persons, including health care workers, to get vaccinated (CDC, 2011).
- ▲ Influenza: Teach symptoms of influenza and importance of vaccination for influenza.

Risk for Injury

NANDA-I Definition

Vulnerable to physical damage due to environmental conditions interacting with the individual's adaptive and defensive resources, which may compromise health

Risk Factors

External

Alteration in cognitive functioning; alteration in psychomotor functioning; compromised nutritional source (e.g., vitamins, food types); exposure to pathogen; exposure to toxic chemical; immunization level within community; nosocomial agent; physical barrier (e.g., design, structure, arrangement of community, building, equipment); unsafe mode of transport

Internal

Abnormal blood profile; alteration in affective orientation; alteration in sensation (resulting from, e.g., spinal cord injury, diabetes mellitus); autoimmune dysfunction; biochemical dysfunction; effector dysfunction; extremes of age; immune dysfunction; impaired primary defense mechanisms (e.g., broken skin); malnutrition; sensory integration dysfunction; tissue hypoxia

Client Outcomes

Client Will (Specify Time Frame)

- Remain free of injuries
- Explain methods to prevent injuries
- Demonstrate behaviors that decrease the risk for injury

• = Independent   ▲ = Collaborative

Nursing Interventions

Prevent iatrogenic harm to the hospitalized client by following the National Patient Safety goals:

* Accuracy of Client Identification
  ○ Use at least two methods (e.g., client's name and medical record number or birth date) to identify the client upon initial entrance to a client's room and before administering medications, blood products, treatments, or procedures.
  ○ Before beginning any invasive or surgical procedure, have a final verification to confirm the correct client, the correct procedure, and the correct site for the procedure using active communication techniques.
  ○ Label containers used for blood and other specimens in the presence of the client.
* Effectiveness of Communication Among Care Staff
  ○ Verbal or telephone orders should be written and then read back for verification to the individual giving the order. Avoid verbal or telephone orders whenever possible.
  ○ Standardize use of abbreviations, acronyms, symbols, and dose designations that are used in the institution.
  ○ Ensure critical test results and values are recorded and reported in a timely manner.
  ○ Use a standardized approach of "handing off" communications, including opportunities to ask and answer questions.
  ○ Use only approved abbreviations.
  ○ Staff should always wear hospital nametags.
* Medication Safety
  ○ Standardize and limit the number of drug concentrations used by the institution (e.g., concentrations of medications such as morphine in client-controlled analgesia pumps).
  ○ Label all medications and medication containers (e.g., syringes, medication cups, or other solutions on or off the surgical field).
  ○ Identify all of the client's current medications upon admission to a health care facility, and ensure that all health care staff have access to the information.
  ○ Ensure that accurate medicine information is sent with the client throughout their care.
  ○ Reconcile all medication at admission and discharge, and provide list to the client.

- ○ Improve the effectiveness of alarm systems in the clinical area.
- ○ Standardize a list of medications that look alike or sound alike. This list needs to be updated yearly.
- ○ Identify and take extra care with clients who are on anticoagulants.
- Infection Control
  - ○ Reduce the risk of infections by following the Centers for Disease Control and Prevention (CDC, 2014) hand hygiene guidelines.
  - ○ Document clearly when clients obtain injuries or die of infectious disease.
  - ○ Use proven guidelines to prevent infections that are difficult to treat.
  - ○ Use proven guidelines to prevent infection of the blood from central lines.
  - ○ Use safe practices to treat the surgical site of the client.
  - ○ Use proven guidelines to prevent catheter-associated urinary tract infections.
- Fall Prevention
  - ○ Evaluate all clients for fall risk daily and take appropriate actions to prevent falls.
- Client Involvement in Care
  - ○ Educate the client and family on how to recognize and report concerns about safety issues.
- Identify Clients with Safety Risks
  - ○ Identify which clients are at risk for harming themselves.
- Identify Clients Who Are Susceptible to Changes in Health Status
  - ○ Educate staff on how to recognize changes in client condition, how to respond quickly, and how to alert specially trained staff to intervene if needed.
  - ○ Prevent errors in surgery by following established protocols. Update protocols yearly.
  - ○ Standardize steps to educate staff so documents for surgery are ready before surgery.
  - ○ Educate staff to mark the body part scheduled for surgery and engage the client in this process as well.
- See care plan for Risk for **Falls.**
- Avoid use of physical and chemical restraints if at all possible. Restraint-free is now the standard of care for hospitals and

long-term care facilities. Obtain a health care provider's order if restraints are necessary.
- Consider providing individualized music of the client's choice if a client is agitated.
- Review drug profile for potential side effects and interactions that may increase risk of injury.
- Provide a safe environment
  - ○ Use one fourth– to one half–length side rails only, and maintain bed in a low position. Ensure that wheels are locked on bed and commode. Keep dim light in room at night.
  - ○ Remove all possible hazards in environment such as razors, medications, room clutter, wet floors, and matches.
  - ○ Place a client who is at risk for injury in a room that is near the nurse's station.
- Assist clients to sit in a stable chair with armrests. Avoid use of wheelchairs and geri-chairs except for transportation.
- If the client has a new onset of confusion (delirium), refer to the care plan for Acute **Confusion.** If the client has chronic confusion, see the care plan for Chronic **Confusion.**
- Involve family in helping to provide a culture of safety.
- ▲ Refer the client for physical therapy for strengthening as needed.
- ▲ Use nonphysical forms of behavior management for the agitated psychotic client.

Pediatric
- Teach parents the need for close supervision of young children playing near water.
- If child has an underlying medical problem that puts them at risk for drowning, it is recommended that they be given showers, not tub baths. No unsupervised swimming is ever allowed.
- Assess the client's socioeconomic status because financial hardship may correlate with increased rates of injury.
- Never leave young children unsupervised around cooking or open flames.
- Teach parents and children the need to maintain safety for the exercising child, including wearing helmets when biking.
- Encourage parents to insist on safety precautions in all phases of participation sports involving children.
- Provide parents of children with traumatic brain injury with written instruction and emergency phone numbers. Ensure that instructions

• = Independent   ▲ = Collaborative

are understood before the child is discharged from a health care setting. Instruct parents to observe for the following symptoms: nausea, mild headache, dizziness, irritability, lethargy, poor concentration, loss of appetite, and insomnia.
• Teach both parents and children the need for gun safety; refer to hunting safety courses.
• Educate parents regarding proper car safety seat use.

Geriatric
• Encourage the client to wear glasses and hearing aids and to use walking aids, including nonslip footwear when ambulating.
• Assess for orthostatic hypotension when getting up, teach methods to decrease dizziness, such as rising slowly, remaining seated several minutes before standing, flexing feet upward several times while sitting, sitting down immediately if feeling dizzy, and trying to have someone present when standing.
• Discourage driving at night.

Multicultural
• Acknowledge racial/ethnic differences at the onset of care.
• Evaluate the influence of culture on the client's perceptions of risk for injury.
• Evaluate whether exposure to community violence is a contributor to a client's risk for injury.
• Use culturally relevant injury prevention programs when possible. Validate the client's feelings and concerns related to environmental risks.

Home Care and Client/Family Teaching and Discharge Planning
• See Risk for **Trauma** for additional interventions.

Risk for corneal Injury
NANDA-I Definition

Vulnerable to infection or inflammatory lesion in the corneal tissue that can affect superficial or deep layers, which may compromise health

Risk Factors

Blinking less than five times per minute; exposure of the eyeball; Glasgow Coma Scale score <7; intubation; mechanical ventilation; periorbital edema; pharmaceutical agent; prolonged hospitalization; tracheotomy; use of supplemental oxygen

• = Independent   ▲ = Collaborative

Client Outcomes

Client Will (Specify Time Frame)

- Demonstrate relaxed facial expressions
- Remain as independent as possible
- Remain free of physical harm resulting from vision injury risk
- Demonstrate improvement in visual acuity

Nursing Interventions

Emergency Department Visits or Primary Care Office Visit

▲ Perform a standard ophthalmic exam or examine eye with a slit lamp using fluorescein stain to optimize visualization of the abrasion injury if available.

- Attempt visual acuity measuring using the Snellen eye chart (corrected with glasses).
- Ensure immunization status is current, namely tetanus-diphtheria-pertussis status (every 10 years).
- Teach the client that fingernail induced corneal abrasions are one of the most common eye injuries and are at risk for complications (Lin et al, 2014).
- Provide analgesia as needed/prescribed.
- Injuries that penetrate the cornea are more serious. The outcome depends on the specific injury.

Hospitalization

- Assess for perioperative corneal abrasion risks, including advanced age, general anesthesia, greater blood loss, eye taping during surgery, prone and Trendelenburg positions, and supplemental oxygen use (Segal et al, 2014).

▲ Corneal abrasion is the most common ophthalmological complication that occurs during general anesthesia for nonocular surgery and can lead to sight-threatening microbial keratitis and permanent scarring.

- Assess for corneal abrasion and eye dryness, which are common problems in clients in the intensive care unit. Eye dryness is the main risk factor for the development of corneal abrasions.

Client/Family Teaching and Discharge Planning

▲ First aid principles should be reinforced in the event of an eye injury. Clients should not attempt to remove any object in the eye. Reserve this for the health care provider. A referral to an ophthalmologist may be required (Jacobs, 2014).

• = Independent   ▲ = Collaborative

- Teach clients to use caution when using household cleaners. Many household products contain strong acids, alkalis, or other chemicals. Drain and oven cleaners are particularly dangerous. They can lead to blindness if not used correctly (Vorvick, 2014).
- If chemical exposure has occurred, flush the eye immediately with clean water for 10 minutes. Seek prompt health care attention.
- Wear safety goggles at all times when using hand or power tools or chemicals, during high-impact sports, or in other situations when eye injury is more likely.
- Wear sunglasses that screen ultraviolet light when outdoors, even in winter.
- Pain is usually improved within 3 days. If pain becomes intolerable, an analgesic may be prescribed short term. Seek medical attention if pain is not resolving.
- Driving should be restricted for safety until client's visual acuity is evaluated.

Risk for urinary tract Injury
NANDA-I Definition

Vulnerable to damage of the urinary tract structures from use of catheters, which may compromise health

NOTE: This nursing diagnosis overlaps with other diagnoses such as Risk for **Trauma,** Impaired **Urinary** elimination, and Risk for **Infection.** Refer to care plans for these diagnoses if appropriate.

Risk Factors

Condition preventing ability to secure catheter (e.g., burn, trauma, amputation); long-term use of urinary catheter; multiple catheterizations; retention balloon inflated to ≥30 mL; use of large-caliber urinary catheter

Client Outcomes

Client Will (Specify Time Frame)

- Remain free of urinary tract injury
- State absence of pain with catheter care and during urination
- Experience unobstructed urination after removal of catheter

Nursing Interventions

- Monitor urinary elimination, including frequency, consistency, odor, volume, and color, as appropriate; teach client signs and symptoms of urinary tract infection.

• = Independent   ▲ = Collaborative

- Assess for proper placement of a urinary catheter. Urinary catheters are among the most widely used medical devices. Proper placement is necessary to prevent trauma to the urinary tract structure as well as infections (e.g., catheter-associated urinary tract infection [CAUTI] and urosepsis).
▲ To prevent injury, educate the client/family as to the reason for the indwelling urinary catheter to prevent harm (Scott et al, 2014).
- Assess clinical indication for urinary catheter daily.
- To avoid catheterizations, evaluate alternative strategies for managing urine output for the client.
- If an indwelling urinary catheter is determined to be clinically indicated in the care of a client, proper selection of the right catheter, technique during insertion, and evidence-based care management are needed to reduce infection and injury to the urinary tract structures.
  - ○ Selecting the smallest catheter size (e.g., smaller than 18 French) reduces irritation and inflammation of the urethra and reduces infection risk (Gray, 2010; Hooten et al, 2010).
  - ○ Insert the catheter using aseptic technique. Wash hands and use sterile technique when opening the catheterization kit and cleansing the urethral meatus and perineal area with an antiseptic solution. Insert the catheter using a no-touch technique (Gray, 2010; Lo et al, 2014).
  - ○ Provide routine hygiene care; once a urinary catheter is placed, optimal management includes care of the urethral meatus according to "routine hygiene" (e.g., daily cleansing of the meatal surface during bathing with soap and water and as needed, e.g., following a bowel movement) (Hooten et al, 2010; Watts et al, 2011). Cleansing with antiseptics, creams, lotions, or ointment has been found to irritate the meatus, possibly increasing the risk of infection (Lo et al, 2014; Watts et al, 2011).
  - ○ Secure the catheter after placement to reduce friction from movement (Hooten et al, 2010; Watts et al, 2011; Clarke et al, 2013).
  - ○ Maintain a closed catheter system to reduce the risk of infection (Hooten et al, 2010; Lo et al, 2014; Memorial Sloan Kettering, 2015).
  - ○ Maintaining the urine collection bag below the level of the bladder minimizes reflux into the catheter itself, preventing

• = Independent   ▲ = Collaborative

retrograde flow of urine and risk for infection (Hooten et al, 2010; Watts et al, 2011; Memorial Sloan Kettering, 2015; Clarke et al, 2013).

○ Establish workflow protocols to routinely empty the drainage bag frequently and before transport to reduce urine reflux and opportunities for infection.

○ Use an ultrasound bladder scanner to determine the estimated urine volume in the bladder and the need to insert or reinsert a urinary catheter (Saint et al, 2013).

Home Care and Client/Family Teaching and Discharge Planning

- Teach the client/family proper technique for inserting a urinary catheter. Instruct the client/family to never forcefully advance the catheter. Contact a health care provider if resistance is experienced (Herter et al, 2010; Watts et al, 2011).

- Develop a personalized plan of care to teach the client/family proper catheterization technique. Consider developing a routine bladder draining schedule to avoid bladder distention or other complications (Watts et al, 2011).

- Cleanse the catheter and surrounding area during a shower (avoid tub baths) using mild soap; dry catheter and skin. Ensure catheter and drainage bag are secured to thigh and lower leg (Memorial Sloan Kettering, 2015).

- Teach the client/family methods to keep the urinary tract healthy. Refer to Client/Family Teaching in the care plan for Readiness for enhanced **Urinary** elimination.

Insomnia

NANDA-I Definition

A disruption in amount and quality of sleep that impairs functioning

Defining Characteristics

Alteration in affect; alteration in concentration; alteration in mood; alteration in sleep pattern; compromised health status; decrease in quality of life; difficulty initiating sleep; difficulty maintaining sleep; dissatisfaction with sleep; early awakening; increase in absenteeism; increase in accidents; insufficient energy; nonrestorative sleep pattern (i.e., due to caregiver responsibilities, parenting practices, sleep partner); sleep disturbance producing next-day consequences

• = Independent   ▲ = Collaborative

Related Factors (r/t)

Alcohol consumption; anxiety, average daily physical activity is less than recommended for gender and age; depression; environmental barrier (e.g., ambient noise, daylight/darkness exposure, ambient temperature/humidity, unfamiliar setting); fear; frequent naps; grieving; hormonal change; inadequate sleep hygiene; pharmaceutical agent; physical discomfort; stressors

Client Outcomes

Client Will (Specify Time Frame)

- Verbalize plan to implement sleep-promoting routines
- Fall asleep with less difficulty a minimum of four nights out of seven
- Wake up less frequently during night a minimum of four nights out of seven
- Sleep a minimum of 6 hours most nights and more if needed to meet next stated outcome
- Awaken refreshed and not be fatigued during day most of the time

Nursing Interventions

- Obtain a sleep history including time needed to initiate sleep, duration of awakenings after the first sleep onset, total nighttime sleep amounts, and satisfaction with sleep amounts. Also explore bedtime routines, use of medications and stimulants, and use of complementary/alternative therapies for stress management (e.g., herbal agents) and relaxation before bedtime.
- From the history, assess the degree and chronic nature of insomnia.
- Avoid negative associations with ability to sleep.
- If feasible, have client arise from bed to participate in calming activities whenever anxious about failure to fall asleep.
- Avoid a focus on the clock and subsequent worry about sleep time lost to sleeplessness.
- Focus on positive aspects of life.
- ▲ Assist clients with chronic insomnia to limit use of sleeping agents and to select nights for sleeping pill use if complete discontinuance of sleeping pills is not feasible.
- ▲ For clients with chronic insomnia, refer to a health care provider trained in cognitive behavioral therapies.
- ▲ Assess pain medication use and, when feasible, recommend pain medications that promote rather than interfere with sleep (see Acute **Pain** and Chronic **Pain** care plans).

• = Independent   ▲ = Collaborative

▲ Assess level of anxiety. If chronic insomnia is accompanied by anxiety, use relaxation techniques. (See further nursing interventions for **Anxiety.**)

▲ Assess for signs of depression: depressed mood state, statements of hopelessness, poor appetite. Refer for counseling as appropriate.

▲ Assess for signs of sleep apnea and restless leg syndrome; if present, refer to an accredited sleep clinic for evaluation. If the client is waking frequently during the night, other primary sleep disorders may be the cause (Gooneratne et al, 2014; Matthews, 2011).

▲ Assess for signs of substance overuse/abuse including prescription, over-the-counter, and illicit drugs, as well as alcohol, caffeine, and theophylline use. Suggest lifestyle change and refer for addiction counseling as appropriate.

▲ Evaluate noise and interruptions during the delivery of care of clients.

• Supplement other interventions with teaching about sleep and sleep promotion. (See further nursing interventions for Readiness for enhanced **Sleep.**)

Geriatric

• Assessment of medications used for pain and other symptoms in older adults is important because pain medications may be interfering with the client's ability to initiate and maintain sleep (Matthews, 2011; Gooneratne et al, 2014).

• Clients with heart failure, pulmonary disease, and dementia have a higher risk of sleep apnea, which may be undiagnosed. Consult with a health care provider to evaluate the client for sleep apnea in the older adult (Gooneratne et al, 2014).

• Exercise enhances sleep. Older adults should be encouraged to participate in routine exercise to enhance quality of sleep (Melancon et al, 2014).

• Most interventions discussed previously may be used with geriatric clients. In addition, see the care plan for Readiness for enhanced **Sleep.**

Home Care

• Assessments and interventions discussed previously may be adapted for use in home care.

• In addition, see the interventions for Readiness for enhanced **Sleep.**

• = Independent   ▲ = Collaborative

Client/Family Teaching and Discharge Planning

- Teach family about normal sleep and promote adoption of behaviors that enhance it. See nursing interventions for Readiness for enhanced **Sleep.**
- Teach family about sleep deprivation and how to avoid it. See nursing interventions for **Sleep** deprivation.
- Advise family of importance of not disrupting sleep of others unnecessarily. See nursing interventions for Disturbed **Sleep** pattern.
- Advise family of importance of minimizing noise and light, including light from electronic devices in the sleep environment. See nursing interventions for Disturbed **Sleep** pattern.
- Help family differentiate insomnia from externally caused sleep disruption and resultant sleep deprivation. Family members may have direct control over interruptions in sleep and thus may help limit sleep deprivation directly.

Decreased Intracranial adaptive capacity

NANDA-I Definition

Intracranial fluid dynamic mechanisms that normally compensate for increases in intracranial volumes are compromised, resulting in repeated disproportionate increases in intracranial pressure (ICP) in response to a variety of noxious and non-noxious stimuli

Defining Characteristics

Baseline intracranial pressure (ICP) ≥10 mm Hg; disproportionate increases in intracranial pressure (ICP) following stimuli; elevated P2 ICP waveform; repeated increase in intracranial pressure (ICP) ≥10 mm Hg for ≥5 minutes following external stimuli; volume-pressure response test variation (volume:pressure ratio 2, pressure-volume index ≤10); wide-amplitude ICP waveform

Related Factors

Brain injury (e.g., cerebrovascular impairment, neurological illness, trauma, tumor); decreased cerebral perfusion ≥50-60 mm Hg; sustained increase in intracranial pressure (ICP) of 10 to 15 mm Hg; systemic hypotension with intracranial hypertension

• = Independent ▲ = Collaborative

Client Outcomes

Client Will (Specify Time Frame)

- Experience fewer than five episodes of disproportionate increases in intracranial pressure (DIICP) in 24 hours
- Have neurological status changes that are not triggered by episodes of DIICP
- Have cerebral perfusion pressure (CPP) remaining greater than 60 to 70 mm Hg in adults

Nursing Interventions

▲ To assess ICP and CPP effectively:
  ○ Monitor and display ICP and CPP in clients with severe traumatic brain injury (TBI) and spontaneous intracranial hemorrhage (ICH).
  ○ Maintain ICP less than 20 mm Hg and CPP greater than 60 mm Hg.
  ○ Monitor neurological status frequently (hourly in acute situations) determining both pupillary size and reaction to light and the Glasgow Coma Scale (GCS) score, noting changes in eye opening, motor response to painful stimuli, and awareness of self, time, and place.
  ○ Monitor brain tissue oxygen ($PbtO_2$).
▲ To prevent harmful increases in ICP:
  ○ Elevate head of bed 30 to 45 degrees with head in midline position.
  ○ Administer sedation per collaborative protocol.
  ○ Maintain glycemic control per collaborative protocol.
  ○ Maintain optimal oxygenation and ventilation, applying positive end-expiratory pressure (PEEP) as needed and avoiding hyperventilation.
  ○ Provide hyperbaric oxygen/normobaric hyperoxia if available during the acute phase of severe TBI.
▲ To prevent and treat harmful decreases in CPP:
  ○ See care plan for Risk for ineffective **Cerebral** tissue perfusion.
▲ To treat sustained intracranial hypertension (ICP greater than 20 mm Hg):
  ○ Remove or loosen rigid cervical collars.
  ○ Administer hypertonic saline (bolus or continuous infusion) per collaborative protocol.

• = Independent   ▲ = Collaborative

○ Drain cerebrospinal fluid (CSF) from an intraventricular catheter system per collaborative protocol.
○ Induce moderate hypothermia (32° C to 34° C) per collaborative protocol.

Neonatal Jaundice

NANDA-I Definition

The yellow-orange tint of the neonate's skin and mucous membranes that occurs after 24 hours of life as a result of unconjugated bilirubin in the circulation

Defining Characteristics

Abnormal blood profile; bruised skin; yellow mucous membranes; yellow sclera; yellow-orange skin color

Related Factors (r/t)

Age <7 days; deficient feeding pattern; delay in meconium passage; infant experiences difficulty making the transition to extrauterine life; weight loss >10%

Client Outcomes

Client (Infant) Will (Specify Time Frame)

- Establish effective feeding pattern (breast or bottle)
- Receive bilirubin assessment and screening within the first week of life to identify potentially harmful levels of serum bilirubin
- Receive appropriate therapy to enhance indirect bilirubin excretion
- Receive nursing assessments to determine risk for severity of jaundice
- Maintain hydration: moist buccal membranes, 4 to 6 wet diapers in 24-hour period, weight loss no greater than 10% of birth weight
- Evacuate stool within 48 hours of birth, and pass 3 or 4 stools per 24 hours by day 4 of life

Client (Parent[s]) Will (Specify Time Frame)

- Receive information on neonatal jaundice prior to discharge from birth hospital
- Verbalize understanding of physical signs of jaundice prior to discharge
- Verbalize signs requiring immediate health practitioner notification: sleepy infant who does not awaken easily for feedings, fewer than 4 to

• = Independent   ▲ = Collaborative

6 wet diapers in 24-hour period by day 4, fewer than 3 to 4 stools in 24 hours by day 4, breastfeeds fewer than 8 times per day
- Demonstrate ability to operate home phototherapy unit if prescribed

Nursing Interventions

- Evaluate maternal and delivery history for risk factors for neonatal jaundice (RhD, ABO, G6PD deficiency, direct Coombs).
- Perform neonatal gestational age assessment once the newborn has had an initial period of interaction with mother and father.
- Encourage breastfeeding within the first hour of the neonate's life.
- Encourage skin-to-skin mother-newborn contact shortly after delivery.
- Assess infant's skin color at birth and every 8 hours thereafter until birth hospital discharge for the appearance of jaundice.
- Encourage and assist mother with frequent breastfeeding (at least 8 to 12 times per day in the first week of life).
- Assist parents with bottle-feeding neonate.
- Avoid feeding supplements such as water, dextrose water, or any other milk substitutes in breastfeeding neonate.
- Assess neonate's stooling pattern in first 48 hours of life.
- ▲ Collect and evaluate laboratory blood specimens as prescribed or per unit protocol.
- ▲ Monitor transcutaneous bilirubin level in jaundiced neonate per unit protocol or at least once every 8 hours.
- Perform hour-specific total serum bilirubin risk assessment before newborn's birth center discharge and document the results.
- Monitor newborn for signs of inadequate breast milk or formula intake: dry oral mucous membranes, fewer than 4 to 6 wet diapers per 24 hours, no stool in 24 hours, body weight loss greater than 10%.
- Assess late preterm infant (born between 34 weeks and 36 6/7 weeks' gestation) for ability to breastfeed successfully and adequate intake of breast milk.
- Assist mother with breastfeeding and assess latch-on.
- Encourage alternate methods for providing expressed breast milk if maternal health status is compromised (use of expressed breast milk) and assist mother with collection of breast milk via use of breast pump or hand expression.

• = Independent   ▲ = Collaborative

- Encourage father's participation in newborn care by changing diapers, helping position newborn for breastfeeding, and holding newborn while mother rests.
- Weigh newborn daily.
- ▲ When phototherapy is ordered, place seminude infant (diaper only) under prescribed amount of phototherapy lights.
- Protect infant's eyes from phototherapy light source with eye shields. Remove eye shields periodically when infant is removed from light source for feeding and parent-infant interaction.
- Monitor infant's hydration status, fluid intake, skin status, and body temperature while undergoing phototherapy.
- ▲ Collect and evaluate laboratory blood specimens (total serum bilirubin) while infant is undergoing phototherapy.
- Encourage continuation of breastfeeding and brief infant care activities such as changing diapers while infant is being treated with phototherapy; phototherapy may be interrupted for breastfeeding.
- Provide emotional support for parents of infants undergoing phototherapy.

Multicultural
- Assess infants of Asian ethnicity for early rising bilirubin levels, especially when breastfeeding.
- Encourage early and exclusive breastfeeding among Chinese and other Asian newborns.
- Assess Chinese and other Asian newborns suspected of being jaundiced with a serum bilirubin level or transcutaneous monitor.

Client/Family Teaching and Discharge Planning
- Teach the breastfeeding mother and support persons about the appearance of jaundice.
- Teach parents regarding the signs of inadequate milk intake: fewer than 3 to 4 stools by day 4, fewer than 4 to 6 wet diapers in 24 hours, and dry oral mucous membranes; additional danger signs include a sleepy baby who does not awaken for breastfeeding or appears lethargic (decreased activity level from usual newborn pattern).
- ▲ Teach parents about the importance of medical follow-up in the first several days of life for the evaluation of jaundice.
- Teach parents about the use of phototherapy (hospital or home, as prescribed), the proper use of the phototherapy equipment, feedings, and assessment of hydration, body temperature, skin status, and urine and stool output.

• = Independent   ▲ = Collaborative

Quality and Safety in Nursing

- **Client safety:** Minimizes risk of harm to client
- Knowledge: Nurses continually assess newborns for risk factors associated with the development of jaundice
- Skills: Nurses use transcutaneous and serum bilirubin measurements to determine the newborn's bilirubin risk according to the hour-specific nomogram
- Attitudes: Nurses appreciate their role as one of promoting safety for the newborn at risk for developing jaundice
- Knowledge: Nurses implement client-focused strategies to promote serum bilirubin reduction; these include but are not limited to placing the newborn to mother's breast in first hours of life and encouraging frequent breastfeeding or no less than 10 to 12 feedings per 24 hours
- Skills: Nurses identify individual clinical risk factors in the neonate that place him/her at risk for jaundice
- Attitudes: Nurses value their role as a health care team member to promote the safe care of the newborn at discharge from the birth center and beyond
- Knowledge: Nurses understand use of phototherapy to reduce levels of indirect bilirubin
- Skills: Nurses use phototherapy lights appropriately
- Skills: Nurses assess infant for untoward effects of phototherapy
- Attitudes: Nurses appreciate the role of phototherapy as a treatment
- Attitudes: Nurses value their role in the promotion of safety with the use of phototherapy
- Quality and Safety Education for Nurses: http://www.qsen.org/ksas_graduate.php#safety and http://www.qsen.org/about_qsen.php

Risk for neonatal Jaundice
NANDA-I Definition

Vulnerable to the yellow-orange tint of the neonate's skin and mucous membranes that occur after 24 hours of life as a result of unconjugated bilirubin in the circulation, which may compromise health

Risk Factors

Abnormal weight loss >10%; age <7 days; delay in meconium passage; feeding pattern not well established; infant experiences difficulty making the transition to extrauterine life; prematurity (≤37 weeks)

• = Independent   ▲ = Collaborative

Client Outcomes

- Neonatal total serum bilirubin (TSB) will be monitored and there will be no undetected TSB values in the high-risk (95th percentile or greater) or high-intermediate risk (75th to 94th percentile) zones (as determined by the hour-specific nomogram)
- Newborn will receive appropriate therapies to enhance bilirubin excretion
- Newborn will remain free of undetected signs of acute bilirubin neurotoxicity
- Establish effective feeding pattern (breast or bottle)
- Receive bilirubin assessment and screening within the first week of life to detect increasing levels of serum bilirubin
- Receive nursing assessments to determine risk for severity of jaundice prior to discharge from birth hospital
- Maintain hydration: moist buccal membranes, 4 to 6 wet diapers in 24-hour period, weight loss no greater than 10% of birth weight
- Evacuate stool within 48 hours of birth, and pass 3 to 4 stools per 24 hours by day 4 of life

Nursing Interventions

- Identify clinical risk factors that place the infant at greater risk for development of neonatal jaundice: exclusive breastfeeding, isoimmune or hemolytic disease, preterm birth (38⅞ weeks' gestation or less), weight loss of 10% or more from birth weight, previous sibling with jaundice, East Asian ethnicity, and significant bruising or cephalhematoma.
- Weigh daily the late preterm infant, early term, and term newborn who is at high risk for inadequate caloric intake for the first week of life.

Multicultural

Refer to care plan for Neonatal **Jaundice** for additional interventions.

Client/Family Teaching and Discharge Planning

- ▲ Teach parents about the importance of medical follow-up in the first several days of life for the evaluation of jaundice, especially in the late preterm infant.
- Refer to care plan for Neonatal **Jaundice** for additional interventions.

Quality and Safety in Nursing

- Refer to care plan for Neonatal **Jaundice** for additional interventions.

• = Independent   ▲ = Collaborative

Deficient Knowledge

NANDA-I Definition

Absence or deficiency of cognitive information related to a specific topic

Defining Characteristics

Inaccurate follow through of instruction; inaccurate performance on a test; inappropriate behavior (e.g., hysterical, hostile, agitated, apathetic); insufficient knowledge

Related Factors (r/t)

Alteration in cognitive functioning; alteration in memory; insufficient information; insufficient interest in learning; insufficient knowledge of resources; misinformation presented by others

Client Outcomes

Client Will (Specify Time Frame)

- Explain disease state, recognize need for medications, and understand treatments
- Describe the rationale for therapy/treatment options
- Incorporate knowledge of health regimen into lifestyle
- State confidence in one's ability to manage health situation and remain in control of life
- Demonstrate how to perform health-related procedure(s) satisfactorily
- Identify resources that can be used for more information or support after discharge

Nursing Interventions

- Consider the health literacy and the readiness to learn for all clients and caregivers (e.g., mental acuity, ability to see or hear, existing pain, emotional readiness, motivation, and previous knowledge).
- Focus on the nature of spoken and written communication when teaching clients and caregivers, especially those who may have health literacy needs.
- Consider the context, timing, and order of how information is presented.
- Use client-centered approaches that engage clients and caregivers as active vs. passive learners.
- Reinforce learning through frequent repetition and follow-up sessions.
- Use technological and multimedia methods of disbursing information as appropriate.
- Help the client and caregivers locate appropriate post-discharge groups and resources.

• = Independent   ▲ = Collaborative

- Encourage clients and caregivers to maintain and/or expand supportive social networks as self-care learning resources when appropriate.

Pediatric

- Use family-centered approaches when teaching children and adolescents.
- Guide children and adolescents to credible information about their condition.
- Use teaching strategies to enhance learning that are uniquely tailored for the information needs of children and/or adolescents.

Geriatric

- Educate all older clients on safety issues, including fall prevention and medication management.
- Consider using teaching methods and materials appropriate for older adults, especially those with cognitive challenges.
- Assess readiness of older adults for use of technological resources.

Multicultural

- Use educational interventions that are culturally tailored to the health literacy needs of the client.
- Assess for cultural/ethnic self-care practices.
- Consider the potential influence of medical interpreters in information sharing and decision-making and of the possible difficulties for clients when using medical interpreters.
- Consider involving bilingual members of a community who are considered outside the traditional health care system who may assist in the teaching of community health issues.

Home Care

- All of the previously mentioned interventions are applicable to the home setting.
- Use telehealth and technology-enhanced practices as appropriate.

Readiness for enhanced Knowledge

NANDA-I Definition

A pattern of cognitive information related to a specific topic or its acquisition, which can be strengthened

Defining Characteristics

Expresses desire to enhance learning

• = Independent ▲ = Collaborative

Client Outcomes
Client Will (Specify Time Frame)
- Meet personal health-related goals
- Explain how to incorporate new health regimen into lifestyle
- List sources to obtain information

Nursing Interventions
- Assume a facilitator role vs. authority role when engaging clients seeking health-related knowledge.
- Consider "health coaching" and motivational interviewing techniques when focusing on health-related goals, priorities, and preferences.
- Seek teachable moments for those with chronic conditions to enhance their knowledge of health promotion.
- ▲ Refer clients to lifestyle and health promotion resources delivered in the workplace or community sites outside traditional health care environments.
- Refer clients to interactive and Web-based technological resources as appropriate.
- Refer to Deficient **Knowledge** care plan.

Pediatric
- Consider the use of mobile text messaging as a resource for delivery of health promotion information.
- Incorporate health promotion education that reflects the unique cultural interests and values of diverse groups.
- Involve children and especially adolescents in designing health promotion programs and teaching methods.
- Consider settings outside traditional health care centers and interdisciplinary approaches for engaging children and adolescents in preventive health care.
- Provide a developmentally appropriate environment when addressing health education needs of adolescents.
- Refer to Deficient **Knowledge** care plan.

Geriatric and Multicultural
- Discuss healthy lifestyle changes that promote safety, health promotion, and health maintenance for older clients.
- Consider involving bilingual members of a community who are considered outside the traditional health care system who may assist in the teaching of community health issues.
- Refer to Deficient **Knowledge** care plan.

• = Independent ▲ = Collaborative

Latex Allergy response

NANDA-I Definition

A hypersensitive reaction to natural latex rubber products

Defining Characteristics

Life-Threatening Reactions Occurring Less Than 1 Hour After Exposure to Latex

Protein

Bronchospasm; cardiac arrest; contact urticaria progressing to generalized symptoms; dyspnea; edema of the lips; edema of the throat; edema of the tongue; edema of the uvula; hypotension; respiratory arrest; syncope; tightness in chest; wheezing

Orofacial Characteristics

Edema of eyelids; edema of sclera; erythema of the eyes; facial erythema; facial itching; itching of the eyes; oral itching; nasal congestion; nasal erythema; nasal itching; rhinorrhea; tearing of the eyes

Gastrointestinal/Characteristics

Abdominal pain; nausea

Generalized Characteristics

Flushing; generalized discomfort; generalized edema; increasing complaint of total body warmth; restlessness

Type IV Reactions Occurring More Than 1 Hour After Exposure to Latex Protein

Discomfort reaction to additives such as thiuram and carbamates; eczema; irritation; redness

Related Factors (r/t)

Hypersensitivity to natural latex rubber protein

Client Outcomes

Client Will (Specify Time Frame)

- Identify presence of natural rubber latex (NRL) allergy
- List history of risk factors
- Identify type of reaction
- State reasons not to use or to have anyone use latex products
- Experience a latex-safe environment for all health care procedures
- Avoid areas where there is powder from NRL gloves
- State the importance of wearing a medical alert bracelet and wear one
- State the importance of carrying an emergency kit with a supply of nonlatex gloves, antihistamines, and an autoinjectable epinephrine syringe (EpiPen), and carry one

• = Independent   ▲ = Collaborative

Nursing Interventions

- Identify clients at risk: those persons who are most likely to exhibit sensitivity to NRL that may result in varying degrees of reactivity. Consider the following client groups:
  - Persons with neural tube defects including spina bifida, myelomeningocele/meningocele.
  - Children with spinal cord injuries.
  - Clients with history of multiple surgeries or other latex-exposing procedures.
  - Children who have experienced three or more surgeries, particularly as a neonate, and adults who have undergone multiple surgeries.
  - Atopic individuals (persons with a tendency to have multiple allergic conditions) including allergies to food products. Particular allergies to fruits and vegetables including bananas, avocado, celery, fig, chestnut, papaya, potato, tomato, melon, and passion fruit are significant.
  - Persons who possess a known or suspected NRL allergy by having exhibited an allergic or anaphylactic reaction, positive skin testing, or positive IgE antibodies against latex.
  - Persons who have had an ongoing occupational exposure to NRL, including health care workers, rubber industry workers, bakers, laboratory personnel, food handlers, hairdressers, janitors, policemen, and firefighters.
  - Latex sensitization is also prevalent in older adults but they are often overlooked as a high-risk population.
- Take a thorough history of the client at risk.
- Have management protocols in place for treating anaphylaxis.
- Question the client about associated symptoms of itching, swelling, and redness after contact with rubber products such as rubber gloves, balloons, and barrier contraceptives, or swelling of the tongue and lips after dental examinations.
- Consider the use of a provocation test (cutaneous, sublingual, mucous, conjunctival) for latex allergy diagnosis confirmation.
- Consider a blood test to measure serum IgE levels.
- All latex-sensitive clients are treated as if they have NRL allergy.
- Clients with spina bifida and others with a positive history of NRL sensitivity or NRL allergy should have all medical/surgical/dental procedures performed in a latex-controlled environment.

L

• = Independent   ▲ = Collaborative

- In select high-risk atopic individuals, a specific immunotherapy regimen should be discussed with their health care provider.
▲ The most effective approach to preventing NRL anaphylaxis is complete latex avoidance.
▲ Materials and items that contain NRL must be identified and latex-free alternatives must be found.
▲ In health care settings, general use of latex gloves having negligible allergen content, powder-free latex gloves, and non-latex gloves and medical articles should be considered to minimize exposure to latex allergen.
▲ If latex gloves are chosen for protection from blood or body fluids, a reduced-protein, powder-free glove should be selected.

Home Care

- Assess the home environment for presence of NRL products (e.g., balloons, condoms, gloves, and products of related allergies, such as bananas, avocados, and poinsettia plants).
- At onset of care, assess client history and current status of NRL allergy response.
▲ Seek medical care as necessary.
- Do not use NRL products in caregiving.
- Assist the client in identifying and obtaining alternatives to NRL products.

Client/Family Teaching and Discharge Planning

- Provide written information about NRL allergy and sensitivity.
▲ Instruct the client to inform health care professionals if he or she has an NRL allergy, particularly if the client is scheduled for surgery.
- Teach the client what products contain NRL and to avoid direct contact with all latex products and foods that trigger allergic reactions.
- Teach the client to avoid areas where powdered latex gloves are used, as well as where latex balloons are inflated or deflated.
- Instruct the client with NRL allergy to wear a medical identification bracelet and/or carry a medical identification card.
- Instruct the client to carry an emergency kit with a supply of nonlatex gloves, antihistamines, and an autoinjectable epinephrine syringe (EpiPen).

Risk for Latex Allergy response
NANDA-I Definition
Risk of hypersensitivity to natural latex rubber products
Risk Factors
Allergies to avocados; allergies to bananas; allergies to chestnuts; allergies to kiwis; allergies to poinsettia plants; allergies to tropical fruits; history of allergies; history of asthma; history of reaction to latex; multiple surgical procedures, especially from infancy; professions with daily exposure to latex

Client Outcomes
Client Will (Specify Time Frame)
- State risk factors for natural rubber latex (NRL) allergy
- Request latex-free environment
- Demonstrate knowledge of plan to treat NRL allergic reaction

Nursing Interventions
- Clients at high risk need to be identified, such as those with frequent bladder catheterizations, occupational exposure to latex, past history of atopy (hay fever, asthma, dermatitis, or food allergy to fruits such as bananas, avocados, papaya, chestnut, or kiwi); those with a history of anaphylaxis of uncertain etiology, especially if associated with surgery; health care workers; and women exposed to barrier contraceptives and routine examinations during gynecological and obstetrical procedures.
- Clients with spina bifida are a high-risk group for NRL allergy and should remain latex free from the first day of life.
- Children who require regular medical treatments at home (e.g., catheterization, home ventilation) should be assessed for NRL allergy.
- Assess for NRL allergy in clients who are exposed to "hidden" latex.
- See care plan for **Latex Allergy** response.

Home Care
▲ Ensure that the client has a medical plan if a response develops. Prompt treatment decreases potential severity of response.
- See care plan for **Latex Allergy** response. Note client history and environmental assessment.

Client/Family Teaching and Discharge Planning
▲ A client who has had symptoms of NRL allergy or who suspects he or she is allergic to latex needs to give this information to health care providers.

• = Independent   ▲ = Collaborative

▲ Provide written information about latex allergy and sensitivity.
• Health care workers should avoid the use of latex gloves and seek alternatives such as gloves made from nitrile.
• Health care institutions should develop prevention programs for the use of latex-free gloves and the absence of powdered gloves; they should also establish latex-safe areas in their facilities and emergency management plans for anaphylaxis episodes.
• Institute measures that reduce or completely avoid any latex exposure to clients.

Risk for impaired Liver function

NANDA-I Definition

Vulnerable to a decrease in liver function, which may compromise health

Risk Factors

HIV co-infection; pharmaceutical agent; substance abuse; viral infection

Client Outcomes

Client Will (Specify Time Frame)

• State the upper limit of the amount of acetaminophen safely taken per day
• Verbalize understanding that over-the-counter (OTC) medications may contain acetaminophen (e.g., OTC cold medicines)
• Have normal liver enzymes, serum and urinary bilirubin levels, white blood cell count, and red blood cell count
• Be free of unexplained weight loss, jaundice, pruritus, bruising, petechiae, gastrointestinal bleeding, and hemorrhage
• Be free of abdominal tenderness/pain, increased abdominal girth, and have normal-colored stool and urine
• Be able to eat frequent small meals per day without nausea and/or vomiting
• If alcohol abuse is factor, state relationship between abuse and worsening gastrointestinal and liver disease

Nursing Interventions

▲ Watch for signs of liver dysfunction including fatigue, nausea, jaundice of the eyes or skin, pruritus, gastrointestinal bleeding, coagulopathy, infections, increasing abdominal girth, fluid overload, shortness of breath, mental status changes, light-colored stools, dark urine, and increased serum and urinary bilirubin levels.

▲ Evaluate liver function tests. Standard liver panels include the serum enzymes aspartate transaminase (AST), alanine transaminase (ALT), alkaline phosphatase, and γ-glutamyltransferase; total, direct, and indirect serum bilirubin; and serum albumin.

▲ Discuss with the client/family preparations for other diagnostic studies, such as ultrasound, computed tomography, and magnetic resonance imaging exams (Beaumont & Leadbeater, 2011).

▲ Evaluate coagulation studies such as international normalized ratio, prothrombin time, and partial thromboplastin time, especially when there is bleeding of the mouth or gums.

• Monitor for signs of hemorrhage, especially in the upper gastrointestinal tract, as it is the most frequent site.

• Obtain a list of all medications, including OTC nonsteroidal antiinflammatory drugs, acetaminophen, and herbal remedies. Review risk of drug-induced liver disease. The list includes some antibiotics, anticonvulsants, antidepressants, antiinflammatory drugs, antiplatelets, antihypertensives, calcium channel blockers, cyclosporine, lipid-lowering drugs, chemotherapy drugs, oral hypoglycemics, and tranquilizers, among others (Dienstag, 2012). If client is taking either OTC medications or herbals, discuss signs and symptoms of toxic hepatitis.

▲ In clients receiving drugs associated with liver injury, review risk factors to prevent potentially severe drug reactions.

▲ Determine the total amount of acetaminophen the client is taking per day. The amount of acetaminophen ingested should not exceed 3.25 g per day, or even lower in the client with chronic alcohol intake (Dienstag, 2012).

▲ Evaluate the serum acetaminophen-protein adducts in the client with possible liver failure from excessive intake of acetaminophen.

▲ If the client is on statin medications, ensure that liver enzyme testing is done at intervals. Liver enzymes can become elevated from taking statin medications; it is uncommon, but possible for statins to cause actual liver damage (Zamor & Russo, 2011).

▲ If the client is an alcoholic, refer to a cessation program. It is essential the client stop drinking as soon as possible to allow the liver to heal. Alcoholism is associated with malnutrition, which is harmful to the liver (O'Shea et al, 2010). Alcoholism is also associated with formation of proteins called cytokines, which cause

• = Independent   ▲ = Collaborative

inflammation and resultant damage to the liver (Dienstag, 2012). See care plans for Ineffective **Denial** and Dysfunctional **Family** processes.

▲ Provide frequent smaller meals for easier digestion. Provide diet with optimal carbohydrates, proteins, and fats. Consult with a registered dietitian to discuss best nutritional support.

▲ Recognize that severe malnutrition may result in acute liver failure, which is reversible with improved nutrition.

▲ Review medical history with the client, recognizing that obesity and type 2 diabetes, along with hypertriglyceridemia and polycystic ovarian syndrome, are major risk factors in the development of liver disease, specifically nonalcoholic fatty liver disease.

• Encourage vaccinations for hepatitis A and B for all ages.

• Measure abdominal girth if individual presents with abdominal distention and pain.

• Assess for tenderness and/or pain level in the right upper quadrant.

• Use standard precautions for handling of blood and body fluids. Review sterile techniques when giving intravenous solution and/or medications.

▲ Observe for signs and symptoms of mental status changes such as confusion from encephalopathy. Assess ammonia level if mental changes occur (Dienstag, 2012).

Pediatric/Parents

▲ Prescreen pregnant women for hepatitis B surface antigens. If found, recommend nursing case management during pregnancy.

▲ Recommend implementation of postexposure prophylaxis, including the hepatitis B virus vaccine for an infant born to a hepatitis B surface antigen–positive woman (CDC, 2015b).

• Encourage vaccinations for hepatitis A and B for all ages.

▲ Recognize that children can develop fatty liver disease, which can result in liver failure. Most children are asymptomatic, but others complain of malaise, fatigue, or vague recurrent abdominal pain (Marzuillo et al, 2014).

▲ During a well-baby visit, assess for signs of potential liver problems. Observe for prolonged jaundice, pale stools, and urine that is anything other than colorless. Consult with health care provider to order a split bilirubin as needed (CDC, 2015b).

• = Independent   ▲ = Collaborative

Home Care

- Encourage rest, optimal nutrition (high carbohydrates, sufficient protein, essential vitamins and minerals) during initial inflammatory processes of the liver.

Client/Family Teaching and Discharge Planning

- Teach the client and family to examine all medications the client is taking, looking for acetaminophen as an ingredient, and reinforce the 3.25-g upper limit of intake of acetaminophen to protect liver function (Dienstag, 2012).
- For the caregiver or client with hepatitis A, B, or C, teach the need for careful handwashing, use of gloves, and other precautions to prevent spread of any of these diseases.
- Teach avoidance of high-risk behaviors that cause hepatitis and ways to avoid those behaviors.
- Educate clients and their caregivers about treatment options and interventions for hepatitis. Recommend other informational support: risk factors, side effects of the different treatment options, and dietary advice.
- Recommend psychological support if possible during education sessions.
- For those clients with mental health problems, collaborate with outreach programs to teach signs/symptoms of hepatitis, risk factors, and factors that increase transmission.

Risk for Loneliness

NANDA-I Definition

Vulnerable to experiencing discomfort associated with a desire or need for more contact with others, which may compromise health

Risk Factors

Affectional deprivation; emotional deprivation; physical isolation; social isolation

Client Outcomes

Client Will (Specify Time Frame)

- Maintain one or more meaningful relationships (growth-enhancing versus codependent or abusive in nature)
- Sustain relationships that allow self-disclosure and demonstrate a balance between emotional dependence and independence

• = Independent ▲ = Collaborative

- Participate in personally meaningful activities and interactions that are ongoing, positive, and relevant socially
- Demonstrate positive use of time alone when socialization is not possible

Nursing Interventions

- Assess the client's perception of loneliness. (Is the person alone by choice, or are there other factors that contribute to the feelings of loneliness? Is the client in one of the at-risk populations for loneliness?)
- Refer to care plan for **Social** isolation.
- Use active listening skills. Establish a therapeutic relationship and spend quality time with the client.
- Assess how unmet needs challenge the client. NOTE: See care plan for Disturbed **Body Image** if loneliness is associated with chronic illness and/or afflictions (e.g., multiple sclerosis, skin disturbance, mental illness).
- ▲ Assess the bereaved client for risk of suicide and make appropriate referrals as necessary. Refer to care plan for Risk for **Suicide.**
- Assess the client who is alone for substance abuse and make appropriate referrals.
- Evaluate the client's desire for social interaction.
- Assess the client for feelings of loneliness.
- Explore ways to increase the client's support systems.
- Show respect for the client's personal attributes.

Adolescents

- Assess the client's social support system.
- Evaluate the family stability of adolescent clients.
- Evaluate peer relationships.
- Encourage social support for clients with disabilities.
- Encourage relationships with peers and involvement with groups and organizations.

Geriatric

- Evaluate the client for any health deviations that may limit or decrease his/her ability to interact with others.
- Assess family caregivers of older persons with chronic conditions for depression related to loneliness.
- Identify support systems for older adults.
- When relocation is necessary for older adults, evaluate relocation stress as a contributing factor to loneliness.

• = Independent   ▲ = Collaborative

- Identify risk factors for loneliness in older persons.
- Encourage support for the client when the decision to stop driving must be made.
- Provide activities that are pleasurable to the client. Refer to the care plan for **Social** isolation for additional interventions.

Multicultural
- Refer to the care plan for **Social** isolation.

Home Care
▲ The preceding interventions may be adapted for home care use.
▲ Assess for depression with the lonely older client and make appropriate referrals.
- If the client has unexplained somatic complaints, evaluate these complaints to ensure that physical needs are being met, and assess for a possible relationship between somatic complaints and loneliness.
- Evaluate alternatives to being alone.
- Refer to the care plan for **Social** isolation.

Client/Family Teaching and Discharge Planning
- Identify the type of loneliness that the client is experiencing: emotional and/or social.
- Encourage family members' involvement, if possible, in helping alleviate client's loneliness.
- Include the family, if possible, in all client-teaching activities, and give them accurate information.
- Provide appropriate education for clients and their support persons about disease transmission and treatment if applicable.
- Refer to the care plan for **Social** isolation for additional interventions.

M

Risk for disturbed Maternal–Fetal dyad

NANDA-I Definition

Vulnerable to disruption of the symbiotic maternal–fetal dyad as a result of comorbid or pregnancy-related conditions, which may compromise health

Risk Factors

Alteration in glucose metabolism (e.g., diabetes mellitus, steroid use); compromised fetal oxygen transport (due to anemia, asthma, cardiac

• = Independent   ▲ = Collaborative

disease, hypertension, seizures, premature labor, hemorrhage); inadequate prenatal care; pregnancy complication (e.g., premature rupture of membranes, placenta previa/abruption, multiple gestations); presence of abuse (e.g., physical, psychological, sexual); substance abuse; treatment regimen

Client Outcomes

Client Will (Specify Time Frame)

- Cope with discomforts of high-risk pregnancy until delivery of baby
- Adhere to prescribed regimens to maintain homeostasis during pregnancy

Nursing Interventions

- Standardize internal and external transport forms using SBAR format (situation, background, assessment, recommendation) to provide safe and efficient transport of a high-risk pregnant client.
- Arrange for psychotherapeutic support when woman expresses intense fear related to high-risk pregnancy and fetal outcomes. Encourage verbalization of feelings, beliefs, and concerns about fetal well-being, maternal health, and family functioning.
- Screen all antepartum clients for depression using a tool that evaluates the biopsychosocial-spiritual dimensions in a culturally sensitive way.
- Offer flexible visiting hours, private space for families, and nursing support for management of family stressors; provide distractors such as music, TV, and laptops with Internet access when a woman is hospitalized with a high-risk pregnancy.
- Focus on the abilities of a woman with disabilities by encouraging her to identify her support system, resources, and needs for modification of her environment.
- Recognize patterns of physical abuse in all pregnant and postpartum women, regardless of age, race, and socioeconomic status.
- Perform accurate blood pressure readings at each client's clinic encounter.
- Provide educational materials and support for personal autonomy about genetic counseling and testing options before pregnancy, that is, preimplantation genetic testing, or during pregnancy, that is, fetal nuchal translucency ultrasound, quadruple screen, cystic fibrosis.
- Identify adherence barriers and assist with meal selections to maintain optimal nutrition and safe pregnancy weight gain (25 to 35 pounds; 15 to 25 pounds if overweight). Identify cultural beliefs and

• = Independent   ▲ = Collaborative

nutritional patterns. A prenatal vitamin with 400 mcg of folate should also be strongly recommended.
• Teach pregnant women diagnosed with gestational diabetes about management and treatment.
• Use the five A's (tobacco cessation interventions) to treat tobacco use and dependence in pregnant women.
• When questioning at-risk clients regarding recreational drug use, ask if they have used substances such as marijuana or cocaine within the last month, instead of questioning whether they have used within the last few days.
• Refer clients who self-report drug abuse or have positive toxicology screens to a comprehensive addiction program designed for the pregnant woman. Children born to addicted mothers often have poor neonatal outcomes.
• Encourage pregnant women to use electronic resources, such as Text4Baby or whattoexpect.com, to track pregnancy progress and provide education and motivation to make healthy lifestyle choices (abstinence from poor nutrition, smoking, alcohol).

M

Impaired Memory

NANDA-I Definition

Inability to remember or recall bits of information or behavioral skills

Defining Characteristics

Forgetfulness; forgets to perform a behavior at scheduled time; inability to learn new skill; inability to perform a previously learned skill; inability to recall events; inability to recall factual information; inability to recall if a behavior was performed; inability to retain new information

Related Factors (r/t)

Alterations in fluid volume; anemia; decrease in cardiac output; distractions in the environment; electrolyte imbalance; hypoxia; neurological impairment (e.g., positive EEG, head trauma, seizure disorders)

Client Outcomes

Client Will (Specify Time Frame)

• Demonstrate use of techniques to help with memory loss
• State he or she has improved memory for everyday concerns

• = Independent   ▲ = Collaborative

Nursing Interventions

- Assess overall cognitive function and memory. The emphasis of the assessment is everyday memory, the day-to-day operations of memory in real-world ordinary situations. A screening instrument such as the Mini-Mental State Examination (MMSE) is useful as a first level of evaluation.
- Determine whether onset of memory loss is gradual or sudden. If memory loss is sudden, refer the client to a health care provider or neuropsychologist for evaluation.
- Determine amount and pattern of alcohol intake.
- ▲ Note the client's current medications and intake of any mind-altering substances, such as benzodiazepines, ecstasy, marijuana, cocaine, or glucocorticoids.
- ▲ Note the client's current level of anxiety and stress. Ask if there has been a recent traumatic event (Luijten et al, 2014).
- Encourage the client to develop an aerobic exercise program.
- Determine the client's sleep patterns. If sleep quantity and quality is insufficient, refer to care plan for Disturbed **Sleep** pattern.
- ▲ Determine the client's blood sugar levels. If they are elevated, refer to health care provider for treatment and encourage healthy diet and exercise.
- ▲ If signs of depression such as weight loss, insomnia, or sad affect are evident, refer the client for psychotherapy.
- ▲ Question the client about cholesterol level. If it is high, refer to health care provider or dietitian for help in lowering. Encourage the client to eat a healthy diet, avoiding saturated fats and trans-fat acids.
- Suggest clients use cues, including alarm watches, electronic organizers, calendars, lists, or pocket computers, to trigger certain actions at designated times.
- Encourage the client to participate in a multicomponent cognitive rehabilitation program that recommends stress and relaxation training, physical activity, and external memory devices, such as a calendar for appointments and reminder lists.
- Help the client set up a medication box that reminds him/her to take medication at prescribed times; assist the client with refilling the box at intervals if necessary.
- If safety is an issue with certain activities (e.g., the client forgets to turn off stove after use or forgets emergency telephone numbers),

• = Independent   ▲ = Collaborative

suggest alternatives such as using a microwave or a whistling teakettle for heating water and programming emergency numbers in the telephone so that they are readily available.

▲ Refer the client to a memory clinic (if available), a neuropsychologist, or an occupational therapist.

• For clients with memory impairments associated with dementia, see care plan for Chronic **Confusion.**

Geriatric

• Assess for signs of depression.

• Perform a nutritional assessment. If nutritional status is marginal, confer with a dietitian and primary health care practitioner to evaluate whether the client needs supplementation with foods or vitamins. Teach the client the need to eat a healthy diet with adequate intake of whole grains, fruits, and vegetables to decrease cerebrovascular infarcts.

• Evaluate all medications that the client is taking to determine whether they are causing the memory loss. Evaluate all herbal and/or nutraceutical products that the individual might be using to improve memory function, particularly Ginkgo biloba (Diamond & Bailey, 2013).

• Recommend that older clients maintain a positive attitude and active involvement with the world around them and that they maintain good nutrition.

• Encourage older adults to believe in themselves and to work to improve their memory. Negative attitudes and beliefs may decrease motivation and impair everyday memory function.

• Refer the client to a memory improvement class that focuses on helping older adults learn memory strategies.

Multicultural

• Assess for the influence of cultural beliefs, norms, and values on the family or caregiver's understanding of impaired memory.

• When assessing memory in Mexican Americans, the MMSE has been used with success.

• Inform the client's family or caregiver of meaning of and reasons for common behaviors observed in the client with impaired memory.

• Attempt to validate family members' feelings regarding the impact of the client's behavior on family lifestyle.

M

• = Independent ▲ = Collaborative

Home Care

- The above interventions may be adapted for home care use.
- Assess the client's need for outside assistance with recall of treatment, medications, and willingness/ability of family to provide needed support.
- Identify a checking-in support system (e.g., Lifeline or significant others). Checking in ensures the client's safety.
- Keep furniture placement and household patterns consistent. Change increases risk of impaired memory and decreased functioning.

Client/Family Teaching and Discharge Planning

- When teaching the client, determine what the client knows about memory techniques and then build on that knowledge.
- When teaching a skill to the client, set up a series of practice attempts that will enhance motivation. Begin with simple tasks so the client can be positively reinforced and progress to more difficult concepts.
- Teach clients to use memory techniques such as concentrating and attending, repeating information, making mental associations, and placing items in strategic places so that they will not be forgotten.

Impaired bed Mobility

NANDA-I Definition

Limitation of independent movement from one bed position to another

Defining Characteristics

Impaired ability to move between long sitting and supine positions; impaired ability to move between prone and supine positions; impaired ability to move between sitting and supine positions; impaired ability to reposition self in bed; impaired ability to turn from side to side

Related Factors

Alteration in cognitive functioning; environmental barrier (e.g., bed size, bed type, equipment, restraints); insufficient knowledge of mobility strategies; insufficient muscle strength; musculoskeletal impairment; neuromuscular impairment; obesity; pain; pharmaceutical agent; physical deconditioning

Client Outcomes

Client Will (Specify Time Frame)

- Demonstrate optimal independence in positioning, exercising, and performing functional activities in bed

• = Independent   ▲ = Collaborative

- Demonstrate ability to direct others on how to do bed positioning, exercising, and functional activities

Nursing Interventions

- Choose therapeutic bed positions based on client's history and risk profile; assess to determine if positioning for one condition may negatively affect another; use critical thinking skills for risk-benefit analysis.
- Assess risk for aspiration; if present, elevate head of bed (HOB) to 30 to 45 degrees unless contraindicated and elevate HOB to 90 degrees during oral intake of fluids, solids, and oral medications.
- Raise HOB to 30 degrees for clients with acute increased intracranial pressure and brain injury. Refer to care plan for Decreased **Intracranial** adaptive capacity.
▲ Consult health care provider for HOB elevation for acute stroke and monitor response. Refer to care plan for Decreased **Intracranial** adaptive capacity.
- Raise HOB as close to 45 degrees as possible for critically ill ventilated clients to prevent pneumonia (this height may place clients at higher risk for pressure ulcers). Elevating the HOB decreases regurgitation and risk for aspiration of gastric contents.
- Assist client with dysphagia to sit as upright as possible for oral intake, including solids, fluids, and oral medications. Refer to care plan for Impaired **Swallowing.**
- Periodically sit client as upright as tolerated in bed; dangle client, if vital signs and oxygen saturation levels remain stable.
- To prevent pressure ulcers, maintain HOB at lowest elevation that is medically possible and raise the foot of the bed to prevent shear-related injury. Assess the client's sacrum, ischial tuberosities, and heels at least every 2 hours.
- Try prone positioning for clients with acute respiratory distress syndrome (ARDS), acute lung injury (ALI), and amputation and monitor their tolerance/response.
- Assess client's risk for falls using a valid fall risk assessment tool, such as the Morse Fall Scale (Morse et al, 1987).
- Beds should be kept locked and in the lowest position when occupied. Specialty low beds in which mattresses are approximately 8 to 12 inches from the floor are helpful for clients at risk for falls. Cushioned mats, 2 to 3 inches thick, with beveled edges lined

M

• = Independent ▲ = Collaborative

with reflective tape and covered by a rubberized material are also helpful.

▲ Bed rails and restraints must be prescribed by a health care provider.

▲ While placing all four bed rails up is considered a form of restraint and requires a health care provider's order, two and even three rails up can be a support for bed mobility.

• Place frequently used items within client's reach; demonstrate use of call bell (Hill & Fauerbach, 2014).

• Use a formalized screening tool to identify clients who are at high risk for thromboembolism, or deep venous thrombosis.

▲ Implement thromboembolism prophylaxis and treatment as prescribed (e.g., anticoagulants, antiembolic stockings, elastic leg wraps, sequential compression devices, feet/ankle exercises, and hydration). Refer to care plan for Ineffective peripheral **Tissue Perfusion.**

• Use a valid and reliable tool to assess a client's risk for pressure ulcers.

• Implement the following interventions to prevent pressure ulcers and complications of immobility:
  ○ Position sitting clients with special attention to the individual's anatomy, postural alignment, distribution of weight, and foot support.
  ○ Placing a client who is generally immobilized in a recliner is a good alternative to the bed (Gefen et al, 2013).
  ○ Turn (logroll) clients at high risk for pressure/shear/friction frequently and regularly.

• Pressure redistribution surfaces cannot replace turning and repositioning.
  ○ Use static/dynamic bed surfaces and assess for "bottoming out" under susceptible bony areas (body sinks into mattress, thus the recommended 1 inch between mattress/bones is absent). Refer to care plan for Risk for impaired **Skin** integrity.
  ○ Use heel protection devices that completely float or offload heels (National Pressure Ulcer Advisory Panel, 2011).
  ○ Implement a 2-hour on/off schedule for heel protector boots or high-top tennis shoes with socks underneath in clients with paralyzed feet, and check condition of heels when removed.

• = Independent   ▲ = Collaborative

○ Strictly maintain leg abduction in persons with a surgical hip pinning or replacement by placing an abductor splint/pillow between legs as prescribed.

○ Place bariatric beds along a corner wall, which helps keep the bed from moving during repositioning.

○ Identify/modify hospital beds with large gaps between bed rail/mattress that create an entrapment hazard. Ensure that mattress fits the bed; install gap fillers/rail inserts, then monitor effectiveness.

• Use devices such as trapeze, friction-reducing slide sheets, mechanical lateral transfer aids, and ceiling-mounted or floor lifts to move (rather than drag) dependent or obese clients in bed to prevent injury to staff.

○ Use special beds and equipment to move bariatric (very obese) clients, such as mattress overlay, sliding/roller board, trapeze, stirrup, and pulley attached to overhead traction system (holds one leg up during pericare).

○ Place bariatric clients in free-standing or ceiling-mounted lifts with padded slings while changing bed linen.

• Apply elbow pads to comatose and/or restrained clients and to those who use their elbows to prop or scoot up in bed. Apply nocturnal elbow splint as ordered if ulnar nerve palsy exists or if painful elbow with paresthesia in ulnar side of fourth/fifth fingers develops.

• Explain importance of exhaling versus holding one's breath (Valsalva maneuver) and straining during bed activities.

• Reassess pain level, especially before movement and/or exercising, and accept clients' pain rating and level they think is appropriate for comfort. Administer analgesics based on clients' pain rating. Refer to Acute **Pain** or Chronic **Pain.**

Exercise

• Test strength in bilateral grips, arms at elbow flexion and extension, bilateral arm abduction and adduction, bilateral leg or thigh raise (one at a time in bed or chair), and quadriceps and hamstring strength to extend and flex at knee to assess baseline and interval strength gains.

• Perform passive range of motion (ROM) of three repetitions, at least twice a day, to immobile joints.

• Range or move a hemiplegic arm with the shoulder slightly externally rotated (hand up).

• = Independent   ▲ = Collaborative

▲ Encourage client's practice of exercises taught by therapists (muscle setting, strengthening, contraction against resistance, and weight lifting).

Bed Positioning

• Incorporate the following measures to promote normal tone and prevent complications in clients with neurological impairment:
  ○ Use a flat head pillow when clients are supine. Use a small pillow behind the head and/or between shoulder blades if neck extension occurs.
  ○ Abduct the shoulders of clients with high paraplegia or quadriplegia horizontally to 90 degrees briefly two to three times a day while client is supine.
  ○ Position a hemiplegic shoulder fairly close to the client's body.

▲ Elevate a client's paralyzed forearms on a pillow when client is supine and apply Isotoner gloves. Elevate edematous legs on a pillow supporting the knees to prevent hyperextension. Apply elastic wraps and compression garments as prescribed.

• Tilt hemiplegics onto both unaffected and affected sides with the affected shoulder slightly forward (e.g., move/lift the affected shoulder, not the forearm/hand).

▲ Apply resting wrist, hand, and foot/ankle splints or other devices. Range joints before applying splints. Adhere to on/off schedule as prescribed by the physical therapist.

▲ Recognize that components of normal bed mobility include rolling, bridging, scooting, long sitting, and sitting upright. Activity starts with the client supine, flat in bed, and promotes normal movements that are bilateral, segmental, well timed, and involve set positions such as weight bearing and trunk centering. Refer to a physical therapist (PT) for individualized instructions and mobility strategies.

Geriatric

• Assess caregiver's strength, health history, and cognitive status to predict ability/risk for assisting bed-bound clients at home. Refer to care plan for **Caregiver Role Strain.**

• Assess the client's stamina and energy level during bed activities/exercises; if limited, spread out activities and allow rest breaks.

Home Care

▲ Collaborate with nurse case managers, care coordinators, social workers, and physical/occupational therapists to assess home support systems and needs, and to provide for home modifications, durable medical equipment, assistive technology, and home health services.

- Encourage use of the client's bed unless contraindicated. Raise HOB with commercial blocks or grooved-out pieces of wood under legs; set bed against walls in a corner. Emotionally, clients may benefit from sleeping in their own beds with familiar partners.

- Stress psychological/physical benefits of clients being as self-sufficient as possible with bed mobility/care even though it may be time-consuming. Allowing independence and autonomy may help prevent disuse syndromes and feelings of helplessness and low self-esteem.

- Offer emotional support and help client identify usual coping responses to help with adjustment and loss issues. The home environment may trigger the reality of lost function and disability.

- Discuss support systems available for caregivers to help them cope. Refer to care plan for **Caregiver Role Strain.**

▲ In the presence of medical disorders, institute case management for frail older adult to support continued independent living.

- Refer to the home care interventions in the care plan for Impaired physical **Mobility.**

Client/Family Teaching and Discharge Planning

- Use various sensory modalities to teach client/caregivers correct range of motion, exercises, positioning, self-care activities, and use of devices. Readiness and learning styles vary but may be enhanced with visual/auditory/tactile/cognitive stimulus as follows:
  - ○ Provide visual information such as demonstrations, sketches, instructional videos, written directions/schedules, notes.
  - ○ Provide auditory information such as verbal instructions, recorded audiotapes, timers, reading aloud written directions, and self-talk during activities.
  - ○ Use tactile stimulation such as motor task practice/repetition, return demonstrations, note taking, manual guidance, or staff's hand-on-client's-hand technique.

▲ Schedule time with family/caregivers for education and practice for nursing, physical therapy, and occupational therapy. Suggest family come prepared with questions and wear comfortable, safe clothing/shoes. Practice provides opportunity for learning; repetition helps memory retention.

M

• = Independent   ▲ = Collaborative

▲ Implement safe approaches for caregivers/home care staff and reinforce adequate number of people and handling equipment (e.g., friction pads, slide boards, lifts) during bed mobility, exercise, toileting, and bathing to decrease risk of injury.

▲ Coordinate evaluations for bariatric equipment for home use before discharge, including a weight-rated bed, a wheelchair or mobility device (scooter), and lift device. Doorways may need to be widened, floors reinforced, and ramps added for safety.

Impaired physical Mobility
NANDA-I Definition

Limitation in independent, purposeful physical movement of the body or of one or more extremities

Defining Characteristics

Alteration in gait; decrease in fine motor skills; decrease in gross motor skills; decrease in range of motion; decrease in reaction time; difficulty turning; discomfort; engages in substitutions for movement (e.g., attention to other's activity, controlling behavior, focus on pre-illness activity); exertional dyspnea; movement-induced tremor; postural instability; slowed movement; spastic movement; uncoordinated movement

Related Factors (r/t)

Activity intolerance; alteration in bone structure integrity; alteration in cognitive functioning; alteration in metabolism; anxiety; body mass index >75th percentile for age; contractures; cultural belief regarding appropriate activity; decrease in endurance; decrease in muscle control; decrease in muscle mass; decrease in muscle strength; depression; developmental delay; disuse; insufficient environmental support (e.g., physical, social); insufficient knowledge of value of physical activity; joint stiffness; malnutrition; musculoskeletal impairment; neuromuscular impairment; pain; pharmaceutical agent; physical deconditioning; prescribed movement restrictions; reluctance to initiate movement; sedentary lifestyle; sensory-perceptual impairment

Client Outcomes

Client Will (Specify Time Frame)

- Meet mutually defined goals of increased ambulation and exercise that include individual choice, preference, and enjoyment in the exercise prescription
- Verbalize feeling of increased strength and ability to move

• = Independent   ▲ = Collaborative

- Verbalize less fear of falling and pain with physical activity
- Demonstrate use of adaptive equipment (e.g., wheelchairs, walkers, gait belts, weighted walking vests) to increase mobility
- Increase exercise to 20 minutes per day for those who were previously sedentary (less than 150 minutes per week). NOTE: Light to moderate intensity exercise may be beneficial in deconditioned persons. In very deconditioned individuals, exercise bouts of less than 10 minutes are beneficial.
- Increase pedometer step counts by 1000 steps per day every 2 weeks to reach a daily step count of at least 7000 steps per day, with a daily goal for most healthy adults of 10,000 steps per day (approximately 5 miles)
- Perform resistance exercises that involve all major muscle groups (legs, hips, back, chest, abdomen, shoulders, and arms) performed 2 or 3 days per week
- Perform flexibility exercise (stretching) for each of the major muscle-tendon groups 2 days per week for 10 to 60 seconds to improve joint range of motion; greatest gains occur with daily exercise
- Engage in neuromotor exercise 20 to 30 minutes per day including motor skills (e.g., balance, agility, coordination, and gait), propriocep-tive exercise training, and multifaceted activities (e.g., tai chi and yoga) to improve and maintain physical function and reduce falls in those at risk for falling (older persons)
- Engage in purposeful moderate-intensity cardiorespiratory (aerobic) exercise for 30 to 60 minutes per day at least 5 days per week for a total of 2 hours and 30 minutes (150 minutes) per week

Nursing Interventions

- Adults with disabilities should follow the adult guidelines; however, if not possible, these persons should be as physically active as their abilities allow and avoid inactivity (U.S. Department of Health & Human Services, 2008). Use "start low and go slow" approach for intensity and duration of physical activity if client highly deconditioned, functionally limited, or has chronic conditions affecting performance of physical tasks. When progressing client's activities, use an individualized and tailored approach based on client's tolerance and preferences (American College of Sports Medicine [ACSM], 2014).
- Screen for mobility skills in the following order: (1) bed mobility; (2) supported and unsupported sitting; (3) transition movements

• = Independent   ▲ = Collaborative

such as sit to stand, sitting down, and transfers; and (4) standing and walking activities.

- Screen for additional measures of physical function to assess strength of muscle groups, including unassisted leg stand, use of a balance platform, elbow flexion and knee extension strength, grip strength, timed chair stands, and the 6-minute walk.

- Assess the client for cause of impaired mobility. Determine whether cause is physical, psychological, or motivational. Refer to care plans for Risk for **Falls**, Acute **Pain**, Chronic **Pain**, Ineffective **Coping**, or **Hopelessness**.

- Use Self-Efficacy for Exercise Scale (Resnick & Jenkins, 2000) and the Outcome Expectation for Exercise Scale (Resnick et al, 2001) to determine client's self-efficacy and outcome expectations toward exercise (Resnick & D'Adamo, 2011).

- Function-focused care should be used, such as encouraging self performance of bathing, walking to the bathroom instead of using a bedpan/urinal, and taking the older adult to an exercise class (Resnick & Galik, 2013).

- Monitor and record the client's ability to tolerate activity and use all four extremities; note pulse rate, blood pressure, dyspnea, and skin color before and after activity. Refer to the care plan for **Activity** intolerance.

▲ Before activity, observe for and, if possible, treat pain with massage, heat pack to affected area, or medication. Ensure that the client is not oversedated.

▲ Consult with physical therapist for further evaluation, strength training, gait training, and development of a mobility plan.

- Before the activity begins, obtain any assistive devices needed for activity, such as gait belt, weighted vest, walker, cane, crutches, or wheelchair; ergonomic shower chairs; ceiling and floor-based lifts; and air-assisted lateral transfer devices.

- If the client is immobile, perform passive range-of-motion (ROM) exercises at least twice a day unless contraindicated; repeat each maneuver three times.

▲ If the client is immobile, consult with health care provider for a safety evaluation before beginning an exercise program; if program is approved, begin with the following exercises:
  ○ Active ROM exercises using both upper and lower extremities (e.g., flexing and extending at ankles, knees, hips)

• = Independent   ▲ = Collaborative

○ Chin-ups and pull-ups using a trapeze in bed (may be contraindicated in clients with cardiac conditions)
○ Strengthening exercises such as gluteal or quadriceps sitting exercises
- If client is immobile, consider use of vertical transfer techniques such as air-assisted lateral transfer devices or gait belt pending weight-bearing status and client cooperation.
- Help the client achieve mobility and start walking as soon as possible if not contraindicated.
- Use a gait-walking belt when ambulating the client.
▲ Apply any ordered brace before mobilizing the client. Braces support and stabilize a body part, allowing increased mobility.
- Initiate a "no lift" policy where appropriate assistive devices are used for manual lifting.
- Increase independence in ADLs, encouraging self-efficacy and discouraging helplessness as the client gets stronger.
▲ If the client has osteoarthritis or rheumatoid arthritis, ask for a referral to a physical therapist to begin an exercise program that includes aerobic exercise, resistance exercise, and flexibility exercise (stretching).
▲ If client has had a cerebrovascular accident (CVA) with hemiparesis, consider use of constraint-induced movement therapy, wherein the functional extremity is purposely constrained and the client is forced to use the involved extremity.
- If the client has had a CVA, recognize that balance and mobility are likely impaired, and engage client in fall prevention strategies and protect from falling.
- If the client does not feed or groom self, sit side-by-side with the client, put your hand over the client's hand, support the client's elbow with your other hand, and help the client feed self; use the same technique to help the client comb hair.

Geriatric
- Assess ability to move using valid and reliable criterion-referenced standards for fitness testing (e.g., senior fitness test) designed for older adults that can predict the level of capacity associated with maintaining physical independence into later years of life (e.g., get up and go test).
- Help the mostly immobile client achieve mobility as soon as possible, depending on physical condition.

• = Independent   ▲ = Collaborative

- For a client who is mostly immobile, minimize cardiovascular deconditioning by positioning the client in the upright position several times daily.
▲ Refer the client to physical therapy for resistance exercise training as able, involving all major muscle groups (e.g., abdominal crunch, leg press, leg extension, leg curl, and calf press) (ACSM, 2014).
- Use the FFC rehabilitative philosophy of care in older adults in residential nursing facilities to prevent avoidable functional decline. The primary goals of FFC are to alter how direct care workers provide care to residents to maintain and improve time spent in physical activity and improve or maintain function.
- If client is scheduled for an elective surgery that will result in admission into the intensive care unit and immobility, or recovery from a joint replacement, for example, initiate a prehabilitation program that includes warm-up, aerobic activity, strength, flexibility, neuromotor, and functional task work.
▲ Evaluate the client for signs of depression (flat affect, insomnia, anorexia, frequent somatic complaints), anxiety, or cognitive impairment (use Mini-Mental State Exam [MMSE]). Refer for treatment and counseling as needed.
- Watch for orthostatic hypotension when mobilizing older clients. Have the client dangle at the side of the bed with legs hanging over the edge of the bed, flex and extend feet several times after sitting up, then stand up slowly with someone holding the client. If client becomes lightheaded or dizzy, return client to bed immediately.
- Do not routinely assist with transfers or bathing activities unless necessary.
- Use gestures and nonverbal cues when helping clients move if they are anxious or have difficulty understanding and following verbal instructions.
- Recognize that wheelchairs are not a good mobility device and often serve as a mobility restraint.
- Ensure that chairs fit clients. Chair seat should be 3 inches above the height of the knee. Provide a raised toilet seat if needed.
- If the client is mainly immobile, provide opportunities for socialization and sensory stimulation (e.g., television and visits). Refer to the care plan for Deficient **Diversional** activity.
- Recognize that immobility and a lack of social support and sensory input may result in confusion or depression in older adults

• = Independent   ▲ = Collaborative

(American Academy of Nursing's Expert Panel on Acute and Critical Care, 2012). Refer to nursing interventions for Acute **Confusion** or **Hopelessness** as appropriate.

Home Care

- The preceding interventions may be adapted for home care use.
- ▲ Begin discharge planning as soon as possible with a personal health navigator (e.g., nurse care coordinator or case manager) to assess need for home support systems, assistive devices, and community or home health services (Paulus et al, 2008).
- ▲ Assess home environment for factors that create barriers to physical mobility. Refer to occupational therapy services if needed to assist the client in restructuring home environment and daily living patterns.
- ▲ Refer to home health aide services to support the client and family through changing levels of mobility. Reinforce need to promote independence in mobility as tolerated.
- ▲ Refer to physical therapy for gait training, strengthening, and balance training. Physical therapists can provide direct interventions as well as assess need for assistive devices (e.g., cane, walker).
- Discuss with client and caregiver the possibility of a service dog to support the more immobile client.
- Assess skin condition at every visit. Establish a skin care program that enhances circulation and maximizes position changes.
- Once the client is able to walk independently, suggest the client enter an exercise program, or walk with a friend.
- Provide support to the client and family/caregivers during long-term impaired mobility. Refer to the care plan for **Caregiver Role Strain.**
- ▲ Institute a personal health navigator (e.g., nurse care coordinator or case manager) and transitional care management of frail older adults to support continued independent living (Paulus et al, 2008).

Client/Family Teaching and Discharge Planning

- Consider using motivational interviewing techniques when working with both children and adult clients to increase their activity. Refer to the care plan for **Sedentary** lifestyle.
- Teach the client progressive mobilization (e.g., dangle legs, get out of bed slowly when transferring from the bed to the chair).
- Teach the client relaxation techniques such as deep breathing and stretching to use during activity.

M

• = Independent   ▲ = Collaborative

- Teach the client to use assistive devices such as a cane, walker, gait belt, weighted vest, or crutches or wheelchair to increase mobility (Yeom et al, 2009).
- Teach family members and caregivers to work with clients actively during self-care activities using a restorative care philosophy for eating, bathing, grooming, dressing, and transferring to restore the client to maximum function and independence (Resnick et al, 2009).
- Work with the client using self-efficacy interventions using single or multiple methods. Teach client and family members to assess fear of falling and develop strategies to mitigate its effect on mobility progression.
- Work with the client using theory-based interventions (e.g., social cognitive theoretical components such as self-efficacy; transtheoretical model).

M

Impaired wheelchair Mobility
NANDA-I Definition

Limitation of independent operation of wheelchair within environment

Defining Characteristics

Impaired ability to operate power wheelchair on a decline; impaired ability to operate power wheelchair on an incline; impaired ability to operate power wheelchair on curbs; impaired ability to operate power wheelchair on even surface; impaired ability to operate power wheelchair on uneven surface

Related Factors

Alteration in cognitive functioning; alteration in mood; decrease in endurance; environmental barrier (e.g., stairs, inclines, uneven surfaces, obstacles, distance); impaired vision; insufficient knowledge of wheelchair use; insufficient muscle strength; musculoskeletal impairment; neuromuscular impairment; obesity; pain; physical deconditioning

Client Outcomes

Client Will (Specify Time Frame)

- Demonstrate independence in operating and moving a wheelchair or other device with wheels
- Demonstrate the ability to direct others in operating and moving a wheelchair or other device

• = Independent ▲ = Collaborative

- Demonstrate therapeutic positioning, pressure relief, and safety principles while operating and moving a wheelchair or other device equipped with wheels

Nursing Interventions

- ▪ Assist client to put on and take off equipment (e.g., braces, orthoses, abdominal binders, compression stockings) in bed.
- ▪ Inspect skin where orthoses, braces, and other equipment rested once they are removed.
- ▲ Refer to physical and occupational therapy or wheelchair seating clinic.
- ▪ Recognize that use of support surfaces on chairs and beds redistributes pressure and should be used for at-risk clients as an adjunct to reduce risk of pressure ulcer. However, using support surfaces does not replace the need for repositioning the client on a regular schedule (i.e., weight shifts) (Sprigle & Sonenbaum, 2011; Requejo et al, 2015).
- ▪ Intervene to maintain continence or use absorbent diapers/underpads to help prevent skin breakdown due to excessive moisture and macerated skin. Some wheelchair cushions have moisture-wicking characteristics.
- ▪ Routinely assess client's sitting posture and frequently reposition him/her into alignment.
- ▪ Sit dysphagic clients as upright as possible in individualized wheelchair versus geri-chair when eating. See care plan for Risk for **Aspiration.**
- ▪ Implement use of friction-coated projection hand rims and leather gloves for clients to propel manual wheelchairs.
- ▪ Manually guide or explain to the client to push forward on both wheel rims to move ahead, push the right rim to turn left and vice versa, and pull backward on both wheel rims to back up.
- ▪ Recommend that clients back wheelchair into an elevator. If entering face first, instruct them to turn chair around to face the elevator doors.
- ▲ In conjunction with physical therapy for teaching and assessment, reinforce principle of descending a curb backward ("popping a wheelie") if balance, trunk control, strength, and timing are adequate.
- ▪ Ascend curbs in a forward position by popping a wheelie or having someone aid in tilting the chair back, place front wheels over curb, and roll chair up. If surface is muddy or sandy, ascend backward.

- During assisted wheelies, helper must hold wheelchair until all four wheels are back on the ground and client has control of wheelchair.
▲ Follow therapist's recommendations for how clients should propel manual wheelchairs to prevent upper extremity pain and joint degeneration.
- Inform clients that ultra-lightweight, push-rim-activated, power-assisted, or electric wheelchairs may be more therapeutic than manual ones.
- Help clients transition from a manual to a powered wheelchair/scooter if progressive disability occurs.
▲ Reduce floor clutter and establish safety rules for drivers of electric/power mobility devices; make referrals to physical or occupational therapy for driver reevaluations if accidents occur or client's health deteriorates.
- Request and receive client's permission before moving unoccupied wheelchair in room or out to hallway.
- Reinforce compensatory strategies for unilateral neglect and agnosia (e.g., visual scanning, self-talk, self-questioning as to what could be wrong) as clients propel wheelchair through doorways and around obstacles. Refer to care plan for **Unilateral Neglect.**
- Offer support to help clients cope with issues related to physical disability. Refer to care plan for Ineffective **Role** performance.
- Provide information on support group and reliable Internet resource options.
- Provide information about advocacy, accessibility, assistive technology, and issues under the Americans with Disabilities Act.
▲ Make social service or wheelchair clinic referral to educate clients on financial coverage/regulations of third-party payers and Health Care Financing Association for wheelchairs.
- Recommend that clients test-drive wheelchairs and try out cushions/postural supports with the advice of a qualified seating professional before purchasing them.

Pediatric
▲ Help client/family transition from a manual to a powered wheelchair/scooter if disability is severe.

Geriatric
- Avoid using restraints on fidgeting clients who slide down in a wheelchair; rather, assess for deformities, spinal curvatures, abnormal tone, discomfort, and limited joint range.

• = Independent   ▲ = Collaborative

- Ensure proper seat depth/leg positioning and use custom foot rests (not elevated leg rests) to prevent older adults from sliding down in wheelchairs.
▲ Assess for side effects of medications and potential need for dosage readjustments to increase wheelchair tolerance. Give prescribed hydration and medications to treat orthostatic hypotension. Consider leg wraps. Client should perform warm-up bed exercises.
- Allow client to propel wheelchair independently at his/her own speed.

Home Care

▲ Establish a support system for emergency and contingency care (e.g., remote monitoring, emergency call system, alert local emergency medical system).
- Recommend the following changes to the home to accommodate the use of a wheelchair:
  ○ Arrange traffic patterns so they are wide enough to maneuver a wheelchair.
  ○ Recognize a 5-foot turning space is necessary to maneuver wheelchairs; doorways need to have 32 to 36 inches clear width; and entrance ramps/path slope should be assessed before permanent ramps are installed because standardized slopes may not be appropriate. Temporary ramps are cost-effective and easier to adjust (Sofka, 2011).
  ○ Replace door hardware with fold-back hinges, remove doorway encasements (if too narrow), remove/replace thresholds (if too high), hang wall-mounted sinks/handrails, grade floors in showers for roll-in chairs, use nonskid/nonslip floor coverings (e.g., nonwaxed wood, linoleum, or Berber carpet).
  ○ Rearrange room functions, furniture, and storage so that toileting, sleeping, bathing, and preparing/eating meals can safely take place on one level of the home.
  ○ Refer to the Easter Seals Summary on Home Accessibility for further details: http://www.easterseals.com/shared-components/document-library/easy_access_housing.pdf.
▲ Request physical and occupational therapy referrals to evaluate wheelchair fitting, skills, safety, and maintenance. Suggest community resources for servicing and tuning up wheelchairs and/or locating parts so clients can service their own chairs; an annual tune-up is recommended.

• = Independent   ▲ = Collaborative

Client/Family Teaching and Discharge Planning

▲ Assess pain levels of long-term wheelchair users and make referrals to therapists or wheelchair clinics for modifications as needed.

• Instruct and have client return demonstrate reinflation of pneumatic tires; encourage client to monitor tire pressure every 2 to 3 weeks.

• Instruct family/clients to remove large wheelchair parts (leg rests, arm rests) when lifting wheelchair into car for transport; when reassembling, check that all parts are fastened securely and temperature is tepid.

• Teach the critical importance of using seatbelts and secure chair tie-downs when riding in motor vehicles in a wheelchair. Never transport a client in an unsecured wheelchair in any kind of vehicle.

• For further information, refer to care plan for Impaired **Transfer** ability.

M

Impaired Mood regulation
NANDA-I Definition

A mental state characterized by shifts in mood or affect and that comprises a constellation of affective, cognitive, somatic, and/or physiological manifestations varying from mild to severe

Defining Characteristics

Changes in verbal behavior; disinhibition; dysphoria; excessive guilt; excessive self-awareness; excessive self-blame; flight of thoughts; hopelessness; impaired concentration; influenced self-esteem; irritability; psychomotor agitation; psychomotor retardation; sad affect; withdrawal

Related Factors

Alteration in sleep pattern; anxiety; appetite change; chronic illness; functional impairment; hypervigilance; impaired social functioning; loneliness; pain; psychosis; recurrent thoughts of death; recurrent thoughts of suicide; social isolation; substance misuse; weight change

Client Outcomes

Client Will (Specify Time Frame)

• State feelings related to changes in mood
• Eat appropriate diet for height and weight
• Follow exercise plan
• Have no attempts at self-harm

• = Independent   ▲ = Collaborative

Nursing Interventions

- Provide nutritional intake for a client who is unable to feed self.
- Encourage regular physical exercise to maintain or advance to a higher level of fitness and health.
- Reduce the risk of self-inflicted harm for a client in crisis or severe depression with a planned treatment program.
- Facilitate the safe and effective use of prescription and over-the-counter drugs.

Client/Network Interventions

- Provide a treatment involving the cooperation of several aide workers in neighborhood teams and provide customized treatment at the place where the client resides.

Moral Distress

M

NANDA-I Definition

Response to the inability to carry out one's chosen ethical/moral decision/action

Defining Characteristics

Anguish about acting on one's moral choice (e.g., powerlessness, anxiety, fear)

Related Factors (r/t)

Conflict among decision makers; conflicting information available for ethical decision-making; conflicting information available for moral decision-making; cultural incongruence; end-of-life decisions; loss of autonomy; physical distance of decision maker; time constraint for decision-making; treatment decision

Client Outcomes

Client Will (Specify Time Frame)

- Be able to act in accordance with values, goals, and beliefs
- Regain confidence in the ability to make decisions and/or act in accord with values, goals, and beliefs
- Express satisfaction with the ability to make decisions consistent with values, goals, and beliefs
- Have choices respected

Nursing Interventions

- Assess if moral distress is present and its relationship to intrinsic or extrinsic factors.
- Affirm the distress, commitment "to take care of yourself," and your obligations. Validate feelings and perceptions with others.
- Implement strategies to change situations causing moral distress.
- Assess sources and severity of distress.
- Give voice/recognition to moral distress and express concerns about constraints to supportive individuals.
- Engage in healthy problem-solving.
- Engage in interdisciplinary problem-solving forums including family meeting and/or interdisciplinary rounds.
- Implement multidisciplinary interventions/strategies to address moral distress.
- Identify/use a support system.
- Initiate an ethics consult or ethics committee review.

Pediatric

- Consider the developmental age of children when evaluating decisions and conflict.

Multicultural

- Acknowledge and understand cultural differences that may influence a client's moral choices.

Geriatric and Home Care

- Previous interventions may be adapted for geriatric or home care use.

Nausea

NANDA-I Definition

A subjective phenomenon of an unpleasant feeling in the back of the throat and stomach, which may or may not result in vomiting

Defining Characteristics

Aversion to food; gagging sensation; increase in salivation; increase in swallowing; nausea; sour taste

Related Factors

Biophysical

Biochemical dysfunction (e.g., uremia, diabetic ketoacidosis); esophageal disease; exposure to toxin; gastric distention; gastrointestinal irritation; increase in intracranial pressure; intra-abdominal tumors; labyrinthitis; liver capsule stretch; localized tumors (e.g., acoustic neuroma, brain tumor,

• = Independent   ▲ = Collaborative

bone metastasis); Ménière's disease; meningitis; motion sickness; pancreatic disease; pregnancy; splenetic capsule stretch; treatment regimen

Situational

Anxiety; fear; noxious environmental stimuli; noxious taste; psychological disorder; unpleasant visual stimuli

Client Outcomes

Client Will (Specify Time Frame)

• State relief of nausea
• Explain methods clients can use to decrease nausea and vomiting (N&V)

Nursing Interventions

▲ Determine cause or risk for N&V (e.g., medication effects, infectious causes [viral and bacterial gastroenteritis], disorders of the gut and peritoneum [mechanical obstruction, motility disorders, or other intra-abdominal causes], central nervous system causes [including anxiety], endocrine and metabolic causes [including pregnancy], postoperative-related status).

▲ Evaluate and document the client's history of N&V, with attention to onset, duration, timing, volume of emesis, frequency of pattern, setting, associated factors, aggravating factors, and past medical and social histories.

• Document each episode of nausea and/or vomiting separately, as well as effectiveness of interventions. Consider an assessment tool for consistency of evaluation.

• Identify and eliminate contributing causative factors. This may include eliminating unpleasant odors or medications that may be contributing to nausea.

▲ Implement appropriate dietary measures such as NPO status as appropriate; small, frequent meals; and low-fat meals. It may be helpful to avoid foods that are spicy, fatty, or highly salty. Reverting to previous practices when ill in the past and consuming "comfort foods" may also be helpful at this time.

▲ Recognize and implement interventions and monitor complications associated with N&V. This may include administration of intravenous fluids and electrolytes.

▲ Administer appropriate antiemetics, according to emetic cause, by most effective route, considering the side effects of the medication, with attention to and coverage for the timeframes that the nausea is anticipated.

N

• = Independent   ▲ = Collaborative

- Consider nonpharmacological interventions such as acupressure, acupuncture, music therapy, distraction, and slow, deliberate movements.
- Provide oral care after the client vomits. Oral care helps remove the taste and smell of vomitus, thus reducing the stimulus for further vomiting.

Nausea in Pregnancy

- Early recognition and conservative measures are recommended to successfully manage nausea in pregnancy, and to prevent progression to hyperemesis gravidarum. Dietary and lifestyle modifications should be implemented before pharmacological interventions. Avoidance of any aversive odors or foods is recommended. Eating multiple small meals per day is also recommended to have some food in the stomach at all times, thereby avoiding hypoglycemia and gastric overdistention. Foods with higher protein and carbohydrate and lower fat content are helpful. Drinking smaller volumes of liquids at multiple times throughout the day is recommended.
- ▲ Due to the high incidence of coexisting gastroesophageal reflux disease (GERD), it is important to assess and manage these symptoms of heartburn, belching, and indigestion.
- ▲ It is well established that *Helicobacter pylori (H. Pylori)* infection is associated with hyperemesis gravidarum.
- ▲ Coexisting psychosocial factors may also influence the severity of N&V with pregnancy. Symptoms of anxiety and depression can occur in early pregnancy, especially when N&V is severe and can make the treatment of the N&V more challenging and even ineffective.
- ▲ The American Congress of Obstetricians & Gynecologists (ACOG) currently recommends a combination of oral pyridoxine hydrochloride (vitamin B6, 25 mg) and doxylamine succinate (antihistamine 12.5 mg) be used as first-line treatment for N&V of pregnancy after failure of pyridoxine alone. This combination agent (Diclegis) is the only U.S. Food and Drug Administration pregnancy Category A approved therapy for N&V of pregnancy. There are, however, several pharmacological treatments outlined by the ACOG.

Nausea Following Surgery

- ▲ Evaluate for risk factors for postoperative nausea and vomiting (PONV).

• = Independent   ▲ = Collaborative

▲ Reduction of risk factors associated with PONV is beneficial for both adults and children.

▲ Medicate the client prophylactically for nausea as ordered, throughout the period of risk.

▲ Alleviate postoperative pain using ordered analgesic agents (refer to care plan for Acute **Pain**).

• Consider the use of nonpharmacological techniques, such as P6 acupoint stimulation, as an adjunct for controlling PONV, which has been shown to be effective.

• Include client education on the management of PONV for all outpatients and discuss key assessment criteria (Odom-Forren et al, 2014).

Nausea Following Chemotherapy

• Perform risk assessment before chemotherapy administration. Risk factors include female gender, younger age, history of low alcohol consumption, history of morning sickness during pregnancy, anxiety, previous history of chemotherapy, client expectancy of nausea, and emetic potential of the regimen.

▲ Initiate antiemetic strategy prophylactically or when N&V occurs in accordance with evidence-based guidelines.

▲ Drug classes that are recommended for practice include the serotonin receptor antagonists, the neurokinin (NK-1) receptor antagonists, and cannabinoids.

▲ Consider the use of progressive muscle relaxation and guided imagery with antiemetics.

• Consider managing client expectations about CINV.

Geriatric

• There are no specific guidelines that address the prophylaxis of CINV specifically in older adults. Risk still needs to be assessed, although many older clients are often treated with less emetic chemotherapy. Chemotherapy, however, can cause increased toxicity due to age-related decreases in organ function, comorbidities, and drug-drug interactions secondary to polypharmacy. Additionally, adherence may be an issue, due to cognitive decline, impaired senses, and economic issues.

Pediatric

• Interventions for CINV should be implemented before and after chemotherapy.

• = Independent   ▲ = Collaborative

- Relatively few studies exist examining the antiemetic medications used for CINV in children. It appears that 5-HT$_3$ antagonists combined with dexamethasone are better than older agents (Basch et al, 2011).

Home Care

- Previously mentioned interventions may be adapted for home care use.

▲ In hospice care clients, assess for causes of nausea, such as constipation, bowel obstruction, adverse effects of medications, and onset of increased intracranial pressure. Refer the client to a primary health care provider if needed.

- Assist the client and family with identifying and avoiding irritants in the home that exacerbate nausea (e.g., strong odors from food, plants, perfume, and room deodorizers). All medications except antiemetics should be given after meals to minimize the risk of nausea.

Client/Family Teaching and Discharge Planning

- Teach the client techniques to use before and after chemotherapy, including antiemetics/medication management schedules and dietary approaches, such as eating smaller meals, avoiding spicy and fatty foods, and avoiding an empty stomach before chemotherapy (Irwin & Johnson, 2014).

Noncompliance

NANDA-I Definition

Behavior of person and/or caregiver that fails to coincide with a health-promoting or therapeutic plan agreed on by the person (and/or family and/or community) and health care professional; in the presence of an agreed-on, health-promoting, or therapeutic plan, person's or caregiver's behavior is fully or partially nonadherent and may lead to clinically ineffective or partially ineffective outcomes

Defining Characteristics

Behavior indicative of failure to adhere; evidence of development of complications; evidence of exacerbation of symptoms; failure to keep appointments; failure to progress; objective tests (e.g., physiological measures, detection of physiological markers)

• = Independent   ▲ = Collaborative

Related Factors (r/t)

Health System

Access to care; communication skills of the provider; convenience of care; credibility of provider; difficulty in client-provider relationship; individual health coverage; provider continuity; provider regular follow-up; provider reimbursement; satisfaction with care; teaching skills of the provider

Health Care Plan

Complexity; cost; duration; financial flexibility of plan; intensity

Individual Factors

Cultural influences; developmental abilities; health beliefs; deficient knowledge relevant to the regimen behavior; individual's value system; motivational forces; personal abilities; significant others; skill relevant to the regimen behavior; spiritual values

Network

Involvement of members in health plan; perceived beliefs of significant others; social value regarding plan

NOTE: The nursing diagnosis **Noncompliance** is judgmental and places blame on the client for some things the client has no control over. The authors recommend use of the diagnosis Ineffective **Health** management in place of the diagnosis **Noncompliance.** The diagnosis Ineffective **Health** management has interventions that are developed by both health care providers and the client. It is a more respectful and efficacious nursing diagnosis.

Client Outcomes, Nursing Interventions, and Client/Family Teaching and Discharge Planning

Refer to care plans for Ineffective **Health** management.

Readiness for enhanced Nutrition

NANDA-I Definition

A pattern of nutrient intake that can be strengthened

Defining Characteristics

Expresses desire to enhance nutrition

Client Outcomes

Client Will (Specify Time Frame)

- Explain how to eat according to the U.S. Dietary Guidelines
- Design dietary modifications to meet individual long-term goal of health, using principles of variety, balance, and moderation
- Maintain weight within normal range for height and age

• = Independent   ▲ = Collaborative

Nursing Interventions

- Assess the meaning and importance of food in the client's life.
- Counsel the client to measure regularly consumed foods periodically. Help the client learn usual portion sizes.
- Help the client determine his/her body mass index (BMI) and understand the significance of the result. Use a chart or a website such as http://www.cdc.gov/healthyweight/assessing/bmi/index.html (Centers for Disease Control and Prevention [CDC], 2014).
- Recommend the client follow the U.S. Dietary Guidelines to determine foods to eat, which can be found at http://www .choosemyplate.gov/weight-management-calories/weight -management/better-choices/amount-calories.html.
- Recommend the client use Super Tracker (http://www .choosemyplate.gov/food-groups) to determine the number of calories to eat and gain more information on how to eat in a healthy fashion. To lose weight, the client must eat fewer calories (U.S. Department of Agriculture, 2014).
- Recommend the client eat a healthy breakfast every morning.
- Recommend the client avoid eating in fast-food restaurants.
- Demonstrate the use of food labels to make healthful choices. Alert the client/family to focus on serving size, total fat, and simple carbohydrates.

Carbohydrates/Sugars

- Encourage the client to decrease intake of sugars, including intake of soft drinks, desserts, and candy. Limit sugar intake to 6.5 teaspoons of added sugars for women and 9.5 teaspoons of added sugar for men daily.
- Share with client the names of sugars including glucose, dextrose, corn syrup, maple syrup, brown sugar, molasses, evaporated cane juice, sucrose, honey, orange juice concentrate, grape juice concentrate, apple juice concentrate, brown rice syrup, high-fructose corn syrup, agave, and fructose (Nutrition Action, 2011).
- Limit intake of fruit juice to 1 cup per day.
- Recommend the client eat whole grains whenever possible, and explain how to find whole grains using the food label.
- Assess the client's usual intake of fiber. Recommended intake is 25 g per day for women and 38 g per day for men. Increase intake of whole grains, beans, fruits, and vegetables to obtain needed fiber. Wheat bran is an excellent source of fiber, but cannot be tolerated by

all people; beans are the second-best source of fiber (Nutrition Action, 2011).

- Recommend the client eat five to nine fruits and vegetables per day, with a minimum of two servings of fruit and three servings of vegetables. Encourage client to eat a rainbow of fruits and vegetables because bright colors are associated with increased nutrients.

Fats

- Recommend the client limit intake of saturated fats and avoid trans fatty acids completely; instead increase intake of vegetable oils such as polyunsaturated and monounsaturated oils.
- Recommend client use low-fat choices when selecting and cooking meat, and also when selecting dairy products.
- Recommend that the client eat cold-water fish such as salmon, tuna, or mackerel at least two times per week to ensure adequate intake of omega-3 fatty acids. If client is unwilling to eat fish, suggest sources such as flaxseed, soy, or walnuts. NOTE: Fish oil capsules should be taken cautiously; some brands can be contaminated with mercury or pesticides. Intake of excessive omega-3 fatty acids can result in bleeding.

Protein

- Recommend the client decrease intake of red meat and processed meats, and instead eat more poultry, fish, soy, and dairy sources of protein.
- Recommend the client eat meatless meals at intervals and try alternative sources of protein, including nuts, especially almonds (one handful), and nut butters.
- Recommend the client eat beans and soy as an alternative to animal proteins at intervals. Introduce the client to soy products such as flavored soy milk and tofu.

Fluid and Electrolytes

- Recommend the client choose and prepare foods with less salt, aiming for a maximum of 2300 mg per day (Harvard Health Letter, 2012).
- If the client drinks alcohol, encourage him or her to drink in moderation—no more than one drink per day for women and two drinks per day for men.
- Recommend client increase intake of water to at least 2000 mL or 2 quarts per day. A guideline is 1 to 1.5 mL of fluid for each calorie needed, so an average intake would be between 2000 and 3000 mL/day or at least 8 cups of fluid.

N

• = Independent   ▲ = Collaborative

Supplements

- Recommend that clients use dietary supplements such as vitamins and minerals only after consulting with their primary health care provider (Mayo Clinic Health Letter, 2012).

Pediatric

- Recommend that families eat together for at least one meal per day.
- Recommend involving the family in planning meals and food preparation. Children can learn about nutrition as they help plan and make meals.
- Suggest that parents work at being good role models of healthy eating.
- Recommend that the family try new foods, either a new food or recipe every week.
- Suggest the parents keep healthy snacks on hand. Store the snacks in a purse, the car, a desk drawer.
- Plan ahead before eating out.

Geriatric

- Use a nutritional screening tool designed for older adults, such as the Mini Nutrition Assessment (MNA), the Malnutrition Universal Screening Tool (MUST), or the Nutrition Risk Screening (NRS).
- Assess changes in lifestyle and eating patterns. Older clients need to decrease portion size as they age because they do not burn as many calories as when they were younger.
- Assess fluid intake. Recommend routine drinks of water regardless of thirst. Monitor older adults for deficient fluid volume carefully, noting new onset of weakness, dizziness, and postural hypotension.
- Observe for socioeconomic factors that influence food choices (e.g., funds, cooking facilities, food insecurity).

Multicultural

- Assess for the influence of cultural beliefs, norms, and values on the client's nutritional knowledge.
- Tailor nutritional interventions to be consistent with cultural beliefs, norms, and values.
- Offer tailored lifestyle counseling via the telephone.

Client/Family Teaching and Discharge Planning

- The majority of the preceding interventions involve teaching.
- Work with family members regarding information on how to improve nutritional status.

• = Independent ▲ = Collaborative

Imbalanced Nutrition: less than body requirements

NANDA-I Definition

Intake of nutrients insufficient to meet metabolic needs

Defining Characteristics

Abdominal cramping; abdominal pain; alteration in taste sensation; body weight 20% or more below ideal weight range; capillary fragility; diarrhea; excessive loss of hair; food aversion; food intake less than recommended daily allowance; hyperactive bowel sounds; insufficient information; insufficient interest in food; insufficient muscle tone; misinformation; misperception; pale mucous membranes; perceived inability to ingest food; satiety immediately upon ingesting food; sore buccal cavity; weakness of muscles required for mastication; weakness of muscles required for swallowing; weight loss with adequate food intake

Related Factors (r/t)

Biological factors; economically disadvantaged; inability to absorb nutrients; inability to digest food; inability to ingest food; insufficient dietary intake; psychological factors

Client Outcomes

Client Will (Specify Time Frame)

- Progressively gain weight toward desired goal
- Weigh within normal range for height and age
- Recognize factors contributing to being underweight
- Identify nutritional requirements
- Consume adequate nourishment
- Be free of signs of malnutrition

Nursing Interventions

▲ Conduct a nutrition screen on all clients within 24 hours of admission and refer to a dietitian as deemed necessary.

▲ The screening tool should be based on the client population, and the validity and reliability of the screening tool. The 3-Minute Nutrition Screening (3-MinNS) tool, for example, assesses weight loss, dietary intake, and muscle wasting.

- Recognize the importance of rescreening and monitoring oral intake in hospitalized individuals to help facilitate the early identification and prevention of nutritional decline.

- Recognize the characteristics that classify individuals as malnourished and refer to a dietitian for a complex nutritional assessment and intervention.

• = Independent   ▲ = Collaborative

- Recognize clients who are likely to experience malnutrition in the context of social or environmental circumstances, characterized by pure chronic starvation and anorexia nervosa without the presence of an inflammatory process (White et al, 2012).
  - ○ Chronic disease-related malnutrition: those with organ failure, pancreatic cancer, rheumatoid arthritis, sarcopenic obesity
  - ○ Acute disease or injury-related malnutrition: those with major infection, burns, trauma, closed head injuries accompanied by a marked inflammatory response (White et al, 2012).
- ▲ Note laboratory values cautiously; albumin and prealbumin may be indicators of the inflammatory response that often accompanies acute malnutrition.
- Weigh the client daily in acute care, weekly to monthly in extended care at the same time (usually before breakfast), with same amount of clothing.
- Observe for potential barriers to eating such as willingness, ability, and appetite.

NOTE: If the client is unable to feed self, refer to nursing interventions for Feeding **Self-Care** deficit. If the client has difficulty swallowing, refer to nursing interventions for Impaired **Swallowing.** If the client is receiving tube feedings, refer to the nursing interventions for Risk for **Aspiration.**

- Advocate for the implementation of a feeding protocol, if not already in place, to avoid unnecessary and/or prolonged nothing per os (mouth)/clear liquid (NPO/CL) status in hospitalized clients.
- For the client with anorexia nervosa, consider offering high-calorie foods and snacks often.
- For the client who is able to eat but has a decreased appetite, try the following activities:
  - ○ Offer oral nutritional supplements (ONS) early after admission and continue to encourage intake of ONS throughout the hospital stay.
  - ○ Avoid interruptions during mealtimes and offer companionship; meals should be eaten in a calm and peaceful environment.
  - ○ Allow for access to meals or snacks during "off times" if the client is not available at time of meal delivery, monitor food and ONS intake, and communicate with dietitian/health care provider.
  - ○ If the client lacks endurance, schedule rest periods before meals, and open packages and cut up food for the client.

• = Independent   ▲ = Collaborative

- For the client with fracture due to fall, consider the need for vitamin D supplementation.
- For the client who has had a stroke, repeat nutritional screenings weekly and provide timely interventions for those at risk or who may already be malnourished.
- Recognize the importance of offering high-protein foods to most hospitalized individuals (use caution with those with compromised renal/liver function).
- Monitor state of oral cavity (gums, tongue, mucosa, teeth). Provide good oral hygiene before each meal.
- ▲ Administer antiemetics and pain medications as ordered and needed before meals.
- Anorexia. If client is nauseated, remove cover of food tray before bringing it into the client's room.
- Work with the client to develop a plan for increased activity.

Critical Care

- Recognize the need to begin enteral feeding within 24 to 48 hours of admission to the critical care environment, once the client is free of hemodynamic compromise, if the client is unable to eat.
- Recognize that it is important to administer feedings to the client and that frequently checking for gastric residual and fasting clients for procedures can be a limiting factor to adequate nutrition in the tube-fed client.

Pediatric

- ▲ Use a nutritional screening tool designed for nurses such as the Paediatric Yorkhill Malnutrition Score (PYMS) tool, and if the child has a score of 2 or more, make a referral to a dietitian.
- Watch for symptoms of malnutrition in the child including short stature, thin arms and legs, poor condition of skin and hair, visible vertebrae and rib cage, wasted buttocks, wasted facial appearance, lethargy, and, in extreme cases, edema.
- Weigh and measure the length (height) of the child, and use a growth chart to help determine growth pattern, which reflects nutrition.
- ▲ Refer to a health care provider and a dietitian a child who is underweight for any reason.
- Work with the child and parents to develop an appropriate weight gain plan.

• = Independent   ▲ = Collaborative

- Recognize that a large percentage of girls and teenagers are dieting, which can result in nutritional problems.

Geriatric
- Screen for malnutrition in older clients.
- Screen for dysphagia in all older clients.
- Recognize that geriatric clients with moderate or severe cognition impairment have a significant risk for developing malnutrition.
▲ Interpret laboratory findings cautiously. Watch the color of urine for an indication of fluid balance; darker urine demonstrates dehydration. Low axillary moisture could indicate mild to moderate dehydration.
- Consider using dining assistants, trained non-nursing staff, to provide feeding assistance care in extended care facilities to ensure adequate time for feeding clients as needed.
- Consider offering healthy snacks such as yogurt, which is a good source of protein, calcium, zinc, B vitamins, and probiotics.
- Encourage high-protein foods for the older client, unless medically contraindicated by organ failure.
- Encourage physical activity throughout the day as tolerated.
- Recognize the implications of malnutrition on client strength and mobility.
- Consider the need for a multivitamin if food intake is low.
- Monitor for onset of depression.
- Consider offering nutritional supplement drinks served in a glass rather than with a straw inserted directly into the container.
- Recommend to families that enteral feedings may or may not be indicated for clients with dementia (Chang and Roberts, 2011).

NOTE: If the client is unable to feed self, refer to nursing interventions for Feeding **Self-Care** deficit. If client has impaired physical function, malnutrition, depression, or cognitive impairment, refer to care plan for **Frail Elderly** syndrome.
- Emphasize importance of good oral care in the older client.
- Consult the dietitian if the client has pressure ulcers.

Home Care
- The preceding interventions may be adapted for home care use.
- Screen for malnutrition using the MUST, which is easy and simple. Recognize that the client may also use MUST as a self-screening tool in the home setting.

- Monitor food intake. Instruct the client in intake of small frequent meals of foods with increased calories and protein.
- Assess the client's willingness to eat.
- Consider social factors that may interfere with nutrition (e.g., lack of transportation, inadequate income, lack of social support).
- Continue to encourage intake of ONS to help optimize oral intake.
▲ Recognize that the client on home parenteral nutrition requires regularly scheduled lab work for electrolyte monitoring.

Client/Family Teaching and Discharge Planning

- Help the client/family identify the area to change that will make the greatest contribution to improved nutrition.
- Build on the strengths in the client/family's food habits. Adapt changes to their current practices.
- Select appropriate teaching aids for the client/family's background.
- Implement instructional follow-up to answer the client/family's questions.
- Recommend that clients discuss with their primary health care provider before taking any supplements such as vitamins and minerals.
- Suggest community resources, such as Meals on Wheels and community centers, as suitable food sources.
- Teach the client and family how to manage tube feedings or parenteral therapy at home as needed.

Obesity
NANDA-I Definition

A condition in which an individual accumulates abnormal or excessive fat for age and gender that exceeds overweight

Defining Characteristics

ADULT: Body mass index (BMI) >30 kg/m^2; CHILD <2 years: term not used with children at this age; CHILD 2 to 18 years: BMI >30 kg/m^2 or >95th percentile for age and gender

Related Factors

Average daily physical activity is less than recommended for gender and age; consumption of sugar-sweetened beverages; disordered eating behaviors; disordered eating perceptions; economically disadvantaged; energy expenditure below energy intake based on standard assessment (e.g., WAVE assessment [weight, activity, variety in diet, excess]); excessive alcohol consumption; fear regarding lack of food supply; formula- or mixed-fed infants; frequent snacking; genetic disorder; heritability of interrelated factors (e.g., adipose tissue distribution, energy expenditure, lipoprotein lipase activity, lipid synthesis, lipolysis); high disinhibition and restraint eating behavior score; high frequency of eating restaurant or fried food; low dietary calcium intake in children; maternal diabetes mellitus; maternal smoking; overweight in infancy; parental obesity; portion sizes larger than recommended; premature pubarche; rapid weight gain during childhood; rapid weight gain during infancy, including the first week, first 4 months, and first year; sedentary behavior occurring more than 2 hours per day; shortened sleep time; sleep disorder; solid foods as major food source in infants younger than 5 months of age

Client Outcomes

Client Will (Specify Time Frame)

- Explain how to eat according to the U.S. Dietary Guidelines
- Design dietary modifications to meet individual long-term goal of health, using principles of variety, balance, and moderation
- Maintain weight within normal range for height and age

Nursing Interventions

- Assess the meaning and importance of food in the client's life.
- Counsel the client to eat breakfast daily.
- Assess the client with a Patient Readiness Scale to determine if the client is ready to discuss weight loss and/or would like weight loss information.
- Assess the client's current nutrition through a 1- to 3-day food diary in which everything ingested orally is recorded. Analyze the following areas:
  - Intake of food and beverage calories and fat
  - Portion sizes
  - Underconsumption or overconsumption of nutrients
  - Use of supplements
  - Use of meal replacements
  - Timing/consistency of meals and snacks
- Counsel the client to measure regularly consumed foods periodically. Help the client to learn usual portion sizes.
- Assist the client to develop a system of self-management, which may include self-monitoring of weight, BMI, and food intake; interpreting food labels; portion control; recipe modification; restaurant and social food negotiation; and physical activity.

• = Independent   ▲ = Collaborative

- Document the client's height and weight and teach significance of his/her BMI in relationship to current health.
- Assist the client to use Super Tracker (http://www.choosemyplate .gov/food-groups) to determine the number of calories to eat and gain more information on how to eat in a healthy fashion.
- Encourage the client to engage in regular physical activity for at least 150 minutes weekly.
- Recommend the client eat a healthy breakfast every morning.
- Recommend the client avoid eating in fast-food restaurants.
- Assist the client to reframe slips in weight loss or physical activity behavior as lapses that are a single event and not a full return to previous unhealthy behaviors.
- Teach problem-solving strategies to deal with barriers to changing eating and physical activity patterns.
- Assist clients to engage their social support systems in ways that facilitate weight loss, as well as eating and physical activity behavior change.
- Assist the client to reframe the goal focus from outcome (weight loss) to process (eating behaviors) for weight loss.
- Assist the client to develop stimulus control techniques designed to reduce environmental cues associated with eating behaviors. Specifically, clients should be taught to limit the presence of high-calorie/high-fat foods in the home; to reduce the visibility of unhealthy food choices in the home; to limit where and when they eat; to avoid distractions like reading, using the computer, or watching television when eating; and to eat more slowly.
- Use the motivational interviewing technique when working with clients to promote healthy eating and weight loss.
- Refer the client to tailored weight management programs that provide opportunities for ongoing support.
- Refer the client to a weight-loss–related therapy group.
- Recommend that clients use dietary supplements such as vitamins and minerals after consulting with their primary health care provider.
- Behavior methods of losing weight are diverse and effective for weight loss through developing methods to control eating behavior, changing habits, and mindset.

Pediatric

- Offer obese or overweight adolescents healthy methods for weight loss.

• = Independent   ▲ = Collaborative

- Offer families of obese or overweight children prejudice-free, individually accepting, and supportive interventions to address weight loss.
- Use motivational interviewing counseling techniques to implement weight loss interventions.
- Recommend that families eat together for at least one meal per day.
- Recommend involving the family in planning meals and food preparation. Children can learn about nutrition as they help plan and make meals.
- Suggest that parents work at being good role models of healthy eating.
- Recommend that the family try new foods, either a new food or recipe every week.
- Suggest the parents keep healthy snacks on hand. Store the snacks in a purse, the car, a desk drawer.

Geriatric

- Recognize that it is generally not appropriate to have an older client on a calorie-restrictive diet.
- Observe for socioeconomic factors that influence food choices (e.g., funds, cooking facilities, food insecurity).

Multicultural

- Tailor nutritional interventions to be consistent with cultural beliefs, norms, and values.
- Offer tailored lifestyle counseling via the telephone.
- Integrate weight loss and weight maintenance interventions with church faith based concepts for cultural congruence with African American clients.

Client/Family Teaching and Discharge Planning

- The majority of the preceding interventions involve teaching.
- Work with the family members regarding information on how to support and promote weight loss and healthy intakes.

Impaired Oral Mucous Membrane

NANDA-I Definition

Injury to the lips, soft tissue, buccal cavity, and/or oropharynx

Defining Characteristics

Bad taste in mouth; bleeding; cheilitis; coated tongue; decrease in taste sensation; desquamation; difficulty eating; difficulty speaking; enlarged tonsils; exposure to pathogen; fissures; geographic tongue; gingival hyperplasia; gingival pallor; gingival recession; halitosis; hyperemia; impaired ability to swallow; macroplasia; mucosal denudation; oral discomfort; oral edema; oral fissure; oral lesion; oral mucosal pallor; oral nodule; oral pain; oral papule; oral ulcer; oral vesicles; presence of mass (e.g., hemangioma); purulent oral-nasal drainage; purulent oral-nasal exudates; smooth atrophic tongue; spongy patches in mouth; stomatitis; white patches in mouth; white plaque in mouth; white, curd-like oral exudate; xerostomia

Related Factors (r/t)

Alcohol consumption; allergy; alteration in cognitive functioning; autoimmune disease; autosomal disorder; barrier to dental care; barrier to oral self-care; behavior disorder (e.g., attention deficit, oppositional defiant); chemical injury agent (e.g., burn, capsaicin, methylene chloride, mustard agent); cleft lip; cleft palate; decrease in hormone level in women; decrease in platelets; decrease in salivation; dehydration; depression; immunodeficiency; immunosuppression; infection; insufficient knowledge of oral hygiene; insufficient oral hygiene; loss of oral support structure; malnutrition; mechanical factor (e.g., ill-fitting dentures, braces, endotracheal/nasogastric tube, oral surgery); mouth breathing; nil per os (NPO) more than 24 hours; oral trauma; smoking; stressors; syndrome (e.g., Sjögren's); treatment regimen

Client Outcomes

Client Will (Specify Time Frame)

- Maintain intact, moist oral mucous membranes that are free of ulceration, inflammation, infection, and debris
- Demonstrate measures to maintain or regain intact oral mucous membranes

Nursing Interventions

- ▲ Inspect the oral cavity/teeth at least once daily and note any discoloration, presence of debris, amount of plaque buildup, presence of lesions such as white lesions or patches, edema, or bleeding, and intactness of teeth. Refer to a dentist or periodontist as appropriate.
- • If the client does not have a bleeding disorder and is able to swallow, encourage the client to brush the teeth with a soft toothbrush using fluoride-containing toothpaste at least twice per day.
- • Recommend the client use a powered toothbrush if desired for removal of dental plaque and prevent gingivitis.

• = Independent   ▲ = Collaborative

- Use foam sticks to moisten the oral mucous membranes, clean out debris, and swab out the mouth of the edentulous client. **Do not use foam sticks to clean the teeth** unless the platelet count is very low and the client is prone to bleeding gums. Foam sticks are useful for cleansing the oral cavity of a client who is edentulous.
- If the client does not have a bleeding disorder, encourage the client to floss once per day or use an interdental cleaner.
- Use an antimicrobial mouthwash as ordered or tap water or saline only for a mouth rinse. Do not use commercial mouthwashes containing alcohol or hydrogen peroxide. Also, do not use lemon-glycerin swabs.
- Provide oral hygiene if the client is unable to care for himself/herself. The nursing diagnosis Bathing **Self-Care** deficit is then applicable.
- If the client is unable to brush own teeth, follow this procedure:
  ○ Position the client sitting upright or on side.
  ○ Use a soft bristle toothbrush.
  ○ Use fluoride toothpaste and tap water or saline as a solution.
  ○ Brush teeth in an up-and-down manner.
  ○ Suction as needed.
- Monitor the client's nutritional and fluid status to determine if it is adequate. Refer to the care plan for Deficient **Fluid** volume or Imbalanced **Nutrition:** less than body requirements if applicable.
- Encourage fluid intake of up to 3000 mL/day if not contraindicated by the client's medical condition.
- Determine the client's usual method of oral care and address any concerns regarding oral hygiene.
▲ If the client has a dry mouth (xerostomia):
  ○ Recognize that more than 500 medications may cause xerostomia, and at times the medication can be discontinued to increase the client's comfort (Schub et al, 2010a).
  ○ Provide saliva substitutes as ordered.
  ○ Suggest the client chew sugarless gum or sugarless sour candy to promote salivary flow.
  ○ Examine the oral cavity for signs of mucositis ulceration and oral candidiasis.
- Recommend the client decrease or preferably stop intake of soft drinks. Sugar-containing soft drinks can cause cavities, and the low pH of the drink can cause erosion in teeth (ADA, 2015a).

• = Independent   ▲ = Collaborative

- If client has halitosis, review good oral care with the client including brushing teeth, using floss, and brushing the tongue. Halitosis can be a beginning sign of gingivitis and can be eradicated by a good program of dental hygiene (ADA, 2015b).
- Instruct the client with halitosis to clean the tongue when performing oral hygiene; brush tongue with tongue scraper or toothbrush and follow with a mouth rinse.
▲ Assess the client for underlying medical condition that may be causing halitosis.
- Keep the lips well lubricated using a lip balm that is water- or aloe-based.

Client Receiving Chemotherapy/Radiation

- Ensure that the client receives a comprehensive oral examination before initiation of chemotherapy or radiation, with aggressive preventive dental care given as needed (Radvansky et al, 2013).
- Provide both verbal and written instruction about the need for and method of providing frequent oral care to the client before radiation therapy or chemotherapy. Assess the condition of the oral cavity daily in the client receiving radiation or chemotherapy (Radvansky et al, 2013).
- For measurement of presence or severity of mucositis, use the Oral Mucositis Assessment Scale (OMAS).
- Use a protocol to prevent/treat mucositis that includes the following:
  ○ Use a soft toothbrush that is replaced on a regular basis; brush teeth at least two times a day and for at least 90 seconds.
  ○ Continue to floss teeth daily.
  ○ Use a bland, alcohol-free rinse to remove debris and moisten the oral cavity. Rinse the mouth often (every 2 hours while awake) if the client has mouth sores.
  ○ Avoid tobacco, alcohol, and irritating foods (hot, rough, acidic, or spicy).
  ○ Use a valid and reliable pain assessment tool and treatment of pain as needed.
- Help the client use a mouth rinse of normal saline or salt and soda every 1 to 2 hours for prevention and treatment of stomatitis. A typical mixture is 1 teaspoon of salt or sodium bicarbonate per pint of water. Clients are directed to take a tablespoon of the rinse and swish it in the mouth for 30 seconds, then expectorate.

• = Independent ▲ = Collaborative

▲ If the mouth is severely inflamed and it is painful to swallow, contact the health care provider for a topical anesthetic or analgesic order. Modification of oral intake (e.g., soft or liquid diet) may also be necessary to prevent friction trauma. The nursing diagnosis Imbalanced **Nutrition:** less than body requirements may apply.

• If the client's platelet count is lower than 50,000/mm^3 or the client has a bleeding disorder, use a specially made toothbrush designed for sensitive or diseased tissue, or a toothette that is not soaked in glycerin or flavorings; if the client cannot tolerate a toothbrush or a toothette, a piece of gauze wrapped around a finger can be used to remove plaque and debris (Radvansky et al, 2013).

Critical Care—Client on a Ventilator

• Use a soft toothbrush to brush teeth to clean the client's teeth at least every 12 hours; use suction to remove secretions. Provide oral moisturizer to oral mucosa and lips every 4 hours. Recognize that good oral care is paramount in the prevention of ventilator-associated events (VAE) and ventilator-associated pneumonia (VAP).

▲ Apply chlorhexidine gluconate mouthwash or gel in the oral cavity after performing tooth brushing, which may reduce the risk of the client developing VAE and VAP.

Geriatric

• Determine the functional ability of the client to provide his/her own oral care. Refer to Bathing **Self-Care** deficit.

• Provide appropriate oral care to older adults with a self-care deficit, brushing the teeth after breakfast and in the evening.

• If the client has dementia or delirium and exhibits care-resistant behavior such as fighting, biting, or refusing care, use the following method:

  ○ Ensure client is in a quiet environment such as own bathroom, sitting or standing at the sink to prime memory for appropriate actions.

  ○ Approach the client at eye level within his/her range of vision.

  ○ Approach with a smile and begin conversation with a touch of the hand and gradually move up.

  ○ Use mirror-mirror technique, standing behind the client, and brush and floss teeth.

  ○ Use respectful adult speech, not elder speak—sing-song voice, calling "dearie," "honey," and so forth.

• = Independent   ▲ = Collaborative

    ○   Promote self-care where client brushes own teeth if possible.
    ○   Use distractors when needed, such as singing, talking, reminiscing, or use of a teddy bear.
- Carefully observe the oral cavity and lips for abnormal lesions such as white or red patches, masses, ulcerations with an indurated margin, or a raised granular lesion.
- Ensure that dentures are removed and cleaned regularly, preferably after every meal and before bedtime.

Home Care

- The interventions described previously may be adapted for home care use.
▲ Instruct the client in ways to soothe the oral cavity (e.g., cool beverages, Popsicles, viscous lidocaine).
▲ If necessary, refer for home health aide services to support the family in oral care and observation of the oral cavity.

Client/Family Teaching and Discharge Planning

- Teach the client how to inspect the oral cavity and monitor for signs and symptoms of infection or complications and when to call the health care provider (Radvansky et al, 2013; Eilers et al, 2014).
- Recommend the client not smoke, use chewing tobacco, or drink excessive amounts of alcohol.
- Teach the client and family if necessary how to perform appropriate mouth care. Use the motivational interviewing technique.

Risk for impaired Oral Mucous Membrane

NANDA-I Definition

Vulnerable to injury to the lips, soft tissues, buccal cavity, and/or oropharynx, which may compromise health

Risk Factors

Alcohol consumption; allergy; alteration in cognitive functioning; autoimmune disease; autosomal disorder; barriers to dental care; barrier to oral self-care; behavior disorder (e.g., attention deficit, oppositional defiant); chemotherapy; decrease in hormone level in women; economically disadvantaged; immunodeficiency; immunosuppression; inadequate nutrition; infection; insufficient knowledge of oral hygiene; insufficient oral hygiene; mechanical factor (e.g., orthodontic appliance, device for ventilation or food, ill-fitting dentures); radiation therapy; smoking; stressors; surgical procedure; syndrome (e.g., Sjögren's); trauma

Client Outcomes, Nursing Interventions, and Client/Family Teaching and Discharge Planning

Refer to care plan for Impaired **Oral Mucous Membrane.**

Overweight
NANDA-I Definition

A condition in which an individual accumulates abnormal or excessive fat for age and gender

Defining Characteristics

Children age 2 or younger

Weight-for-length percentiles >95th percentile

Childhood (age 2 to 18 years)

Body mass index (BMI) >85th but <95th percentile or kg/m² (whichever is smaller)

Adult

BMI >25 kg/m²

Related Factors

Average daily physical activity is less than recommended for gender and age; consumption of sugar-sweetened beverages; disordered eating behaviors (e.g., binge eating, extreme weight control); disordered eating perceptions; economically disadvantaged; energy expenditure below energy intake based on standard assessment (e.g., weight, activity, variety in diet, excess [WAVE] assessment); excessive alcohol consumption; fear regarding lack of food supply; formula or mixed fed infants; frequent snaking; genetic disorder heritability of interrelated factors (e.g., adipose tissue distribution, energy expenditure, lipoprotein lipase activity, lipid synthesis, lipolysis); high disinhibition and restraint eating behavior score; high frequency of restaurant or fried food; low dietary calcium intake in children; maternal diabetes mellitus; maternal smoking; obesity in childhood; parental obesity; portion sizes larger than recommended; premature pubarche; rapid weight gain during childhood; rapid weight gain during infancy, including the first week, first 4 months, and first year; sedentary behavior occurring for >2 hours/day; shortened sleep time; sleep disorder; solid foods as major food source at <5 months of age

• = Independent ▲ = Collaborative

Nursing Interventions

- Assess the meaning and importance of food in the client's life.
- Counsel the client to eat breakfast daily.
- Assess the client with a Patient Readiness Scale to determine if the client is ready to discuss weight loss and/or would like weight loss information.
- Assess the client's current nutrition through a 1- to 3-day food diary in which everything ingested orally is recorded. Analyze the following areas:
  - Intake of food and beverage calories and fat
  - Portion sizes
  - Underconsumption or overconsumption of nutrients
  - Use of supplements
  - Use of meal replacements
  - Timing/consistency of meals and snacks
- Counsel the client to measure regularly consumed foods periodically. Help the client learn usual portion sizes. Measuring food alerts the client to normal portion sizes. Estimating amounts can be extremely inaccurate.
- Assist the client to develop a system of self-management, which may include self-monitoring of weight, BMI, and food intake; interpreting food labels; portion control; recipe modification; restaurant and social food negotiation; and physical activity.
- Document the client's height and weight and teach significance of his/her BMI in relationship to current health. Use a chart or a website such as http://www.cdc.gov/healthyweight/assessing/bmi/index.html.
- Assist the client to use Super Tracker (http://www.choosemyplate.gov/food-groups) to determine the number of calories to eat and gain more information on how to eat in a healthy fashion. To lose weight, the client must eat fewer calories.
- Encourage the client to engage in regular physical activity for at least 150 minutes weekly.
- Recommend the client eat a healthy breakfast every morning.
- Recommend the client avoid eating in fast-food restaurants.
- Assist the client to reframe slips in weight loss or physical activity behavior as lapses that are a single event and not a full return to previous unhealthy behaviors.

O

• = Independent ▲ = Collaborative

- Teach problem-solving strategies to deal with barriers to changing eating and physical activity patterns.
- Assist clients to engage their social support systems in ways that facilitate weight loss, as well as eating and physical activity behavior change.
- Assist the client to reframe the goal focus from outcome (weight loss) to process (eating behaviors) for weight loss.
- Assist the client to develop stimulus control techniques designed to reduce environmental cues associated with eating behaviors. Specifically clients should be taught to limit the presence of high-calorie/high-fat foods in the home; to reduce the visibility of unhealthy food choices in the home; to limit where and when they eat; to avoid distractions like reading, using the computer, or watching television when eating; and to eat more slowly.
- Use the motivational interviewing technique when working with clients to promote healthy eating and weight loss.
- Refer the client to tailored weight management programs that provide opportunities for ongoing support.
- Refer the client to a weight-loss–related therapy group.
- Recommend that clients use dietary supplements such as vitamins and minerals after consulting with their primary health care provider.
- Behavior methods of losing weight are diverse and effective for weight loss through developing methods to control eating behavior, changing habits, and mindset.

Pediatric

- Offer obese or overweight adolescents healthy methods for weight loss.
- Offer families of obese or overweight children prejudice-free, individually accepting, and supportive interventions to address weight loss.
- Recommend that families eat together for at least one meal per day.
- Recommend involving the family in planning meals and food preparation. Children can learn about nutrition as they help plan and make meals.
- Suggest that parents work at being good role models of healthy eating.
- Recommend that the family try new foods, either a new food or recipe every week.

• = Independent   ▲ = Collaborative

- Suggest the parents keep healthy snacks on hand. Store the snacks in a purse, the car, and a desk drawer.

Geriatric
- Recognize that it is generally not appropriate to have an older client on a calorie-restrictive diet.
- Observe for socioeconomic factors that influence food choices (e.g., funds, cooking facilities, food insecurity).

Multicultural
- Tailor nutritional interventions to be consistent with cultural beliefs, norms, and values.
- Offer tailored lifestyle counseling via the telephone.
- Integrate weight loss and weight maintenance interventions with church faith based concepts for cultural congruence with African American clients.

Client/Family Teaching and Discharge Planning
- The majority of the preceding interventions involve teaching.
- Work with the family members regarding information on how to support and promote weight loss and healthy intakes.

0

Risk for Overweight*

NANDA-I Definition

Vulnerable to abnormal or excessive fat accumulation for age and gender, which may compromise health

Risk Factors

ADULT: Body mass index (BMI) approaching 25 kg/m^2; average daily physical activity is less than recommended for gender and age; CHILD older than 2 years: weight for length approaching 95th percentile; CHILD 2 to 18 years: BMI approaching 85th percentile, or 25 kg/m^2 (whichever is smaller); children who are crossing BMI percentiles upward; children with high BMI percentiles; consumption of sugar-sweetened beverages; disordered eating behaviors (e.g., binge eating, extreme weight control); disordered eating perceptions; eating in response to external cues (e.g., time of day, social situations); eating in response to internal cues other than hunger (e.g., anxiety); economically disadvantaged; energy expenditure below energy intake based on standard assessment (e.g., WAVE

---

*Previously Risk for imbalanced Nutrition: more than body requirements

• = Independent   ▲ = Collaborative

[weight, activity, variety in diet, excess]); excessive alcohol consumption; fear regarding lack of food supply; formula- or mixed-fed infants; frequent snacking; genetic disorder; heritability of interrelated factors (e.g., adipose tissue distribution, energy expenditure, lipoprotein lipase activity, lipid synthesis, lipolysis); high disinhibition and restraint eating behavior score; high frequency of eating restaurant or fried food; higher baseline weight at beginning of each pregnancy; low dietary calcium intake in children; maternal diabetes mellitus; maternal smoking; obesity in childhood; parental obesity; portion sizes larger than recommended; premature pubarche; rapid weight gain during childhood; rapid weight gain during infancy, including the first week, first 4 months, and the first year; sedentary behavior occurring for more than 2 hours per day; shortened sleep time; sleep disorder; solid foods as major food sources of less than 5 months of age

Nursing Interventions

- Assess the meaning and importance of food in the client's life.
- Counsel the client to eat breakfast daily.
- Assess the client with a Patient Readiness Scale to determine if the client is ready to discuss weight loss and/or would like weight loss information.
- Assess the client's current nutrition through a 1- to 3-day food diary in which everything ingested orally is recorded. Analyze the following areas:
  ○ Intake of food and beverage calories and fat
  ○ Portion sizes
  ○ Underconsumption or overconsumption of nutrients
  ○ Use of supplements
  ○ Use of meal replacements
  ○ Timing/consistency of meals and snacks
- Counsel the client to measure regularly consumed foods periodically. Help the client learn usual portion sizes.
- Assist the client to develop a system of self-management, which may include self-monitoring of weight, BMI, and food intake; interpretation of food labels; portion control; recipe modification; restaurant and social food negotiation; and physical activity.
- Document the client's height and weight and teach significance of his/her BMI in relationship to current health.

• = Independent   ▲ = Collaborative

- Assist the client to use Super Tracker (http://www.choosemyplate.gov/food-groups) to determine the number of calories to eat and gain more information on how to eat in a healthy fashion.
- Encourage the client to engage in regular physical activity for at least 150 minutes weekly.
- Recommend the client eat a healthy breakfast every morning.
- Recommend the client avoid eating in fast-food restaurants.
- Assist the client to reframe slips in weight loss or physical activity behavior as lapses that are a single event and not a full return to previous unhealthy behaviors.
- Teach problem-solving strategies to deal with barriers to changing eating and physical activity patterns.
- Assist clients to engage their social support systems in ways that facilitate weight loss, as well as eating and physical activity behavior change.
- Assist the client to reframe the goal focus from outcome (weight loss) to process (eating behaviors) for weight loss.
- Assist the client to develop stimulus control techniques designed to reduce environmental cues associated with eating behaviors. Specifically, clients should be taught to limit the presence of high-calorie/high-fat foods in the home; to reduce the visibility of unhealthy food choices in the home; to limit where and when they eat; to avoid distractions like reading, using the computer, or watching television when eating; and to eat more slowly.
- Use the motivational interviewing technique when working with clients to promote healthy eating and weight loss.
- Refer the client to tailored weight management programs that provide opportunities for ongoing support.
- Refer the client to a weight-loss–related therapy group.
- Recommend that clients use dietary supplements such as vitamins and minerals after consulting with their primary health care provider.
- Use behavioral methods to control eating behavior and change habits and mindset.

Pediatric
- Offer obese or overweight adolescents healthy methods for weight loss.
- Offer families of obese or overweight children prejudice-free, individually accepting, and supportive interventions to address weight loss.

- Use motivational interviewing counseling techniques to implement weight loss interventions.
- Recommend that families eat together for at least one meal per day.
- Recommend involving the family in planning meals and food preparation. Children can learn about nutrition as they help plan and make meals.
- Suggest that parents work at being good role models of healthy eating.
- Recommend that the family try new foods, either a new food or recipe every week.
- Suggest the parents keep healthy snacks on hand. Store the snacks in a purse, the car, a desk drawer.

Geriatric
- Recognize that it is generally not appropriate to have an older client on a calorie-restrictive diet.
- Observe for socioeconomic factors that influence food choices (e.g., funds, cooking facilities, food insecurity).

Multicultural
- Tailor nutritional interventions to be consistent with cultural beliefs, norms, and values.
- Offer tailored lifestyle counseling via the telephone.
- Integrate weight loss and weight maintenance interventions with church faith based concepts for cultural congruence with African American clients.

Client/Family Teaching and Discharge Planning
- The majority of the preceding interventions involve teaching.
- Work with the family members regarding information on how to support and promote weight loss and healthy intakes.

Acute Pain
NANDA-I Definition

An unpleasant sensory and emotional experience associated with actual or potential tissue damage, or described in terms of such damage (International Association for the Study of Pain, 1979); sudden or slow onset of any intensity from mild to severe with an anticipated or predictable end

Defining Characteristics

Appetite change; change in physiological parameter (e.g., blood pressure, heart rate, respiratory rate, oxygen saturation, and end-tidal CO_2);

• = Independent   ▲ = Collaborative

diaphoresis; distraction behavior; evidence of pain using standardized pain behavior checklist for those unable to communicate verbally (e.g., Neonatal Infant Pain Scale, Pain Assessment Checklist for Seniors with Limited Ability to Communicate); expressive behavior (e.g., restlessness, crying, vigilance); facial expression of pain (e.g., eyes lack luster, beaten look, fixed or scattered movement, grimace); guarding behavior; hopelessness; narrowed focus (e.g., time, perception, thought processes, interaction with people and environment); positioning to ease pain; protective behavior; proxy report of pain behavior/activity changes (e.g., family member, caregiver); pupil dilation; self-focused; self-report of intensity using standardized pain scale (e.g., Wong-Baker FACES scale, visual analog scale, numerical rating scale); self-report of pain characteristics using standardized pain instrument (e.g., McGill Pain Questionnaire, Brief Pain Inventory)

Related Factors (r/t)

Biological injury agent (e.g., infection, ischemia, neoplasm); chemical injury agent (e.g., burn, capsaicin, methylene chloride, mustard agent); physical injury agent (e.g., abscess, amputation, burn, cut, heavy lifting, operative procedure, trauma, overtraining)

Client Outcomes

Client Will (Specify Time Frame)

For the client who is able to provide a self-report

- Use a self-report pain tool to identify current pain intensity level and establish a comfort-function goal
- Report that pain management regimen achieves comfort-function goal without side effects
- Describe nonpharmacological methods that can be used to help achieve comfort-function goal
- Perform activities of recovery or activities of daily living (ADLs) easily
- Describe how unrelieved pain will be managed
- State ability to obtain sufficient amounts of rest and sleep
- Notify member of the health care team promptly for pain intensity level that is consistently greater than the comfort-function goal, or occurrence of side effects

For the client who is unable to provide a self-report

- Decrease in pain-related behaviors
- Perform activities of recovery or ADLs easily as determined by client condition
- Demonstrate the absence of side effects of analgesics

• = Independent   ▲ = Collaborative

- No pain-related behaviors will be evident in the client who is completely unresponsive; a reasonable outcome is to demonstrate the absence of side effects related to the prescribed pain treatment plan

Nursing Interventions

- During the initial assessment and interview, if the client is experiencing pain, conduct and document a comprehensive pain assessment, using appropriate pain assessment tools. Implement or request orders to implement pain management interventions to achieve a satisfactory level of comfort. Components of this initial assessment include location, quality, onset/duration, temporal profile, intensity, aggravating and alleviating factors, and effects of pain on function and quality of life. **(Please refer to the Hierarchy of Pain Measures presented later for assessment approach in clients who are unable to provide self-report of pain.)**
- Assess if the client is able to provide a self-report of pain intensity, and if so, assess pain intensity level using a valid and reliable self-report pain tool, such as the 0-10 numerical pain rating scale.
- Ask the client to describe prior experiences with pain, effectiveness of pain management interventions, responses to analgesic medications including occurrence of side effects, and concerns about pain and its treatment (e.g., fear about addiction, worries, or anxiety) and informational needs.
- Using a self-report pain tool, ask the client to identify a comfort-function goal that will allow the client to perform necessary or desired activities easily.
- ▲ Describe the adverse effects of unrelieved pain.
- Use the Hierarchy of Pain Measures as a framework for pain assessment (McCaffery et al, 2011): (1) attempt to obtain the client's self-report of pain; (2) consider the client's condition and search for possible causes of pain (e.g., presence of tissue injury, pathological conditions, or exposure to procedures/interventions that are thought to result in pain); (3) observe for behaviors that may indicate pain presence (e.g., facial expressions, crying, restlessness, and changes in activity); (4) evaluate physiological indicators, with the understanding that these are the least sensitive indicators of pain and may be related to conditions other than pain (e.g., shock, hypovolemia, anxiety); and (5) conduct an analgesic trial.
- Assume that pain is present if the client is unable to provide a self-report and has tissue injury, a pathological condition, or has

• = Independent ▲ = Collaborative

undergone a procedure that is thought to produce pain, and conduct an analgesic trial.

▲ Obtain and review an accurate and complete list of medications the client is taking or has taken.

▲ Explain to the client the pain management approach, including pharmacological and nonpharmacological interventions, the assessment and reassessment process, potential side effects, and the importance of prompt reporting of unrelieved pain.

▲ Manage acute pain using a multimodal approach.

▲ Select the route for administration of analgesics based upon client condition and pain characteristics.

▲ Provide perineural infusions and intraspinal analgesia when appropriate and available.

▲ Use diverse analgesic delivery methods such as PCA to increase client's satisfaction with pain management, to lower cost, and to decrease occurrence of adverse reactions.

▲ Administer a nonopioid analgesic for mild to moderate pain and add an opioid analgesic if indicated for moderate to severe acute pain.

• Administer analgesics around-the-clock for continuous pain (expected to be present approximately 50% of the day, such as postoperative pain) and PRN (as needed) for intermittent or breakthrough pain.

• Prevent pain by administering analgesia before painful procedures whenever possible (e.g., endotracheal suctioning, wound care, heel puncture, venipunctures, and peripherally inserted intravenous catheters).

• Administer supplemental analgesic doses as ordered to keep the client's pain level at or below the comfort-function goal, or desired outcome based on clinical judgment or behaviors if client is unable to provide a self-report.

• Perform nursing care during the peak effect of analgesics to optimize client comfort and participation in care.

▲ Discuss the client's fears of undertreated pain, side effects, and addiction.

• The assessment of clients with acute pain on opioids should be done at regular intervals and include frequent assessment of pain level, assessment of respiratory status (including rate, rhythm, noisiness, depth), and systematic assessment of sedation level using a sedation scale (Pasero, 2009b).

• = Independent   ▲ = Collaborative

▲ Provide the client with a stool softener and stimulant to prevent/treat opioid-related constipation, and ask about other opioid related side effects including nausea, pruritus, lack of appetite, and changes in rest and sleep.

- Review the client's pain flow sheet and medication administration record to evaluate effectiveness of pain relief, previous 24-hour opioid requirements, and occurrence of side effects.

- Advocate for the use of "as needed" opioid range orders to provide effective and appropriate pain relief.

- Choose analgesic and dose based on orders that reflect the client's report of pain severity and response to the previous dose in terms of pain relief, occurrence of side effects, and ability to perform the activities of recovery or ADLs.

▲ When converting opioids from parenteral doses to oral doses (the preferred route when the client can tolerate and absorb oral medications), use equianalgesic dosing charts and carefully monitor the client's response to the new medication route and dose.

- Support the client's use of nonpharmacological methods to supplement pharmacological analgesic approaches to help control pain, such as distraction, imagery, music therapy, simple massage, relaxation, and application of heat and cold.

- Assist client to identify resources for coping with psychological impact of pain.

- Teach and implement nonpharmacological interventions when pain is relatively well controlled with pharmacological interventions.

Pediatric

- Assess for the presence of pain using a valid and reliable pain scale based on age, cognitive development, and the child's ability to provide a self-report.

▲ Administer prescribed analgesics using a multimodal approach to treat pain in children, infants, and neonates.

- Prevent procedural pain in neonates, infants, and children by using opioid analgesics and anesthetics, as indicated, in appropriate dosages.

- Use a topical local anesthetic such as *eutectic* mixture of local anesthetics (EMLA) cream or LMX-4 before performing venipuncture in neonates, infants, and children.

- For the neonate, use oral sucrose and nonnutritional sucking (NNS) or human milk for pain of short duration such as heel stick or

venipuncture. Neonates, especially preterm neonates, are more sensitive to pain than older children.
- Recognize that breastfeeding has been shown to reduce behavioral indicators of pain.

As with adults, use nonpharmacological analgesic interventions to supplement, not replace, pharmacological interventions in pediatric clients.

Geriatric
- Refer to the nursing interventions in the care plan for Chronic **Pain**.

Multicultural
- Refer to the nursing interventions in the care plan for Chronic **Pain**.

Home Care
- ▲ Develop the treatment plan with the client and caregivers.
- ▲ Assess the client's full medication profile, including medications prescribed by all health care providers and all over-the-counter medications for drug interactions, and instruct the client to refrain from mixing medications without health care provider approval.
- ▲ Assess the client/family's knowledge of side effects and safety precautions associated with pain medications.
- If medication is administered using highly technological methods, assess the home for the necessary resources (e.g., electricity) and ensure that there will be responsible caregivers available to assist the client with administration.
- Assess the knowledge base of the client and family with regard to highly technological medication administration and provide necessary education, including the procedure to follow if analgesia is unsatisfactory.

Client/Family Teaching and Discharge Planning
NOTE: To avoid the negative connotations associated with the words "drugs" and "narcotics," use the term "pain medicine" when teaching clients.
- Discuss the various discomforts encompassed by the word "pain" and ask the client to give examples of previously experienced pain. Explain the pain assessment process and the purpose of the pain rating scale.
- Teach the client to use the self-report pain tool to rate the intensity of past or current pain. Ask the client to set a comfort-function goal

• = Independent   ▲ = Collaborative

by selecting a pain level on the self-report tool that will allow performance of desired or necessary activities of recovery with relative ease (e.g., turn, cough, deep breathe, ambulate, participate in physical therapy). If the pain level is consistently above the comfort-function goal, the client should take action that decreases pain or notify a member of the health care team so that effective pain management interventions may be implemented promptly.

• Provide written educational materials on various aspects of pain control to improve client understanding of pain and pain-related interventions.

• Discuss and evaluate the client's understanding about the total plan for pharmacological and nonpharmacological treatment, including the medication plan for around-the-clock administration and supplemental doses, and the use of supplies and equipment.

• Teach basic principles of pain management using a variety of educational strategies, and evaluate learning.

▲ Reinforce the importance of taking pain medications to maintain the comfort-function goal.

▲ Reinforce that taking opioids for pain relief is not addiction and that addiction is very unlikely to occur.

▲ Demonstrate the use of appropriate nonpharmacological approaches in addition to pharmacological approaches to help control pain, such as application of heat and/or cold, distraction techniques, relaxation breathing, visualization, rocking, stroking, listening to music, and watching television.

Chronic Pain
NANDA-I Definition

Unpleasant sensory and emotional experience associated with actual or potential tissue damage, or described in terms of such damage (International Association for the Study of Pain, 1979); sudden or slow onset of any intensity from mild to severe, constant or recurring without an anticipated or predictable end and a duration of greater than 3 months

Defining Characteristics

Alteration in ability to continue previous activities; alteration in sleep pattern; anorexia; evidence of pain using standardized pain behavior checklist for those unable to communicate verbally (e.g., Neonatal Infant Pain Scale, Pain Assessment Checklist for Seniors with Limited Ability

• = Independent   ▲ = Collaborative

to Communicate); facial expression of pain (e.g., eyes lack luster, beaten look, fixed or scattered movement, grimace); proxy report of pain behavior/activity changes (e.g., family member, caregiver); self-focused; self-report of intensity using standardized pain scale (e.g., Wong-Baker FACES scale, visual analog scale, numerical rating scale); self-report of pain characteristics using standardized pain instrument (e.g., McGill Pain Questionnaire, Brief Pain Inventory)

Related Factors (r/t)

Age older than 50 years; alteration in sleep pattern; chronic musculoskeletal condition; contusion; crush injury; damage to the nervous system; emotional distress; fatigue; female gender; fracture; genetic disorder; history of abuse (e.g., physical, psychological, sexual); history of genital mutilation; history of indebtedness; history of static work postures; history of substance abuse; history of vigorous exercise; imbalance of neurotransmitters, neuromodulators, and receptors; immune disorder (e.g., HIV-associated neuropathy, varicella-zoster virus); impaired metabolic functioning; increase in body mass index; ineffective sexuality pattern; injury agent (may be present, but not required; pain may be of unknown etiology); ischemic condition; malnutrition; muscle injury; nerve compression; post-trauma related condition (e.g., infection, inflammation); prolonged computer use (>20 hours/week); prolonged increase in cortisol level; repeated handling of heavy loads; social isolation; spinal cord injury; tumor infiltration; whole-body vibration

Client Outcomes

Client Will (Specify Time Frame)

For the client who is able to provide a self-report

- Provide a description of the pain experience including physical, social, emotional, and spiritual aspects
- Use a self-report pain tool to identify current pain level and establish a comfort-function goal
- Report that the pain management regimen achieves comfort-function goal without the occurrence of side effects
- Describe nonpharmacological methods that can be used to supplement, or enhance, pharmacological interventions and help achieve the comfort-function goal
- Perform necessary or desired activities at a pain level less than or equal to the comfort-function goal
- Demonstrate the ability to pace activity, taking rest breaks before they are needed
- Describe how unrelieved pain will be managed

• = Independent   ▲ = Collaborative

- State the ability to obtain sufficient amounts of rest and sleep
- Notify a member of the health care team for pain level consistently greater than the comfort-function goal or occurrence of side effect

For the client who is unable to provide a self-report

- Demonstrate decreased or resolved pain-related behaviors
- Perform desired activities as determined by client condition
- Demonstrate the absence of side effects
- No pain-related behaviors will be evident in the client who is completely unresponsive; a reasonable outcome is to demonstrate the absence of side effects related to the prescribed pain treatment plan

Nursing Interventions

▲ During the initial assessment and interview, if the client is experiencing pain, conduct and document a comprehensive pain assessment, using appropriate pain assessment tools.

▲ Determine the quality of the pain and whether the pain has persisted beyond the usual duration for tissue healing. **Please refer to the acute Pain section for the Hierarchy of Pain Measures for assessment approach in clients who are unable to provide self-report of pain.**

▲ Assess pain intensity level in a client using valid and reliable self-report pain tools, such as the 0-10 numerical pain rating scale (NRS), pain relief scale (PRS), or chronic pain grade scale.

▲ Ask the client to describe prior experiences with pain, effectiveness of pain management interventions, responses to analgesic medications including occurrence of side effects, and concerns about pain and its treatment (e.g., fear about addiction, worries, or anxiety) and informational needs.

• Using a self-report tool, ask the client to identify a comfort-function goal that will allow the client to perform necessary or desired activities easily. Assess the client for the presence of acute pain (see care plan for Acute **Pain**).

▲ Assess chronic pain regularly including the impact of chronic pain on activity, sleep, eating habits, social conditions including relationships, finances, and employment.

▲ Assess the client for the presence of psychiatric conditions, including anxiety and depression.

▲ If opioid therapy is considered, assist the provider with aspects of an opioid risk assessment, which includes a comprehensive client interview and examination with a pain focus, mental health screening, use of an opioid risk assessment tool, examination of prescription drug monitoring program results, and urine drug screening.

▲ For the client who is receiving outpatient opioid therapy, at each visit, assess effect of opioids on pain status, function, goal achievement, and presence of side effects including sleep disturbance and sexual dysfunction; assessment for signs of opioid misuse, abuse, and addiction should be included, which may involve the use of random urine drug toxicology screening, pill counts, and review of prescription monitoring database.

• Ask the client to maintain a diary (if able) of pain ratings, timing, precipitating events, medications, and effectiveness of pain management interventions.

▲ Obtain and review an accurate and complete list of medications the client is taking or has taken.

▲ Explain to the client the pain management approach that has been ordered or revised, including therapies, medication administration, side effects, and complications.

• Discuss the client's fears of undertreated pain, addiction, and overdose.

▲ Manage chronic pain using an individualized, multimodal approach.

▲ Select the route of administration of analgesics based on client condition and pain characteristics.

▲ When chronic pain has a neuropathic component, treat with adjuvant analgesics, such as anticonvulsants, antidepressants, and topical local anesthetics.

▲ Administer a nonopioid analgesic for mild to moderate chronic pain and as a component of the treatment for all levels of pain for clients with cancer pain.

▲ Recognize that opioid therapy may be indicated for some clients experiencing chronic pain.

▲ Administer analgesics around-the-clock for continuous pain and PRN (as needed) for intermittent or breakthrough pain as may be experienced by clients with cancer pain.

▲ At regular intervals, assess inpatient clients with chronic pain for opioid-related adverse events and include frequent assessment of pain level, assessment of respiratory status (including rate, rhythm, noisiness, depth), and systematic assessment of sedation level using a sedation scale.

• = Independent   ▲ = Collaborative

▲ Provide the client with a stool softener and stimulant to prevent/treat opioid-related constipation. Ask about other opioid-related side effects including nausea, pruritus, lack of appetite, and changes in rest and sleep.

▲ Question the client about any disruption in sleep.

▲ In addition to administering analgesics, support the client's use of nonpharmacological methods to help control pain, such as distraction, imagery, relaxation, and application of heat and cold.

• Teach and implement nonpharmacological interventions when pain is relatively well controlled with pharmacological interventions.

▲ Encourage the client to plan activities around periods of greatest comfort whenever possible.

▲ Explore appropriate resources for management of pain on a long-term basis (e.g., hospice, pain care center).

▲ If the client has progressive cancer pain, assist the client and family with handling issues related to death and dying and provide access to palliative care programs and hospice services.

Pediatric

• Assess for the presence of pain using a valid and reliable pain scale based on age, cognitive development, and the child's ability to provide a self-report.

▲ Administer prescribed analgesics using a multimodal approach to treat pain in children, infants, and neonates.

• As with adults, use nonpharmacological analgesic interventions to supplement, not replace, pharmacological interventions in pediatric clients.

Geriatric

▲ An older client's report of pain should be taken seriously and assessed and treated.

• When assessing pain, speak clearly, slowly, and loudly enough for the client to hear, ensure hearing aids and glasses are in place as appropriate; enlarge pain scales and written materials; and repeat information as needed.

• Handle the client's body gently and allow the client to move at his or her own speed.

▲ Use nonopioid analgesics for mild to moderate pain.

▲ Use opioids cautiously in the older client with moderate to severe pain.

▲ Avoid the use of meperidine (Demerol) in older clients.

• = Independent   ▲ = Collaborative

▲ Use nonpharmacological approaches in addition to analgesics.
▲ Monitor for signs of depression in older clients and refer to specialists with relevant expertise.

Multicultural
▲ Assess for pain disparities among racial and ethnic minorities.
▲ Assess for the influence of cultural beliefs, norms, and values on the client's perception and experience of pain.
▲ Assess for the effect of fatalism on the client's beliefs regarding the current state of comfort.
▲ Use a family-centered approach to care.
• Use culturally relevant pain scales to assess pain in the client.

Home Care
• The interventions previously described may be adapted for home care use. Refer to the nursing interventions in the care plan for Acute **Pain.**

Client/Family Teaching and Discharge Planning
NOTE: To avoid the negative connotations associated with the words "drugs" and "narcotics," use the term "pain medicine" when teaching clients.

• Discuss the various discomforts encompassed by the word "pain" and ask the client to give examples of previously experienced pain. Explain the pain assessment process and the purpose of the pain rating scale.
• Teach the client that if the pain level is consistently above the comfort-function goal, the client should take action that decreases pain or should notify a member of the health care team so that effective pain management interventions may be implemented promptly. (See information on teaching clients to use the pain rating scale.)
• Provide educational materials on various aspects of pain control to improve client understanding of pain and pain-related interventions.
• Discuss and evaluate the client's understanding about the total plan for pharmacological and nonpharmacological treatment, including the medication plan for around-the-clock administration and supplemental doses, the maintenance of a pain diary, and the use of supplies and equipment.
• Reinforce the importance of taking pain medications to maintain the comfort-function goal.

• = Independent ▲ = Collaborative

▲ Reinforce that taking opioids for pain relief is not addiction and that addiction is very unlikely to occur.

• Demonstrate the use of appropriate nonpharmacological approaches in addition to pharmacological approaches for helping control pain, such as application of heat and/or cold, distraction techniques, relaxation breathing, visualization, rocking, stroking, listening to music, and watching television. Teach these methods when pain is relatively well controlled, because pain interferes with cognition.

▲ Emphasize to the client the importance of participating in a structured, individualized pacing activity and taking rest breaks before they are needed.

• Teach nonpharmacological methods when pain is relatively well controlled.

Labor Pain
NANDA-I Definition

Sensory and emotional experience that varies from pleasant to unpleasant, associated with labor and childbirth

Defining Characteristics

Alteration in blood pressure; alteration in heart rate; alteration in muscle tension; alteration in neuroendocrine functioning; alteration in respiratory rate; alteration in sleep pattern; alteration in urinary functioning; decrease in appetite; diaphoresis; distraction behavior; expressive behavior; facial expression of pain (e.g., eyes lack luster, beaten look, fixed or scattered movement, grimace); increase in appetite; narrowed focus; nausea; pain; perineal pressure; positioning to ease pain; protective behavior; pupil dilation; self-focused; uterine contraction; vomiting

Related Factors (r/t)

Cervical dilation; fetal expulsion

Client Outcomes, Nursing Interventions, and Client/Family Teaching and Discharge Planning

Refer to care plan for Acute **Pain.**

Chronic Pain syndrome
NANDA-I Definition

Recurrent or persistent pain that has lasted at least 3 months and that significantly affects daily functioning or well-being

• = Independent   ▲ = Collaborative

Defining Characteristics

Anxiety; constipation; deficient knowledge; disturbed sleep pattern; fatigue; fear; impaired mood regulation; impaired physical mobility; insomnia; obesity; social isolation; stress overload

Client Outcomes, Nursing Interventions, and Client/Family Teaching and Discharge Planning

Refer to care plan for Acute **Pain** and Chronic **Pain.**

Impaired Parenting

NANDA-I Definition

Inability of the primary caretaker to create, maintain, or regain an environment that promotes the optimum growth and development of the child

Defining Characteristics

Infant/Child

Behavioral disorders (e.g., attention deficit, oppositional defiant); delay in cognitive development; diminished separation anxiety; failure to thrive; frequent accidents; frequent illness; history of abuse (e.g., physical, psychological, sexual); history of trauma (e.g., physical, psychological, sexual); impaired social functioning; insufficient attachment behavior; low academic performance; runaway

Parental

Abandonment; decrease in ability to manage child; decrease in cuddling; deficient parent-child interaction; frustration with child; history of childhood abuse (e.g., physical, psychological, sexual); hostility; inadequate child health maintenance; inappropriate caretaking skills; inappropriate childcare arrangements; inappropriate stimulation (e.g., visual, tactile, auditory); inconsistent behavior management; inconsistent care; inflexibility in meeting needs of child; neglects needs of child; perceived inability to meet child's needs; perceived role inadequacy; punitive; rejection of child; speaks negatively about child; unsafe home environment

Related Factors (r/t)

Infant/Child

Alteration in perceptual abilities; behavior disorder (e.g., attention deficit, oppositional defiant); chronic illness; developmental delay; difficult temperament; disabling condition; gender other than desired; multiple births; parent-child separation; prematurity; temperament conflicts with parental expectations

• = Independent   ▲ = Collaborative

Knowledge

Alteration in cognitive functioning; ineffective communication skills; insufficient cognitive readiness for parenting; insufficient knowledge about child development; insufficient knowledge about child health maintenance; insufficient knowledge about parenting skills; insufficient response to infant cues; low educational level; preference for physical punishment; unrealistic expectation

Physiological

Physical illness

Psychological

Alteration in sleep pattern; closely spaced pregnancies; depression; difficult birthing process; disability condition; high number of pregnancies; history of mental illness; history of substance abuse; insufficient prenatal care; sleep deprivation; young parental age

Social

Change in family unit; compromised home environment; conflict between partners; economically disadvantaged; father of child not involved; history of abuse (e.g., physical, psychological, sexual); history of being abusive; inability to put child's needs before own; inadequate childcare arrangements; ineffective coping strategies; insufficient family cohesiveness; insufficient parental role model; insufficient problem-solving skills; insufficient resources (e.g., financial social, knowledge); insufficient social support; insufficient transportation; insufficient valuing of parenthood; legal difficulty; low self-esteem; mother of child not involved; relocation; single parent; social isolation; stressors; unemployment; unplanned pregnancy; unwanted pregnancy; work difficulty

Client Outcomes

Client Will (Specify Time Frame)

- Initiate appropriate measures to develop a safe, nurturing environment
- Acquire and display attentive, supportive parenting behaviors and child supervision
- Identify appropriate strategies to manage a child's inappropriate behaviors
- Identify strategies to protect child from harm and/or neglect and initiate action when indicated

• = Independent   ▲ = Collaborative

Nursing Interventions

- Use the Parenting Sense of Competence (PSOC) scale to measure parental self-efficacy.
- Examine the characteristics of parenting style and behaviors. Consider dysfunctional child-centered and parent-centered cognitions as potentially critical correlates of abusive behavior.
- ▲ Institute abuse/neglect protection measures if evidence exists of an inability to cope with family stressors or crisis, signs of parental substance abuse are observed, or a significant level of social isolation is apparent.
- ▲ For a mother with a toddler, assess maternal depression. Make appropriate referral.
- Appraise the parent's resources and the availability of social support systems. Determine the single mother's particular sources of support, especially the availability of her own mother and partner. Encourage the use of healthy, strong support systems. Provide education to at-risk parents on behavioral management techniques such as looking ahead, giving good instructions, providing positive reinforcement, redirecting, planned ignoring, and instituting time-outs.
- Promotion of better quality relationships between parents and children is an effective strategy that can lead to enhanced learning. Good quality parenting leads to improved cognitive and social skills for children.
- Support parents' competence in appraising their infant's behavior and responses.
- Aim supportive interventions at minimizing parents' experience of strain.
- Model age-appropriate and cognitively appropriate caregiver skills by doing the following: communicating with the child at an appropriate cognitive level of development, giving the child tasks and responsibilities appropriate to age or functional age/level, instituting safety considerations such as the use of assistive equipment, and encouraging the child to perform activities of daily living as appropriate.
- Encourage mothers to understand and capitalize on their infant's capacity to interact, particularly in the early months of life.
- ▲ Provide programs for homeless mothers with severe mental illness who have lost physical custody of their children.

P

• = Independent   ▲ = Collaborative

▲ Provide a recovery program that includes instruction in parenting skills and child development for mothers who are addicted to cocaine.

• Refer to Readiness for enhanced **Parenting** for additional interventions.

Multicultural

• Acknowledge that value conflicts from acculturation stresses may contribute to increased anxiety and significant conflict with children.

• Approach individuals of color with respect, warmth, and professional courtesy.

• Clarify parents' feelings, expectations, perceptions, and availability regarding participation in the care of their sick child.

• Carefully assess meaning of terms used to describe health status when working with Native Americans.

• Provide support for Chinese families caring for children with disabilities.

• Facilitate modeling and role playing to help the family improve parenting skills.

Home Care

• The interventions previously described may be adapted for home care use.

• Assess parenting stress at each home visit to provide appropriate support and anticipatory guidance to families of children with a chronic disease.

▲ Assess the single mother's history regarding childhood and partner abuse and current status regarding depressive symptoms, abusive parenting attitudes (lack of empathy, favorable opinion of corporal punishment, parent-child role reversal, and inappropriate expectations). Refer for mental health services as indicated.

• Provide a parenting program of Planned Activities Training (PAT).

• Provide follow-up support for the PAT via cell phone and text messaging.

Client/Family Teaching and Discharge Planning

• Consider individual and/or group-based parenting programs for teenaged mothers.

• Consider group-based parenting programs for parents of children younger than 3 years with emotional and behavioral problems.

• Consider group-based parenting programs for parents with anxiety, depression, and/or low self-esteem.

• = Independent   ▲ = Collaborative

- ▲ Refer adolescent parents for comprehensive psychoeducational parenting classes.
- • Parent training is one of the most effective interventions for behavior problems in young children.
- ▲ Initiate referrals to community agencies, parent education programs, stress management training, and social support groups. Consider the use of technology and the media.
- • Provide information regarding available telephone counseling services and Internet support. Refer to the care plans for Risk for disproportionate **Growth,** Risk for delayed **Development,** Risk for impaired **Attachment,** and Readiness for enhanced **Parenting** for additional teaching interventions.

Readiness for enhanced Parenting
NANDA-I Definition

A pattern of providing an environment for children or other dependent persons to nurture growth and development, which can be strengthened

Defining Characteristics

Children express desire to enhance home environment; children express desire to enhance parenting; parent expresses desire to enhance emotional support of children; parent expresses desire to enhance emotional support of other dependent person

Client Outcomes

Client/Family Will (Specify Time Frame)

- • Affirm desire to improve parenting skills to further support growth and development of children
- • Demonstrate loving relationship with children
- • Provide a safe, nurturing environment
- • Assess risks in home/environment and take steps to prevent possibility of harm to children
- • Meet physical, psychosocial, and spiritual needs or seek appropriate assistance

Nursing Interventions

- • Use family-centered care and role modeling for holistic care of families.
- • Assess parents' feelings when dealing with a child who has a chronic illness.

- Promote low-technology interventions, such as massage and multisensory interventions (maternal voice, eye-to-eye contact, and rocking) and music to reduce maternal and infant stress and improve mother-infant relationship.
- Support kangaroo care for infants at risk at birth; keep infants in an upright position in skin-to-skin contact.
- When the person who is ill is the parent, use family-centered assessment skills to determine the impact of an adult's illness on the child, and then guide the parent through those topics that are most likely to be of concern.
- Provide practical and psychological assistance for parents of clients with psychiatric diagnoses, such as schizophrenia.
- Refer to the care plan for Impaired **Parenting** for additional interventions.

Multicultural

- Assess the influence of cultural beliefs, norms, and values on the client's perception of parenting.
- Acknowledge racial and ethnic differences at the onset of care and provide appropriate health information and social support.
- Support programs for parents of young children in specific cultural communities.
- Clarify parents' feelings, expectations, perceptions, and availability regarding participation in the care of their sick child.
- Acknowledge and praise parenting strengths noted.

Home Care

- The nursing interventions previously described should be used in the home environment with adaptations as necessary.
- ▲ Refer to a parenting program to facilitate learning of parenting skills.

Client/Family Teaching and Discharge Planning

- Refer to Client/Family Teaching and Discharge Planning for Impaired **Parenting** for suggestions that may be used with minor adaptations.
- Teach parents home safety: reduction of hot water temperature, proper poison storage, use of smoke alarms, and installation of safety gates for stairs.
- Teach parents and young teens conflict resolution by using a hypothetical conflict solution with and without a structured conflict resolution guide. Support self-direction of families with minimal therapist intervention.

• = Independent   ▲ = Collaborative

- Refer mothers of children with type 1 diabetes for community support in babysitting, child care, or respite.
- Teach families the importance of monitoring television viewing and limiting exposure to violence.
- Promotion of better quality relationships between parents and children is an effective strategy that can lead to enhanced learning. Good quality parenting leads to improved cognitive and social skills for children.

Risk for impaired Parenting

NANDA-I Definition

Vulnerable to inability of the primary caretaker to create, maintain, or regain an environment that promotes the optimum growth and development of the child, which may compromise the well-being of the child

Risk Factors

Infant or Child

Altered perceptual abilities; behavior disorder (e.g., attention deficit, oppositional defiant); developmental delay; difficult temperament; disabling condition; gender other than desired; illness; multiple births; prematurity; prolonged separation from parent; temperament conflicts with parental expectations

Knowledge

Alteration in cognitive functioning; ineffective communication skills; insufficient cognitive readiness for parenting; insufficient knowledge about child development; insufficient knowledge about child health maintenance; insufficient knowledge about parenting skills; insufficient response to infant cues; low educational level; preference for physical punishment; unrealistic expectations

Physiological

Physical illness

Psychological

Closely spaced pregnancies; depression; difficult birthing process; disabling condition; high number of pregnancies; history of mental illness; history of substance abuse; nonrestorative sleep pattern (i.e., due to caregiver responsibilities, parenting practices, sleep partner); sleep deprivation; young parental age

Social

Change in family unit; compromised home environment; conflict between partners; economically disadvantaged; father of child not involved; history

P

of abuse (e.g., physical, psychological, sexual); history of being abusive; inadequate child care arrangements; ineffective coping strategies; insufficient access to resources; insufficient family cohesiveness; insufficient parental role model; insufficient prenatal care; insufficient problem-solving skills; insufficient resources (e.g., financial, social, knowledge); insufficient social support; insufficient transportation; insufficient valuing of parenthood; late-term prenatal care; legal difficulty; low self-esteem; mother of child not involved; parent-child separation; relocation; role strain; single parent; social isolation; stressors; unemployment; unplanned pregnancy; unwanted pregnancy; work difficulty

Client Outcomes, Nursing Interventions, and Client/Family Teaching and Discharge Planning

Refer to care plans for Readiness for enhanced **Parenting** and Impaired **Parenting**.

Risk for Perioperative Positioning injury

NANDA-I Definition

Vulnerable to inadvertent anatomical and physical changes as a result of posture or equipment used during an invasive/surgical procedure, which may compromise health

Risk Factors

Disorientation; edema; emaciation; immobilization; muscle weakness; obesity; sensory-perceptual disturbance from anesthesia

Client Outcomes

Client Will (Specify Time Frame)

- Demonstrate unchanged skin condition, with exception of the incision, throughout the perioperative experience
- Demonstrate resolution of redness of the skin at points of pressure within 30 minutes after pressure is eliminated
- Remain injury-free related to surgical positioning, including intact skin and absence of pain and/or numbness associated with surgical positioning
- Demonstrate unchanged or improved physical mobility from preoperative status
- Demonstrate unchanged or improved peripheral sensory integrity from preoperative status

• = Independent   ▲ = Collaborative

Nursing Interventions

General Interventions for Any Surgical Client

- Assess the client's skin integrity throughout the perioperative process to avoid skin breakdown during surgical/invasive procedures.

Prevention of Pressure Ulcers

- Complete a preoperative assessment to identify physical alterations that may require additional precautions for procedure-specific positioning and to identify specific procedural positioning needs, type of anesthesia, and so on.
- Identify risk factors such as length and type of surgery, potential for intraoperative hypotensive episodes, low core temperatures, and decreased mobility on postoperative day 1.
- Recognize that all surgical clients should be considered at high risk for pressure ulcer development, because pressure ulcers can develop in as little as 20 minutes in the operating room.
- Protect the heels during surgery by elevating the heels completely.
- Use pressure-reducing devices and pressure-relieving mattresses as necessary to prevent ulcer formation.
- Avoid using rolled sheets and towels as positioning devices; they tend to produce high and inconsistent pressures. Special positioning devices are available that redistribute pressure.
- Avoid covering positioning devices or placing extra blankets on top of a pressure-reducing surface.
- The nurse should demonstrate knowledge not only of the equipment, but also of anatomy and the application of physiological principles in order to properly position the client.
- Monitor pressure being applied to the client intraoperatively by staff, equipment, and/or instruments (AORN, 2015a).
- Pad all bony prominences.
- Recognize that reddened areas or areas injured by pressure should not be massaged.
- Implement measures to prevent inadvertent hypothermia.

Positioning the Perioperative Client

- Ensure that linens on the operating room table are free of wrinkles.
- Lock the operating room table, cart, or bed and stabilize the mattress before transfer/positioning the client. Monitor the client while on the operating room table at all times.

- Lift rather than pull or slide the client when positioning to reduce the incidence of skin injury from shearing and/or friction.
- Ensure that appropriate numbers of personnel are present to assist in positioning the client.
- Recognize that, optimally, clients (especially those with limited range of motion/mobility) should be asked to position themselves under the nurse's guidance before induction of anesthesia so that he/she can verify that a position of comfort has been obtained.
- Ensure that nerves are protected by positioning extremities carefully.
- Use slow and smooth movements during positioning to allow the circulatory system to readjust.
- Reassess the client after positioning and periodically during the procedure to maintain proper alignment and skin integrity.
- Frequently assess the eyes and/or monitor intraocular pressure, especially when client is in prone or knee-chest position.
- Position hips in proper alignment with knees flexed. Unaligned hips can cause pressure to the low back and hip joints.
- Position the arms extended on arm boards so that they do not extend beyond a 90-degree angle. Do not position arms at sides unless surgically necessary.
- Protect the client's skin surfaces from injury by preventing pooling of preparative solutions, blood, irrigation, urine, and feces. Keep the client appropriately covered during the procedure.
- When positioning the client prone, care should be taken to ensure the head and neck are properly positioned.
- Recognize that clients positioned in lithotomy position should be kept in this position for as short a time as possible.
- The lowest heel position should be used in the lithotomy position.
- Position the client's legs parallel and uncrossed.
- Maintain normal body alignment.
- When applying body supports and restraint straps (safety belt), apply loosely and secure over waist or mid-thigh at least 2 inches above knees; avoid bony prominences by placing a blanket between the strap and the client.
- Assess the client's skin integrity immediately postoperatively.
- Ensure that complete, concise, accurate documentation of client assessment and use of positioning devices is in the client's medical record.

• = Independent   ▲ = Collaborative

Risk for Peripheral Neurovascular dysfunction

NANDA-I Definition

Vulnerable to disruption in the circulation, sensation, and motion of an extremity, which may compromise health

Risk Factors

Burns; fractures; immobilization; mechanical compression (e.g., tourniquet, cane, cast, brace, dressing, restraint); orthopedic surgery; trauma; vascular obstruction

Client Outcomes

Client Will (Specify Time Frame)

- Maintain circulation, sensation, and movement of an extremity within client's own normal limits
- Explain signs of neurovascular compromise

Nursing Interventions

▲ Recognize situations listed in the Risk Factors that may result in peripheral neurovascular dysfunction. Compartment syndrome may be due to increased volume of the contents of a compartment, or reduced capacity of the compartment sheath. Reduced capacity is associated with tight dressings, bandages, or casts (Mabvuure et al, 2012).

▲ Assess for the early onset of compartment syndrome, and report to health care provider promptly. Perform neurovascular assessment every 15 minutes to every 4 hours as ordered or needed based on client's condition. Use the five Ps of assessment as outlined below.

  ○ Pain: Assess severity (on a scale of 1 to 10), quality, radiation, and relief by medications. Pain is usually "out of proportion" to the injury, requiring strong opiates, and is often described as burning, feeling deep in the muscle or structure, and elicited with passive stretching of the compartment (Donaldson et al, 2014).

  ○ Pulses: Check the pulses distal to the injury.

  ○ Pallor: Check color and temperature changes below the injury site. Check capillary refill.

  ○ Paresthesia (change in sensation): Check by lightly touching the skin proximal and distal to the injury. Ask if the client has any unusual sensations such as hypersensitivity, tingling, prickling, decreased feeling, or numbness. Check nerve function (e.g.,

P

• = Independent   ▲ = Collaborative

whether the client can feel a touch to the area of concern, such as the first web space of the foot [deep peroneal nerve] with tibial fracture).

    ○ Paralysis: Ask the client to perform appropriate range-of-motion exercises in the unaffected and then the affected extremity.

    ○ Pressure: Check by feeling the extremity; note new onset of firmness or swelling of the extremity, as well as a firm "wooden" feeling upon deep palpation.

▲ All of the Ps may not be present, and they are not specific for compartment syndrome. Have a high index of suspicion for any of the Ps. Noting two or more of the Ps increases the probability of compartment syndrome. Monitor the client for compartment syndrome of the nonoperated leg as well as the operated leg.

• Monitor appropriate application and function of corrective device (e.g., cast, splint, traction) every 1 to 4 hours as needed.

▲ For prevention of deep vein thrombosis (DVT), nursing care of DVT, and pulmonary embolism, refer to the interventions on DVT prevention and treatment in the care plan for Ineffective peripheral **Tissue Perfusion**.

Risk for Poisoning
NANDA-I Definition

Vulnerable to accidental exposure to, or ingestion of, drugs or dangerous products in sufficient doses that may compromise health

Risk Factors

External

• Access to dangerous product
• Access to illicit drugs potentially contaminated by poisonous additives
• Access to large supply of pharmaceutical agents in house
• Access to pharmaceutical agent

Internal

• Alteration in cognitive functioning
• Emotional disturbance
• Inadequate precautions against poisoning
• Insufficient knowledge of pharmacological agents
• Insufficient knowledge of poisoning prevention
• Occupational setting without adequate safeguards

       • = Independent   ▲ = Collaborative

- Reduced vision
- Addiction

Client Outcomes
Client Will (Specify Time Frame)
- Prevent inadvertent ingestion of or exposure to toxins or poisonous substances
- Explain and undertake appropriate safety measures to prevent ingestion of or exposure to toxins or poisonous substances
- Verbalize appropriate response to apparent or suspected toxic ingestion or poisoning

Nursing Interventions
- When a client comes to the hospital with possible poisoning, begin care following the ABCs and administer oxygen if needed.
- ▲ It is important for the triage nurse to call the poison control center. The poison control hotline is 1-800-222-1222. Poison centers are a valuable tool for medical consultations. They are staffed by nurses, pharmacists, toxicologists, and other specialists in poisons and toxins who can recommend treatment advice (American Association of Poison Control Centers, 2014).
- Obtain a thorough history of what was ingested, how much, and when, and ask to look at the containers. Note the client's age, weight, medications, medical conditions, and any history of vomiting, choking, coughing, or change in mental status. Also take note of any interventions performed before seeking treatment.
- Carefully inspect for signs of ingestion of poisons, including an odor on the breath, a trace of the substance on the clothing, burns, or redness around the mouth and lips, as well as signs of confusion, vomiting, or dyspnea.
- ▲ Note results of toxicology screens, arterial blood gases, blood glucose levels, and any other ordered laboratory tests.
- ▲ Initiate any ordered treatment for poisoning quickly. The poison control center will specify any treatment or medications that need to be administered.

Safety Guidelines for Medication Administration
- Prevent iatrogenic harm to the hospitalized client by following these guidelines for administering medications:
  - Use at least two methods to identify the client before administering medications or blood products, such as the client's name and medical record number or birth date. Do not use the

---

• = Independent   ▲ = Collaborative

client's room number. Use bar code scanning system for client identification if used by your facility.

○ When taking verbal or telephone orders, the orders should be written down and read back for verification to the individual giving the order. The health care provider who gave the orders for the medication then needs to confirm the information that was read back.

• Standardize use of abbreviations, acronyms, symbols, and dose designations and eliminate those that are prone to cause errors. (Refer to The Joint Commission, Critical Access Hospital National Patient Safety Goals for list of abbreviations, acronyms, symbols, and dose designations that should not be used.)

○ Be aware of the medications that look/sound alike and ensure that the correct medication is ordered and administered.

○ Use the eight rights of medication administration to decrease the potential for error:

○ Right client, right medication, right reason, right dose, right frequency, right route, right site, and right time (College of Nurses of Ontario, 2014). Take high-alert medications off the nursing unit, such as potassium chloride. Standardize concentrations of medications such as morphine in patient-controlled analgesia pumps.

○ Follow agency policy/procedures for medications that require two-person check and co-signature.

○ Label all medications and medication containers or other solutions that are on or off a sterile field for a procedure. Label them when they are first taken out of the original packaging to another container. Label with medication name, strength, amount, and expiration date/time. Review the labels whenever there is a change of personnel.

○ Use only intravenous (IV) pumps that prevent free flow of IV solution when the tubing is taken out of the pump.

• Identify all the client's current medications on admission to a health care facility and compare the list with the current ordered medications. Reconcile any differences in medications. Use the expertise of the pharmacy department if there is any uncertainty regarding the accuracy of the client's medications.

• = Independent   ▲ = Collaborative

- Reconcile the list of medications if the client is transferred from one unit to another, when there is a handoff to the next provider of care, and when the client is discharged.
- Detect possible interactions and cumulative or other adverse effects among prescribed medications, self-administered over-the-counter products, culturally based home treatments, herbal remedies, and foods. Medication reconciliation is an important safety issue due to the number of people taking multiple medications and involves determining what medications the person should be taking, medications they are actually taking, and resolving discrepancies (The Joint Commission, 2014).

Pediatric

▲ Evaluate lead exposure risk and consult the health care provider regarding lead screening measures as indicated (public/ambulatory health).

- Provide guidance for parents and caregivers regarding age-related safety measures, including the following:
  - ○ Store prescription and over-the-counter medications, vitamins, herbs, and alcohol in a locked cabinet far from children's reach.
  - ○ Do not take medications in front of children (Rodgers et al, 2012).
  - ○ Store cleaning products including things like dishwashing liquids in a high cabinet, out of children's reach.
  - ○ Use safety latches on cabinets that contain poisonous substances.
  - ○ Store potentially harmful substances in the original containers with safety closures intact.
  - ○ Recognize that no container is completely childproof.
  - ○ Do not store medications or toxic substances in food containers or near or with food products.
  - ○ Do not leave alcoholic drinks, cosmetics, or toiletries where children can reach them.
  - ○ Remove poisonous houseplants from the home. Teach children not to put leaves or berries in their mouths (Oerther, 2011).
  - ○ Do not suggest that medications are candy.
  - ○ If interrupted when using a harmful product, take it with you; children can get into it within seconds.
  - ○ Store poisonous automotive or gardening supplies in a locked area.

• = Independent   ▲ = Collaborative

- ○ Use extreme caution with pesticides and gardening materials close to children's play areas.
- ○ When visitors enter the home, place their handbags or backpacks up high where children are unable to reach them, and ask about any potential poisonous substances.
- Children naturally put things in their mouths and experience new taste sensations as a part of child development. Prevention of this is unrealistic, and interventions should target environmental and caregiver behaviors to reduce harm (Rosenberg et al, 2011).
- Advise families that syrup of ipecac is no longer recommended to be kept and used in the home. Previous studies have shown unreliable performance with ipecac, and the number of poison control centers that have stopped recommending ipecac use for poisonings has increased significantly over the last decades (Gutierrez et al, 2011). Advise families that over-the-counter cough and cold suppressant medications are not recommended and are no longer considered safe for children 2 or younger (U.S. Food and Drug Administration, 2014).
- Recognize that some children may have been exposed to methamphetamines or the components used to make methamphetamines.

Geriatric

- Caution the client and family to avoid storing medications with similar appearances close to one another (e.g., nitroglycerin ointment near toothpaste or denture creams).
- Remind older clients to store medications out of reach when young children come to visit. Childhood poisonings are common events that involve exposure to both prescription and nonprescription pharmaceuticals in the home, resulting in an increased number of serious outcomes (Spiller et al, 2013).
- Perform medication reconciliation in all older clients entering the health care system as well as upon discharge.

Home Care

- The interventions previously described may be adapted for home care use.
- Provide the client and/or family with a poison control poster to be kept on the refrigerator or a bulletin board. Ensure that the telephone number for local poison control information is readily available and/or preprogrammed into household telephones.

• = Independent ▲ = Collaborative

- Pre-pour medications for a client who is at risk for ingesting too much of a given medication because of mistakes in preparation. Delegate this task to the family or caregivers if possible.
- Identify poisonous substances in the immediate surroundings of the home, such as a garage or barn, including paints and thinners, fertilizers, rodent and bug control substances, animal medications, gasoline, and oil. Label with the name, a poison warning sign, and a poison control center number. Lock out of the reach of children.
- Identify the risk of toxicity from environmental activities such as spraying trees or roadside shrubs. Contact local departments of agriculture or transportation to obtain material safety data sheets or to prevent the activity in desired areas.
- To prevent carbon monoxide poisoning, instruct the client and family in the importance of using a carbon monoxide detector in the home and changing it every 6 months, having the home heating system serviced every year by a qualified technician, and ensuring proper installation and venting of all combustion equipment. Carbon monoxide results from fumes produced by portable generators, stoves, lanterns, gas ranges, running vehicles, or burning charcoal and wood, which can build up in enclosed or partially enclosed spaces and result in harm or death for people and animals exposed (Centers for Disease Control and Prevention, 2014).

P

Multicultural

- Assess housing for pathways of lead poisoning.
- Prompt caregivers to take action to prevent lead poisoning.
- If children live in a high-lead environment, teach the need for handwashing before each meal, annual blood testing for lead levels, and avoidance of high lead areas.
- Work with immigrant Mexican families to implement medication, household cleaners, and carbon monoxide safety interventions in the home to prevent accidental poisoning in children. Use the Hispanic social network.

Client/Family Teaching and Discharge Planning

- Teach parents that any substance that is absorbed by the body by a variety of means and can affect health and cause mortality is considered a poison. The increasing use of medications and home cleaning products puts children at risk for poison due to the potential for access in the home environment.

• = Independent   ▲ = Collaborative

Safety Guidelines

- Counsel the client and family members regarding the following points of medication safety:
  - Avoid sharing prescriptions.
  - Always use good light when preparing medication. Do not dispense medication during the night without a light on.
  - Read the label before you open the bottle, after you remove a dose, and again before you give it.
  - Always use child-resistant caps and lock all medications away from your child or confused older adult.
  - Give the correct dose. *Never* guess.
  - Do not increase or decrease the dose without calling the health care provider.
  - Always follow the weight and age recommendations on the label.
  - Avoid making conversions. If the label calls for 2 tsp and you have a dosing cup labeled only with ounces, do not use it.
  - Be sure the health care provider knows if you are taking more than one medication at a time.
  - Never let young children take medication by themselves.
  - Read and follow labeling instructions on all products; adjust dosage for age.
  - Avoid excessive amounts and/or frequency of doses. ("If a little does some good, a lot should do more.")
- Every day in the United States, about 165 children are treated in emergency departments after getting into medication. Unintentional ingestion of medications is the leading cause of child poisoning among young children, and the number of children dying of poisoning has more than doubled since 1999 (Safekids.org, 2014).
- Advise the family to post first-aid charts and poison control center instructions in an accessible location. Poison control center telephone numbers should be posted close to each telephone and the number programmed into cell phones.
- Advise family when calling the poison control center to do the following:
  - Give as much information as possible, including your name, location, and telephone number, so that the poison control operator can call back in case you are disconnected or summon help if needed.

- ○ Give the name of the potential poison ingested and, if possible, the amount and time of ingestion. If the bottle or package is available, give the trade name and ingredients if they are listed.
  - ○ Be prepared to divulge the child's height, weight, age, and medical history.
  - ○ Describe the state of the poisoning victim. Is the victim conscious? Does he or she have any symptoms? What is the person's general appearance, skin color, respiration, breathing difficulties, mental status (alert, sleepy, unusual behavior)? Is the person vomiting? Having convulsions?
- Encourage the client and family to take first-aid and other types of safety-related programs.
- ▲ Initiate referrals to peer group interventions, peer counseling, and other types of substance abuse prevention/rehabilitation programs when substance abuse is identified as a risk factor.
- Teach parents and other caregivers that cough and cold medications bought over the counter are not safe for children younger than 2 unless specifically ordered by a health care provider. Analysis of exposures to cough/cold preparations supports the concept that poisoning exposure occurs in children with substances that they can easily access (Spiller et al, 2013).
- Teach parents about home prevention strategies to prevent accidental poisonings (Gutierrez et al, 2011).
- Teach parents that they can be a source of lead exposure for their children via contaminated work clothing from a lead-related occupation such as transportation workers or automobile repair or if they engage in certain hobbies such as stained glass or ceramics (Schnur & John, 2014). Precautions should be taken to eliminate the risk of exposure.

P

Post-Trauma syndrome
NANDA-I Definition

Sustained maladaptive response to a traumatic, overwhelming event
Defining Characteristics

Aggression; alienation; alteration in concentration; alteration in mood; anger; anxiety; avoidance behaviors; compulsive behavior; denial; depression; dissociative amnesia; enuresis; exaggerated startle response; fear; flashbacks; gastrointestinal irritation; grieving; guilt; headache; heart

• = Independent   ▲ = Collaborative

palpitations; history of detachment; hopelessness; horror; hypervigilance; intrusive dreams; intrusive thoughts; irritability; neurosensory irritability; nightmares; panic attacks; rage; reports feeling numb; repression; shame; substance abuse

Related Factors

Destruction of one's home; event outside the range of usual human experience; exposure to disaster (natural or man-made); exposure to epidemic; exposure to event involving multiple deaths; exposure to war; history of abuse (e.g., physical, psychological, sexual); history of being a prisoner of war; history of criminal victimization; history of torture; self-injurious behavior; serious accident (e.g., industrial, motor vehicle); serious injury to loved one; serious threat to loved one; serious threat to self; witnessing mutilation; witnessing violent death

Client Outcomes

Client Will (Specify Time Frame)

- Return to pretrauma level of functioning as quickly as possible
- Acknowledge traumatic event and begin to work with the trauma by talking about the experience and expressing feelings of fear, anger, anxiety, guilt, and helplessness
- Identify support systems and available resources and be able to connect with them
- Return to and strengthen coping mechanisms used in previous traumatic event
- Acknowledge event and perceive it without distortions
- Assimilate event and move forward to set and pursue life goals

Nursing Interventions

- Observe for a reaction to a traumatic event in all clients regardless of age or sex.
- After a traumatic event, assess for intrusive memories, avoidance and numbing, and hyperarousal.
- Remain with the client and provide support during periods of overwhelming emotions.
- Help the individual try to comprehend the trauma if possible.
- Use touch with the client's permission (e.g., a hand on the shoulder, holding a hand).
- Explore and enhance available support systems.
- Help the client regain previous sleeping and eating habits.
- ▲ Provide the client pain medication if he/she has physical pain.
- ▲ Assess the need for pharmacotherapy.

• = Independent   ▲ = Collaborative

▲ Refer for appropriate psychotherapy: cognitive therapy, exposure therapy, eye movement desensitization and reprocessing (EMDR), and CBT.

• Help the client use positive cognitive restructuring to reestablish feelings of self-worth.

• Provide the means for the client to express feelings through therapeutic drawing.

• Encourage the client to return to the normal routine as quickly as possible.

• Talk to and assess the client's social support after a traumatic event.

Pediatric

• Refer to nursing care plan for Risk for **Post-Trauma** syndrome.

▲ Carefully assess children exposed to disasters and trauma. Note behavior specific to developmental age. Refer for therapy as needed.

Geriatric

• Carefully screen older adults for signs of PTSD, especially after a disaster.

• Consider using the Horwitz Impact of Event Scale, an appropriate instrument to measure the subjective response to stress in the older population.

▲ Monitor the client for clinical signs of depression and anxiety; refer to a health care provider for medication if appropriate.

• Instill hope.

Multicultural

• Assess the influence of cultural beliefs, norms, and values on the client's ability to cope with a traumatic experience.

• Acknowledge racial and ethnic differences at the onset of care.

▲ Carefully assess refugees for PTSD and refer for treatment as appropriate; encourage them to learn the language of their new residence.

• Use a family-centered approach when working with Latin, Asian, African American, and Native American clients.

• When working with Asian American clients, provide opportunities by which the family can save face.

• Incorporate cultural traditions as appropriate.

Home Care

▲ Assess family support and the response to the client's coping mechanisms. Refer the family for medical social services or other counseling as necessary.

• = Independent   ▲ = Collaborative

- Assess the impact of the trauma on significant others (e.g., a father may have to take over his partner's parenting responsibility after she has been raped and injured). Provide empathy and caring to significant others. Refer for additional services as necessary.

Client/Family Teaching and Discharge Planning

- Teach positive coping skills and avoidance of negative coping skills.
- Teach stress reduction methods such as deep breathing, visualization, meditation, and physical exercise. Encourage their use especially when intrusive thoughts or flashbacks occur.
- Encourage other healthy living habits of proper diet, adequate sleep, regular exercise, family activities, and spiritual pursuits.
- Refer the client to peer support groups.
- Consider the use of complementary and alternative therapies.

Risk for Post-Trauma syndrome

NANDA-I Definition

Vulnerable to sustained maladaptive response to a traumatic, overwhelming event, which may compromise health

Risk Factors

Diminished ego strength; displacement from home; duration of traumatic event; environment not conducive to needs; exaggerated sense of responsibility; human service occupations (e.g., police, fire, rescue, corrections, emergency room, mental health); insufficient social support; perceives event as traumatic; survivor role

Client Outcomes

Client Will (Specify Time Frame)

- Identify symptoms associated with PTSD and seek help
- Acknowledge event and perceive it without distortions
- Identify support systems and available resources and be able to connect with them
- State that he/she is not to blame for the event

Nursing Interventions

- Assess for PTSD in a client who has chronic/critical illness, anxiety, or personality disorder; was a witness to serious injury or death; or experienced sexual molestation.
- Consider the use of a self-reported screening questionnaire.

• = Independent ▲ = Collaborative

- Assess for ongoing symptoms of dissociation, avoidance behavior, hypervigilance, and reexperiencing.
- Assess for past experiences with traumatic events.
- Consider screening for PTSD in a client who is a high user of medical care.
▲ Provide deployed combat veterans with previous history of low mental or physical health status before deployment with appropriate referral after deployment.
- Provide peer support to contact co-workers experiencing trauma to remind them that others in the organization are concerned about their welfare.
- Provide post-trauma debriefings. Effective post-trauma coping skills are taught, and each participant creates a plan for his/her recovery. During the debriefing, the facilitators assess participants to determine their needs for further services in the form of post-trauma counseling. For maximal effectiveness, the debriefing should occur within 2 to 5 days of the incident (Guess, 2006).
- Provide post-trauma counseling. Counseling sessions are extensions of debriefings and include continued discussion of the traumatic event and post-trauma consequences and the further development of coping skills.
- Consider exposure therapy for civilian trauma survivors following a nonsexual assault or motor vehicle crash.

Things to Try: Critical Incident Stress Debriefing
- Instruct the client to use the following critical incident stress management techniques:
  ○ Within the first 24 to 48 hours, engage in periods of appropriate physical exercise alternated with relaxation to alleviate some of the physical reactions; structure your time; keep busy; you are normal and are having normal reactions; do not label yourself as "crazy"; talk to people; talk is the most healing medicine; be aware of numbing the pain with overuse of drugs or alcohol; you do not need to complicate the stress with a substance abuse problem; reach out; people do care; maintain as normal a schedule as possible; spend time with others; help your co-workers as much as possible by sharing feelings and checking out how they are doing; give yourself permission to feel rotten and share your feelings with others; keep a journal; write your way through those sleepless hours; do things that feel good to

you; realize that those around you are under stress; do not make any big life changes; do make as many daily decisions as possible to give you a feeling of control over your life (e.g., if someone asks you what you want to eat, answer the person even if you are not sure); get plenty of rest; recurring thoughts, dreams, or flashbacks are normal; do not try to fight them because they will decrease over time and become less painful; eat well-balanced and regular meals (even if you do not feel like it).

▲ Assess for a history of life-threatening illness such as cancer and provide appropriate counseling. The physical and psychological impact of having a life-threatening disease, undergoing cancer treatment, and living with recurring threats to physical integrity and autonomy constitute traumatic experiences for many cancer clients (National Cancer Institute, 2013).

Pediatric

- Children with cancer should continue to be assessed for PTSD into adulthood.

- Provide protection for a child who has witnessed violence or who has had traumatic injuries. Help the child acknowledge the event and express grief over the event.

- Assess for a medical history of anxiety disorders.

▲ Assess children of deployed parents for PTSD and provide appropriate referrals.

- Consider implementation of a school-based program for children to decrease PTSD after catastrophic events.

Geriatric and Multicultural

- Refer to the care plan for **Post-Trauma** syndrome.

Home Care

▲ Evaluate the client's response to a traumatic or critical event. If screening warrants, refer to a therapist for counseling/treatment.

- Refer to the care plan for **Post-Trauma** syndrome.

Client/Family Teaching and Discharge Planning

- Instruct family and friends to use the following critical incident stress management techniques:

▲ Listen carefully; spend time with the traumatized person; offer your assistance and a listening ear, even if the person has not asked for help; help the person with everyday tasks such as cleaning, cooking, caring for the family, and minding children; give the person some private time; do not take the individual's anger or other feelings

• = Independent   ▲ = Collaborative

personally, and do not tell the person that he/she is "lucky it wasn't worse"; such statements do not console traumatized people. Instead, tell the person that you are sorry such an event has occurred and you want to understand and assist him or her (National Interagency Fire Center, CISM Information Sheets, 2014).

▲ After exposure to trauma, teach the client and family to recognize symptoms of PTSD and seek treatment for "recurrent and intrusive distressing recollections of the traumatic event," insomnia, irritability, difficulty concentrating, hypervigilance.

• Provide education to explain that acute stress disorder symptoms are normal when preparing combatants for their role in deployment. Instruct clients to seek help if the symptoms persist.

Readiness for enhanced Power

NANDA-I Definition

A pattern of participating knowingly in change for well-being, which can be strengthened

Defining Characteristics

Expresses desire to enhance awareness of possible changes; expresses desire to enhance identification of choices that can be made for change; expresses desire to enhance independence with actions for change; expresses desire to enhance involvement in change; expresses desire to enhance knowledge for participation in change; expresses desire to enhance participation in choices for daily living; expresses desire to enhance participation in choices for health; expresses desire to enhance power

Client Outcomes

Client Will (Specify Time Frame)

• Describe power resources
• Identify realistic perceptions of control
• Develop a plan of action based on power resources
• Seek assistance as needed

Nursing Interventions

• Develop partnerships for shared power.
• Focus on the positive aspects of power, rather than prevention of powerlessness.
• Listen with intent.

- Collaborate with and encourage the person to identify resources to put a plan into action.
- Assess the meaning of the event to the person.
- Identify the client's health literacy and provide access to information.
- Facilitate trust in self and others.
- Help client to mobilize social supports, a power resource.
- Support beliefs of power and perceptions of behavioral control.
- Promote the client's optimum level of physical functioning.
- Reframe professional image, role, and values to incorporate a vision of clients as the experts in their own care.

Home Care

- The preceding interventions may be adapted for home care use.

Client/Family Teaching and Discharge Planning

- Assess motivation to learn specific content.

Powerlessness

NANDA-I Definition

The lived experience of lack of control over a situation, including a perception that one's actions do not significantly affect an outcome

Defining Characteristics

Alienation; dependency; depression; doubt about role performance; frustration about inability to perform previous activities; inadequate participation in care; insufficient sense of control; shame

Related Factors

Complex treatment regimen; dysfunctional institutional environment; insufficient interpersonal interactions

Client Outcomes

Client Will (Specify Time Frame)

- State feelings of powerlessness and other feelings related to powerlessness (e.g., anger, sadness, hopelessness)
- Identify factors that are uncontrollable
- Participate in planning and implementing care; make decisions regarding care and treatment when possible
- Ask questions about care and treatment
- Verbalize hope for the future and sense of participation in planning and implementing care

• = Independent ▲ = Collaborative

Nursing Interventions

NOTE: Before implementation of interventions in the face of client powerlessness, nurses should examine their own philosophies of care to ensure that control issues or lack of faith in client capabilities will not bias the ability to intervene sincerely and effectively.

- Observe for factors contributing to powerlessness (e.g., immobility, hospitalization, unfavorable prognosis, lack of support system, misinformation about situation, inflexible routine, chronic illness, addiction, history of trauma, gender). Help clients channel their behaviors in an effective manner.
- Engage with clients using respectful listening and questioning to develop an awareness of clients' most important concerns.
- Assess the client's locus of control related to his or her health.
- Establish a therapeutic relationship with the client by spending one-on-one time with him or her, assigning the same caregiver, keeping commitments (e.g., saying, "I will be back to answer your questions in the next hour"), providing encouragement and social support, and being empathetic.
- Encourage the client to share his or her beliefs, thoughts, and expectations about his or her illness.
- Help the client assist in planning care and specify the health goals he or she would like to achieve, prioritizing those goals with regard to immediate concerns and identifying actions that will achieve the goals. Goals may need to be small to be attainable (e.g., dangle legs at bedside for 2 days, then sit in chair 10 minutes for 2 days, then walk to window).
- Encourage the client in goal-directed activities that promote a sense of accomplishment, especially regular exercise.
- Empower clients by providing access to health education in conjunction with counseling and opportunities for discussion.
- Encourage the client to take control of as many activities of daily living (ADLs) as possible; keep the client informed of all care that will be given. Keep items the client uses and needs within reach (e.g., a urinal, tissues, telephone, and television controls).
- Give realistic and sincere praise for accomplishments.
- Use a Rehabilitative Behavioral Learning Model that assists clients to understand how the mechanisms of habit and ritual work to reinforce powerlessness in their lives.

• = Independent ▲ = Collaborative

- Consider using one of the measures of powerlessness that are available for general and specific client groups:
  - ○ Measure of Powerlessness for Adult Patients (De Almeida & Braga, 2006)
  - ○ Personal Progress Scale—Revised, tested with women (Johnson et al, 2005)
  - ○ Life Situation Questionnaire—Powerlessness subscale, tested with stroke caregivers (Larson et al, 2005)
  - ○ Making Decisions Scale, tested in clients with mental illness (Hansson & Bjorkman, 2005)
- Refer to the care plans for **Hopelessness** and **Spiritual** distress.

Pediatric

- Assess for power differentials in the dating relationships of female adolescent clients and provide teaching that addresses relationship power and dating violence.
- Provide nursing care that shifts the focus from the illness to the child.

Geriatric

- In addition to the preceding interventions as appropriate:
  - ○ Assist older adults to retain a sense of power and control as they are making the transition to residential care.
  - ○ Initiate focused assessment questioning and education of client and caregivers regarding syndromes common in older adults, including dementia.
  - ○ Assess for the presence of elder abuse. Initiate referral to Adult Protective Services and help client regain a sense of safety and control.

Multicultural

- In addition to the preceding interventions as appropriate:
  - ○ Assess for the influence of communication patterns, cultural differences in medical consultations, and client perceptions of inequalities in care quality as contributors to client feelings of powerlessness.

Home Care

- In addition to the preceding interventions as appropriate:
  - ○ Develop a therapeutic relationship in the home setting that respects the client's domain.
  - ○ Empower the client by encouraging the client to guide specifics of care such as wound care procedures and dressing and

grooming details. Confirm the client's knowledge and document in the chart that the client is able to guide procedures. Document in the home and in the chart the preferred approach to procedures. Orient the family and caregivers to the client's role.

○ Assess the affective climate within the family and family support system, including other caregivers. Instruct the family in appropriate expectations of the client and in the specifics of the client's illness. Assist the family and caregivers to assert personal needs and develop closer proximity to health care providers.

○ Evaluate the powerlessness of caregivers to ensure they continue their ability to care for the client. Provide assistance using interventions from this care plan.

○ Assist family caregivers, especially fathers, to take an active role in the client's care.

○ Assess for denial in clients with cancer and provide support for caregivers.

○ Be aware of and assist clients with potential needs for help in negotiating the health care system.

○ Teach stress reduction, relaxation, and imagery. Many audio recordings are available on relaxation and meditation.

○ Teach cognitive-behavioral activities, such as active problem solving, reframing (reappraising the situation from a different perspective), or thought stopping (in response to a negative thought, such as picturing a large stop sign and replacing the image with a prearranged positive alternative). Teach the client to confront his or her own negative thought patterns (cognitive distortions).

○ Identify the strengths of the caregiver and efforts to gain control of unpredictable situations. Help the caregiver stay connected with a client who may be behaving differently than usual to make life as routine as possible, help the client set goals and sustain hope, and allow the client space to experience progress.

Client/Family Teaching and Discharge Planning

• The preceding interventions may be adapted for home care use.

• = Independent   ▲ = Collaborative

Risk for Powerlessness

NANDA-I Definition

Vulnerable to the lived experience of lack of control over a situation, including a perception that one's actions do not significantly affect the outcome, which may compromise health

Risk Factors

Anxiety; caregiver role; economically disadvantaged; illness; ineffective coping strategies; insufficient knowledge to manage a situation; insufficient social support; low self-esteem; pain; progressive illness; social marginalization; stigmatization; unpredictability of illness trajectory

Client Outcomes, Nursing Interventions, and Client/Family Teaching and Discharge Planning

See the care plan for **Powerlessness.**

Risk for Pressure ulcer

NANDA-I Definition

Vulnerable to localized injury to the skin and/or underlying tissue usually over a bony prominence as a result of pressure, or pressure in combination with shear

Risk Factors

Adult

Braden scale score <18; alteration in cognitive functioning; alteration in sensation; American Society of Anesthesiologist (ASA) Physical Status classification score ≥2; anemia; cardiovascular disease

Child

Braden Q scale ≤16; decrease in mobility; decrease in serum albumin level; decrease in tissue oxygenation; decrease in tissue perfusion; dehydration; dry skin; edema; elevated skin temperature by 1° C to 2° C; extended period of immobility on hard surface (e.g., surgical procedure ≥2 hours); extremes of age; extremes of weight; female gender; hip fracture; history of cerebral vascular accident; history of pressure ulcer; history of trauma; hyperthermia; impaired circulation; inadequate nutrition; incontinence; insufficient caregiver knowledge of pressure ulcer prevention; low score on Risk Assessment Pressure Sore (RAPS) scale; lymphopenia; New York Heart Association (NYHA) functional classification ≥2; nonblanchable erythema; pharmaceutical agents (e.g., general anesthesia, vasopressors, antidepressant, norepinephrine); physical immobilization; pressure over bony prominence; reduced triceps skin fold thickness; scaly skin; self-care

• = Independent ▲ = Collaborative

deficit; shearing forces; skin moisture; smoking; surface friction; use of linens with insufficient moisture-wicking property

Client Outcomes

Client Will (Specify Time Frame)

- Report any altered sensation or pain at site of tissue impairment
- Skin, without redness over bony prominences and capillary refill of less than 6 seconds over areas of redness
- Be repositioned off of bony prominences frequently if risk for pressure ulcers is high (e.g., Braden scale score <18)
- Demonstrate understanding of plan to reduce pressure ulcer risk
- Describe measures to protect the skin

Nursing Interventions

- Routinely assess clients for risk of pressure ulcers using a valid and reliable risk assessment tool (NPUAP/EPUAP, 2014).
- Pressure ulcer risk assessment should be completed on admission, daily, and after procedures or changes in the client's condition (Kelleher et al, 2012; NPUAP/EPUAP, 2014).
- Inspect the skin daily, especially bony prominences and dependent areas for pallor, redness, and breakdown In addition to assessing pressure ulcer risk, client-specific interventions should be implemented to prevent tissue injury. Implement interventions to prevent tissue breakdown:
  - Assist client to turn at least every 2 hours unless contraindicated
  - Position client properly; use pressure-reducing or pressure-relieving devices (e.g., pillows, gel or foam cushions, alternating pressure mattress, air-fluidized bed, kinetic bed) if indicated
  - Lift and move client carefully using a turn sheet and adequate assistance; keep bed linens dry and wrinkle-free
  - Perform actions to keep client from sliding down in bed (e.g., bend knees slightly when head of bed is elevated 30 degrees or higher) in order to reduce the risk of skin surface abrasion and shearing
  - Instruct or assist client to shift weight at least every 30 minutes
  - Keep client's skin clean; thoroughly dry skin after bathing and as often as needed, paying special attention to skin folds and opposing skin surfaces (e.g., axillae, perineum, beneath breasts); pat skin dry rather than rub; use a mild soap for bathing and apply moisturizing lotion at least once a day

P

• = Independent ▲ = Collaborative

- ○ Protect the skin from contact with urine and feces (e.g., keep perineal area clean and dry, apply a protective ointment or cream to perineal area)
- ○ Encourage a fluid intake of 2500 mL/day unless contraindicated
- ○ Apply a protective covering such as a hydrocolloid or transparent membrane dressing to areas of the skin susceptible to breakdown (e.g., coccyx, heels, elbows)
- ○ Consult with nutrition/dietary specialist to evaluate client's nutritional status
- ○ Increase activity as allowed
- A medical device–related pressure ulcer (MDRPU) is a localized injury to the skin or underlying tissue as a result of sustained pressure from a medical device. The tissue injury will often have the same configuration as the device (NPUAP 2014; Baharestani, 2013; Black, 2010).
  - ○ The head/face/neck, heel/ankle/foot, coccyx/buttocks, abdomen, and extremities are common body regions for MDRPU.
  - ○ Common devices associated with pressure-related tissue injury include oxygen delivery and monitoring devices (e.g., face mask, nasal cannula, pulse oximetry, BiPAP mask); feeding tubes (e.g., nasogastric, gastric, jejunal tubes); endotracheal devices (oral and/or nasal endotracheal tubes, tracheostomy tubes); urinary and bowel elimination (indwelling urinary catheter, fecal containment catheter); musculoskeletal (cervical collar, splints, braces).
  - ○ Assess and evaluate the purpose and function of the medical device
  - ○ Assess proper fit of the medical device and securement to prevent rubbing, torque, or pulling on the device and skin
  - ○ Protect the skin below and around the device to reduce pressure
- Critically ill clients are at increased risk for pressure ulcers, often requiring frequent skin risk assessment and preventive interventions.
- If tissue breakdown occurs, notify a health care provider or wound care specialist. See care plan for Impaired **Skin** integrity for additional interventions if a pressure ulcer occurs.

Pediatric

- Perform an age-appropriate pressure ulcer risk assessment using a valid and reliable tool.

• = Independent   ▲ = Collaborative

- Implement a comprehensive plan to reduce the client's risk of skin breakdown from pressure. Assessment should include the following:
  - ○ Client independent activity and mobility levels
  - ○ Body mass index and/or birth weight; lower weight may increase client risk of pressure-associated skin breakdown
  - ○ Skin maturity
  - ○ Adequate nutritional and hydration status
  - ○ Perfusion and oxygenation
  - ○ Presence of external devices
  - ○ Duration of hospital stay
- Select an age-appropriate support surface for premature neonates and pediatric clients at high risk for pressure ulcers.
- Document risk assessment and interventions implemented to reduce the client's risk for pressure ulcer development.

Geriatric
- Consider the older client's cognitive status when assessing the skin and in developing a comprehensive plan of care to prevent pressure ulcers (NPUAP/EPUAP, 2014).
- Aging skin, medications (e.g., steroids), and moisture place the older client at increased risk for pressure-associated skin breakdown.
- For older clients with continence concerns, develop and implement an individualized continence management program (NPUAP/EPUAP, 2014).

Home Care
- The interventions described previously may be adapted for home care use.
- Instruct and assist the client and caregivers in how to assess the skin for excessive pressure. Provide written instructions for actions they can implement to reduce the risk of pressure ulcer development.
- Educate client and caregivers on proper nutrition and when to call the agency and/or health care provider with concerns.
- ▲ It may be beneficial to initiate a consultation in a case assignment with a wound, ostomy, continence nurse (or wounds specialist) to establish a comprehensive plan for pressure ulcer risk reduction for clients at high risk for skin breakdown.

P

• = Independent   ▲ = Collaborative

Ineffective Protection

NANDA-I Definition

Decrease in the ability to guard self from internal or external threats such as illness or injury

Defining Characteristics

Alteration in clotting; alteration in perspiration; anorexia; chills; coughing; deficient immunity; disorientation; dyspnea; fatigue; immobility; insomnia; itching; maladaptive stress response; neurosensory impairment; pressure ulcer; restlessness; weakness

Related Factors (r/t)

Abnormal blood profiles; cancer; extremes of age; immune disorder (e.g., HIV-associated neuropathy, varicella zoster virus); inadequate nutrition; pharmaceutical agent; substance abuse; treatment regimen)

Client Outcomes

Client Will (Specify Time Frame)

- Remain free of infection while in contact with health care provider
- Remain free of any evidence of new bleeding as evident by stable vital signs
- Explain precautions to take to prevent infection including hand hygiene
- Explain precautions to take to prevent bleeding including fall prevention

Nursing Interventions

- Take temperature, pulse, and blood pressure (e.g., every 1 to 4 hours).
- ▲ Observe nutritional status (e.g., weight, serum protein and albumin levels, muscle mass, and usual food intake). Work with the dietitian to improve nutritional status if needed.
- Observe the client's sleep pattern; if altered, see nursing interventions for Disturbed **Sleep** pattern.
- Identify stressors in the client's life. If stress is uncontrollable, see nursing interventions for Ineffective **Coping**.

Prevention of Infection

- ▲ Monitor for and report any signs of infection (e.g., fever, chills, flushed skin, drainage, edema, redness, abnormal laboratory values, and pain) and notify the health care provider promptly.

• = Independent   ▲ = Collaborative

- If white blood cell count is severely decreased (i.e., absolute neutrophil count of less than 1000/mm³), initiate the following precautions:
  - ○ Take vital signs every 2 to 4 hours
  - ○ Complete a head-to-toe assessment twice daily, including inspection of oral mucosa, invasive sites, wounds, urine, and stool; monitor for onset of new reports of pain
- ▲ Avoid any invasive procedures, including catheterization, injections, and rectal or vaginal procedures unless absolutely necessary.
  - ○ Consider warming the client before elective surgery.
- ▲ Administer granulocyte growth factor as ordered.
  - ○ Take meticulous care of all invasive sites; use chlorhexidine gluconate for cleansing.
  - ○ Provide frequent oral care.
  - ○ Follow Standard Precautions, especially when performing hand hygiene to prevent health care–associated infections.
- ▲ Refer for appropriate prophylactic antifungal treatment and avoid pathogen exposure (through air filtration, regular hand hygiene, and avoidance of plants and flowers).
  - ○ Have the client wear a mask when leaving the room.
  - ○ Help the client bathe daily.
  - ○ Practice food safety; a neutropenic diet may not be necessary.
  - ○ Ensure that the client is well nourished. Provide food with protein, and consider vitamin supplements. If appetite is suppressed, institute a dietary referral. Keep track of serum albumin levels, as well as transferrin and prealbumin levels.
  - ○ Help the client cough and practice deep breathing regularly. Maintain an appropriate activity level.
  - ○ Obtain a private room for the client. Use high-energy particulate air filters if available and appropriate. Protective isolation is not recommended. Recognize that cotton cover gowns may not be effective in decreasing infection.
- ▲ Watch for signs of sepsis, including change in mental status, fever, shaking, chills, and hypotension. If present, notify the health care provider promptly.
- Refer to care plan for Risk for **Infection.**
- Refer to care plan for Readiness for enhanced **Nutrition** for additional interventions.

• = Independent   ▲ = Collaborative

Pediatric

- Suggest kangaroo care, frequent and exclusive or nearly exclusive breastfeeding, and early discharge from hospital for low-birth-weight infants.
- Assess postoperative fever in pediatric oncology clients promptly.
- For hand hygiene with low-birth-weight infants, use alcohol hand rub and gloves.

Geriatric

- If not contraindicated, promote exercise to improve quality of life in older adults.
- Refer to the care plan for Risk for **Infection** for more interventions related to the prevention of infection.

Prevention of Bleeding

- ▲ Monitor the client's risk for bleeding; evaluate results of clotting studies and platelet counts.
- Watch for hematuria, melena, hematemesis, hemoptysis, epistaxis, bleeding from mucosa, petechiae, and ecchymoses.
- ▲ Give medications orally or intravenously only; avoid giving intramuscularly, subcutaneously, or rectally (Shuey, 1996).
- Apply pressure for a longer time than usual to invasive sites, such as venipuncture or injection sites.
- Take vital signs often; watch for changes associated with fluid volume loss. Excessive bleeding causes decreased blood pressure and increased pulse and respiratory rates.
- Monitor menstrual flow if relevant; have the client use pads instead of tampons.
- Have the client use a moistened toothette or a very soft child's toothbrush instead of an adult toothbrush. Follow the dentist's recommendation for flossing and appropriate rinses to use. Control gum bleeding by applying pressure to gums with gauze pad soaked in ice water.
- Ask the client either to not shave or to use only an electric razor.
- ▲ To decrease risk of bleeding, avoid administering salicylates or nonsteroidal antiinflammatory drugs (NSAIDs) if possible.

Home Care

- Some of the interventions previously described may be adapted for home care use.

• = Independent   ▲ = Collaborative

▲ Consider using a nurse-led client-centered medical home (PCMH) for monitoring anticoagulant therapy.

• For terminally ill clients, teach and institute all of the aforementioned noninvasive precautions that maintain quality of life. Discuss with the client, family, and health care provider the consequences of contracting infection. Determine which precautions do not maintain quality of life and should not be used (e.g., physical assessment twice daily or multiple vital sign assessments).

Client/Family Teaching and Discharge Planning
Depressed Immune Function

• Teach the client and family how to take a temperature. Encourage the family to take the client's temperature between 3 PM and 7 PM at least once daily.

• Teach precautions to use to decrease the chance of infection (e.g., avoiding uncooked fruits and vegetables, using appropriate self-care including good hand hygiene, and ensuring a safe environment). Teach the client to avoid crowds and contact with persons who have infections. Teach the need for good nutrition, avoidance of stress, and adequate rest to maintain immune system function.

Bleeding Disorder

• Teach the client to wear a medical alert bracelet and notify all health care personnel of the bleeding disorder. Teach the client and family the signs of bleeding, precautions to take to prevent bleeding, and action to take if bleeding begins. Caution the client to avoid taking over-the-counter medications without the permission of the health care provider. *Medications containing salicylates can increase bleeding.*

• Teach the client to wear loose-fitting clothes and avoid physical activity that might cause trauma.

Rape-Trauma syndrome
NANDA-I Definition

Sustained adaptive response to a forced, violent sexual penetration against the victim's will and consent

Defining Characteristics

Aggression; agitation; anger; anxiety; change in relationships; confusion; denial; dependence; depression; disorganization; dissociative disorders;

• = Independent   ▲ = Collaborative

embarrassment; fear; guilt; helplessness; humiliation; hyperalertness; impaired decision-making; loss of self-esteem; mood swings; muscle spasms; muscle tension; nightmares; paranoia; phobias; physical trauma; powerlessness; revenge; self-blame; sexual dysfunction; shame; shock; sleep disturbances; substance abuse; suicide attempts; vulnerability

Related Factors (r/t)

Rape

Client Outcomes

Client Will (Specify Time Frame)

- Share feelings, concerns, and fears
- Recognize that the rape or attempt was not client's own fault
- State that, no matter what the situation, no one has the right to assault another
- Describe medical/legal treatment procedures and reasons for treatment
- Report absence of physical complications or pain
- Identify support resources and attend psychotherapy/group assistance in coping with the trauma and effects of the traumatic experience
- Function at same level as before crisis, including sexual functioning
- Recognize that it is normal for full recovery to take a minimum of 1 year

R Nursing Interventions

- Escort the client to a treatment room immediately upon arrival to the emergency department. Stay with (or have a trusted person stay with) the client.
- Assure the client of confidentiality.
- ▲ Provide a sexual assault response team (SART), if available, that includes a sexual assault nurse examiner (SANE), rape counseling advocate, and representative of law enforcement for best possible outcomes.
- Observe for signs of physical injury.
- Document the client's chief complaint and request an event history of the sexual assault in her/his own words.
- Encourage the client to verbalize her/his feelings.
- Make sure that the victim understands everything you are doing.
- Explain to the client that all or some of the client's clothing may be kept for evidential purposes and photographs may be taken (with consent) to document the client's injuries.

• = Independent   ▲ = Collaborative

▲ If a law enforcement interview is permitted, provide support by staying with the client at her/his request.

• Use the sexual assault evidence collection kits that have been reviewed by the SART members and provided by your state to collect adequate and accurate evidence for analysis by a forensic laboratory.

▲ Discuss the possibility of pregnancy and sexually transmitted infections (STIs) and the treatments available.

▲ Encourage the client to report the sexual assault to law enforcement agency.

▲ For those interested in a spiritual connection, make the appropriate recommendation.

▲ Stress the necessity of follow-up care with a mental health professional to recognize and intervene with problems associated with the effects of rape-trauma/sexual assault.

• Stress the importance of awareness throughout the community of the scope and severity of the effects of sexual abuse as a means of additional healing empowerment.

Geriatric

• Build a trusting relationship with the client.

• All examinations should be done on older adults as they would be done on any adult client after sexual assault, with modifications for comfort if necessary.

• Assess for mobility limitations and cognitive impairment.

• Explain and encourage the client to report sexual abuse.

• Observe for psychosocial distress. Consider arrangements for safe housing.

Multicultural

• Assess for the influence of cultural beliefs, norms, and values on the client's ability to cope with the trauma of the rape experience.

• Assess to determine if physically abused women are also victims of sexual assault.

Home Care

• Some of the interventions described previously may be adapted for home care use.

• Corroborate the client's feelings of self-worth. A study has proposed that the feeling of self-worth moderates the effects of violence—especially violent loss—on PTSD and depression (Mancini et al, 2011).

• = Independent ▲ = Collaborative

- Assist the client with realistically assessing the home setting for safety and/or selecting a safe environment in which to live.
▲ Ensure that the client has systems in place for long-term support.
▲ Design a practical discharge plan to include a safe shelter if needed, follow-up care for physical injury, and follow-up referral for psychological support.
▲ Assess for other client vulnerabilities such as mental health issues or addiction and refer client to social agencies for implementation of a therapeutic regimen.

Client/Family Teaching and Discharge Planning

- Emphasize the client's need for safety and to decrease the opportunities for repeat attacks.
- NOTE: PTSD has a high probability of being a psychological sequela to rape. Research demonstrated two effective treatments for improvement of PTSD in rape victims: prolonged exposure and stress inoculation training. Prolonged exposure involves reliving the rape experience; by imagining it as vividly as possible, describing it aloud in the present tense, taping this description, and listening to the tape at least once daily. Stress inoculation training uses breathing exercises to diminish anxiety and instruction in coping skills, thought stopping, cognitive restructuring, self-dialogue, and role playing. Research suggests that a combination of both treatments may provide the optimal effect. Furthermore, for those who reported the assault to police, lower levels of legal system success and satisfaction were linked to higher levels of perceived control over present recovery.

R

Ineffective Relationship
NANDA-I Definition

A pattern of mutual partnership that is insufficient to provide for each other's needs

Defining Characteristics

Delay in meeting of developmental goals appropriate for family life-cycle stage; dissatisfaction with complementary relationship between partners; dissatisfaction with emotional need fulfillment between partners; dissatisfaction with idea sharing between partners; dissatisfaction with information sharing between partners; dissatisfaction with physical need fulfillment between partners; inadequate understanding of partner's compromised

• = Independent   ▲ = Collaborative

functioning (e.g., physical, psychological social); insufficient balance in autonomy between partners; insufficient balance in collaboration between partners; insufficient mutual respect between partners; insufficient mutual support in daily activities between partners; partner not identified as support person; unsatisfying communication with partner

Related Factors

Alteration in cognitive functioning in one partner; developmental crisis; history of domestic violence; incarceration of one partner; ineffective communication skills; stressors; substance abuse; unrealistic expectations

Client Outcomes, Nursing Interventions, and Client/Family Teaching and Discharge Planning

Refer to care plan for Readiness for enhanced **Relationship.**

Readiness for enhanced Relationship

NANDA-I Definition

A pattern of mutual partnership to provide for each other's needs, which can be strengthened

Defining Characteristics

Expresses desire to enhance autonomy between partners; expresses desire to enhance collaboration between partners; expresses desire to enhance communication between partners; expresses desire to enhance emotional need fulfillment for each partner; expresses desire to enhance mutual respect between partners; expresses desire to enhance satisfaction with complementary relationship between partners; expresses desire to enhance satisfaction with emotional need fulfillment for each partner; expresses desire to enhance satisfaction with idea sharing between partners; expresses desire to enhance satisfaction with information sharing between partners; expresses desire to enhance satisfaction with physical need fulfillment for each partner; expresses desire to enhance understanding of partner's functional deficit (e.g., physical, psychological social)

Client Outcomes

Family/Client Will (Specify Time Frame)

• Share thoughts and feelings with each other
• Communicate openly with each other
• Assist in performing family roles and tasks
• Provide support for each other
• Obtain appropriate assistance

• = Independent   ▲ = Collaborative

Nursing Interventions

▲ Assess for signs of depression in the family when one partner is depressed, and make appropriate referrals.

▲ Assist couples to identify sources of their own perceived dyadic empathy in the relationship.

• Assist families to identify sources of gratitude in their lives.

• Assist clients to identify sources of gratitude in their lives using a future-oriented focus.

• Support "relationship talk" between couples (talking with a partner about the relationship, what one needs from one's partner, and/or the relationship implications of a shared stressor). Such discussions in couples with lung cancer have been shown to help partners better define their relationships and repair relationships that are functioning poorly (Badr et al, 2008).

• Encourage couples to participate and share in exciting and satisfying leisure activities and to share stories.

• Assist couples in establishing boundaries between work and home.

• Assist couples in regulating negative emotions.

• Assist couples in dealing with anger and communication when the diagnosis is cancer.

R

• Refer to care plans for Readiness for enhanced **Family** processes and Readiness for enhanced family **Coping**.

Pediatric

• Provide guidance and information on communication techniques for teenagers, especially those involved in intimate relationships.

• Encourage supportive relationships among parents and teenagers.

Geriatric

▲ Assess for spousal depression when one partner has cardiovascular disease, and make appropriate referrals.

▲ Assess for depression and anxiety, and make appropriate referrals for "prewidows" caring for spouses with chronic life-limiting conditions.

• Support older couples' positive collaborative communication.

• Encourage collaborative coping (i.e., spouses pooling resources and problem solving jointly) among older adults.

Multicultural

• Provide culturally tailored community-level interventions to raise awareness about HIV and bisexuality, and decrease HIV and sexual orientation stigma.

• = Independent   ▲ = Collaborative

Home Care
- Provide home-based psychoeducation to assist new parent couples with parenting and their couple relationship.

Client/Family Teaching and Discharge Planning
- Encourage clients and spouses to participate together in interventions to lower low-density lipoprotein cholesterol (LDL-C).
- Teach spouses how to provide emotional and instrumental support, allow clients to decide which component of the intervention they would like to receive, and have clients determine their own goals and action plans.
- Provide telephone calls to clients and spouses separately. During each client telephone call, client progress is reviewed, and clients create goals and action plans for the upcoming month. During spouse telephone calls, which occur within 1 week of client calls, spouses are informed of clients' goals and action plans and devise strategies to increase emotional and instrumental support.

Risk for Ineffective Relationship

R

NANDA-I Definition
Vulnerable to developing a pattern that is insufficient for providing a mutual partnership to provide for each other's needs

Risk Factors
Alteration in cognitive functioning in one partner; developmental crisis; history of domestic violence; incarceration of one partner; ineffective communication skills; stressors; substance abuse; unrealistic expectations

Client Outcomes, Nursing Interventions, and Client/Family Teaching and Discharge Planning
Refer to care plan for Ineffective **Relationship.**

Impaired Religiosity

NANDA-I Definition
Impaired ability to exercise reliance on beliefs and/or participate in rituals of a particular faith tradition

Defining Characteristics
Desire to reconnect with previous belief pattern; desire to reconnect with previous customs; difficulty adhering to prescribed religious beliefs; difficulty adhering to prescribed religious beliefs; difficulty adhering to

prescribed religious rituals (e.g., ceremonies, regulations, clothing, prayer, services, holiday observances); distress about separation from faith community; questioning of religious belief patterns; questioning of religious customs

Related Factors (r/t)

Developmental and Situational

Aging; end-stage life crises; life transitions

Physical

Illness; pain

Psychological

Anxiety; fear of death; history of religious manipulation; ineffective coping strategies; insufficient social support; personal crisis

Sociocultural

Cultural barriers to practicing religion; environmental barriers to practicing religion; insufficient social integration; insufficient sociocultural interaction

Spiritual

Spiritual crises; suffering

Client Outcomes

Client Will (Specify Time Frame)

- Express satisfaction with the ability to express religious practices
- Express satisfaction with access to religious materials and rituals
- Demonstrate balance between religious practices and healthy lifestyles
- Avoid high-risk, controlling religious relationships that inflict physical, sexual, or emotional harm and/or exploitation

Nursing Interventions

- Recognize when clients integrate religious practices in their life.
- Encourage and/or coordinate the use of and participation in usual religious rituals or practices that support coping.
- Encourage the use of prayer or meditation, as appropriate.
- Promote family coping using religious practices to help cope with loss, as appropriate.
- ▲ Refer to religious leader, professional counseling, or support group as needed.

Geriatric

- Promote established religious practices in older adults.

Multicultural

- Promote religious practices that are culturally appropriate.

• = Independent ▲ = Collaborative

Readiness for enhanced Religiosity

NANDA-I Definition

A pattern of reliance on religious beliefs and/or participation in rituals of a particular faith tradition, which can be strengthened

Defining Characteristics

Expresses desire to enhance belief patterns used in past; expresses desire to enhance connection with a religious leader; expresses desire to enhance forgiveness; expresses desire to enhance participation in religious experiences; expresses desire to enhance participation in religious practices (e.g., ceremonies, regulations, clothing, prayer, services, holiday observances); expresses desire to enhance religious customs used in the past; expresses desire to enhance religious options; expresses desire to enhance use of religious material

Client Outcomes, Nursing Interventions, and Client/Family and Discharge Planning

See care plan for Impaired **Religiosity.**

Pediatric

- Provide spiritual care for children based on developmental level.
  - **Infants:** Have the same nurse care for the child on a daily basis. Encourage holding, cuddling, rocking, playing with, and singing to the infant.
  - **Toddlers:** Provide consistency in care and familiar toys, music, stories, clothing, blankets, pillows, and any other individual object of contentment. Schedule home religious routines into the plan of care, and support home routines regarding good and bad behavior.
  - **School-age children and adolescents:** Encourage both groups to express their feelings regarding spirituality. Ask them, "Do you wish to pray, and what do you want to pray about?" Offer age-appropriate complementary therapies such as music, art, videos, and connectedness with peers through cards, letters, and visits.

Risk for impaired Religiosity

NANDA-I Definition

Vulnerable to an impaired ability to exercise reliance on religious beliefs and/or participate in rituals of a particular faith tradition, which may compromise health

Risk Factors

Developmental

Life transitions

Environmental

Barriers to practicing religion; lack of transportation

Physical

Hospitalization; illness; pain

Psychological

Depression; ineffective caregiving; ineffective coping strategies; insecurity; insufficient social support

Sociocultural

Cultural barrier to practicing religion; insufficient social interaction

Spiritual

Suffering

Client Outcomes and Nursing Interventions

Refer to care plan for Impaired **Religiosity.**

Relocation stress syndrome

NANDA-I Definition

Physiological and/or psychosocial disturbance following transfer from one environment to another

Defining Characteristics

Alienation; aloneness; alteration in sleep pattern; anger; anxiety; concern about relocation; dependency; depression; fear; frustration; increase in illness; increase in physical symptoms; increase in verbalization of needs; insecurity; loneliness; loss of identity; loss of self-worth; low self-esteem; pessimism; unwillingness to move; withdrawal; worried

Related Factors (r/t)

Compromised health status; history of loss; impaired psychosocial functioning; ineffective coping strategies; insufficient predeparture counseling; insufficient support system; language barrier; move from one environment to another; powerlessness; social isolation; unpredictability of experience

Client Outcomes

Client Will (Specify Time Frame)

- Recognize and know the name of at least one staff member or new neighbor within 1 week of relocating
- Express concern about move when encouraged to do so during individual contacts within 24 hours of awareness of impending relocation

• = Independent ▲ = Collaborative

- Carry out activities of daily living (ADLs) in usual manner
- Maintain previous mental and physical health status (e.g., nutrition, elimination, sleep, social interaction, physical activity) within 2 months of relocating

Nursing Interventions

- Be aware that relocation to supportive housing may be a positive change.
- Begin relocation planning as early in the decision process as possible.
- Obtain a history, including the reason for the move, the client's usual coping mechanisms, history of losses, and family support for the client.
- Identify to what extent the client can participate in the relocation decisions and advocate for this participation.
- Assess client's readiness to relocate and relocation self-efficacy.
- Consult an evidence-based practice guide for relocation.
- Assess family members' perceptions of client's ability to participate in relocation decisions. Particularly in cases of dementia, be alert to care workers' involvement in making the decision to relocate. They may need support and encouragement through the process.
- Consider the client's and family's cultural and ethnic values as much as possible when choosing roommates, foods, and other aspects of care.
- Promote clear communication between all participants in the relocation process.
- Observe the following procedures if the client is being transferred to an extended care facility or assisted living facility:
  - Facilitate the client's participation in decisions and choice of placement, and arrange a preadmission visit if possible.
  - If the client cannot visit the new facility, arrange for a visit or telephone call by a member of the staff to welcome the client and show a videotape or at least provide pictures of the new care facility.
  - Have a familiar person accompany the client to the new facility.
  - Recommend that the caregiver write a journal of thoughts and feelings regarding the relocation of his/her loved one.
  - Continue to assess caregiver psychological distress during a 6-month period following relocation.

R

• = Independent   ▲ = Collaborative

- Identify previous routines for ADLs. Try to maintain as much continuity with the previous schedule as possible.
- Bring in familiar items from home (e.g., pictures, clocks, afghans). Familiarity eases transition and symbolizes safeness.
- Establish the way the client would like to be addressed (Mr., Mrs., Miss, first name, nickname).
- Thoroughly orient the client and the family to the new environment and routines; repeat directions as needed.
- Spend one-to-one time with the client. Allow the client to express feelings and convey acceptance of them; emphasize that the client's feelings are real and individual and that it is acceptable to be sad or angry about moving.
- Allocate a caring staff member to help the client adjust to the move. Assign the same staff members to the client for care if compatible with client; maintain consistency in the personnel with whom the client interacts.
- Ask the client to state one positive aspect of the new living situation each day. Helping the client focus on the positive aspects of the move can help change attitude and reframe the situation in a positive fashion.
- Monitor the client's health status and provide appropriate interventions for problems with social interaction, nutrition, sleep, new onset of infection, or elimination problems.
- If the client is being transferred within a facility, have staff members from the new unit visit the client before transfer.
- Work with the caregivers and family members helping them deal with stages of "making the best of it," "making the move," and "making it better."
- If a client is being transferred from the intensive care unit (ICU), have previous staff make occasional visits until the client is comfortable in the new surroundings. Ensure that the family is told relevant information.
- Watch for coping problems (e.g., withdrawal, regression, angry behavior, impaired sleeping, refusal to eat, flat affect, anxiety) and intervene immediately.
- Encourage the client to express grief for the loss of the old situation; explain that it is normal to feel sadness over change and loss.
- Pay special attention to assessing and giving psychosocial care.

• = Independent   ▲ = Collaborative

- Encourage the client to participate in care as much as possible and make own decisions when possible (e.g., placement of the bed, choice of roommate, bathing routines).

Pediatric

- Assess family history and contact information from children relocated to rescue shelters.
- Be aware that community relocation may be beneficial for children, and assess community resources of new location.
- Provide support for a child and family who must relocate to be near a transplant center.
- In divorce situations, recommend alternative dispute resolution versus traditional litigated settlement.
- Encourage child to verbalize concerns in divorce situations when they and/or a parent relocate.
- Assess presence of allergies before and after relocation.
- If the client is an adolescent, try to avoid a move in the middle of the school year, find a newcomers' club for the adolescent to join, and refer for counseling if needed.
- Assess adolescents' perceptions of their acceptance by peers.
- Help parents recognize that relocation stress syndrome may persist for prolonged periods (e.g., 2 years) in adolescents.
- Be aware that young people may cope with the transition by exerting control in particular domains.
- The effects of frequent relocation may not manifest immediately and may have long-term impacts on physical and mental health.

Geriatric

- Monitor the need for transfer and transfer only when necessary.
- Implement discharge planning early so that it is not rushed.
- Protect the client from injuries such as falls.
- Utilize technologies such as sensing devices to measure average in-home gait speed (AIGS) as a predictor of fall risk.
- Implement a registered nurse (RN) care coordination model to restore older adults' health, maintain their independence, and reduce care costs.
- After the transfer, determine the client's mental status.
- Facilitate visits from companion animals.
- Encourage reminiscence of happy times.
- Refer for music therapy.
- Monitor for neuroleptic prescriptions.

R

• = Independent   ▲ = Collaborative

Client/Family Teaching and Discharge Planning
- Teach family members and remind direct care staff about relocation stress syndrome. Encourage them to monitor for signs of the syndrome.
- Help significant others learn how to support the client in the move by setting up a schedule of visits, arranging for holidays, bringing familiar items from home, and establishing a system for contact when the client needs support.
- Assist family members and the relocating older adult to use webcam technology for interaction to supplement in-person visits.

Risk for Relocation stress syndrome

NANDA-I Definition

Vulnerable to physiological and/or psychosocial disturbance following transfer from one environment to another that may compromise health

Risk Factors

Compromised health status; deficient mental competence; history of loss; ineffective coping strategies; insufficient predeparture counseling; insufficient support system; move from one environment to another; powerlessness; significant environmental change; unpredictability of experience

Client Outcomes, Nursing Interventions, and Client/Family Teaching and Discharge Planning

Refer to care plan for **Relocation** stress syndrome.

Risk for ineffective Renal perfusion

NANDA-I Definition

Vulnerable to a decrease in blood circulation to the kidney that may compromise health

Risk Factors

Abdominal compartment syndrome; alteration in metabolism; bilateral cortical necrosis; burns; cardiac surgery; cardiopulmonary bypass; diabetes mellitus; exposure to nephrotoxin; extremes of age; female gender; glomerulonephritis; hypertension; hypovolemia; hypoxemia; hypoxia; infection; interstitial nephritis; malignancy; malignant hypertension; polynephritis; renal disease (e.g., polycystic kidney, renal artery stenosis, failure); smoking; substance abuse; systemic inflammatory response syndrome; trauma; treatment regimen; vascular embolism; vasculitis

Client Outcomes

Client Will (Specify Time Frame)

- Maintain normal blood urea nitrogen and serum creatinine levels
- Maintain urine output of 0.5 mL/kg/hr
- Maintain urine output that is yellow and clear
- Maintain serum electrolytes (K^+, PO_4, Na^+) within normal limits
- Maintain glomerular filtration rate of 60 to 89 mL/min/1.73 m^2
- Maintain normal fluid balance

Nursing Interventions

▲ Be aware of major risk factors that increase the risk for decreased renal perfusion.

▲ Be aware of the RIFLE classification system used to indicate progression in severity of acute kidney injury in adults.

• Review client's medical and social history for evidence of chronic conditions such as hypertension and diabetes, exposure to tropical disease, and exposure to nephrotoxins at work, home, or recreation.

• Assess clients for fluid imbalance by examining 24-hour fluid intake and output measurements.

• Assess vital signs, carefully noting new onset of hypertension, hypotension, or dysrhythmia; communicate findings promptly to health care provider.

• Assess for early signs of fluid deficit (skin turgor, tongue turgor, thirst, decreased urinary output).

• Assess for early signs of fluid overload.

• Assess for early changes in mental status (irritability, drowsiness, headache, muscle weakness, difficulty concentrating, disorientation, confusion). Refer to care plan for Acute **Confusion.**

▲ Monitor at-risk clients for increasing levels of serum creatinine and decreasing glomerular filtration rate and urine output.

▲ Use isotonic crystalloids rather than colloids (albumin or starches) to provide expansion of intravascular volume in hypovolemic clients who are at risk for or have acute kidney injury.

▲ Maintain normal to somewhat increased levels of glucose in critically ill patients with insulin therapy.

▲ Communicate to radiology departments when clients scheduled for testing with contrast media had contrast media testing within the last 24 hours or recently received cisplatin or high-dose methotrexate.

▲ Monitor that peak and trough serum levels of aminoglycosides are within acceptable ranges when multiple daily dosing is administered for more than 24 hours.

• Ensure that at-risk clients having diagnostic testing with contrast media are well hydrated with intravenous isotonic sodium chloride or sodium bicarbonate solutions as ordered before and after the procedure. Refer to care plan for Risk for adverse reaction to iodinated **Contrast Media.**

• Collect a 24-hour urine specimen for examination as ordered.

▲ Note the results of diagnostic studies such as renal ultrasound, radionuclide scanning, abdominal/pelvic computed tomography (CT), magnetic resonance angiography, magnetic resonance imaging (MRI), and arteriography.

• Monitor results of serum and urine tests of kidney function as ordered or per protocol and promptly notify health care provider of abnormal results.

Geriatric

• Be aware that advanced age is a risk factor that increases the probability of ineffective renal perfusion.

• Assess for signs of dehydration in older adults who have less thirst and consume less fluid than young adults when experiencing fluid deprivation. Refer to care plan for Deficient **Fluid** volume.

• Ensure older clients receive sufficient fluids to prevent dehydration and hypovolemia (Pinto & Schub, 2013).

Pediatric

• Be aware that renal development in infants and neonates may be adversely affected by nephrotoxic drugs.

▲ Be aware of the pediatric RIFLE classification system used to indicate progression in severity of acute kidney injury in children.

Client/Family Teaching and Discharge Planning

• Instruct at-risk clients and families to inform health care professionals about their kidney status if scheduled for a CT scan, MRI scan, or angiogram (National Kidney Foundation, 2013a).

• Instruct at-risk clients to avoid overuse of analgesics such as acetaminophen and nonsteroidal antiinflammatory drugs (NSAIDs).

• = Independent   ▲ = Collaborative

- Instruct clients about risk factors for renal insufficiency or acute renal failure including signs and symptoms of acute renal failure and lifestyle changes that can improve renal function.
▲ Instruct at-risk clients to alert health care providers about renal status before obtaining new medication prescriptions.
▲ Encourage smoking cessation. Effects of nicotine include increased pulse and blood pressure and constriction of blood vessels; vasoconstriction and atherosclerosis exacerbate existing problems with kidney perfusion (National Kidney Foundation, 2013b).

Impaired Resilience
NANDA-I Definition
Decreased ability to sustain a pattern of positive responses to an adverse situation or crisis
Defining Characteristics
Decreased interest in academic activities; decreased interest in vocational activities; depression; guilt; impaired health status; ineffective coping strategies; low self-esteem; renewed elevation of distress; shame; social isolation
Related Factors (r/t)
Community violence; demographics that increase chance of maladjustment; economically disadvantaged; ethnic minority status; exposure to violence; female gender; inconsistent parenting; insufficient impulse control; large family size; low intellectual ability; low maternal educational level; parental mental illness; perceived vulnerability; psychological disorder; substance abuse
Client Outcomes
Client Will (Specify Time Frame)
- Demonstrate reduced or cessation of drug and alcohol usage
- State effective life events on feelings about self
- Seek help when necessary
- Verbalize or demonstrate cessation of abuse
- Adapt to unexpected crises or challenges
- Verbalize positive outlook on illness, family, situation, and life
- Use available resources to meet coping needs
- Identify role models
- Identify available assets and resources
- Be able to verbalize meaning of one's life

• = Independent   ▲ = Collaborative

R

Nursing Interventions

- Encourage positive, health-seeking behaviors.
- Ensure access to biological, psychological, and spiritual resources.
- Foster communication skills through basic communication skill training.
- Foster cognitive skills in decision-making.
- Assist client in cognitive restructuring of negative thought processes.
- Facilitate supportive family environments and communication.
- Promote engagement in positive social activities.
- Assist client to identify strengths, and reinforce these.
- Help the client identify positive emotions in the midst of adverse situations.
- Build on supportive counseling and therapy.
- Identify protective factors such as assets and resources to enhance coping.
- Provide positive reinforcement and emotional support during the learning process.
- Encourage mindfulness, a conscious attention and awareness of self.
- Educate and encourage the use of stress reduction techniques such as guided imagery in which the client focuses on positive images and emotions.
- Enhance knowledge and use of self-care strategies.
- Assist the client to have an optimistic world view.

Pediatric

- The preceding interventions may be adapted for the pediatric client.
- Promote nurturing, supportive relationships with family.
- Support the seeking of opportunities to improve cognitive abilities, such as tutoring and other resources; the development of positive and supportive relations, such as family, community members, or mentors; and the improvement of general health.
- Promote the development of positive mentor relationships.
- ▲ Consider referral to appropriate community resources, such as faith-based communities for children who have had adverse childhood experiences.

• = Independent   ▲ = Collaborative

Readiness for enhanced Resilience

NANDA-I Definition

A pattern of positive responses to an adverse situation or crisis, which can be strengthened

Defining Characteristics

Demonstrates positive outlook; exposure to crisis; expresses desire to enhance available resources; expresses desire to enhance communication skills; expresses desire to enhance environmental safety; expresses desire to enhance goal setting; expresses desire to enhance involvement in activities; expresses desire to enhance own responsibility for action; expresses desire to enhance progress toward goal; expresses desire to enhance relationships with others; expresses desire to enhance resilience; expresses desire to enhance self-esteem; expresses desire to enhance sense of control; expresses desire to enhance support system; expresses desire to enhance use of conflict management strategies; expresses desire to enhance use of coping skills; expresses desire to enhance use of resource

Client Outcomes

Client Will (Specify Time Frame)

- Adapt to adversities and challenges
- Communicate clearly and appropriately for age
- Take responsibility for own actions
- Make progress towards goals
- Use effective coping strategies
- Express emotions

Nursing Interventions

- Listen to and encourage expressions of feelings and beliefs.
- Establish a therapeutic relationship based on trust and respect.
- Assist client in rating current level of resilience: www.resiliencescale.com.
- Facilitate supportive family environments and communication.
- Assist client to identify and reinforce strengths.
- Enhance skills associated with social and executive functioning.
- Provide positive reinforcement and emotional support during implementation of care.
- ▲ Facilitate the development of mentorship and volunteer opportunities.
- Determine how family behavior affects the client.
- Promote use of mindfulness and other stress reduction techniques.

• = Independent   ▲ = Collaborative

Pediatric
- The preceding interventions may be adapted for the pediatric client.
- Encourage the promotion of protective factors by fostering the seeking of opportunities to improve cognitive abilities, such as tutoring and other resources; the development of positive and supportive relations such as family, community members, or mentors; and the improvement of general health.

Multicultural
- Use teaching strategies that are culturally and age appropriate.

Risk for impaired Resilience

NANDA-I Definition

Vulnerable to decreased ability to sustain a pattern of positive response to an adverse situation or crisis, which may compromise health

Risk Factors

Chronicity of existing crisis; multiple coexisting adverse situations: new crisis (e.g., unplanned pregnancy, loss of housing, death of family member)

Client Outcomes

Client Will (Specify Time Frame)
- Identify available community resources
- Propose practical, constructive solutions for disputes
- Identify and access community resources for assistance
- Accept assistance with activities of daily living from family and friends
- Verbalize an enhanced sense of control
- Verbalize meaningfulness of one's life

Nursing Interventions

- Determine how family behavior affects client.
- Help identify personal rights, responsibilities, and conflicting norms.
- Encourage consideration of values underlying choices and consequences of the choice.
- Help client practice conversational and social skills.
- Assist client to prioritize values.
- Create an accepting, nonjudgmental atmosphere.
- Help identify self-defeating thoughts.
- ▲ Refer to community resources/social services as appropriate.
- ▲ Help clarify problem areas in interpersonal relationships.

• = Independent   ▲ = Collaborative

▲ Promote a sense of an individual's autonomy and control over choices to be made in one's environment. Identify and enroll high-risk families in follow-up programs.

Parental Role conflict
NANDA-I Definition
Parent's experience of role confusion and conflict in response to crisis
Defining Characteristics
Anxiety; concern about family (e.g., functioning, communication, health); disruption in caregiver routines; fear; frustration; guilt; perceived inadequacy to provide for child's needs (e.g., physical, emotional); perceived loss of control over decisions relating to child; reluctance to participate in usual caregiver activities
Related Factors (r/t)
Change in marital status; home care of a child with special needs; interruptions in family life due to home care regimen (e.g., treatments, caregivers, lack of respite); intimidated by invasive modalities (e.g., intubation); intimidation by restrictive modalities (e.g., isolation); living in nontraditional setting (e.g., foster, group or institutional care); parent-child separation

R

Client Outcomes
Client Will (Specify Time Frame)
• Express feelings and perceptions regarding impacts of illness, disability, and/or hospitalization on parental role
• Participate in hospital and home care as much as able given the availability of resources and support systems
• Exhibit assertiveness and responsibility in active family decision-making regarding care of the child
• Describe and select available resources to support parental management of the child's and family's needs
Nursing Interventions
• Assess and support parent's previous coping behaviors.
• Determine parent/family sources of stress, usual methods of coping, and perceptions of illness/condition. Maximize the identified strengths.

• = Independent   ▲ = Collaborative

- Evaluate the family's perceived strength of its social support system, including religious beliefs. Encourage the family to use social support.
- Determine the older childbearing woman's support systems and expectations for motherhood.
- Consider the use of family-centered theory as the conceptual foundation to help guide interventions.
- Be available to accept and support parents by listening and discussing concerns.
▲ Maintain parental involvement in shared decision-making with regard to care by using the following steps: incorporate parents' information concerning the child's typical routines, behaviors, fears, likes, and dislikes; provide clear and direct firsthand information concerning the child's condition and progress; normalize the home/hospital environment as much as possible; collaborate in care by providing choices when possible.
- Seek and support parental participation in care.
- Provide support for each parent's primary coping strategies and needs.
▲ Inform parents of financial resources, respite care, and home support to assist them in maintaining sufficient energy and personal resources to continue caregiving responsibilities.
- Encourage the parent to meet his/her own needs for rest, nutrition, and hygiene. Provide bed space so that the parent may stay with the sick child.
- Provide family-centered care: allow parents to touch and talk to the child, and assist in the handling of medical equipment; offer a comfortable chair, preferably a rocking chair. Provide opportunities and offer praise for successful caregiving.
- Refer parents to available telephone and/or Internet support groups.
- Involve new mother's partner or parents in clinical encounters and invite family members to discuss their expectations and parenting experiences.

Multicultural
- Acknowledge racial/ethnic differences at the onset of care.
- Assess for the influence of cultural beliefs, norms, and values on the client's perceptions of the parental role.

• = Independent   ▲ = Collaborative

- Acknowledge that value conflicts arising from acculturation stresses may contribute to increased anxiety and significant conflict with the parental role.
- Promote the female parenting role by providing a treatment environment that is culturally based and woman-centered.
- Support the client's parenting role in her usual setting via social exchange, including online support.

Home Care

- The interventions described previously may be adapted for home care use.
- Assess family adjustment prenatally and postpartum; assist new parents to renegotiate parenting roles and responsibilities with co-parenting. Encourage the father to take an active role in infant care with the mother's support.

Client/Family Teaching and Discharge Planning

- Offer family-led education interventions to improve participants' knowledge about their condition and its treatment and to decrease their information needs.
- For children and their parents involved in bereavement support groups, identify the family's positive way of coping.
- ▲ Refer parents of children with behavioral problems to parenting programs.
- Involve parents in formal and/or informal social support situations, such as Internet support groups.
- Teach the client about available community resources (e.g., therapists, ministers, counselors, self-help groups).
- Encourage parents with chronic illnesses to implement custody plans for their children.

R

Ineffective Role performance

NANDA-I Definition

Patterns of behavior and self-expression that do not match the environmental context norms and expectations

Defining Characteristics

Alteration in role perceptions; anxiety; change in capacity to resume role; change in other's perception of role; change in self-perception of role; change in usual patterns of responsibility; depression; discrimination; domestic violence; harassment; inappropriate developmental expectations;

• = Independent ▲ = Collaborative

ineffective adaptation to change; ineffective coping strategies; ineffective role performance; insufficient confidence; insufficient external support for role enactment; insufficient knowledge of role requirements; insufficient motivation; insufficient opportunity for role enactment; insufficient self management; insufficient skills; pessimism; powerlessness; role ambivalence; role conflict; role confusion; role denial; role dissatisfaction; role strain; system conflict; uncertainty

Related Factors (r/t)

Knowledge

Insufficient role model; insufficient role preparation (e.g., role transition, skill rehearsal, validation); low education level; unrealistic role expectations

Physiological

Alteration in body image; depression; fatigue; low self-esteem; mental health issue (e.g., depression, psychosis, personality disorder, substance abuse); neurological defect; pain; physical illness; substance abuse

Social

Conflict; developmental level inappropriate for role expectation; domestic violence; economically disadvantaged; inappropriate linkage with the health care system; insufficient resources (e.g., financial, social, knowledge); insufficient rewards; insufficient role socialization; insufficient support system; stressors; young age

Client Outcomes

Client Will (Specify Time Frame)

- Identify realistic perception of role
- State personal strengths
- Acknowledge problems contributing to inability to carry out usual role
- Accept physical limitations regarding role responsibility and consider ways to change lifestyle to accomplish goals associated with role performance
- Demonstrate knowledge of appropriate behaviors associated with new or changed role
- State knowledge of change in responsibility and new behaviors associated with new responsibility
- Verbalize acceptance of new responsibility

Nursing Interventions

Social

- Assess the client's level of resilience and implement nursing actions that increase client resilience.

• = Independent   ▲ = Collaborative

- Assess the impact of uncertainty on the client's role.
- Ask the client direct questions regarding new roles and how the health care system can help him or her continue in roles.
▲ Allow the client to express feelings regarding the role change; refer for support as needed.
▲ Assist the client to identify rewards associated with his or her roles.
▲ Refer for support as needed for home caregivers of military families during the deployment of spouses. Refer the client to Acceptance and Commitment Therapy (ACT).
- Reinforce the client's strengths and internalized values.
- Support the client's religious practices.

Physiological
- Identify ways to compensate for physical disabilities (e.g., have a ramp built to provide access to house, put household objects within the client's reach from wheelchair), and provide technological assistance when available.
- Refer to the care plans for Readiness for enhanced family **Coping,** Readiness for enhanced **Decision-Making,** Impaired **Home** maintenance, Impaired **Parenting,** Risk for **Loneliness,** Readiness for enhanced community **Coping,** Readiness for enhanced **Self-Care,** and Ineffective **Sexuality** pattern.

R

Pediatric
- Assist new parents to adjust to changes in workload associated with childbirth. Mothers may need additional support.
- Assess mothers who present with depressive symptoms in the postpartum period for evidence of role performance distress.
▲ Refer teen parents and families to a community-based, multifamily group intervention strategy (e.g., Families and Schools Together babies).
▲ Refer to home health agency for home visits when there is an infant who has excessive crying.
- Provide parents with coping skills when the role change is associated with a critically and chronically ill child.
▲ Assist families how to manage day-to-day needs of a child with cerebral palsy (CP). Teach family members to value the small things children do, connect with other families, locate community resources, and understand the short- and long-term needs of the child.
- Consider the use of media-based behavioral treatments for children with behavioral disorders.

• = Independent   ▲ = Collaborative

Geriatric

- Assess older adults' choices regarding their care and enable them to live as they wish and receive the help they want by carefully listening to their stories.
- Provide support and practice for older adults to use assistive devices.
- Support the client's religious beliefs and activities and provide appropriate spiritual support persons.
- Explore community needs after assessing the client's strengths. Encourage older adults to participate in volunteer programs.
- Provide educational materials for older clients who are recovering from hip surgery or fractures to promote early mobility.
- ▲ Refer to appropriate support groups for mental stress related to role changes.
- ▲ Refer clients to therapeutic recreation programs that use humor.
- Provide music of choice for clients with Alzheimer's disease.
- Provide support for grandparents raising grandchildren.

Multicultural

- Assess for the influence of cultural beliefs, norms, values, and expectations on the individual's role.
- Assess for conflicts between the caregiver's cultural role, obligations, and competing factors, such as employment or school.
- Negotiate with the client regarding the aspects of their role that can be modified and still honor cultural beliefs.
- Encourage family to use support groups or other service programs to assist with role changes.
- Refer new moms to a new mothers' Internet-based social support network.

Home Care

- The preceding interventions may be adapted for home care use.
- ▲ Offer a referral to medical social services to assist with assessing the short- and long-term impacts of role change.

Client/Family Teaching and Discharge Planning

- Provide educational materials to family members on client behavior management plus caregiver stress-coping management.
- Help the client identify resources for assistance in caring for a disabled or aging parent (e.g., adult day care, nursing home placement).
- Consider pet therapy for college students in a new role, their first semester away from home.

• = Independent   ▲ = Collaborative

Sedentary lifestyle

NANDA-I Definition

Reports a habit of life that is characterized by a low physical activity level

Defining Characteristics

Average daily physical activity is less than recommended for gender and age; physical deconditioning; preference for activity low in physical activity

Related Factors (r/t)

Insufficient interest in physical activity; insufficient knowledge of health benefits associated with physical exercise; insufficient motivation for physical activity; insufficient resources for physical activity; insufficient training for physical exercise

Client Outcomes

Client Will (Specify Time Frame)

- Engage in purposeful moderate-intensity cardiorespiratory (aerobic) exercise for 30 to 60 minutes per day on 5 or more days per week for a total of 2 hours and 30 minutes (150 minutes) per week
- Increase exercise to 20 minutes per day (less than 150 minutes per week); light to moderate intensity exercise may be beneficial in deconditioned persons
- Increase pedometer step counts by 1000 steps per day every 2 weeks to reach a daily step count of at least 7000 steps per day, with a daily goal for most healthy adults of 10,000 steps per day
- Perform resistance exercises that involve all major muscle groups (legs, hips, back, chest, abdomen, shoulders, and arms) performed on 2 to 3 days per week
- Perform flexibility exercise (stretching) for each of the major muscle-tendon groups 2 days per week for 10 to 60 seconds to improve joint range of motion; greatest gains occur with daily exercise
- Engage in neuromotor exercise 20 to 30 minutes per day including motor skills (e.g., balance, agility, coordination, and gait), proprioceptive exercise training, and multifaceted activities (e.g., tai chi and yoga) to improve and maintain physical function and reduce falls in those at risk for falling (older persons)
- Meet mutually defined goals of exercise that include individual choice, preference, and enjoyment in the exercise prescription (American College of Sports Medicine [ACSM], 2011b)

• = Independent   ▲ = Collaborative

Nursing Interventions

- Observe the client for cause of sedentary lifestyle. Determine whether cause is physical, psychological, social, or ecological. See care plans for Ineffective **Coping** or **Hopelessness.**
- ▲ Assess for reasons why the client would be unable to participate in an exercise program; refer for evaluation by a primary health care provider as needed.
- Use the Self-Efficacy for Exercise Scale (Resnick & Jenkins, 2000) and the Outcome Expectation for Exercise Scale (Resnick et al, 2001) to determine client's self-efficacy and outcome expectations toward exercise (Resnick & D'Adamo, 2011).
- Recommend the client enter an exercise program with a person who supports exercise behavior (e.g., friend or exercise buddy).
- Recommend the client begin a walking program using the following criteria:
  - ○ Obtain a pedometer by purchase or from community/public health resources.
  - ○ Determine common times when brisk walking for at least 10-minute intervals can be incorporated into lifestyle and daily activities.
  - ○ Set incremental walking goal and increase it by 1000 steps per day every 2 weeks for a minimum of 7,000 steps per day with a daily goal for most healthy adults of 10,000 steps per day (approximately 5 miles) (ACSM, 2011a).
  - ○ Toward the end of day, if client has not met walking goal, look for opportunities to increase activity level (e.g., park farther from destination; use stairs) or go for a walk indoors or outdoors until designated goal of 7000 to 10,000 steps per day is reached (ACSM, 2011a).
- Encourage prescriptive resistance exercise of each major muscle group (hips, thighs, legs, back, chest, shoulders, and abdomen) using a variety of exercise equipment such as free weights, bands, stair climbing, or machines 2 to 3 days per week. Involve the major muscle groups for 8 to 12 repetitions to improve strength and power in most adults; 10 to 15 repetitions to improve strength in middle-aged and older persons starting exercise; 15 to 20 repetitions to improve muscular endurance. Intensity should be between moderate (5 to 6) and hard (7 to 8) on a scale of 0 to 10 (ACSM, 2014, 2011b).

S

• = Independent   ▲ = Collaborative

- Encourage gradual progression of greater resistance, more repetitions per set, and/or increasing frequency using concentric, eccentric, and isometric muscle actions. Perform bilateral and unilateral single and multiple joint exercises. Optimize exercise intensity by working large before small muscle groups, multiple joint exercises before single-joint exercises, and higher intensity before lower intensity exercises (ACSM, 2009b, 2011b).

Pediatric
- Children and adolescents should participate in 60 minutes (1 hour) or more of physical activity daily.
- Aerobic: Sixty or more minutes a day should be either moderate- or vigorous-intensity aerobic physical activity, and should include vigorous-intensity physical activity at least 3 days a week.
- Muscle-strengthening: As part of daily physical activity, children and adolescents should include muscle-strengthening physical activity on at least 3 days of the week.
- Bone-strengthening: As part of daily physical activity, children and adolescents should include bone-strengthening physical activity on at least 3 days of the week.
- Providing activities that are age appropriate, enjoyable, and offer a variety will encourage young people to participate in physical activities (U.S. Department of Health and Human Services, 2012).
- Encourage child to increase the amount of walking done per day; if child is willing, ask him/her to wear a pedometer to measure number of steps.
- Recommend the child decrease television viewing, watching movies, and playing video games. Ask parents to limit television to 1 to 2 hours per day maximum.

Geriatric
- Use valid and reliable criterion-referenced standards for fitness testing (e.g., Senior Fitness Test) designed for older adults that can predict the level of capacity associated with maintaining physical independence into later years of life (e.g., Get Up and Go test).
- Recommend the client begin a regular exercise program, even if generally active.
- ▲ Refer the client to physical therapy for resistance exercise training, as able, involving all major muscle groups.

• = Independent   ▲ = Collaborative

- Use the Function-Focused Care (FFC) rehabilitative philosophy of care with older adults in residential nursing facilities to prevent avoidable functional decline.
- Recommend the client practice tai chi.
- If client is scheduled for an elective surgery that will result in admission into the intensive care unit and immobility, or recovery from a joint replacement, for example, initiate a prehabilitation program that includes a warm-up followed by aerobic, strength, flexibility, neuromotor, and functional task work.

Home Care
- The preceding interventions may be adapted for home care use.
▲ Assess home environment for factors that create barriers to mobility. Refer to physical and occupational therapy services if needed to assist the client in restructuring home environment and daily living patterns. Use home safety assessment tool to prevent falls and improve mobility and function such as the tool found at http://agingresearch.buffalo.edu/hsst/index.htm.

Client/Family Teaching and Discharge Planning
- Work with the client using theory-based interventions (e.g., social, cognitive, theoretical components such as self-efficacy; transtheoretical model).
- Recommend the client use the Exercise Assessment and Screening for You (EASY) tool to help determine appropriate exercise for the older adult client. This tool is available online at http://www.easyforyou.info (Resnick, 2009).
- Consider using motivational interviewing techniques when working with both children and adult clients to increase their activity.

Readiness for enhanced Self-Care
NANDA-I Definition

A pattern of performing activities for oneself to meet health-related goals, which can be strengthened

Defining Characteristics

Expresses desire to enhance independence with health; expresses desire to enhance independence with life; expresses desire to enhance independence with personal development; expresses desire to enhance independence with well-being; expresses desire to enhance knowledge of self-care strategies; expresses desire to enhance self-care

　　　• = Independent　　　　　▲ = Collaborative

Client Outcomes

Client Will (Specify Time Frame)

- Evaluate current levels of self-care as optimum for abilities
- Express the need or desire to continue to enhance levels of self-care
- Seek health-related information as needed
- Identify strategies to enhance self-care
- Perform appropriate interventions as needed
- Monitor level of self-care
- Evaluate the effectiveness of self-care interventions at regular intervals

Nursing Interventions

- For assessment of self-care, use a valid and reliable screening tool if available for specific characteristics of the person, such as arthritis, diabetes, stroke, heart failure, or dementia.
- Conduct mutual goal setting with the person.
- Support the person's awareness that enhanced self-care is an achievable, desirable, and positive life goal.
- Show respect for the person, regardless of characteristics and/or background.
- Promote trust and enhanced communication between the person and health care providers.
- Promote opportunities for spiritual care and growth.
- Promote social support through facilitation of family involvement.
- Provide opportunities for ongoing group support through establishment of self-help groups on the Internet.
- Help the person identify and reduce the barriers to self-care.
- Provide literacy-appropriate education for self-care activities.
- Facilitate self-efficacy by ensuring the adequacy of self-care education.
- Provide alternative mind-body therapies such as reiki, guided imagery, yoga, and self-hypnosis.
- Promote the person's hope to maintain self-care.

Pediatric

- Assess and evaluate a child's level of self-care and adjust strategies as needed.
- Assist families to engage in and maintain social support networks.
- Encourage activities that support or enhance spiritual care.

• = Independent ▲ = Collaborative

Multicultural

- Identify cultural beliefs, values, lifestyle practices, and problem-solving strategies when assessing the client's level of self-care.
- Enhance cultural knowledge by seeking out information regarding different cultural or ethnic groups.
- Recognize the impact of culture on self-care behaviors.
- Provide culturally competent care.
- Support independent self-care activities.

Home Care

- The nursing interventions described previously may also be used in home care settings.
- Support the new sense of self that may occur with complex health problems.
- Assist individuals and families to prevent exacerbations of chronic illness symptoms so rehospitalization is not necessary.
- In complex chronic illnesses such as heart failure, help individuals and families to accept continued functional disabilities and work toward maintenance of optimum functional status, considering the reality of illness status.
- Use educational guidelines for stroke survivors.
- Ensure appropriate interdisciplinary communication to support client safety.
- Enhance individual and family coping with chronic illnesses.
- Implement a community care management program.

Client/Family Teaching and Discharge Planning

- Teach clients how to regularly assess their level of self-care.
- Instruct clients that a variety of interventions may be needed to enhance self-care.
- Help clients to understand that enhanced self-care is an achievable goal.
- Empower clients.
- Teach clients about the decision-making process and self-care activities needed to manage their illness state and promote well-being.
- Continuously stress that all self-care activities must be regularly evaluated to ensure that enhanced levels of self-care can be maintained.

• = Independent ▲ = Collaborative

Bathing Self-Care deficit

NANDA-I Definition

Impaired ability to perform or complete bathing activities for self

Defining Characteristics

Impaired ability to dry body; impaired ability to access bathroom; impaired ability to access water; impaired ability to gather bathing supplies; impaired ability to regulate bath water; impaired ability to wash body

Related Factors (r/t)

Alteration in cognitive functioning; anxiety; decrease in motivation; environmental barrier; impaired ability to perceive body part; impaired ability to perceive spatial relationships; musculoskeletal impairment; neuromuscular impairment; pain; perceptual impairment; weakness

Client Outcomes

Client Will (Specify Time Frame)

- Remain free of body odor and maintain intact skin
- State satisfaction with ability to use adaptive devices to bathe
- Use methods to bathe safely and effectively with minimal difficulty
- Bathe with assistance of caregiver as needed and report satisfaction and dignity maintained during bathing experience
- Bathe with assistance of caregiver as needed without exhibiting defensive (aggressive) behaviors

Nursing Interventions

S

- **QSEN (Patient-Centered):** Ask patients their bathing preferences, which can increase patient privacy and satisfaction.
- **QSEN (Safety):** Warm bathing area above 25.1° C (77.18° F) while bathing, especially on cold days.
- **QSEN (Safety):** Use chlorhexidine-impregnated cloths rather than soap and water for daily patient bathing.
- **QSEN (Safety):** Consider using a prepackaged bath, especially for patients at high risk for infection (older adult, immunocompromised, invasive procedures, wounds, catheters, drains), to avoid patient exposure to multidrug-resistant pathogens from contaminated bath basins.
- **QSEN (Safety):** Use chlorhexidine gluconate for bath basin bathing.
- **QSEN (Patient-Centered):** Use patient-centered bathing interventions: plan for patient's comfort and bathing preferences, show respect in communications, critically think to solve issues that arise, and use a gentle approach.

• = Independent   ▲ = Collaborative

▲ Provide pain relief measures, such as ice packs, heat, and analgesics for sore joints 45 minutes before bathing; move extremities slowly and carefully; and inform the client before movements associated with pain occur (walking; transferring to a new location; moving joints; and washing genitals, face, and between toes and under arms). Have the client wash painful areas; recognize indicators of pain and apologize for any pain caused.

• Use a comfortable padded shower chair with foot support, or adapt a chair: pad it with towels/washcloths, cover the cold back with dry towels, and cover the arms with foam pipe insulation.

• Ensure that bathing assistance preserves client dignity through use of privacy with a traffic-free bathing area and posted privacy signs, timeliness of personal care, and conveyance of honor and recognition of the deservedness of respect and esteem of all persons.

• For cognitively impaired clients, avoid upsetting factors associated with bathing: instead of using the terms *bath, shower,* or *wash,* use comforting words, such as *warm, relaxing,* or *massage.* Start at the client's feet and bathe upward; bathe the face last after washing hands and using a clean cloth. Use a beautician/barber or wash hair at another time to avoid water dripping in the face.

• Use towel bathing to bathe client in bed, a bath blanket, and warm towels to keep the client covered the entire time. Warm and moisten towels/washcloths and place in plastic bags to keep them warm. Use the towels to massage large areas (front, back) and one washcloth for facial areas and another one for genital areas. No rinsing or drying is needed as is commonly thought for bathing.

• QSEN (Patient-Centered): For shower bathing: use patient-centered techniques; keep patient covered with towels and cleanse under the towels, use no-rinse products, use favorite bathing items, and use a handheld shower with adjustable spray.

▲ QSEN (Teamwork and Collaboration): Request referral of patient who has had a stroke to rehabilitation services.

▲ QSEN (Patient-Centered): Use a wrapped warm footbath for relaxation in patients with cancer.

Geriatric

• QSEN (Patient-Centered, Safety): Advocate for the use of the Bathing Without a Battle educational program for patients with dementia.

- **QSEN** (Patient-Centered): Provide nighttime bathing options for nursing home residents.
- Design the bathing environment for comfort: **Visual.** Reduce clutter and use partitions to hide equipment storage. Laminate and put artwork or decorative objects in bather's view, or place cue cards to bathing process (wall, ceiling, shower). Stand or sit in bather's position to experience what he/she sees. Decrease glare from tiles, white walls, and artificial lights. Use contrasting colors and soft but adequate lighting on a dimming switch for adjustment.
- Arrange the bathing environment to promote sensory comfort: **Auditory.** Reduce noise of voices and water. Do not allow traffic into bathing room. Add fabric to absorb sound (three to four times the width of the opening for sound-absorbing folds). Play soft music.
- Design the bathing environment for comfort: **Tactile.** Use heat lamps or radiant heat panels to keep the room warm. Use powder-coated grab bars in decorative colors with nonslip grip. Provide a soft rug to stand on. Ensure that flooring is not slippery (a high coefficient of friction, ideally above 80, is desired and obtained through flooring coatings).
- Use music during shower for clients with dementia.
- Train caregivers who bathe clients with dementia to avoid behaviors that can trigger assault: confrontational communication, invalidation of the resident's feelings, failure to prepare a resident for a task, initiating shower spray or touch during bathing without verbal prompts beforehand, washing the hair/face, speaking disrespectfully to the client, and hurrying the pace of the bath.
- Develop awareness of the ethics of presence during bathing to better meet clients' needs. Raholm (2012) found in a phenomenological study of nurses in elder care (N = 7) who discussed bathing that one must go beyond being physically present and enter into a caring relationship in which there is no indifference to the client's unique needs.
- Focus on the abilities of the client with dementia to obtain client's participation in bathing.
- **QSEN** (Patient-Centered): Use a Chinese herb formula in bath water to reduce paraplegia spasm.

Multicultural

- **QSEN** (Patient-Centered): Ask the patient for input on bathing habits and cultural bathing preferences.

• = Independent   ▲ = Collaborative

Home Care

- If in a typical bathing setting for the client, assess the client's ability to bathe self via direct observation using physical performance tests for ADLs.
- **QSEN** (Safety): Turn down temperature of water heater and recommend use of a water temperature-sensing shower valve to prevent scalding.

Client/Family Teaching and Discharge Planning

- Inform clients with extremity casts or bandages of inexpensive options to protect these devices during showering such as with plastic newspaper bags or bread bags. In a case study, Naram et al (2011) report on the use of inexpensive or free cast and bandage protector bags.

Dressing Self-Care deficit

NANDA-I Definition

Impaired ability to perform or complete dressing activities for self

Defining Characteristics

Decrease in motivation; discomfort; environmental barrier; fatigue; impaired ability to choose clothing; impaired ability to fasten clothing; impaired ability to gather clothing; impaired ability to maintain appearance; impaired ability to pick up clothing; impaired ability to put clothing on lower body; impaired ability to put clothing on upper body; impaired ability to put on various items of clothing (e.g., shirt, socks, shoes); impaired ability to remove clothing item (e.g., shirt, socks, shoes); impaired ability to use assistive device; impaired ability to use zipper; musculoskeletal impairment; neuromuscular impairment; pain

Related Factors (r/t)

Alteration in cognitive functioning; anxiety; perceptual impairment; weakness

Client Outcomes

Client Will (Specify Time Frame)

- Dress and groom self to optimal potential
- Use assistive technology to dress and groom
- Explain and use methods to enhance strengths during dressing and grooming
- Dress and groom with assistance of caregiver as needed

• = Independent   ▲ = Collaborative

Nursing Interventions

▲ **QSEN** (Teamwork and Collaboration): Assess functional impairment and report functional changes to health care provider to aid in earlier cancer diagnosis.

• **QSEN** (Patient-Centered): Assess a patient's range of movement, upper limb strength, balance, coordination, functional grip, dexterity, sensation, and ability to detect limb position.

▲ **QSEN** (Patient-Centered): Assess independence in dressing and bathing skills after rehabilitation to determine the need for follow-up care.

▲ **QSEN** (Teamwork and Collaboration): Refer patients with hand deformities due to rheumatoid arthritis to occupational therapy for self-care rehabilitation.

• **QSEN** (Patient-Centered): Recognize that dressing is a private task; encourage patient to participate as much as possible regardless of length of time needed.

• **QSEN** (Safety): Encourage patient to sit while dressing to reduce exertion and provide safety for poor balance or postural hypotension.

• **QSEN** (Patient-Centered): Dress the affected side first, then the unaffected side; reverse the process for undressing.

• **QSEN** (Patient-Centered): Use adaptive dressing and grooming equipment as needed (e.g., long-handled brushes, long grasping devices, button hooks, elastic shoelaces, Velcro shoes, soap-on-a-rope, suction holders).

Geriatric

• **QSEN** (Patient-Centered): Offer residents choices in what to wear and ensure staff is trained to do so.

• **QSEN** (Patient-Centered): Allow post-stroke patients who are cognitively impaired, especially if unimanual, to practice dressing.

• **QSEN** (Patient-Centered): Maintain resident's individualized style in clothing as select adaptive clothing: loose clothing; elastic waistbands and cuffs; square, large arm holes; seamless or reversible clothing without a specific front or back; dresses that open down the back and short coats (for wheelchair users); Velcro fasteners; larger or magnetic buttons; zipper pulls for grasping; and absorbent scarves for drooling that can be easily changed.

• **QSEN** (Patient-Centered): Lay clothing upon a contrasting color surface for patient selection.

• = Independent   ▲ = Collaborative

- **QSEN** (Patient-Centered): Inform patient that a winter coat with a funnel sleeve design can be easier to put on.
- Use clocks and explanations for the client with dementia to convey that it is morning and time to get ready for the day's activities by dressing.
- Lay clothing out (with label in back facing up) in the order that it will be put on by the client, either one item at a time or in piles with first item on top of pile.

Multicultural

- Consider use of assistive technology versus personal care assistance for Native Americans.

Home Care

- **QSEN** (Patient-Centered): Teach assisted living staff the philosophy and methods to increase resident participation in dressing.
- **QSEN** (Patient-Centered): Refer and encourage patients to participate in occupational therapy home rehabilitation programs.

Client/Family Teaching and Discharge Planning

- **QSEN** (Patient-Centered): Assess previously independent patients upon hospital admission for risk factors for new-onset disability that will require assistance with ADLs to plan preventive disability care and/or discharge care.
- ▲ **QSEN** (Patient-Centered): For clients who have had a stroke, request referral for occupational therapy for dressing rehabilitation.

Feeding Self-Care deficit

NANDA-I Definition

Impaired ability to perform or complete self-feeding activities

Defining Characteristics

Impaired ability to bring food to the mouth; impaired ability to chew food; impaired ability to get food onto utensils; impaired ability to handle utensils; impaired ability to manipulate food in mouth; impaired ability to open containers; impaired ability to pick up cup; impaired ability to prepare food; impaired ability to self-feed a complete meal; impaired ability to self-feed in an acceptable manner; impaired ability to swallow food; impaired ability to swallow sufficient amount of food; impaired ability to use assistive device

Related Factors (r/t)

Alteration in cognitive functioning; anxiety; decrease in motivation; discomfort; environmental barrier; fatigue; musculoskeletal impairment; neuromuscular impairment; pain; perceptual impairment weakness

NOTE: Specify level of independence using a standardized functional scale.

Client Outcomes

Client Will (Specify Time Frame)

- Feed self safely and effectively
- State satisfaction with ability to use adaptive devices for feeding
- Use assistance with feeding when necessary (caregiver)

Nursing Interventions

- QSEN (Safety): Consider assessment of patients in the intensive care unit (ICU) and stepdown patients or of patients with acute stroke for readiness of an oral diet with a 3-oz water swallow challenge by a trained provider.
- QSEN (Patient-Centered): Conduct repeat structured observations of patients at mealtime after a stroke to detect patients with eating difficulties to prevent possible social and functional consequences.
- ▲ QSEN (Patient-Centered): Develop an overriding guideline for assisted feeding so it is less dependent on a caregiver's own beliefs, time pressures, and organizational characteristics.
- ▲ QSEN (Patient-Centered): Prioritize assisted feeding as important in a caregiver's assignment to allow adequate dedicated time to the activity.
- ▲ QSEN (Teamwork and Collaboration): Give priority to continuity in the cooperation between the parties involved in assisted feeding for those who are completely dependent.
- QSEN (Patient-Centered): Consult patient on the benefit or desire to use assistive devices for feeding.
- QSEN (Safety): Presentation of feeding: provide 1 teaspoon of solid food or 10 to 15 mL of liquid at a time; wait until patient has swallowed the prior food/liquid.
- QSEN (Safety): Ensure oral care is provided to all patients regardless of type of feeding.

Geriatric

- QSEN (Safety): Assess for tooth loss in older patients prior to feeding.

• = Independent   ▲ = Collaborative

- **QSEN** (Patient-Centered): Assess the ability of patients with dementia to self-feed, and supervise the feeding of those with moderate dependency by providing verbal or physical assistance.
- **QSEN** (Patient-Centered): Implement Montessori interventions for patients with dementia who have eating problems, such as playing music to signal learning session start for hand-eye coordination, scooping, pouring, and squeezing activities.
- ▲ **QSEN** (Patient-Centered): Reduce interruptions during mealtimes and provide additional feeding assistance for older patients, especially those with cognitive impairment.
- **QSEN** (Patient-Centered): Use high-calorie oral supplements for patients with advanced dementia.
- **QSEN** (Patient-Centered): Provide nutritional supplement drinks in a glass to older adults with cognitive impairment.
- **QSEN** (Patient-Centered): Allow a resident an average of 42 minutes of staff time per meal and 13 minutes per between-meal snack to improve oral intake.
- **QSEN** (Patient-Centered): Discuss meaningful life topics, as identified by family members, with residents with dementia during mealtimes.
- **QSEN** (Patient-Centered): Encourage family visits at mealtimes for patients with dementia.
- **QSEN** (Patient-Centered): Play familiar music during meals for patients with dementia.
- Use aromatherapy with the smell of baking bread for those with dementia.
- ▲ **QSEN** (Teamwork and Collaboration): Provide feeding training and education programs for nursing home staff.

Multicultural

- **QSEN** (Patient-Centered): For those with impaired hand function who use chopsticks, suggest adapted chopsticks.
- **QSEN** (Patient-Centered): Use the simplified Chinese Edinburgh Feeding Evaluation in Dementia scale to measure feeding problems in people with dementia from Mainland China and other Chinese cultural groups.

Home Care

- **QSEN** (Teamwork and Collaboration): Request referral for physical therapy and occupational therapy to assess client's ability to position and self-feed and provide client and caregiver support with feeding.

• = Independent   ▲ = Collaborative

Client/Family Teaching and Discharge Planning

- **QSEN** (Teamwork and Collaboration): Discuss with family caregivers who are involved in the feeding of a family member with advanced dementia the feeding experience to provide support to ensure that the mealtime purpose is preserved.
- ▲ **QSEN** (Patient-Centered): Educate family members that neither insertion of a feeding tube nor timing of its insertion affects client survival for those with advanced dementia who have eating problems.

Toileting Self-Care deficit

NANDA-I Definition

Impaired ability to perform or complete self-toileting activities

Defining Characteristics

Impaired ability to complete toilet hygiene; impaired ability to flush toilet; impaired ability to manipulate clothing for toileting; impaired ability to reach toilet; impaired ability to rise from toilet; impaired ability to sit on toilet

Related Factors (r/t)

Alteration in cognitive functioning; anxiety; decrease in motivation; environmental barrier; fatigue; impaired ability to transfer; impaired mobility; musculoskeletal impairment; neuromuscular impairment; pain; perceptual impairment; weakness

Client Outcomes

Client Will (Specify Time Frame)

- Remain free of incontinence and impaction with no urine or stool on skin
- State satisfaction with ability to use adaptive devices for toileting
- Explain and demonstrate use of methods to be safe and independent in toileting

Nursing Interventions

- **QSEN** (Safety): Assess patients for fall risk using established and valid fall risk assessment tools (Morse, Heindrich) and implement fall prevention interventions for those at risk for falling or in physical restraints.

- **QSEN** (Patient-Centered): Assess patient's prior use of incontinence briefs and avoid use for hospitalized continent but limited mobility patient.
- **QSEN** (Patient-Centered): Assess patients who have had sphincter-saving surgery for self-care strategies to manage bowel symptoms in order to help support these strategies.
- **QSEN** (Safety): Make assistance call button readily available to the client and answer call light promptly.
- **QSEN** (Safety): Provide folding commode chairs in client bathrooms/at bedside.
- **QSEN** (Patient-Centered): Before use of a bedpan, discuss its use with clients.
- **QSEN** (Patient-Centered): Use necessary assistive toileting equipment.
- **QSEN** (Safety): Close toilet lid before flushing toilet and teach patient to do so.

Geriatric

- Assess residents without dementia for risk factors associated with toileting disability: rating health as fair or poor; living in a residence with four or fewer residents or that is for-profit; incontinence; physical, visual, or hearing impairment; and need for ADL or transferring assistance, to guide prevention interventions.
- **QSEN** (Patient-Centered): Consider use of urine alarm systems for patients with dementias.
- **QSEN** (Patient-Centered): Assess the patient's functional ability to manipulate clothing for toileting and, if necessary, modify clothing with Velcro fasteners, elastic waists, drop-front underwear, or slacks.
- **QSEN** (Patient-Centered): Provide patients with dementia access to regular exercise.

Multicultural

- **QSEN** (Patient-Centered): Remove barriers to toileting, support patient's cultural beliefs, and preserve dignity.

Home Care

- **QSEN** (Patient-Centered): To design a bathroom for an older adult, consider adaptable bath fixtures/furniture and safety needs.

Client/Family Teaching and Discharge Planning

- Teach men who perform routine clean intermittent catheterization that a 40-cm intermittent catheter has been found to provide ease of

• = Independent   ▲ = Collaborative

use, instill confidence in bladder emptying, and draining of urine into a receptacle.

- Have the family install a toilet seat of a contrasting color.
- Explain to family and caregivers of clients with dementia that toilet self-care activities decrease when self-awareness is lost.

Readiness for enhanced Self-Concept

NANDA-I Definition

A pattern of perceptions or ideas about the self, which can be strengthened

Defining Characteristics

Acceptance of limitations; acceptance of strengths; actions are congruent with verbal expression; confidence in abilities; expresses desire to enhance role performance; expresses desire to enhance self-concept; satisfaction with body image; satisfaction with personal identity; satisfaction with sense of worth; satisfaction with thoughts about self

Client Outcomes

Client Will (Specify Time Frame)

- State willingness to enhance self-concept
- State satisfaction with thoughts about self, sense of worthiness, role performance, body image, and personal identity
- Demonstrate actions that are congruent with expressed feelings and thoughts
- State confidence in abilities
- Accept strengths and limitations

Nursing Interventions

- Assess and support activities that promote developmental self-concept.
- Engage client in relaxation training.
- Refer to nutritional and exercise programs to support weight loss.
- Refer clients to massage therapy as an adjunct treatment.
- Refer homeless clients to work skills training programs.
- Refer clients receiving government assistance to Welfare to Work programs.
- Support establishing church-based community health promotion programs with the following key elements: partnerships, positive

• = Independent   ▲ = Collaborative

health values, availability of services, access to church facilities, community-focused interventions, health behavior change, and supportive social relationships.

▲ For clients who have had breast surgery and need a prosthesis, provide the appropriate prosthesis before the client leaves the health care facility.

• Offer client choices in clothing while client is hospitalized.

▲ Refer clients with history of childhood sexual abuse for intensive therapy that uses narrative life stories to promote positive sense of self.

Pediatric

• Consider the development of a Healthy Kids Mentoring Program that has four components: (1) relationship building, (2) self-esteem enhancement, (3) goal setting, and (4) academic assistance (tutoring). Mentors met with students twice each week for 1 hour each session on school grounds. During each meeting, mentors devoted time to each program component.

• Provide activities to bolster physical self-concept.

▲ Consider wheelchair dancing for disabled adolescents.

▲ Provide overweight adolescents access to group-based weight control interventions.

▲ Assess and provide referrals to mental health professionals for clients with unresolved worries associated with terrorism.

• Provide an alternative school-based program for pregnant and parenting teenagers.

Geriatric

• Encourage clients to consider a web-based support program when they are in a caregiving situation.

• Encourage activity and a strength, mobility, balance, and endurance training program.

• Provide opportunities for clients to engage in life skills (themed collections of everyday items based upon general activities that residents may have previously carried out).

• Provide information on advance directives.

• Use an approach that reduces the emphasis put on "old age" self-concept attributions when working with older clients.

Multicultural

• Carefully assess each client and allow families to participate in providing care that is acceptable based on the client's cultural beliefs.

• = Independent   ▲ = Collaborative

- Provide education and support for health-promoting behaviors and self-concept for clients from diverse cultures.
- Refer to the care plans for Disturbed **Body Image,** Readiness for enhanced **Coping,** Chronic low **Self-Esteem,** and Readiness for enhanced **Spiritual** well-being.

Home Care

- Previously discussed interventions may be used in the home care setting.

Chronic low Self-Esteem

NANDA-I Definition

Longstanding negative self-evaluating/feelings about self or self-capabilities

Defining Characteristics

Dependent on others' opinions; exaggerates negative feedback about self; excessive seeking of reassurance; guilt; hesitant to try new experiences; indecisive behavior; nonassertive behavior; overly conforming; passivity; poor eye contact; rejection of positive feedback; repeatedly unsuccessful in life events; shame; underestimates ability to deal with situation

Related Factors (r/t)

Cultural incongruence; exposure to traumatic situation; inadequate belonging; inadequate respect from others; ineffective coping with loss; insufficient group membership; psychiatric disorder; receiving insufficient affection; receiving insufficient approval from others; repeated failures; repeated negative reinforcement; spiritual incongruence

Client Outcomes

Client Will (Specify Time Frame)

- Demonstrate improved ability to interact with others (e.g., maintains eye contact, engages in conversation, expresses thoughts/feelings)
- Verbalize increased self-acceptance through positive self-statements about self
- Identify personal strengths, accomplishments, and values
- Identify and work on small, achievable goals
- Improve independent decision-making and problem-solving skills

S

• = Independent   ▲ = Collaborative

Nursing Interventions

- Actively listen to and respect the client.
- Assess the client's environmental and everyday stressors, including physical health concerns and the potential for abusive relationships.
- Assess existing strengths and coping abilities, and provide opportunities for their expression and recognition.
- Assess the client's self-esteem using valid and established tools like the Rosenberg Self-Esteem Scale.
- Reinforce the personal strengths and positive self-perceptions that a client identifies.
- Identify client's negative self-assessments.
- Encourage realistic and achievable goal setting and resources and identify impediments to achievement.
- Demonstrate and promote effective communication techniques; spend time with the client.
- Encourage independent decision-making by reviewing options and their possible consequences with client.
- Assist client to challenge negative perceptions of self and performance.
- Use failure as an opportunity to provide valuable feedback.
- Promote maintaining a level of functioning in the community.
- Assist client with evaluating the effect of family and peer group on feelings of self-worth.
- Support socialization and communication skills.
- Encourage journal/diary writing as a safe way of expressing emotions.
- Encourage clients to develop their artistic abilities.

Pediatric

- Assess children/adolescents with chronic illness for evidence of reduced self-esteem and make needed referrals.
- Encourage mothers of premature infants to use kangaroo care for at least 30 minutes per day.
- Implement interventions that promote and maintain positive peer relations for adolescent patients.
- ▲ Assess children/adolescents with low self-esteem for evidence of cyber bullying either as a victim or an offender.
- ▲ Provide bully prevention programs and include information on cyber bullying.

• = Independent   ▲ = Collaborative

Geriatric
- Support client in identifying and adapting to functional changes.
- Use reminiscence therapy and productive activities.
- Encourage older adult clients to participate in flexibility, toning, and balance exercise.
- Encourage participation in peer group activities.
- Encourage activities in which a client can support/help others.

Multicultural
- Assess for the influence of cultural beliefs, norms, and values on the client's sense of self-esteem.
- Assess socioeconomic issues.
- Assess for drug and alcohol use in individuals with low self-esteem.
- Validate the client's feelings regarding ethnic or racial identity.

Home Care
- Assess a client's immediate support system/family for relationship patterns and content of communication.
- Encourage the client's family to provide support and feedback regarding client value or worth.
- ▲ Refer to medical social services to assist the family in pattern changes that could benefit the client.
- ▲ If a client is involved in counseling or self-help groups, monitor and encourage attendance. Help the client identify the value of group participation after each group encounter.
- ▲ If a client is taking prescribed psychotropic medications, assess for knowledge of medication side effects and reasons for taking medication. Teach as necessary.
- ▲ Assess medications for effectiveness and side effects and monitor client for compliance.

Client/Family Teaching and Discharge Planning
- ▲ Refer to community agencies for psychotherapeutic counseling.
- ▲ Refer to psychoeducational groups on stress reduction and coping skills.
- ▲ Refer to self-help support groups specific to needs.

Risk for chronic low Self-Esteem
NANDA-I Definition

Vulnerable to longstanding negative self-evaluating/feelings about self or self-capabilities, which may compromise health

• = Independent ▲ = Collaborative

Risk Factors

Cultural incongruence; exposure to traumatic situation; inadequate affection received; inadequate group membership; inadequate respect from others; ineffective coping with loss; insufficient feeling of belonging; psychiatric disorder; repeated failures; repeated negative reinforcement; spiritual incongruence

Client Outcomes, Nursing Interventions, and Client/Family Teaching and Discharge Planning

Refer to care plan for Chronic low **Self-Esteem.**

Risk for situational low Self-Esteem

NANDA-I Definition

Vulnerable to developing a negative perception of self-worth in response to a current situation, which may compromise health

Risk Factors

Alteration in body image; alteration in social role; behavior inconsistent with values; decrease in control over environment; developmental transition; functional impairment; history of abandonment; history of abuse (e.g., physical, psychological, sexual); history of loss; history of neglect; history of rejection; inadequate recognition; pattern of failure; pattern of helplessness; physical illness; unrealistic self-expectations

Client Outcomes

Client Will (Specify Time Frame)

- State accurate self-appraisal
- Demonstrate the ability to self-validate
- Demonstrate the ability to make decisions independent of primary peer group
- Express effects of media on self-appraisal
- Express influence of substances on self-esteem
- Identify strengths and healthy coping skills
- State life events and change as influencing self-esteem

Nursing Interventions

- Assess the client's previous experiences with health care and coping with illness to determine the level of education and support needed.
- Assess for low and negative affect (expression of feelings).
- Assess the client's self-esteem using valid and established tools like the Rosenberg Self-Esteem Scale.
- Encourage client to maintain highest level of community functioning.

• = Independent   ▲ = Collaborative

- Treat the client with respect and as an equal to maintain positive self-esteem.
- Help the client identify and encourage use of available resources and social support networks. Make referrals as needed.
- Encourage the client to find a self-help or therapy group that focuses on self-esteem enhancement. Encourage utilization of above.
- Encourage the client to create a sense of competence through short-term goal setting and goal achievement.
▲ Assess the client for symptoms of depression and anxiety. Refer to specialist as needed. Prompt and effective treatment can prevent exacerbation of symptoms or safety risks.
- See care plans for Disturbed personal **Identity,** Situational low **Self-Esteem,** and Chronic low **Self-Esteem.**

Pediatric
- Assess children/adolescents with chronic illness for evidence of reduced self-esteem and make needed referrals.
- Identify environmental and/or developmental factors that increase risk for low self-esteem, especially in children/adolescents, to make needed referrals.
- Assess children/adolescents who are either a victim or an offender of cyber bullying for low self-esteem.
▲ Provide support for children who do not have supportive families, and provide a haven outside of the home.
▲ Encourage a combination of extracurricular activity for adolescents in a safe, supportive, and empowering environment.

Geriatric
- Support humor as a coping mechanism.
- Assist the client in life review and identifying positive accomplishments.
- Help client establish a peer group and structured daily activities.
- See care plans for Situational low **Self-Esteem** and Chronic low **Self-Esteem.**

Home Care
- Assess current environmental stresses and identify community resources.
- Encourage family members to acknowledge and validate the client's strengths.

• = Independent   ▲ = Collaborative

- Assess the need for establishing an emergency plan.
- See care plans for Situational low **Self-Esteem** and Chronic low **Self-Esteem**.

Client/Family Teaching and Discharge Planning

▲ Refer the client/family to community-based self-help and support groups.

▲ Refer the client to educational classes on stress management, relaxation training, and so on.

▲ Refer the client to community agencies that offer support and environmental resources. Make referrals as needed.

- See care plans for Situational low **Self-Esteem** and Chronic low **Self-Esteem**.

Situational low Self-Esteem

NANDA-I Definition

Development of a negative perception of self-worth in response to a current situation

Defining Characteristics

Helplessness; indecisive behavior; nonassertive behavior; purposelessness; self-negating verbalizations; situational challenge to self-worth; underestimates ability to deal with situation

Related Factors (r/t)

Alteration in body image; alteration in social role; behavior inconsistent with values; developmental transition; functional impairment; history of loss; history of rejection; inadequate recognition; pattern of failure

Client Outcomes

Client Will (Specify Time Frame)

- State effect of life events on feelings about self
- State personal strengths
- Acknowledge presence of guilt and not blame self if an action was related to another person's appraisal
- Seek help when necessary
- Demonstrate self-perceptions are accurate given physical capabilities
- Demonstrate separation of self-perceptions from societal stigmas

• = Independent   ▲ = Collaborative

Nursing Interventions

▲ Assess the client for signs and symptoms of depression and potential for suicide and/or violence. If present, immediately notify the appropriate personnel of symptoms. See care plans for Risk for other-directed **Violence** and Risk for **Suicide.**

• Assess the client's environmental and everyday stressors, including evidence of abusive relationships.

▲ Assess the client's self-esteem using valid and established tools like the Rosenberg Self-Esteem Scale. Assess for unhealthy coping mechanisms, such as substance abuse, and make appropriate referrals.

• Assist in the identification of problems and situational factors that contribute to problems, offering options for resolution.

• Mutually identify strengths, resources, and previously effective coping strategies.

• Have client list strengths.

• Accept client's own pace in working through grief or crisis situations.

• Accept the client's own defenses in dealing with the crisis.

• Provide information about support groups of people who have common experiences or interests.

• Teach the client mindfulness techniques to cope more effectively with strong emotional responses.

• Support client's decisions in health care treatment.

• Encourage objective appraisal of self and life events and challenge negative or perfectionist expectations of self.

• Provide psychoeducation to client and family.

• Validate confusion when feeling ill but looking well.

• Acknowledge the presence of societal stigma. Teach management tools.

• Validate the effect of negative past experiences on self-esteem and work on corrective measures.

• See care plan for Chronic low **Self-Esteem.**

Geriatric and Multicultural

• See care plan for Chronic low **Self-Esteem.**

Home Care

• Establish an emergency plan and contract with the client for its use.

• Access supplies that support a client's success at independent living.

• See care plan for Chronic low **Self-Esteem.**

• = Independent   ▲ = Collaborative

Client/Family Teaching and Discharge Planning

- Assess the person's support system (family, friends, and community) and involve them if desired.
- Educate client and family regarding the grief process.
- Teach client and family that the crisis is temporary.
- ▲ Refer to appropriate community resources or crisis intervention centers.
- ▲ Refer to resources for handicap and/or disability services.
- Refer to illness-specific consumer support groups.
- See care plan for Chronic low **Self-Esteem**.

Self-Mutilation

NANDA-I Definition

Deliberate self-injurious behavior causing tissue damage with the intent of causing nonfatal injury to attain relief of tension

Defining Characteristics

Abrading; biting; constricting a body part; cuts on body; hitting; ingestion of harmful substances; inhalation of harmful substances; insertion of object into body orifice; picking at wounds; scratches on body; self-inflicted burn; severing of a body part

Related Factors (r/t)

Absence of family confidant; adolescence; alteration in body image; autism; borderline personality disorder; character disorder; childhood illness; childhood surgery; depersonalization; developmental delay; dissociation; disturbance in interpersonal relationships; eating disorders; emotional disorder; family divorce; family history of self-destructive behaviors; family substance abuse; feeling threatened with loss of significant relationship; history of childhood abuse (e.g., physical, psychological, sexual); history of self-directed violence; impaired self-esteem; impulsiveness; inability to express tension verbally; incarceration; ineffective communication between parent and adolescent; ineffective coping strategies; irresistible urge for self-directed violence; irresistible urge to cut self; isolation from peers; labile behavior; living in nontraditional setting (e.g., foster, group, or institutional care); low self-esteem; mounting tension that is intolerable; negative feeling (e.g., depression, rejection, self-hatred, separation anxiety, guilt, depersonalization); pattern of inability to plan solutions; pattern of inability to see long-term consequences; peers who self-mutilate; perfectionism; psychotic disorder; requires rapid stress reduction; sexual identity crisis;

• = Independent ▲ = Collaborative

substance abuse; use of manipulation to obtain nurturing relationship with others; violence between parental figures

Client Outcomes

Client Will (Specify Time Frame)

- Have injuries treated
- Refrain from further self-injury
- State appropriate ways to cope with increased psychological or physiological tension
- Express feelings
- Seek help when having urges to self-mutilate
- Maintain self-control without supervision
- Use appropriate community agencies when caregivers are unable to attend to emotional needs

Nursing Interventions

NOTE: Before implementing interventions in the face of self-mutilation, nurses should examine their own knowledge base and emotional responses to incidents of self-harm to ensure that interventions will not be based on countertransference reactions.

▲ Provide medical treatment for injuries. Use aseptic technique when caring for wounds. Care for the wounds in a matter-of-fact manner.

• Assess for risk of suicide or other self-damaging behaviors. Refer to the care plan for Risk for **Suicide.**

• Assess for signs of psychiatric disorders, including depression, anxiety, borderline personality disorder, dissociative disorders, eating disorders, and impulsivity.

• Assess for presence of hallucinations. Ask specific questions such as, "Do you hear voices that other people do not hear? Are they telling you to hurt yourself?"

▲ Assure the client that he or she will be safe during hallucinations, and engage supportively. Provide referrals for medication.

▲ Assess for the presence of medical disorders, mental retardation, medication effects, or disorders such as autism that may include self-mutilation. Initiate referral for evaluation and treatment as appropriate.

▲ Case finding and referral by school nurses for psychological or psychiatric treatment are critical.

• Monitor the client's behavior closely, using engagement and support as elements of safety checks while avoiding intrusive overstimulation.

S

• = Independent   ▲ = Collaborative

- Establish trust, listen to client, convey safety, and assist in developing positive goals for the future.
- Recognize that self-mutilation may serve a variety of functions for the client.
- ▲ Refer to family or group psychotherapy as appropriate.
- ▲ Use a collaborative approach to care. A collaborative approach to care is more helpful to the client.
- Refer to the care plan for Risk for **Self-Mutilation** for additional information.

Home Care and Client/Family Teaching and Discharge Planning
- See the care plan for Risk for **Self-Mutilation**.

Risk for Self-Mutilation
NANDA-I Definition
Vulnerable to deliberate self-injurious behavior causing tissue damage with the intent of causing nonfatal injury to attain relief of tension

Risk Factors
Adolescence; alteration in body image; battered child; borderline personality disorders; character disorders; childhood illness; childhood surgery; depersonalization; developmental delay; dissociation; disturbed interpersonal relationships; eating disorders; emotional disorder; family divorce; family history of self-destructive behavior; family substance abuse; feeling threatened with loss of significant relationship; history of childhood abuse (e.g., physical, psychological, sexual); history of self-directed violence; impaired self-esteem; impulsiveness; inability to express tension verbally; incarceration; ineffective coping strategies; irresistible urge for self-directed violence; isolation from peers; living in nontraditional setting (e.g., foster, group, or institutional care); loss of control over problem-solving situation; loss of significant relationship(s); low self-esteem; mounting tension that is intolerable; negative feelings (e.g., depression, rejection, self-hatred, separation anxiety, guilt, depersonalization); pattern of inability to plan solutions; pattern of inability to see long-term consequences; peers who self-mutilate; perfectionism; psychotic disorder; requires rapid stress reduction; sexual identity crisis; substance abuse; use of manipulation to obtain nurturing relationship with others; violence between parental figures

• = Independent   ▲ = Collaborative

Client Outcomes

Client Will (Specify Time Frame)

- Refrain from self-injury
- Identify triggers to self-mutilation
- State appropriate ways to cope with increased psychological or physiological tension
- Express feelings
- Seek help when having urges to self-mutilate
- Maintain self-control without supervision
- Use appropriate community agencies when caregivers are unable to attend to emotional needs

Nursing Interventions

NOTE: Before implementing interventions in the face of self-injury, nurses should examine their own knowledge base and emotional responses to incidents of self-injury to ensure that interventions will not be based on countertransference reactions.

- Assess client's ability to regulate his/her own emotional states, which may be influenced by the client's perception of his or her body.
- Assess client's degree of self-criticism and use of effective coping skills. Self-harm serves as a coping mechanism for clients.
- Assess client's perception of powerlessness. Refer to the care plan for **Powerlessness.**
- Assessment data from the client and family members may have to be gathered at different times; allowing a family member or trusted friend with whom the client is comfortable to be present during the assessment may be helpful.
- Assess for risk factors of self-mutilation described above.
- Perform a thorough skin assessment at least annually and check for behavioral cues of self-harm.
- Assess for co-occurring disorders that require response, specifically childhood abuse, substance abuse, and suicide attempts. Implement reporting or referral as indicated.
- Assess family dynamics and the need for family therapy and community support.
- Assess for the presence of medical disorders, mental retardation, medication effects, or disorders such as autism that may include self-mutilation. Initiate referral for evaluation and treatment as appropriate.

S

• = Independent ▲ = Collaborative

- Be alert to other risk factors of self-mutilation in clients with psychosis, including acute intoxication, dramatic changes in body appearance, preoccupation with religion and sexuality, and anticipated or perceived object loss.
- Monitor the client's behavior closely, using engagement and support as elements of safety checks while avoiding intrusive overstimulation. Offer activities that will serve as a distraction.
- Establish trust, listen to client, convey safety, and assist in developing positive goals for the future. Refer to mental health counseling. Multiple therapeutic modalities are available for treatment. Inform the client of expectations for appropriate behavior and consequences within the unit. Emphasize that the client must comply with the rules. Give positive reinforcement for compliance and minimize attention paid to disruptive behavior while setting limits.
- Clients need to learn to recognize distress as it occurs and express it verbally rather than as a physical action against the self.
- Assist the client to identify the motives/reasons for self-mutilation that have been perceived as positive. Self-harm serves as a defense mechanism.
- Help the client identify cues that precede impulsive behavior.
- Assist clients to identify ways to soothe themselves and generate hopefulness when faced with painful emotions.
- Reinforce alternative ways of dealing with depression and anxiety, such as exercise, engaging in unit activities, or talking about feelings.
- Keep the environment safe; remove all harmful objects from the area. Use of unbreakable glass is recommended for the client at risk for self-injury.
- Anticipate trigger situations and intervene to assist the client in applying alternatives to self-mutilation.
- If self-mutilation does occur, use a calm, nonpunitive approach. Whenever possible, assist the client to assume responsibility for consequences (e.g., dress self-inflicted wound). Refer to the care plan for **Self-Mutilation.**
- If the client is unable to control self-mutilation behavior, provide interactive supervision, not isolation.
- Involve the client in planning his/her care and problem solving, and emphasize that the client can make choices.
- ▲ Refer to protective services if evidence of abuse exists.
- Refer to the care plan for **Self-Mutilation.**

• = Independent   ▲ = Collaborative

Pediatric
- The same dynamics described previously apply to adolescents.
- Maintaining a therapeutic relationship with teens requires explicit assurances of confidentiality, consistency of clinical routines, and a nonjudgmental communication style.
- Encourage expression of painful experiences and provide supportive counseling.
- Multiple treatment modalities may be used in addressing the themes of young people who self-harm.
- Teach coping skills as an important intervention for adolescents.
- Assess for the presence of an eating disorder or substance abuse. Attend to the themes that preoccupy teens with eating disorders who self-mutilate.
- Evaluate for suicidal ideation/suicide risk. Refer to the care plan for Risk for **Suicide** for additional information.
- Be aware that there is not complete overlap between self-mutilation and suicidal behavior. The motivation may be different (coping with difficult feelings rather than ending life), and the method is usually different.
- Use treatment approaches detailed in nursing interventions, with modifications as appropriate for this age group.

Geriatric
- Provide hand or back rubs and calming music when older clients experience anxiety.
- Provide soft objects for older clients to hold and manipulate when self-mutilation occurs as a function of delirium or dementia. Apply mitts, splints, helmets, or restraints as appropriate.
- Be aware that older adults may demonstrate self-neglect. Older adults who show self-destructive behaviors should be evaluated for dementia.

Home Care
- Communicate degree of risk to family/caregivers; assess the family and caregiving situation for ability to protect the client and to understand the client's self-mutilative behavior. Provide family and caregivers with guidelines on how to manage self-harm behaviors in the home environment.
- Establish an emergency plan, including when to use hotlines and 911. Develop a contract with the client and family for use of the

S

• = Independent   ▲ = Collaborative

emergency plan. Role-play access to the emergency resources with the client and caregivers.

• Assess the home environment for harmful objects. Have family remove or lock objects as able.

▲ If client behaviors intensify, institute an emergency plan for mental health intervention. The degree of disturbance and the ability to manage care safely at home determine the level of services needed to protect the client.

▲ Refer for homemaker or psychiatric home health care services for respite, client reassurance, and implementation of therapeutic regimen.

▲ If the client is on psychotropic medications, assess client and family knowledge of medication administration and side effects.

▲ Evaluate the effectiveness and side effects of medications. Accurate clinical feedback improves health care provider's ability to prescribe an effective medical regimen specific to client needs.

Client/Family Teaching and Discharge Planning

• Explain all relevant symptoms, procedures, treatments, and expected outcomes for self-mutilation that is illness based (e.g., borderline personality disorder, autism).

• Assist family members to understand the complex issues of self-mutilation. Provide instruction on relevant developmental issues and on actions that parents can take to avoid media that glorify self-harm behaviors.

• Provide written instructions for treatments and procedures for which the client will be responsible.

• Instruct the client in coping strategies (assertiveness training, impulse control training, deep breathing, progressive muscle relaxation).

• Role play responses to stressful situations (e.g., say, "Tell me how you will respond if someone ignores you").

• Teach cognitive-behavioral activities, such as active problem solving, reframing (reappraising the situation from a different perspective), or thought-stopping (in response to a negative thought, picture a large stop sign and replace the image with a prearranged positive alternative). Teach the client to confront his or her own negative thought patterns (or cognitive distortions), such as catastrophizing (expecting the very worst), dichotomous thinking (perceiving events

• = Independent ▲ = Collaborative

in only one of two opposite categories), or magnification (placing distorted emphasis on a single event).
▲ Provide the client and family with phone numbers of appropriate community agencies for therapy and counseling. Continuous follow-up care should be implemented; therefore, the method to access this care must be given to the client.
▲ Give the client positive things on which to focus by referring to appropriate agencies for job-training skills or education.

Self-Neglect
NANDA-I Definition
A constellation of culturally framed behaviors involving one or more self-care activities in which there is a failure to maintain a socially accepted standard of health and well-being (Gibbons et al, 2006)

Defining Characteristics
Insufficient environmental hygiene; insufficient personal hygiene; nonadherence to health activities

Related Factors (r/t)
Alteration in cognitive functioning; Capgras syndrome; deficient executive function; fear of institutionalization; frontal lobe dysfunction; functional impairment; inability to maintain control; learning disability; lifestyle choice; malingering; psychiatric disorder; psychotic disorder; stressors; substance abuse

Client Outcomes
Client Will (Specify Time Frame)
• Show improvement in mental health problems
• Show improvement in chronic medical problems
• Reveal improvement in cognition (e.g., if reversible and treatable)
• Demonstrate improvement in functional status (e.g., basic and instrumental activities of daily living)
• Demonstrate adherence to health activities (e.g., medications and medical appointments)
• Exhibit improved personal hygiene
• Exhibit improved environmental hygiene
• Have fewer hospitalizations and emergency room visits
• Increase safety of client
• Increase safety of community in which client lives

• = Independent   ▲ = Collaborative

- Agree to necessary personal and environmental changes that eliminate risk/endangerment to self or others (e.g., neighbors)

NOTE: Because self-neglect is a culturally framed and socially defined phenomenon, change in a client's status must occur in such a way that it respects individual rights while ensuring individual health and well-being. This is accomplished through client-nurse partnership as well as interdisciplinary collaboration and team work, and, in some instances, assistance of next of kin and/or adult protective services (APS) may be needed (e.g., a state agency or local social services program).

Nursing Interventions

- Monitor individuals with acute or chronic mental and complex physical illness for defining characteristics for self-neglect.
- Assist individuals with complex mental and physical health issues to adopt positive health behaviors so that they may maintain their health status in the community.
- Assess persons with complex health issues for adequate coping abilities, and assist those with coping problems to maintain their health and well-being in the community.
- Assist individuals with reconnecting with family, friends, and other social networks available to them.
- Assist individuals whose self-care is failing with managing their medication regimen.
- Assess individuals with failing self-care for noncompliance (e.g., diagnostic testing, medication regimen, therapeutic regimen, and safety precautions).
- Assist persons with self-care deficits due to ADL or IADL impairments.
- Assess persons with failing self-care for changes in cognitive function (e.g., dementia or delirium).
- ▲ Refer persons with failing self-care to appropriate specialists (e.g., psychologist, psychiatrist, social work) and therapists (e.g., physical therapy, occupational therapy).
- Use behavioral modification as appropriate to bring about client changes that lead to improvement in personal hygiene, environmental hygiene, and adherence to medical regimen.
- Monitor persons with substance abuse problems (i.e., drugs, alcohol, smoking) for adequate safety.

• = Independent   ▲ = Collaborative

▲ Refer persons with failing self-care who are significantly impaired cognitively or functionally and who are suspected victims of abuse to APS.

• Monitor clients with changes in cognitive function for adequate safety.

• Monitor clients with functional impairments for adequate safety.

• Assist individuals with complex mental and physical health needs with maintaining their health and well-being in the community.

Geriatric

▲ Assess client's socioeconomic status and refer for appropriate support.

▲ Refer persons demonstrating a significant decline in self-care abilities (e.g., posing a threat to themselves or to their community) for evaluation of capacity and executive function.

▲ Obtain the assistance of APS in the case of refusal of professional health care services when there is a clear indication of self-endangerment.

Multicultural

• Deliver health care that is sensitive to the culture and philosophy of individuals whose self-care appears inadequate.

• Awareness that racial differences for self-neglect may exist, putting some older adults more at risk than others.

S

Sexual dysfunction

NANDA-I Definition

A state in which an individual experiences a change in sexual function during the sexual response phases of desire, excitation, and/or orgasm, which is viewed as unsatisfying, unrewarding, or inadequate

Defining Characteristics

Alteration in sexual activity; alteration in sexual excitation; alteration in sexual satisfaction; change in interest toward others; change in self-interest; change in sexual role; decrease in sexual desire; perceived/actual sexual limitation; seeks confirmation of desirability; undesired change in sexual function

Related Factors (r/t)

Absent of privacy; absence of significant other; alteration in body function (due to anomaly, age, disease, medication, pregnancy, radiation, surgery, trauma); alteration in body structure (due to anomaly, disease, pregnancy,

• = Independent ▲ = Collaborative

radiation, surgery, trauma); inadequate role model; insufficient knowledge about sexual function; misinformation about sexual function; presence of abuse (e.g., physical, psychological, sexual); psychosocial abuse (e.g., controlling, manipulation, verbal abuse); value conflict; vulnerability

Client Outcomes

Client Will (Specify Time Frame)

- Identify individual cause of sexual dysfunction
- Identify stressors that contribute to dysfunction
- Discuss alternative, satisfying, and acceptable sexual practices for self and partner
- Identify the degree of sexual interest by the client and partner
- Adapt sexual technique as needed to cope with sexual problems
- Discuss with partner concerns about body image and sex role

Nursing Interventions

- Gather the client's sexual history, noting normal patterns of functioning and the client's vocabulary, and encouraging clients to ask questions or discuss sexual problems experienced.
- ▲ Assess duration and risk factors for sexual dysfunction and explore potential causes such as medications, medical problems, aging process, or psychosocial issues.
- Assess for history of sexual abuse.
- Determine the client and partner's current knowledge and understanding, and validate that it is normal to have sexual concerns.
- ▲ Assess and provide treatment for sexual dysfunction, involving the person's partner in the process, and evaluating pharmacological and nonpharmacological interventions.
- Assess risk factors for sexual dysfunction, especially with varying sexual partners.
- Observe for stress and anxiety as possible causes of dysfunction.
- ▲ Assess for depression as a possible cause of sexual dysfunction, and institute appropriate treatment, as depression is commonly observed in clients with chronic disease and chronic pain.
- Observe for grief related to loss (e.g., amputation, mastectomy, ostomy), as a change in body image often precedes sexual dysfunction. See care plan for Disturbed **Body Image.**
- ▲ Explore physical causes of sexual dysfunction such as diabetes, cardiovascular disease, arthritis, or benign prostatic hypertrophy (BPH).

• = Independent　　　　▲ = Collaborative

- Certain chronic diseases such as cancer often have significant effects on sexual function. Both the disease process and treatment can contribute to sexual dysfunction.
- Consider that neurological diseases such as multiple sclerosis (MS) affect sexual function directly, but with secondary effects due to disability related to the illness, social, and emotional effects.
- Explore behavioral or other causes of sexual dysfunction, such as smoking, dietary factors, or obesity.
▲ Consider medications as a cause of sexual dysfunction.
- Provide privacy when discussing sexual problems and be verbally and nonverbally nonjudgmental.
- Explain the need for the client to share concerns with partner.
▲ Refer to appropriate medical providers for consideration of medication for premature ejaculation, erectile dysfunction, or orgasmic problems.
- Refer women for possible pharmacological intervention for sexual dysfunction.

Geriatric
▲ Carefully assess the sexuality needs and sexual dysfunction of older adults and refer for counseling if needed.
- Teach about normal changes that occur with aging that may be perceived as sexual dysfunction, such as reduction in vaginal lubrication and reduction in duration and resolution of orgasm for women; and for men, increased time required for erection and for subsequent erections, erection without ejaculation, less firm erection, and decreased volume of seminal fluid.
- Explore various sexual gratification alternatives (e.g., caressing, sharing feelings) with the client and partner.
- Discuss the difference between sexual function, sexuality, and sexual dysfunction, including that all individuals possess sexuality from birth to death, regardless of changes occurring over the life span.
- If prescribed, instruct clients with chronic pain to take pain medication before sexual activity.
- See care plan for Ineffective **Sexuality** pattern.

Multicultural
- Evaluate culturally influenced risk factors for sexual dysfunction.
- Validate client feelings and emotions regarding the changes in sexual behavior, letting the client know that the nurse heard and

S

• = Independent   ▲ = Collaborative

understands what was said, and promoting the nurse-client relationship.

Home Care

- Previously discussed interventions may be adapted for home care use.
- ▲ Identify specific sources of concern about sexual dysfunction and provide reassurance and instruction on appropriate expectations as indicated.
- ▲ Confirm that physical reasons for dysfunction have been addressed, and refer for therapy and/or support groups if appropriate.
- Reinforce or teach the client about sexual functioning, alternative sexual practices, and necessary sexual precautions, and update teaching as client status changes.
- See care plan for Ineffective **Sexuality** pattern.

Client/Family Teaching and Discharge Planning

- Provide accurate information for clients concerning sexual activity after a cardiac event; consider using cognitive and behavioral strategies.
- Include the partner/family in discharge instructions, because partner concerns are often overlooked in regard to sexual issues.
- Teach the client and partner about condom use, for those at risk.
- ▲ Teach the client with cardiovascular disease that sexual activity can be resumed within a few weeks for those with minimal symptoms with moderate physical activity, although clients at higher risk or with exercise intolerance may need further evaluation.
- For cardiac clients, discuss being well rested, reporting any cardiac warning signs, using foreplay to determine tolerance for sexual activity, not using alcohol or eating heavy meals before sex, and having sex with a familiar partner and in the usual setting to decrease any stress the couple might feel.
- Provide written educational materials that address sexual issues for clients and families of clients with implantable cardiac defibrillators (ICDs).
- Discuss sexual problems and adaptations needed for sexual activity with spinal cord injury.
- ▲ Refer to appropriate community resources, such as a clinical specialist, family counselor, or cardiac rehabilitation, including the

• = Independent   ▲ = Collaborative

partner if appropriate; for complex issues, a referral to a sex counselor, urologist, gynecologist, or other specialist may be needed.
- Teach the importance of diabetic control and its effect on sexuality to clients with diabetes.
▲ Refer for medical advice when ED lasts longer than 2 months or is recurring.
- Teach the following interventions to decrease the likelihood of ED: limit or avoid the use of alcohol, stop smoking, exercise regularly, reduce stress, get enough sleep, deal with anxiety or depression, and see a health care provider for regular checkups and medical screening tests.
- See care plan for Ineffective **Sexuality** pattern.

Ineffective Sexuality pattern

NANDA-I Definition

Expressions of concern regarding own sexuality

Defining Characteristics

Alterations in relationship with significant other; alteration in sexual activity; alteration in sexual behavior; change in sexual role; difficulty with sexual activity; difficulty with sexual behavior; value conflict

Related Factors (r/t)

Absence of privacy; absence of significant other; conflict about sexual orientation; conflict about variant preference; fear of pregnancy; fear of sexually transmitted infection; impaired relationship with a significant other; inadequate role model; insufficient knowledge about alternatives related to sexuality; skill deficit about alternatives related to sexuality

Client Outcomes

Client Will (Specify Time Frame)
- State knowledge of difficulties, limitations, or changes in sexual behaviors or activities
- State knowledge of sexual anatomy and functioning
- State acceptance of altered body structure or functioning
- Describe acceptable alternative sexual practices
- Identify importance of discussing sexual issues with significant other
- Describe practice of safe sex with regard to pregnancy and avoidance of STIs

Nursing Interventions

- After establishing rapport or therapeutic relationship, give the client permission to discuss issues dealing with sexuality, for example: "Have you been or are you concerned about functioning sexually because of your health status?"
- Use assessment questions and standardized instruments to assess sexual problems, where possible.
▲ Assess any risks associated with sexual activity, particularly coronary risks.
- Include the client's partner in discussing sexual concerns and in providing sexual counseling. Encourage the client to discuss concerns with his or her partner.
- Explore attitudes about sexual intimacy and changes in sexuality patterns.
- Assess psychosocial function such as anxiety, fear, depression, and low self-esteem.
- Discuss alternative sexual expressions for altered body functioning or structure, including closeness and sexual and nonsexual touching as other forms of expression.
- Some clients choose masturbation for sexual release, an acceptable form of sexual expression, and for some with chronic illnesses, it may be an alternative to sexual intercourse when exercise tolerance is low.
- Assess the client's sexual orientation and usual pattern of sexual activities, and discuss prevention of illnesses for which the client may be at increased risk (e.g., anorectal cancer), asking specific questions about sexual orientation, for example, "Do you have sexual relationships with men, women, or both?" Assess use of safer sex practices (e.g., condom use); the frequency of anal intercourse; number of sexual partners in the last year; last HIV screening/results; and use of medications, alcohol, and illicit drugs.
- Specific guidelines for sexual activity for clients who have had total hip arthroplasty include the following: sexual activity can be generally resumed 1 to 2 months after surgery, and a supine position ("missionary") at maximum abduction in extension to prevent hip dislocation, avoiding the lateral decubitus positions, which carry a higher risk of adduction and internal rotation of the hip.
- Specific guidelines for those who have had a myocardial infarction (MI) include the following: sexual activity can generally be resumed

S

• = Independent   ▲ = Collaborative

within a few weeks after MI unless complications are experienced, such as arrhythmias or cardiac arrest; engaging in sexual activity in familiar surroundings with the usual partner; a comfortable room temperature, when well rested to minimize cardiac stress; avoiding heavy meals or alcohol for 2 to 3 hours before sexual activity, and choosing a position of comfort to minimize stress of the cardiac client.

• Specific guidelines for those who had complete coronary revascularization, in addition to those mentioned with MI, including those with successful percutaneous cardiovascular revascularization without complication, can resume sex within a few days; those who have had coronary artery bypass grafting (CABG) or noncoronary open heart surgery may resume sex in 6 to 8 weeks. Incisional pain with sexual activity can be managed by premedicating with a mild pain reliever; and reassurance should be provided to the partner that sexual activity will not harm the sternum as long as direct pressure is avoided.

• Specific guidelines for those with an implantable cardioverter defibrillator (ICD) include assuring the client and partner that fears about being shocked during sexual activity are normal, and sex can be resumed after the ICD is placed as long as strain on the implant site is avoided; if the ICD discharges with sexual activity, the client should stop, rest, and later notify the health care provider that the device fired so that a determination can be made if this was an appropriate shock or not. The client should be instructed to report any dyspnea, chest pain, or dizziness with sexual activity.

• Specific guidelines for those with chronic lung disease include planning for sexual activity when energy level is highest; use of controlled breathing techniques; avoiding physical exertion prior to sexual activity; using positions that minimize shortness of breath, such as a semi-reclining position; engaging in sexual activity when medications are at peak effectiveness; and use of an oxygen cannula, if prescribed, to provide oxygen before, during, or after sex (Steinke, 2013).

• Specific guidelines for those with multiple sclerosis include treatment of symptoms with prescribed medications, assessing changes in body image, and supportive therapies to assist with a more satisfying sexual experience, including treatment of neuropathic pain, sexual positions that are most supportive, discussing changes in

S

• = Independent   ▲ = Collaborative

sensation and stimulation with the partner, use of stretching exercise for tight muscles prior to sexual activity, and avoiding a distended bowl or bladder that may cause discomfort.
- Refer to the care plan for **Sexual** dysfunction for additional interventions.

Pediatric
- Provide age-appropriate information for adolescents regarding HIV/AIDS and sexual behavior, and discuss sexually transmitted infections, particularly human papillomavirus, including the risks of perinatal transmission and methods to reduce risks among HIV-infected adolescents.
- Encourage client and partner communication in HIV prevention strategies.
- Provide age-appropriate information regarding potential for sexual abuse.

Geriatric
- Carefully assess the sexuality needs of the older client and refer for counseling if needed; the ability to form satisfying social relationships and to be intimate with others, including building strong emotional intimate connections, contributes to adaptation and successful aging (Steinke, 2013).
- ▲ Explore possible changes in sexuality related to health status, menopause, medications, and sexual risk, and make appropriate referrals.
- Allow the client to verbalize feelings regarding loss of sexual partner, and acknowledge problems such as disapproving children, lack of available partner for women, and environmental variables that make forming new relationships difficult.
- ▲ Provide a milieu that allows for discussion of sexual issues and a higher level of sexual satisfaction, including allowing couples to room together and the provision of privacy.
- See care plan for **Sexual** dysfunction.

Multicultural
- Assess for the influence of cultural beliefs, norms, and values on client's perceptions of normal sexual behavior.

Home Care
- Previously discussed interventions may be adapted for home care use. Also see care plan for **Sexual** dysfunction.

• = Independent   ▲ = Collaborative

- Help the client and significant other identify a place and time in the home and daily living for privacy in sharing sexual or relationship activity, and if necessary, help the client communicate the need for privacy to family members.
- Confirm that physical reasons for dysfunction have been addressed, and provide support for coping behaviors, including participation in support groups or therapy if appropriate.
- Reinforce or teach about sexual functioning, alternative sexual practices, and necessary sexual precautions, and update teaching as client status changes.

Client/Family Teaching and Discharge Planning

▲ Refer to appropriate community agencies (e.g., certified sex counselor, Reach to Recovery, Ostomy Association, American Association of Sex Educators, Counselors, and Therapists).
- Sexuality education is important to all populations, whether hearing or deaf, sighted or blind, disabled or not disabled. Discuss contraceptive choices as appropriate, and refer to a health professional (e.g., gynecologist, urologist, nurse practitioner).
▲ Teach safe sex to all clients including older adults, including using latex condoms, washing with soap immediately after sexual contact, not ingesting semen, avoiding oral-genital contact, not exchanging saliva, avoiding multiple partners, abstaining from sexual activity when ill, and avoiding recreational drugs and alcohol when engaging in sexual activity.

Risk for Shock
NANDA-I Definition

Vulnerable to an inadequate blood flow to the body's tissues that may lead to life-threatening cellular dysfunction, which may compromise health

Risk Factors

Hypotension; hypovolemia; hypoxemia; hypoxia; infection; sepsis; systemic inflammatory response syndrome (SIRS)

Client Outcomes

Client Will (Specify Time Frame)

- Discuss precautions to prevent complications of disease
- Maintain adherence to agreed upon medication regimens
- Maintain adequate hydration
- Monitor for infection signs and symptoms

• = Independent ▲ = Collaborative

- Maintain a mean arterial pressure above 65 mm Hg
- Maintain a heart rate between 60 and 100 with a normal rhythm
- Maintain urine output greater than 0.5 mL/kg/hr
- Maintain warm, dry skin

Nursing Interventions

- Review data pertaining to client risk status including age, primary diseases, immunosuppression, antibiotic use, and presence of hemodynamic alterations.
- Review client's medical and surgical history, noting conditions that place the client at higher risk for shock, including trauma, myocardial infarction, pulmonary embolism, head injury, dehydration, infection, and complicated pregnancy.
- Complete a full nursing physical examination.
- Monitor circulatory status (e.g., blood pressure [BP], mean arterial pressure [MAP], skin color, skin temperature, heart sounds, heart rate and rhythm, presence and quality of peripheral pulses, Doppler ultrasound, and pulse oximetry).
- Maintain intravenous (IV) access and provide isotonic IV fluids such as 0.9% normal saline or Ringer's lactate as ordered; these fluids are commonly used in the prevention and treatment of shock.
- Monitor for inadequate tissue oxygenation (e.g., apprehension, increased anxiety, changes in mental status, agitation, oliguria, cool/mottled periphery) and determinants of tissue oxygen delivery (e.g., PaO_2, SpO_2, $ScvO_2/SvO_2$, MAP, hemoglobin levels, lactate levels, cardiac output [CO]).
- ▲ Maintain vital signs (BP, pulse, respirations, and temperature) and pulse oximetry within normal parameters.
- ▲ Administer oxygen immediately to maintain SpO_2 greater than 90% and antibiotics and other medications as prescribed to any client presenting with symptoms of early shock.
- ▲ Monitor trends in noninvasive hemodynamic parameters (e.g., MAP) as appropriate.
- ▲ Monitor serum lactate levels, interpreting them within the context of each client.

Critical Care

- ▲ Prepare the client for the placement of an additional IV line, central line, and/or a pulmonary artery catheter as prescribed.
- ▲ Monitor trends in hemodynamic parameters (e.g., CVP, CO, CI, SVR, PAP, and MAP) as appropriate.

• = Independent   ▲ = Collaborative

▲ Monitor electrocardiography. Tachycardia may be present as a result of decreased fluid volume, which will be seen before a decrease in blood pressure as a compensatory mechanism.

▲ Monitor arterial blood gases, coagulation, chemistries, point-of-care blood glucose, cardiac enzymes, blood cultures, and hematology.

▲ Administer vasopressor agents as prescribed.

▲ If the client is in shock, refer to the following care plans: Risk for ineffective **Renal** perfusion, Risk for ineffective **Gastrointestinal** perfusion, Impaired **Gas** exchange, and Decreased **Cardiac** output.

Client/Family Teaching and Discharge Planning

• Instruct the client and family on disease process and rationale for care.

• Instruct clients and their family members on the signs and symptoms of low blood pressure to report to their health care provider (dizziness, lightheadedness, fainting, dehydration and unusual thirst, lack of concentration, blurred vision, nausea, cold, clammy, pale skin, rapid and shallow breathing, fatigue, depression).

• Implement educational initiatives to reduce health care–associated infections (HAIs).

• Promote a culture of client safety and individual accountability.

S

Impaired Sitting

NANDA-I Definition

Limitation of ability to independently and purposefully attain and/or maintain a rest position that is supported by the buttocks and thighs, in which the torso is upright

Defining Characteristics

Impaired ability to adjust position of one or both lower limbs on uneven surface; impaired ability to attain a balanced position of the torso; impaired ability to flex or move both hips; impaired ability to flex or move both knees; impaired ability to maintain the torso in balanced position; impaired ability to stress torso with body weight; insufficient muscle strength

Related Factors

Alteration in cognitive functioning; impaired metabolic functioning; insufficient endurance; insufficient energy; malnutrition; neurological disorder; orthopedic surgery; pain; prescribed posture; psychological disorder; sarcopenia; self-imposed relief posture

• = Independent   ▲ = Collaborative

Client Outcomes

Client Will (Specify Time Frame)

- Verbalize importance of being able to sit as a method to engage in activities of daily living
- Understand somatic physiology of posture control
- Choose health care options that enhance ability to sit
- Engage in physical conditioning exercises to enhance sitting ability
- Understand relationship of posture and emotions
- Control pain to increase ability to sit

Nursing Interventions

- Acknowledge the importance of being able to sit as a method to engage in activities of daily living.
- Understands the somatic physiology of posture control.
- Choose the musculoskeletal options that enhance ability to sit properly.
- Engage in physical conditioning exercises to enhance proper sitting ability.
- Understands the relationship of posture and somatic functioning.
- Understands the relationship of posture and emotions.
- Maintain pain levels below 3 to 4 on a 0- to 10-scale to increase ability to sit.

Pediatric

- Increase cognitive and physical functioning by promoting proper sitting ability.

Geriatric

- Increase cognitive and physical functioning by promoting proper sitting ability.

Multicultural

- Understand the importance of unimpaired sitting to different populations.

Home Care

- Encourage proper sitting posture in the home environment to promote health.

Impaired Skin integrity

NANDA-I Definition

Altered epidermis and/or dermis

• = Independent   ▲ = Collaborative

Defining Characteristics
Alteration in skin integrity; foreign matter piercing skin

Related Factors

External

Chemical injury agent (e.g., burn, capsaicin, methylene chloride, mustard agent); extremes of age; humidity; hyperthermia; hypothermia; mechanical factors (e.g., shearing forces, pressure, physical immobility); moisture; pharmaceutical agent; radiation therapy

Internal

Alteration in fluid volume; alteration in metabolism; alteration in pigmentation; alteration in sensation (e.g., resulting from spinal cord injury, diabetes mellitus); alteration in skin turgor; hormonal change; immunodeficiency; impaired circulation; impaired nutrition; pressure over bony prominence

Client Outcomes

Client Will (Specify Time Frame)

- Regain integrity of skin surface
- Report any altered sensation or pain at site of skin impairment
- Demonstrate understanding of plan to heal skin and prevent reinjury
- Describe measures to protect and heal the skin and to care for any skin lesion

Nursing Interventions

- Assess site of skin impairment and determine cause or type of wound (e.g., acute or chronic wound, burn, dermatological lesion, pressure ulcer, skin tear).
- Use a risk assessment tool to systematically assess client risk factors for skin breakdown due to pressure.
- Determine the extent of the skin impairment (e.g., partial-thickness wound, stage I or stage II pressure ulcer). The following classification system and definition is for pressure ulcers: localized injury to the skin and/or underlying tissue usually over a bony prominence, as a result of pressure, or pressure in combination with shear (Note: Friction is not included in the definition) (NPUAP/EPUAP, 2014).
  - **Category/Stage I:** Intact skin with nonblanchable erythema of a localized area, usually over a bony prominence. Darkly pigmented skin may not have visible blanching. The area may be painful, firm, soft, warmer or cooler than adjacent tissue.

S

• = Independent   ▲ = Collaborative

○ **Category/Stage II:** Partial-thickness skin loss of dermis presenting as a shallow open ulcer with a red pink wound bed, without slough, that may also present as intact or open/ruptured and serum-filled. Presents as a shiny or dry shallow ulcer without slough or bruising.

○ Bruising may indicate suspected deep tissue injury; for wounds deeper into subcutaneous tissue, muscle, or bone (category/stage III or stage IV pressure ulcers), see the care plan for Impaired **Tissue** integrity (NPUAP/EPUAP, 2014).

• Inspect and monitor site of skin impairment at least once a day for color changes, redness, swelling, warmth, pain, or other signs of infection. Determine whether the client is experiencing changes in sensation or pain. Closely assess high-risk areas such as bony prominences, skinfolds, the sacrum, and heels.

• Monitor the client's skin care practices, noting type of soap or other cleansing agents used, temperature of water, and frequency of skin cleansing.

• Consider using normal saline to clean the pressure ulcer or as ordered by the health care provider, but if necessary tap water suitable for drinking may be used to clean the wound.

• Individualize plan according to the client's skin condition, needs, and preferences.

• Monitor the client's continence status, and minimize exposure of skin impairment to other areas of moisture from perspiration or wound drainage.

• If the client is incontinent, implement an incontinence management plan to prevent exposure to chemicals in urine and stool that can damage the skin. Use a skin protectant cream to protect the skin after each incontinence episode. Refer to a continence care specialist, urologist, or gastroenterologist for incontinence assessment (Borchert et al, 2010).

• For clients with limited mobility and activity, use a risk assessment tool to systematically assess immobility and activity-related risk factors.

• Do not position the client on site of skin impairment. If consistent with overall client management goals, reposition the client as determined by individualized tissue tolerance and overall condition. Reposition and transfer the client with care to protect against the

• = Independent   ▲ = Collaborative

adverse effects of external mechanical forces such as pressure, friction, and shear.

- Evaluate for use of support surfaces (specialty mattresses, beds), chair cushions, or devices as appropriate. Maintain the head of the bed at the lowest possible degree of elevation to reduce shear and friction, and use lift devices, pillows, foam wedges, and pressure-reducing devices in the bed (NPUAP/EPUAP, 2014; WOCN, 2010).
- Implement a written treatment plan for topical treatment of the site of skin impairment.
- Select a topical treatment that will maintain a moist wound-healing environment (stage II) and that is balanced with the need to absorb exudate. Stage I pressure ulcers may be managed by keeping the client off of the area and using a protective dressing (Baranoski & Ayello, 2012).
- Avoid massaging around the site of skin impairment and over bony prominences.
- Assess the client's nutritional status. Refer for a nutritional consult and/or institute dietary supplements as necessary.
- Identify the client's phase of wound healing (inflammation, proliferation, maturation) and stage of injury.

Home Care

- The interventions described previously may be adapted for home care use.
- Instruct and assist the client and caregivers in how to change dressings and maintain a clean environment. Provide written instructions and observe the client completing the dressing change before hospital discharge and in the home setting.
- Educate client and caregivers on proper nutrition, signs and symptoms of infection, and when to call the agency and/or health care provider with concerns.
- It may be beneficial to initiate a consultation in a case assignment with a wound, ostomy, continence nurse (or wounds specialist) to establish a comprehensive plan for complex wounds.

Client/Family Teaching and Discharge Planning

- Teach skin and wound assessment and ways to monitor for signs and symptoms of infection, complications, and healing. Early assessment and intervention help prevent serious problems from developing.
- Teach the client why a topical treatment has been selected.

• = Independent ▲ = Collaborative

- If consistent with overall client management goals, teach how to reposition as client condition warrants.
- Teach the client to use pillows, foam wedges, chair cushions, and pressure-redistribution devices to prevent pressure injury.

Risk for impaired Skin integrity

NANDA-I Definition

Vulnerable to alteration in epidermis and/or dermis, which may compromise health

Risk Factors

External

Chemical injury agent (e.g., burn, capsaicin, methylene chloride, mustard agent); excretions; extremes of age; humidity; hyperthermia; hypothermia; mechanical factors (e.g., shearing forces, pressure, physical immobility); moisture; radiation therapy; secretions

Internal

Alteration in metabolism; alteration in pigmentation; alteration in sensation (e.g., resulting from spinal cord injury, diabetes mellitus); alteration in skin turgor; hormonal change; immunodeficiency; impaired circulation; inadequate nutrition; pharmaceutical agent; pressure over bony prominence; psychogenetic factor

NOTE: Risk should be determined by the use of a risk assessment tool (e.g., Norton scale, Braden scale).

Client Outcomes

Client Will (Specify Time Frame)

- Report altered sensation or pain at risk areas as soon as noted
- Demonstrate understanding of personal risk factors for impaired skin integrity
- Verbalize a personal plan for preventing impaired skin integrity

Nursing Interventions

- Identify clients at risk for impaired skin integrity as a result of immobility, chronological age, malnutrition, incontinence, compromised perfusion, immunocompromised status, or chronic medical condition, such as diabetes mellitus, spinal cord injury, or renal failure.
- Inspect and monitor skin condition at least once a day for color or texture changes, redness, localized heat, edema or induration,

pressure damage, dermatological conditions, or lesions and any incontinence-associated dermatitis. Determine whether the client is experiencing loss of sensation or pain.

- Monitor the client's skin care practices, noting type of soap or other cleansing agents used, temperature of water, and frequency of skin cleansing.
- Cleanse the skin gently with pH-balanced cleansers. Avoid harsh cleansing agents, hot water, extreme friction or force, or too-frequent cleansing (WOCN, 2010).
▲ Monitor the client's continence status and minimize exposure of the site of skin impairment (incontinence-associated dermatitis) and other areas to moisture from incontinence, perspiration, or wound drainage. If the client is incontinent, implement an incontinence management plan to prevent exposure to chemicals in urine and stool that can strip or erode the skin. Use a skin barrier product and/ or moisture wicking pads to reduce risk of exposure. Refer to a health care provider (e.g., continence care specialist, urologist, gastroenterologist) for an incontinence assessment (WOCN, 2010).
- For clients with limited mobility, inspect and monitor condition of skin covering bony prominences.
- Implement and communicate a client-specific prevention plan.
- At-risk clients should be frequently repositioning. Frequency of repositioning will be influenced by variables concerning the individual's independent mobility and the support surface in use. Frequency of repositioning should be determined by the individual's tissue tolerance and medical condition (NPUAP/EPUAP, 2014). Reposition the client with care to protect against the adverse effects of external mechanical forces (e.g., pressure, friction, shear) (WOCN, 2010).
- Evaluate for use of specialty mattresses, beds, or devices as appropriate (Brienza et al, 2012; Lippoldt et al, 2014).
- Avoid massaging over bony prominences.
▲ Assess the client's nutritional status; refer for a nutritional consult and/or institute dietary supplements.

Geriatric
- Limit number of complete baths to two or three per week, and alternate them with partial baths. Use a tepid water temperature (between 90°F and 105°F) for bathing or use a no-rinse alternative product.

• = Independent   ▲ = Collaborative

- Use lotions and moisturizers to prevent skin from drying out, especially in the winter.
- Increase fluid intake within cardiac and renal limits to a minimum of 1500 mL per day.
- Increase humidity in the environment, especially during the winter, by using a humidifier or placing a container of water on a warm object.

Home Care

- Assess client and caregiver ability to recognize potential risk for skin breakdown. Provide resources for client/caregiver to contact health care provider with questions/concerns related to skin and incontinence care as needed (Vrtis, 2013).
▲ Initiate a consultation in a case assignment with a wound care specialist or wound, ostomy, or continence nurse to establish a comprehensive plan as soon as possible (Vrtis, 2013).
- See the care plan for Impaired **Skin** integrity.

Client/Family Teaching and Discharge Planning

- Teach the client skin assessment and ways to monitor for impending skin breakdown.
- If consistent with overall client management goals, teach how to turn and reposition the client.
- Teach the client and or caregivers to use pillows, foam wedges, and pressure-reducing devices to prevent pressure injury (WOCN, 2010; NPUAP/EPUAP, 2014).

Readiness for enhanced Sleep

NANDA-I Definition

A pattern of natural, periodic suspension of relative consciousness to provide rest and sustain a desired lifestyle, which can be strengthened

Defining Characteristics

Expresses desire to enhance sleep

Client Outcomes

Client Will (Specify Time Frame)

- Verbalize an interest in what constitutes normal sleep
- Verbalize an interest in nonpharmacological approaches to sleep promotion
- Establish an environment conducive to sleep initiation and maintenance throughout the night

• = Independent   ▲ = Collaborative

Nursing Interventions

- Obtain a sleep history including bedtime routines, sleep patterns, use of medications and stimulants, and use of complementary and alternative medical practices for stress management and relaxation before bedtime.
  - From the history, assess the client's ability to initiate and maintain sleep, obtain adequate amounts of sleep, and manage daytime responsibilities free from fatigue and sleepiness.
- Based on assessment, teach one or more of the listed sleep promotion practices as appropriate.
  - Establish a regular schedule for sleep, exercise, napping, and mealtimes.
  - Avoid long periods of daytime sleep.
  - Limit caffeine.
  - Limit alcohol use.
  - Avoid long-term use of sleeping pills.
  - Engage in relaxing activities before bed.
  - Provide backrub or other forms of massage.
  - Teach relaxation techniques.
  - Teach complementary and alternative interventions as culturally congruent.
  - Lower lighting in sleep area.
  - Mask noise in sleep area when it cannot be eliminated.
  - For anxious clients, consider use of a lavender oil preparation in the health care setting.

Geriatric

- Interventions discussed previously may be adapted for use with geriatric clients.
- Counsel the older adult regarding normal age-related changes in sleep.
- Elicit the older adult's expectations for sleep and correct misconceptions.
- Assess and refer as appropriate if coexisting conditions may be disrupting sleep.
- Discuss appropriate and inappropriate self-help measures for improving sleep.
- Encourage walking and other exercise outdoors unless contraindicated.
- Help older adults engage with others who enjoy similar events.

S

Home Care

- Interventions discussed previously may be adapted for home care use.
- Some complementary and alternative medicine interventions may be more easily tried at home than in health care facilities.
- Assess the conduciveness of the home environment for both caregivers' and clients' sleep.

Sleep deprivation

NANDA-I Definition

Prolonged periods of time without sleep (sustained natural, periodic suspension of relative consciousness)

Defining Characteristics

Agitation; alteration in concentration; anxiety; apathy; combativeness; confusion; decrease in functional ability; decrease in reaction time; drowsiness; fatigue; fleeting nystagmus; hallucinations; hand tremors; heightened sensitivity to pain; irritability; lethargy; listlessness; malaise; perceptual disorders; restlessness; transient paranoia

Related Factors (r/t)

Age-related sleep stage shifts; average daily physical activity less than recommended for gender and age; conditions with periodic limb movement (e.g., restless leg syndrome, nocturnal myoclonus); dementia; environmental barrier; familial sleep paralysis; idiopathic central nervous system hypersomnolence; narcolepsy; nightmares; nonrestorative sleep pattern (e.g., due to caregiver responsibilities, parenting practices, sleep partner); overstimulating environment; prolonged discomfort (e.g., physical, psychological); sleep apnea; sleep terror; sleep walking; sleep-related enuresis; sleep-related painful erections; Sundowner syndrome; sustained circadian asynchrony; sustained inadequate sleep hygiene; treatment regimen

Client Outcomes

Client Will (Specify Time Frame)

- Verbalize plan that provides adequate time for sleep
- Identify actions that can be taken to ensure adequate sleep time
- Awaken refreshed once adequate time is spent sleeping
- Be less sleepy during the day once adequate time is spent sleeping

• = Independent   ▲ = Collaborative

Nursing Interventions

- Obtain a sleep history to identify the specific personal and environmental factors that may be depriving clients of the amount of sleep needed for optimal functioning.
  - o Minimize environmental factors that disturb the client's sleep. See nursing interventions for Disturbed **Sleep** pattern.
  - o Minimize personal factors that disturb the client's sleep. See nursing interventions for **Insomnia.**
- Assess the amount of sleep obtained each night compared with the amount of sleep needed.
- Assess for hypersensitivity to pain.
- When daytime drowsiness occurs despite long, undisturbed periods of sleep, consider sleep apnea as a possible cause.
- Encourage a regular schedule of napping as a way to compensate for sleep deficiency whenever severely restricted sleep amounts cannot be avoided.
- Monitor caffeine intake in clients who may use caffeinated drinks to overcome sleep deficiency.
- If evidence-based interventions are inadequate, consider and carefully evaluate unstudied but commonly used countermeasures for fighting drowsiness.

Pediatric

- Assess the amount of sleep obtained each night compared with the amount of sleep needed.
- Encourage daily schedules that allow for late awakening times for adolescents.
- See the Pediatric section of nursing interventions for: Readiness for enhanced **Sleep,** Disturbed **Sleep** pattern, and **Insomnia.**

Geriatric

- Assess the amount of sleep obtained each night compared with the amount of sleep needed.
- See the Geriatric section of nursing interventions for Disturbed **Sleep** pattern and **Insomnia.**

Multicultural

- Be aware of racial and ethnic disparities in sleep deprivation.

Home Care

- Teach family members about the short-term and long-term consequences of inadequate amounts of sleep for both clients and family caregivers.

• = Independent   ▲ = Collaborative

- Teach client/family caregivers about the need for those with chronic conditions to avoid schedules and commitments that interfere with obtaining adequate amounts of sleep.
- Promote adoption of behaviors that ensure adequate amounts of sleep for all family members. See nursing interventions for Readiness for enhanced **Sleep.**
- Teach family members ways to avoid chronic sleep loss. See nursing interventions for Disturbed **Sleep** pattern.
- Advise against the sleep-deprived client's chronic use of caffeinated drinks to overcome daytime fatigue and or drowsiness; focus on elimination of factors that lead to chronic sleep loss.

Disturbed Sleep pattern
NANDA-I Definition
Time-limited interruptions of sleep amount and quality due to external factors

Defining Characteristics
Alteration in sleep pattern; difficulty in daily functioning; difficulty initiating sleep; dissatisfaction with sleep; feeling unrested; unintentional awakening

Related Factors
Disruption caused by sleep partner; environmental barrier (e.g., ambient noise, daylight/darkness exposure, ambient temperature, humidity, unfamiliar settings); immobilization; insufficient privacy; nonrestorative sleep pattern (e.g., due to caregiver responsibilities, parenting practices, sleep partner)

Client Outcomes
Client Will (Specify Time Frame)
- Verbalize plan to implement sleep promotion routines
- Maintain a regular schedule of sleep and waking
- Fall asleep without difficulty
- Remain asleep throughout the night
- Awaken naturally, feeling refreshed and not be fatigued during day

Nursing Interventions
- Obtain a sleep history to identify (1) noise and light levels in the sleep environment, (2) activities occurring in the sleep environment during hours of sleep, (3) number of times awakened during the

• = Independent ▲ = Collaborative

sleep period, and (4) when during the sleep period, time is available for undisturbed sleep.

- Keep environment quiet during sleep periods.
- Consider masking hospital noise that cannot be eliminated.
- Offer earplugs when feasible.
- Dim the lights during client sleep periods.
- Offer eye covers when lighting cannot be dimmed.
- Be aware that use of eye covers in intubated clients may lead to sensory deprivation and anxiety.
- Consolidate essential care to provide opportunity for uninterrupted sleep the first 3 to 4 hours of the sleep period. Follow with periods of 90 to 110 minutes between interruptions.
- If client must be disturbed the first 3 to 4 hours of the sleep period, attempt to protect 90- to 110-minute blocks of time between awakenings.
- Assess for medications and other stimulants that fragment sleep. Use caution when administering sleep medications. See nursing interventions for **Insomnia.**
- Schedule newly ordered medications to avoid the need to wake the client the first few hours of the night.
- Combine as many of the above interventions as feasible to create a sleep-promotion care bundle.

Pediatric
- Adapt interventions for pediatric clients with caution due to lack of empirical evidence regarding the effects of their use.

Geriatric
- Use of earplugs and eye covers with ataxic clients and clients with dementia may contribute to disorientation.

Multicultural
- Be aware that cultural sleep practices may alter the kinds of environmental sleep disruptors that require management.

Home Care
- Consider the unique characteristics of each home sleep environment when addressing sleep disruption.
- In addition, see the Home Care section of nursing interventions for Readiness for enhanced **Sleep.**

S

• = Independent   ▲ = Collaborative

Impaired Social interaction

NANDA-I Definition

Insufficient or excessive quantity or ineffective quality of social exchange

Defining Characteristics

Discomfort in social situations; dissatisfaction with social engagement (e.g., belonging, caring, interest, shared history); dysfunctional interaction with others; family reports change in interaction (e.g., style, pattern); impaired social functioning

Related Factors (r/t)

Absence of significant others; communication barriers; disturbance in self-concept; disturbance in thought processes; environmental barrier; impaired mobility; insufficient knowledge about how to enhance mutuality; insufficient skills to enhance mutuality; sociocultural dissonance; therapeutic isolation

Client Outcomes

Client Will (Specify Time Frame)

- Identify barriers that cause impaired social interactions
- Discuss feelings that accompany impaired and successful social interactions
- Use available opportunities to practice interactions
- Use successful social interaction behaviors
- Report increased comfort in social situations
- Communicate, state feelings of belonging, demonstrate caring and interest in others
- Report effective interactions with others

Nursing Interventions

- Monitor the client's use of defense mechanisms and support healthy defenses (e.g., the client focuses on the present and avoids placing blame on others for personal behavior).
- Spend time with the client.
- Encourage physical activity, such as aerobics or stretching and toning.
- Have group members support each other in a group setting.
- Model appropriate social interactions and use focused imitation interventions. Give positive verbal and nonverbal feedback for appropriate behavior (e.g., make statements such as, "I'm proud that you made it to work on time and did all the tasks assigned to you"; make eye contact). If not contraindicated, touch the client's arm or hand when speaking.

• = Independent ▲ = Collaborative

- Consider use of social cognition and interaction training (SCIT) combined with social mentoring to improve social functioning.
- Use client-centered humor as appropriate.
- Consider use of animal therapy; arrange for visitation.
- Consider use of videophone or other visual communication devices to promote social interaction in clients with visual impairments.
▲ Refer client for social cognition training to increase social skills.
▲ Refer rehabilitation clients for assistive technologies to increase therapeutic engagement and promote social engagement.
- Refer to care plans for Risk for **Loneliness** and **Social** isolation for additional interventions.

Pediatric
- Encourage social support and counseling for clients with visual and hearing impairments.
- Provide supervised interaction opportunities for children of chronically ill parents.
- Provide computers and Internet access to children with chronic disabilities that limit socialization.
▲ Refer overweight adolescents to group-based weight loss programs.
▲ Refer children with autism for family-centered music therapy (FCMT).
- Consider the use of animal-assisted activities for children on the autistic spectrum.
- Consider the use of theater skills training to facilitate social skills.

Geriatric
- Encourage socialization through education, support groups, and programs for older adults in the community.
- Assess for depression in clients with impaired social functioning.
- Assess cognitive functioning in clients who present with decreased social interaction.
- Assess the communication patterns of clients with verbal domain problems for enactment strategies, paralinguistic features, and nonvocal communication.
- Consider having clients participate in playing Wii.
▲ Refer depressed clients to services for cognitive behavioral therapy (CBT).
- Refer to care plans for **Frail Elderly** syndrome, Risk for **Loneliness,** and **Social** isolation for additional interventions.

S

• = Independent   ▲ = Collaborative

Multicultural

- Assess for the effect of racism on the client's perceptions of social interactions.
- Approach individuals of color with respect, warmth, and professional courtesy.
- Use interpreters as needed.
- Refer to care plan for **Social** isolation for additional interventions.

Home Care

- Previously discussed interventions may be adapted for home care use.
- ▲ Refer clients to or support involvement in supportive groups and counseling.

Client/Family Teaching and Discharge Planning

- ▲ Refer to appropriate social agencies for assistance (e.g., family therapy, self-help groups, creative activities, crisis intervention), especially individuals who are seriously ill.

Social isolation

NANDA-I Definition

Aloneness experienced by the individual and perceived as imposed by others and as a negative or threatening state

Defining Characteristics

Absence of support system; aloneness imposed by others; cultural incongruence; desire to be alone; development delay; developmentally inappropriate interests; disabling condition; feeling different from others; flat affect; history of rejection; hostility; illness; inability to meet expectations of others; insecurity in public; meaningless actions; member of a subculture; poor eye contact; preoccupation with own thoughts; purposelessness; repetitive actions; sad affect; values incongruent with cultural norms; withdrawn

Related Factors (r/t)

Alterations in mental status; alterations in physical appearance; altered state of wellness; developmentally inappropriate interests; factors impacting satisfying personal relationships (e.g., developmental delay); inability to engage in satisfying personal relationships; insufficient personal resources (e.g., poor achievement, poor insight, affect unavailable and poorly controlled); social behavior incongruent with norms; values incongruent with cultural norms; may be present but is not required; pain may be of unknown etiology

• = Independent   ▲ = Collaborative

Client Outcomes

Client Will (Specify Time Frame)

- Identify feelings of isolation
- Practice social and communication skills needed to interact with others
- Initiate interactions with others; set and meet goals
- Participate in activities and programs at level of ability and desire
- Describe feelings of self-worth

Nursing Interventions

- Establish a therapeutic relationship with the client.
- Observe for barriers to social interaction.
- Discuss/assess causes of perceived or actual isolation.
- Allow the client opportunities to describe his/her daily life and to introduce any issues that may be of concern.
- Promote social interactions.
- Assist the client in identifying specific health and social problems; involve him/her in their resolution.
- Assist the client in identifying activities that encourage socialization.
- Identify available support systems and involve those individuals in the client's care.
- ▲ Refer clients and caregivers to support groups as necessary.
- Encourage interactions with others with similar interests.
- See the care plan for Risk for **Loneliness.**

Pediatric

- ▲ Refer obese adolescents for diet, exercise, and psychosocial support.
- ▲ Assess socially isolated adolescents. Refer to appropriate rehabilitation programs as needed.

Geriatric

- ▲ Assess physical and mental status to establish an early baseline for referring at-risk individuals to community resources.
- Assess for hearing.
- Involve client in planning activities.
- Involve nonprofessionals in activities and projects with the client.
- Suggest varied social activities that would decrease isolation and encourage participation.
- ▲ Consider the use of simulated presence therapy (see the care plan for **Hopelessness**).
- Consider using computers and the Internet to alleviate or reduce loneliness and social isolation.

• = Independent ▲ = Collaborative

Multicultural

- Acknowledge racial/ethnic differences at the onset of care.
- Assess for the influence of cultural beliefs, norms, values, and the client's personal cultural needs.
- Use a culturally competent, professional approach when working with clients of various ethnic groups.
- Promote a sense of ethnic attachment.
- Assess the client's feelings regarding social isolation.
- Assist those ethnic minorities who are underserved to access essential health care.

Home Care

- The interventions described previously may be adapted for home care use.
- Confirm that the home setting has health-safety systems in place.
- Consider the use of the computer and Internet to decrease isolation.
- Assess options for living that allow the client privacy, but not isolation.
- Assist clients to interact with neighbors in the community when they move to supported housing.

Client/Family Teaching and Discharge Planning

- Assist the client in initiating contacts with self-help groups, counselors, and therapists.
- Provide information to the client about senior citizen services and community resources.
- Refer socially isolated caregivers to appropriate support groups.
- See the care plan for **Caregiver Role Strain.**

Chronic Sorrow

NANDA-I Definition

Cyclical, recurring, and potentially progressive pattern of pervasive sadness experienced (by parent, caregiver, individual with chronic illness or disability) in response to continual loss throughout the trajectory of an illness or disability

Defining Characteristics

Reports feelings of sadness (e.g., periodic, recurrent); reports feelings that interfere with ability to reach highest level of personal well-being; reports feelings that interfere with ability to reach highest level of social well-being; reports negative feelings (e.g., anger, being misunderstood,

• = Independent ▲ = Collaborative

confusion, depression, disappointment, emptiness, fear, frustration, guilt, helplessness, hopelessness, low self-esteem, being overwhelmed, recurring loss, self-blame)

Related Factors (r/t)

Crisis in management of the disability; crises in management of the illness; crises related to developmental stages; death of a loved one; experiences chronic disability (e.g., physical or mental); experiences chronic illness (e.g., physical or mental); missed opportunities; missed milestones; unending caregiving

Client Outcomes

Client Will (Specify Time Frame)

- Express appropriate feelings of guilt, fear, anger, or sadness
- Identify problems associated with sorrow (e.g., changes in appetite, insomnia, nightmares, loss of libido, decreased energy, alteration in activity levels)
- Seek help in dealing with grief-associated problems
- Plan for the future one day at a time
- Function at normal developmental level

Nursing Interventions

- Determine the client's degree of sorrow.
- Assess for the four discrete stages of grieving in chronic obstructive pulmonary disease (COPD) clients.
- Provide coping strategies for caregivers who may experience chronic sorrow. See care plan for **Caregiver Role Strain.**
- Assess clients for chronic sorrow and provide them with coping strategies.
- Develop a trusting relationship with the client by using empathetic therapeutic communication techniques.
- Help the client understand that sorrow may be ongoing.
- Help the client recognize that although sadness will occur at intervals for the rest of his/her life, it will become bearable.
- Urge the client to use positive coping techniques.

Pediatric

- Encourage the parents of children with uncommon diseases to use online resources to manage their chronic sorrow.
- Educate parents that an increase in chronic sorrow can occur after stressful events.

- Nurses should assess for chronic sorrow and discuss coping strategies with parents of children who have been in the neonatal intensive care unit (NICU).
- Allow children the opportunity to talk about the impending death of a parent or loved one.
- Encourage parents to listen to their child's expression of grief.
- Consider the use of art for children in hospice care who are dying or dealing with the death of a parent, sibling, or other family member.
▲ Refer grieving children and parents to a program to help facilitate grieving.
- Encourage children experiencing grief to participate in bereavement activities and camps.
- Help the adolescent with chronic sorrow determine sources of support and refer for counseling if needed.
- Provide family-centered care to parents of children with disabilities, and encourage parents to attend support groups.
- Encourage parents with chronic sorrow to participate in a support group and learn coping strategies.
- Recognize that mothers who have a miscarriage grieve and experience sorrow because of loss of the child.

Geriatric
- Identify previous losses and assess the client for depression.
- Evaluate the social support system of the older client and refer for bereavement counseling if needed.

Home Care
- In-home bereavement follow-up by nurses should be considered if available.
- Assess the client for depression.
- Refer for mental health services and counseling as indicated.
- Encourage the client to participate in activities that are diversionary and uplifting as tolerated (e.g., outdoor activities, hobby groups, church-related activities, pet care).
- Encourage the client to participate in support groups appropriate to the area of loss or illness.
- Provide empathetic communication for family/caregivers.
- The interventions described previously may be adapted for home care use.
- See the care plans for Chronic low **Self-Esteem,** Risk for **Loneliness,** and **Hopelessness.**

• = Independent ▲ = Collaborative

Spiritual distress

NANDA-I Definition

A state of suffering related to the impaired ability to experience meaning in life through connectedness with self, others, world, or a superior being

Defining Characteristics

Anxiety; crying; fatigue; fear; insomnia; questioning identity; questioning meaning of life; questioning meaning of suffering

Connections to Self

Anger; decrease in serenity; feeling of being unloved; guilt; inadequate acceptance; ineffective coping strategies; insufficient courage; perceived insufficient meaning in life

Connections with Others

Alienation; refuses to interact with spiritual leader; refuses to interact with significant other; separation from support system

Connections with Art, Music, Literature, and Nature

Decrease in expression of previous pattern of creativity; disinterest in nature; disinterest in reading spiritual literature

Connections with Power Greater Than Self

Anger toward power greater than self; feeling abandoned; hopelessness; inability for introspection; inability to experience the transcendent; inability to participate in religious activities; inability to pray; perceived suffering; request for a spiritual leader; sudden change in spiritual practice

S

Related Factors

Actively dying; aging; birth of a child; death of significant other; exposure to death; illness; imminent death; increasing dependence on another; life transition; loneliness; loss of a body part; loss of function of a body part; pain; perception of having unfinished business; receiving bad news; self-alienation; social alienation; sociocultural deprivation; treatment regimen; unexpected life event

Client Outcomes

Client Will (Specify Time Frame)

- Express meaning and purpose in life
- Express sense of hope in the future
- Express sense of connectedness with self
- Express sense of connectedness with family/friends
- Express ability to forgive
- Express acceptance of health status
- Find meaning in relationships with others

• = Independent   ▲ = Collaborative

- Find meaning in relationship with higher power
- Find meaning in personal and health care treatment choices

Nursing Interventions

- Observe clients for cues indicating difficulties in finding meaning, purpose, or hope in life.
- Observe clients with chronic illness, poor prognosis, or life-changing conditions for loss of meaning, purpose, and hope in life.
- Offer spiritual care in disaster relief.
- Promote a sense of love, caring, and compassion in nursing encounters.
- Be physically present and actively listen to the client.
- Help the client find a reason for living; be available for support and promote hope.
- Listen to the client's feelings about suffering and/or death. Be nonjudgmental and allow time for grieving.
- Respect the client's beliefs; avoid imposing your own spiritual beliefs on the client. Be aware of your own belief systems and accept the client's spirituality.
- Monitor and promote supportive social contacts.
- Integrate family into spiritual practices as appropriate.
- Assist family in searching for meaning in client's health care situation.
▲ Refer the client to a support group or counseling.
- Support meditation, guided imagery, journaling, relaxation, and involvement in art, music, or poetry. Support outdoor activities.
▲ Offer or suggest visits with spiritual and/or religious advisors.
- Provide privacy or a "sacred space."
- Allow time and a place for prayer.
- Coordinate or encourage attending spiritual retreats, courses, or programming.

Geriatric

- Identify the client's past spiritual practices that have been helpful. Help the client explore his/her life and identify those experiences that are noteworthy.
- Offer opportunities to practice one's religion.

Pediatric

- Offer adolescents opportunities for reflection and storytelling to express their spirituality.

• = Independent   ▲ = Collaborative

Multicultural

- Recognize the importance of spirituality and provide culturally competent spiritual care to specific populations:
  - ○ Arab Muslims.
  - ○ Chinese elders.
  - ○ Korean immigrants.
  - ○ Latinos.
  - ○ African Americans.
  - ○ Thai.
  - ○ African women.

Veterans of Armed Services

- Recognize the unique spiritual needs of veterans and provide spiritual support or appropriate referrals.

Home Care

- All of the nursing interventions described previously apply in the home setting.

Risk for Spiritual distress

NANDA-I Definition

Vulnerable to an impaired ability to experience and integrate meaning and purpose in life through connectedness within self, literature, nature, and/or a power greater than oneself, which may compromise health

Risk Factors

Developmental

Life transition

Environmental

Environmental change; natural disaster

Physical

Chronic illness; physical illness; substance abuse

Psychosocial

Anxiety; barrier to experiencing love; change in religious ritual; change in spiritual practice; cultural conflict; depression; inability to forgive; ineffective relationships; loss; low self-esteem; racial conflict; separation from support system; stressors

Client Outcomes, Nursing Interventions, and Client/Family Teaching and Discharge Planning

Refer to care plan for **Spiritual Distress.**

• = Independent ▲ = Collaborative

Readiness for enhanced Spiritual well-being

NANDA-I Definition

A pattern of experiencing and integrating meaning and purpose in life through connectedness with self, others, art, music, literature, nature, and/or a power greater than oneself, which can be strengthened

Defining Characteristics

Connections to Self

Expresses desire to enhance acceptance; expresses desire to enhance coping; expresses desire to enhance courage; expresses desire to enhance hope; expresses desire to enhance joy; expresses desire to enhance love; expresses desire to enhance meaning in life; expresses desire to enhance meditative practice; expresses desire to enhance purpose in life; expresses desire to enhance satisfaction with philosophy of life; expresses desire to enhance self-forgiveness; expresses desire to enhance serenity (e.g., peace); expresses desire to enhance surrender; meditation

Connections with Others

Expresses desire to enhance forgiveness from other; expresses desire to enhance interaction with significant other; expresses desire to enhance interaction with spiritual leaders; expresses desire to enhance service to others

Connections with Art, Music, Literature, and Nature

Expresses desire to enhance creative energy (e.g., writing, poetry, music); expresses desire to enhance spiritual reading; expresses desire to enhance time outdoors

Connections with Power Greater than Self

Expresses desire to enhance mystical experiences; expresses desire to enhance participation in religious activity; expresses desire to enhance prayerfulness; expresses desire to enhance reverence

Client Outcomes

Client Will (Specify Time Frame)

- Express hope
- Express sense of meaning and purpose in life
- Express peace and serenity
- Express love
- Express acceptance
- Express surrender
- Express forgiveness of self and others
- Express satisfaction with philosophy of life

• = Independent   ▲ = Collaborative

- Express joy
- Express courage
- Describe being able to cope
- Describe use of spiritual practices
- Describe providing service to others
- Describe interaction with spiritual leaders, friends, and family
- Describe appreciation for art, music, literature, and nature

Nursing Interventions

- Perform a spiritual assessment that includes the client's relationship with God, meaning and purpose in life, religious affiliation, and any other significant beliefs.
- Be present and actively listen to the client.
- Encourage the client to pray or engage in other spiritual meditative practices.
- Coordinate or encourage attending spiritual retreats or courses.
- Promote hope.
- Encourage clients to reflect on what is meaningful to them in life.
- Encourage increased quality of life through social support and family relationships.
- Assist the client in identifying religious or spiritual beliefs that encourage integration of meaning and purpose in the client's life.
- Support meditation, guided imagery, journaling, relaxation, and involvement in art, music, or poetry. Support outdoor activities.
- Encourage outdoor activities.
- Encourage expressions of spirituality.
- Encourage integration of spirituality in healthy lifestyle choices.

Geriatric

- Identify the client's past spiritual practices that have been growth-filled. Help the client explore his or her life and identify those experiences that are noteworthy.
- Offer opportunities to practice one's religion.

Pediatric

- Offer adolescents opportunities for reflection and storytelling to express their spirituality.

Multicultural

- Recognize the importance of spirituality and provide culturally competent spiritual care to specific populations:
  - ○ Arab/Jordanian Muslims.
  - ○ Thai.

S

• = Independent ▲ = Collaborative

- ○ Latinos.
- ○ African Americans.
- ○ Sheltered homeless.
- ○ Chinese.

Home Care

- All of the nursing interventions described previously apply in the home setting.

Impaired Standing

NANDA-I Definition

Limitation of ability to independently and purposefully attain and/or maintain the body in an upright position from feet to head

Defining Characteristics

Impaired ability to adjust position of one or both lower limbs on uneven surface; impaired ability to attain a balanced position of the torso; impaired ability to extend one or both hips; impaired ability to extend one or both knees; impaired ability to flex one or both hips; impaired ability to flex one or both knees; impaired ability to maintain the torso in balanced position; impaired ability to stress torso with body weight; insufficient muscle strength

Related Factors

Circulatory perfusion disorder; emotional disturbance; impaired metabolic functioning; injury to lower extremity; insufficient endurance; insufficient energy; malnutrition; neurological disorder; obesity; pain; prescribed posture; sarcopenia; self-imposed relief posture; surgical procedure

Client Outcomes

Client Will (Specify Time Frame)

- Demonstrate optimal independence and safety when standing
- Demonstrate the proper use of assistive devices
- State benefits of standing

Nursing Interventions

- Encourage clients to stand at intervals throughout the day.
- Advise patients of the physical and psychological benefits of being upright and active.

Geriatric

- Advise older clients who have difficulty standing to use assistive devices.

• = Independent   ▲ = Collaborative

- Encourage trunk exercises after clients have had strokes.
- Encourage clients post-stroke to participate in rehabilitation interventions that promote standing.
- Raise the height of the bed and encourage the use of the client's hands when an older adult is rising from a sitting to standing position.
- Educate older adults who have fallen about the need for balance and muscle training of the ankle joint.
- Educate adults older than age 80 years on the need for vitamin D.

Client/Family Teaching and Discharge Planning

- Educate clients that standing can be beneficial for their health.
- Teach clients about the need to take frequent breaks when standing for long periods.
- Instruct clients about the use of yoga for individuals who have difficulty with standing balance.

Stress overload

NANDA-I Definition

Excessive amounts and types of demands that require action

Defining Characteristics

Excessive stress; feeling of pressure; impaired decision-making; impaired functioning; increase in anger; increase in anger behavior; increase in impatience; negative impact from stress (e.g., physical symptoms, psychological distress, feeling sick); tension

Related Factors (r/t)

Excessive stress; insufficient resources (e.g., financial, social, knowledge); repeated stressors; stressors

Client Outcomes

Client Will (Specify Time Frame)

- Review the amounts and types of stressors in daily living
- Identify stressors that can be modified or eliminated
- Mobilize social supports to facilitate lower stress levels
- Reduce stress levels through use of health promoting behaviors and other strategies

• = Independent ▲ = Collaborative

Nursing Interventions

- Assist client in identification of stress overload during vulnerable life events.
- Listen actively to descriptions of stressors and the stress response.
- In younger adult women, assess interpersonal stressors.
- Categorize stressors as modifiable or nonmodifiable.
- Help clients modify or mitigate stressors identified as modifiable.
- Help clients distinguish among short-term, chronic, and secondary stressors.
- Provide information as needed to reduce stress responses to acute and chronic illnesses.
- ▲ Explore possible therapeutic approaches such as cognitive-behavioral therapy, biofeedback, neurofeedback, acupuncture, pharmacological agents, and complementary and alternative therapies.
- Help the client to reframe his or her perceptions of some of the stressors.
- Assist the client to mobilize social supports for dealing with recent stressors.

Pediatric

- With children, nurses should work with parents to help them to reduce children's stressors.
- Help children to manage their feelings related to self-concept.
- Help children to deal with bullies and other sources of violence in schools and neighborhoods.
- Help children to manage the complexities of chronic illnesses.

Geriatric

- Assess for chronic stress with older adults and provide a variety of stress relief techniques.
- ▲ Encourage older adults to seek appropriate counseling.

Multicultural

- Review cultural beliefs and acculturation level in relation to perceived stressors.

Home Care

- The preceding interventions may be adapted for home care use.
- Develop community-based programs for stress management as needed for groups with increased risk of stress overload (e.g., firefighters, policemen, military personnel, and nurses).
- Support and encourage neighborhood stability.

• = Independent   ▲ = Collaborative

Client/Family Teaching and Discharge Planning

* Diagnose the possibility of stress overload before teaching.
* Establish readiness for learning.
* Provide manageable amounts of information at the appropriate educational level.
* Evaluate the need for additional teaching and learning experiences.

Risk for Sudden Infant Death syndrome

NANDA-I Definition

Vulnerable to unpredicted death of an infant

Risk Factors

Modifiable

Delay in prenatal care; infant overheating; infant overwrapping; infant placed to sleep in the prone position; infants placed to sleep in the side-lying position; bed sharing; lack of prenatal care; smoke exposure; soft underlayment (loose items in the sleep environment)

Potentially Modifiable

Low birth weight; prematurity; young parental age

Nonmodifiable

Ethnicity (e.g., African American or Native American); male gender; season of the year (i.e., winter and fall); infant age of 2 to 4 months

Client Outcomes

Client Will (Specify Time Frame)

* Explain appropriate measures to prevent sudden infant death syndrome (SIDS)
* Demonstrate correct techniques for positioning and blanketing the infant, protecting the infant from harm

Nursing Interventions

* Position the infant supine to sleep during naps and at night; do not position in the prone position or side-lying position (American Academy of Pediatrics [AAP], 2014a).
* Avoid use of bedding, such as blankets and loose sheets, for sleeping. Also keep quilts, pillows, bumpers, sheepskins, and soft toys out of the infant's bed. Dress the child in one-piece sleepers or wearable blankets (AAP, 2014b).

• = Independent   ▲ = Collaborative

- Avoid overbundling, overheating, and swaddling the infant. The infant should not feel hot to touch.
- Provide the infant a certain amount of time in prone position while the infant is awake and observed. Change the direction that the baby lies in the crib from one week to the next; avoid too much time in car seats and carriers.
- Consider offering the infant a pacifier during sleep times.
▲ Use electronic respiratory or cardiac monitors to detect cardiorespiratory arrest only if ordered by the health care provider.

Home Care
- Most of the interventions and client teaching information are relevant to home care.
- Evaluate home for potential safety hazards, such as inappropriate cribs, cradles, or strollers.
- Determine where and how the child sleeps, and provide instructions on safe sleeping positions and environments as needed.

Multicultural
- Encourage pregnant American Indian mothers and native Alaskan Indian mothers to avoid drinking alcohol and to avoid wrapping infants in excessive blankets or clothing.
- Encourage Hispanic and black mothers to find alternatives to bed sharing or placing infants for sleep on adult beds, sofas, or cots, and to avoid placing pillows, soft toys, and soft bedding in the sleep environment.

Client/Family Teaching and Discharge Planning
- Teach the safety guidelines for infant care in the previous interventions.
- Recommend breastfeeding.
- Teach parents the need to obtain a crib that conforms to the safety standards of the Consumer Product Safety Commission (CPSC).
- Teach the need to stop smoking during pregnancy and to not smoke around the infant. Do not allow the infant to be exposed to any secondhand smoke.
- Teach parents, especially mothers, not to use alcohol, medications, or illicit drugs while caring for or bed sharing with an infant.
- Teach parents not to sleep in the same bed with the infant, regardless of alcohol, medications, smoking, or illicit drug use.

• = Independent   ▲ = Collaborative

- Teach parents not to place the infant on a cushion to sleep, or a sofa chair or other soft surface. Infants should sleep in a crib (AAP, 2014a).
- Recommend an alternative to sleeping with an infant of placing the infant's crib near their bed to allow for more convenient breastfeeding and parent contact.
- Recommend that parents with infants in child care make it very clear to the employees that the infant must always be placed in the supine position to sleep, not prone or in a side-lying position (AAP, 2014a).

Risk for Suffocation
NANDA-I Definition
Vulnerable to inadequate air availability for inhalation, which may compromise health
Risk Factors
External
Access to empty refrigerator/freezer; eating large mouthfuls of food; gas leak; low-strung clothesline; pacifier around infant's neck; playing with plastic bag; propped bottle placed in infant's crib; small object in airway; smoking in bed; soft underlayment (e.g., loose items placed near infant); unattended in water; unvented fuel-burning heater; vehicle running in closed garage
Internal
Alteration in cognitive functioning; alteration in olfactory function; emotional disturbance; face/neck disease; face/neck injury; impaired motor functioning; insufficient knowledge of safety precautions
Client Outcomes
Client Will (Specify Time Frame)
- Undertake appropriate measures to prevent suffocation
- Demonstrate correct techniques for emergency rescue maneuvers (e.g., Heimlich maneuver, rescue breathing, cardiopulmonary resuscitation [CPR]), and describe situations that require them

• = Independent   ▲ = Collaborative

Nursing Interventions

* Identify hospitalized clients at particular risk for suffocation, including the following:
  ○ Clients with altered levels of consciousness
  ○ Infants and young children
  ○ Clients with developmental delays
  ○ Clients with mental illness, especially schizophrenia
  ○ Clients who have been physically or chemically restrained

Pediatric

* Counsel families on the following for care of an infant:
  ○ Position infants on their back to sleep; do not position them on their side or prone.
  ○ Obtain a new crib that conforms to the safety standards of the Federal Safety Commission.
  ○ Place the infant in the crib with a properly fitted mattress, only to sleep, not on an adult bed, sofa, chair, baby seat, swing, or playpen.
  ○ Avoid use of loose bedding such as blankets and sheets for sleeping. If blankets are used, they should be tucked in around the crib mattress so the infant's face is less likely to become covered by bedding. The blanket should end at the level of the infant's chest.
* Assess for signs and symptoms of abuse such as Munchausen syndrome by proxy (MSBP).
* Conduct risk factor identification, noting special circumstances in which preventive or protective measures are indicated. Note the presence of environmental hazards, including the following: plastic bags; cribs with slats wider than 2 inches; ill-fitting crib mattresses that can allow the infant to become wedged between the mattress and crib; pillows/loose bedding in crib; placement of crib near windows with blinds or cords; co-sleeping; abandoned large appliances such as refrigerators, dishwashers, or freezers; clothing with cords or hoods that can become entangled; bibs; pacifiers on a string; necklaces in infants and children; drapery cords; pull-toy strings.
* Counsel families to evaluate household furniture for safety, including large dressers, televisions, book shelves, and appliances that may need to be anchored to the wall, to prevent the child from climbing on the furniture, and it falling forward and suffocating the child.

• = Independent   ▲ = Collaborative

- Counsel families to not serve these foods to the child younger than 4 years of age: nuts, seeds, hot dogs, popcorn, pretzels, chips, chunks of meat, hard pieces of fruit or vegetables, raisins, whole grapes, hard candies, gum, chewable vitamins, fish with bones, snacks on toothpicks, and marshmallows.
- Counsel families to keep the following items away from the sight and reach of infants and toddlers:
  - Buttons, beads, jewelry, pins, nails, marbles, coins, stones, magnets, balloons. Choose age-appropriate toys and games for children and check for any small parts that may be a choking hazard because children have the need to put everyday objects in their mouths (safekids.org.2013).
- Stress water and pool safety precautions, including vigilant, uninterrupted parental supervision.
- Underscore the necessity of not allowing children to play with or near electric garage doors and of keeping garage door openers out of the reach of young children.
- For adolescents, watch for signs of depression that could result in suicide by suffocation.

Geriatric
- Assess the status of the swallow reflex. Offer appropriate foods and beverages accordingly.
- Use care in pillow placement when positioning frail older clients who are on bed rest.
- Recognize that older adults in depression may use hanging, strangulation, and suffocation as a means of suicide (Shah & Buckley, 2011).

Home Care
- Assess the home for potential safety hazards in systems that are not likely to be fixed (e.g., faulty pilot lights or gas leaks in gas stoves, carbon monoxide release from heating systems, kerosene fumes from portable heaters).
- Assist the family in having these areas assessed and making appropriate safety arrangements (e.g., installing detectors, making repairs, home safety inspections).

Client/Family Teaching and Discharge Planning
- Recommend that families who are seeking day care or in-home care for children, geriatric family members, or at-risk family members with developmental or functional disabilities inspect the environment

• = Independent ▲ = Collaborative

for hazards and examine the first-aid preparation and vigilance of providers.
- Ensure family members learn and practice rescue techniques, including treatment of choking and lack of breathing, as well as CPR.

Risk for Suicide

NANDA-I Definition

Vulnerable to self-inflicted, life-threatening injury

Related Factors (r/t)

Behavioral

Changing a will; giving away possessions; history of suicide attempt; impulsiveness; making a will; marked change in attitude; marked change in behavior; marked change in school performance; purchase of a gun; stockpiling medication; sudden euphoric recovery from major depression

Demographic

Age (e.g., older people, young adult males, adolescents); divorced status; ethnicity (e.g., white, Native American); male gender; widowed

Physical

Chronic pain; physical illness; terminal illness

Psychological

Family history of suicide; guilt; history of childhood abuse (e.g., physical, psychological, sexual); homosexual youth; psychiatric disorder; substance abuse

Situational

Access to weapon; adolescents living in nontraditional settings (e.g., juvenile detention center, prison, halfway house, group home); economically disadvantaged; institutionalization; living alone; loss of autonomy; loss of independence; relocation; retired

Social

Cluster suicides; disciplinary problems; disrupted family life; grieving; helplessness; hopelessness; insufficient social support; legal difficulty; loneliness; loss of important relationship; social isolation

Verbal

Reports desire to die; threats of killing self

• = Independent   ▲ = Collaborative

Client Outcomes

Client Will (Specify Time Frame)

- Not harm self
- Maintain connectedness in relationships
- Disclose and discuss suicidal ideas if present; seek help
- Express decreased anxiety and control of impulses
- Talk about feelings; express anger appropriately
- Refrain from using mood-altering substances
- Obtain no access to harmful objects
- Yield access to harmful objects
- Maintain self-control without supervision

Nursing Interventions

The American Psychiatric Nurses Association (APNA, 2015) has adapted a set of essential competencies for psychiatric nurses, all of which can be useful for generalist nurses. These competencies have been incorporated below.

- Before implementing interventions in the face of suicidal behavior, nurses should examine their own emotional responses to incidents of suicide to ensure that interventions will not be based on countertransference reactions.
- Pursue an understanding of suicide as a phenomenon at all levels of nursing practice. Elements to be considered include the terminology used with suicidality and self-harm phenomena, the epidemiology of suicide, the risk and protective influences on suicide, and the evidence-based best practices in preventing and responding to suicidality (APNA, 2015).
- Assess for suicidal ideation when the history reveals the following: depression; substance abuse; bipolar disorder; schizophrenia; anxiety disorders; post-traumatic stress disorder; dissociative disorder; eating disorders; substance use disorders; antisocial or other personality disorders; attempted suicide, current or past; recent stressful life events (divorce and/or separation, relocation, problems with children); recent unemployment; recent bereavement; adult or childhood physical or sexual abuse; gay, lesbian, or bisexual gender orientation; family history of suicide; history of chronic trauma. Assess all medical clients and clients with chronic illnesses, traumatic injuries, or pain for their perception of health status and suicidal ideation.

S

• = Independent   ▲ = Collaborative

- Assess the client's ability to enter into a no-suicide contract. Contract (verbally or in writing) with the client for no self-harm if the client is appropriate for a contract; recontract at appropriate intervals.
- Be alert for warning signs of suicide: making statements such as, "I can't go on," "Nothing matters anymore," "I wish I were dead"; becoming depressed or withdrawn; behaving recklessly; getting affairs in order and giving away valued possessions; showing a marked change in behavior, attitudes, or appearance; abusing drugs or alcohol; suffering a major loss or life change.
- Take suicide notes seriously and ask if a note was left in any previous suicide attempts. Consider themes of notes in determining appropriate interventions.
- Question family members regarding the preparatory actions mentioned.
- Determine the presence and degree of suicidal risk. A number of questions will elicit the necessary information: Have you been thinking about hurting or killing yourself? How often do you have these thoughts and how long do they last? Do you have a plan? What is it? Do you have access to the means to carry out that plan? How likely is it that you could carry out the plan? Are there people or things that could prevent you from hurting yourself? What do you see in your future a year from now? Five years from now? What do you expect would happen if you died? What has kept you alive up to now?
- Observe, record, and report any changes in mood or behavior that may signify increasing suicide risk and document results of regular surveillance checks.
- Develop a positive therapeutic relationship with the clients; do not make promises that may not be kept.
- Express desire to help client. Provide education about suicide and the effectiveness of intervention. Validate the client's experience of psychological pain while maintaining a safe environment for the client.
- ▲ Refer for mental health counseling and possible hospitalization if evidence of suicidal intent exists, which may include evidence of preparatory actions (e.g., obtaining a weapon, making a plan, putting affairs in order, giving away prized possessions, preparing a suicide note).

• = Independent   ▲ = Collaborative

- Perform risk assessment for possible suicidality on admission to the hospital and thereafter during hospitalization. Alert treatment team to level of risk.
- Determine client's need for supervision and assign a hospitalized client to a room located near the nursing station.
- Search the newly hospitalized client and the client's personal belongings for weapons or potential weapons and hoarded medications during the inpatient admission procedure, as appropriate. Remove dangerous items.
- Limit access to windows and exits unless locked and shatterproof, as appropriate.
- Monitor the client during the use of potential weapons (e.g., razor, scissors).
- Increase surveillance of a hospitalized client at times when staffing is predictably low (e.g., staff meetings, change of shift report, periods of unit disruption).
- Ensure that all oncoming staff members have adequate information to assist the client, using the acronym SBARR: situation (current status, observations), background (relevant client history), assessment (including nurse's current risk assessment and relevant lab findings), recommendations (what the nurse beliefs is necessary going forward), and response feedback (verification of oncoming staff member's understanding) (APNA, 2015).
▲ If imminent suicide is suspected or an attempt has occurred, call for assistance and do not leave the client alone. Client and staff safety will be served by assistance in the response. The client may attempt additional self-harm if left alone.
- Place the client in the least restrictive, safe, and monitored environment that allows for the necessary level of observation. Assess suicidal risk at least daily and more frequently as warranted.
- Consider strategies to decrease isolation and opportunity to act on harmful thoughts (e.g., use of a sitter).
- Explain suicide precautions and relevant safety issues to the client and family (e.g., purpose, duration, behavioral expectations, and behavioral consequences).
▲ Refer for treatment and participate in the management of any psychiatric illness or symptoms that may be contributing to the client's suicidal ideation or behavior.

S

• = Independent   ▲ = Collaborative

▲ Verify that the client has taken medications as ordered (e.g., conduct mouth checks after medication administration).

▲ Maintain increased surveillance of the client whenever use of an antidepressant has been initiated or the dose increased. Antidepressant medications take anywhere from 2 to 6 weeks to achieve full efficacy.

• Involve the client in treatment planning and self-care management of psychiatric disorders.

• Explore with the client all circumstances and motivations related to the suicidality. Listen to the client's own views on his or her problems.

• Explore with the client all perceived consequences that could act as a barrier to suicide (e.g., effect on family, religious beliefs).

• Keep discussion oriented to the present and future.

• Discuss plans for dealing with suicidal ideation in the future (e.g., how to identify precipitating factors, whom to contact, where to go for help, how to respond to desire for self-harm).

• Assist the client in identifying a network of supportive persons and resources (e.g., clergy, family, care providers).

▲ Refer family members and friends to local mental health agencies and crisis intervention centers if the client has suicidal ideation or if a suspicion of suicidal thoughts exists.

▲ Document client behavior in detail to support outpatient commitment or an overnight psychiatric observation program for an actively suicidal client.

• Utilize cognitive-behavioral techniques that help the client to modify thinking styles that promote depression, hopelessness, and a belief that suicide is a valid means of escaping the current situation.

• Engage the client in group interventions that can be useful to address recurrent suicide attempts.

• With the client's consent, facilitate family-oriented crisis intervention. Family-oriented crisis intervention can clarify stresses and allow assessment of family dynamics.

• Involve the family in discharge planning (e.g., illness/medication teaching, recognition of increasing suicidal risk, client's plan for dealing with recurring suicidal thoughts, community resources).

▲ Before discharge from the hospital, ensure that the client has a supply of ordered medications, has a plan for outpatient follow-up,

• = Independent   ▲ = Collaborative

understands the plan or has a caregiver able and willing to follow the plan, and has the ability to access outpatient treatment.

▲ In the event of successful suicide, refer the family to a therapy group for survivors of suicide. Recommended clinical interventions include addressing psychological distress, normalizing denial as an effective coping strategy, working with concerns about family disintegration, and helping families deal with stigmatization.

• See the care plans for Risk for self-directed **Violence, Hopelessness,** and Risk for **Self-Mutilation.**

Pediatric

• The preceding interventions may be appropriate for pediatric clients.

• Use brief self-report measures to improve clinical management of at-risk cases.

• Recognize that the developmental issues of childhood and adolescence may heighten suicide risks and involve different issues from those with adults. Assess specific stressors for the pediatric client, including bullying.

• Assess for exposure to suicide of a significant other.

• Be alert to the presence of school victimization around lesbian, gay, bisexual, and transgender issues and be prepared to advocate for the client.

• Evaluate for the presence of self-mutilation and related risk factors. Refer to care plan for Risk for **Self-Mutilation** for additional information.

• Be aware that complete overlap does not exist between suicidal behavior and self-mutilation. The motivation may be different (ending life rather than coping with difficult feelings), and the method is usually different.

• Involve the adolescent in multimodal treatment programs.

• Before discharge from the hospital, ensure that the client's parent has a supply of ordered medications, has a plan for outpatient follow-up, has a caregiver who understands the plan or is able and willing to follow the plan, and has the ability to access outpatient treatment.

• Parental education groups can influence suicide risk factors.

• Support the implementation of school-based suicide prevention programs.

Geriatric

- Evaluate the older client's mental and physical health status and financial stressors.
- Explore with client any concerns or pressures (physical and financial) regarding ability to secure support of medical care, especially perceived pressures about being a burden on family.
- Conduct a thorough assessment of client's medications.
- When assessing suicide risk factors, incorporate a higher degree of risk for older men and for some older adults who have lost a loved one in the previous year.
- Explore triggers of and barriers to suicidal behavior, with particular attention to real and perceived losses (e.g., professional role, health).
- An older adult who shows self-destructive behaviors should be evaluated for dementia.
- ▲ Advocate for the older client with other professionals in securing treatment for suicidal states. Primary care providers have been noted to underrecognize and undertreat older adult clients with depression.
- Encourage physical activity in older adults.
- ▲ Refer older adults in primary care settings for care management.
- Consider telephone contacts as an effective intervention for suicidal older adults.

S Multicultural

- Assess for the influence of cultural beliefs, norms, and values on the client's perceptions of suicide, as well as on the nurse's perception and approach to suicide.
- Identify and acknowledge the stresses unique to culturally diverse individuals.
- Identify and acknowledge unique cultural responses to stressors in determining sensitive interventions to prevent suicide.
- Validate the individual's feelings regarding concerns about the current crisis and family functioning.

Home Care

- Communicate the degree of risk to family and caregivers; assess the family and caregiving situation for ability to protect the client and to understand the client's suicidal behavior. Provide the family and caregivers with guidelines on how to manage self-harm behaviors in the home environment.
- Assess risk factors in the home.

• = Independent   ▲ = Collaborative

- If the client's suicidal ideation intensifies, or if a suicide plan with access to means becomes evident, institute an emergency plan for mental health intervention.
- Identify the client's concerns and implement interventions to address the consequences of disability in a client with medical illness. Refer to the care plans for **Hopelessness** and **Powerlessness.**
▲ Refer for homemaker or psychiatric home health care services for respite, client reassurance, and implementation of a therapeutic regimen.
▲ If the client is on psychotropic medications, assess the client's and family's knowledge of medication administration and side effects. Teach as necessary.
▲ Evaluate the effectiveness and side effects of medications and adherence to the medication regimen. Review with the client and family all medications kept in the home; encourage discarding of old prescriptions. Monitor the amount of medications ordered/provided by the physician; limiting the amount of medications to which the client has access may be necessary.

Client/Family Teaching and Discharge Planning

- Establish a supportive relationship with family members.
- Explain all relevant symptoms, procedures, treatments, and expected outcomes for suicidal ideation that is illness based (e.g., depression, bipolar disorder).
- Teach the family how to recognize that the client is at increased risk for suicide (changes in behavior and verbal and nonverbal communication, withdrawal, depression, or sudden lifting of depression).
- Provide written instructions for treatments and procedures for which the client will be responsible.
- Instruct the client in coping strategies (assertiveness training, impulse control training, deep breathing, progressive muscle relaxation).
- Teach cognitive-behavioral activities, such as active problem solving, reframing (reappraising the situation from a different perspective), or thought stopping (in response to a negative thought, picturing a large stop sign and replacing the image with a prearranged positive alternative). Teach the client to confront his or her own negative thought patterns (or cognitive distortions), such as catastrophizing (expecting the very worst), dichotomous thinking (perceiving events

S

• = Independent ▲ = Collaborative

in only one of two opposite categories), or magnification (placing distorted emphasis on a single event).
- Provide the client and family with phone numbers of appropriate community agencies for therapy and counseling. The National Alliance on Mental Illness (NAMI) is an excellent resource for client and family support.

Delayed Surgical recovery
NANDA-I Definition

Extension of the number of postoperative days required to initiate and perform activities that maintain life, health, and well-being

Defining Characteristics

Discomfort; evidence of interrupted healing of surgical area; excessive time required for recuperation; impaired mobility; inability to resume employment; loss of appetite; postpones resumption of work; requires assistance for self-care

Related Factors (r/t)

American Society of Anesthesiologists Physical Status classification score ≥3; diabetes mellitus; edema at surgical site; extensive surgical procedure; extremes of age; history of delayed wound healing; impaired mobility; malnutrition; obesity; pain; perioperative surgical site infection; persistent nausea; persistent vomiting; pharmaceutical agent; postoperative emotional response; prolonged surgical procedure; psychological disorder in postoperative period; surgical site contamination; trauma at surgical site

Client Outcomes

Client Will (Specify Time Frame)
- Have surgical area that shows evidence of healing: no redness, induration, draining, or immobility
- State that appetite is regained
- State that no nausea is present
- Demonstrate ability to move about
- Demonstrate ability to complete self-care activities
- State that no fatigue is present
- State that pain is controlled or relieved after nursing interventions
- Resume employment activities/activities of daily living (ADLs)
- State no depression or anxiety related to surgical procedure

• = Independent   ▲ = Collaborative

Nursing Interventions

- Encourage smoking cessation prior to surgery.
- Preoperatively, perform a thorough assessment of the client, including risk factors. Allow time to be with the client, and actively listen to client's concerns and questions about care, functional status, and recovery. Assess for the presence of medical conditions and treat appropriately before surgery. If the client is diabetic, maintain normal blood glucose levels before surgery.
- Carefully assess client's use of dietary supplements such as feverfew, fish oil, ginkgo biloba, garlic, ginseng, ginger, valerian, kava, St. John's wort, ephedra (Ma huang or metabolite), and echinacea. It is recommended that all clients be advised to stop all dietary supplements at least 1 week before major surgical or diagnostic procedures.
- Play music of the client's choice preoperatively, intraoperatively, and postoperatively.
- Consider using healing touch and other mind-body-spirit interventions such as stress control, therapeutic massage, and imagery in the perianesthesia setting.
- Postoperatively, discuss with surgeon vital sign parameters, signs, and symptoms that could indicate early postoperative infection.
- Use careful aseptic technique when caring for wounds.
- Clients should be allowed to shower after surgery to maintain cleanliness if not contraindicated because of the presence of pacemaker wires.
- The client should be provided with a complete, balanced therapeutic diet after the immediately postoperative period (24 to 48 hours).
- Encourage the client to use prayer as a form of spiritual coping if this is comfortable for the client.
- Carefully assess functional status of client postoperatively using a fall-risk stratification tool such as the Morse Fall Scale to identify clients at high risk for fall.
- See the care plans for **Anxiety,** Acute **Pain, Fatigue,** Risk for deficient **Fluid** volume, Risk for **Perioperative Positioning** injury, Impaired physical **Mobility,** and **Nausea.**

Pediatric

- Encourage children to ask questions about their procedures and postoperative expectations regarding pain, function, and long-term social and emotional care needs.

• = Independent   ▲ = Collaborative

- Teach imagery and encourage distraction for children for postsurgical pain relief.

Geriatric

- Perform a thorough preoperative assessment, including cardiac, social support, and skin assessments.
- Routinely assess pain in postoperative clients using a pain scale that is appropriate for clients with impaired cognition or inability to verbalize.
- Serially evaluate the client's vital signs, including temperature. Know what is normal and abnormal for each client. Check baseline vital signs and monitor trends.
- Provide tools such as clocks, calendars, and other orientation tools to help prevent delirium in the postoperative or extended-stay client. Ensure that hearing aids and glasses are also available as needed.
- Offer spiritual support.

Home Care

- The preceding interventions may be adapted for the home setting.
- Provide supportive telephone calls from nurse to client as a means of decreasing anxiety and providing the psychosocial support necessary for recovery from surgery.

S **Client/Family Teaching and Discharge Planning**

- Provide discharge planning and teaching in language that is appropriate to the client and caregiver's education and literacy level.
- Meet with client and caregivers to create a discharge plan that includes measurable goals for functional activities of daily living and pain levels, discuss expectations for recovery, and address signs and symptoms of postoperative complications.
- Provide individualized teaching plans for the client with an ostomy. Assess client's ability to manage basic needs: (1) maintenance of a pouching seal for a consistent, predictable wear time; (2) maintenance of peristomal skin integrity; and (3) social and professional support of the client. Referrals for home wound care or nursing visits may be necessary to help client maintain hygiene and prevent readmission for complications.

• = Independent   ▲ = Collaborative

Risk for delayed Surgical recovery

NANDA-I Definition

Vulnerable to an extension of the number of postoperative days required to initiate and perform activities that maintain life, health, and well-being, which may compromise health

Risk Factors

American Society of Anesthesiologists Physical Status classification score ≥3; diabetes mellitus; edema at surgical site; extensive surgical procedure; extremes of age; history of delayed wound healing; impaired mobility; malnutrition; obesity; pain; perioperative surgical site infection; persistent nausea; persistent vomiting; pharmaceutical agent; postoperative emotional response; prolonged surgical procedure; psychological disorder in postoperative period; surgical site contamination; trauma at surgical site

Client Outcomes, Nursing Interventions, and Client/Family Teaching and Discharge Planning

See the care plan for Delayed **Surgical** recovery.

Impaired Swallowing

NANDA-I Definition

Abnormal functioning of the swallowing mechanism associated with deficits in oral, pharyngeal, or esophageal structure or function

S

Defining Characteristics

First Stage: Oral

Abnormal oral phase of swallow study; choking prior to swallowing; coughing prior to swallowing; drooling; food falls from mouth; food pushed out of mouth; gagging prior to swallowing; inability to clear oral cavity; incomplete lip closure; inefficient nippling; inefficient suck; insufficient chewing; nasal reflux; piecemeal deglutition; pooling of bolus in lateral sulci; premature entry of bolus; prolonged bolus formation; prolonged mealtime with inefficient consumption; tongue action ineffective in forming bolus

Second Stage: Pharyngeal

Abnormal pharyngeal phase of swallow study; alteration in head position; choking; coughing; delayed swallowing; fevers of unknown etiology; food refusal; gagging sensation; gurgling voice quality; inadequate laryngeal elevation; nasal reflux; recurrent pulmonary infection; repetitive swallowing

• = Independent   ▲ = Collaborative

Third Stage: Esophageal

Abnormal esophageal phase of swallow study; acidic-smelling breath; bruxism; difficulty swallowing; epigastric pain; food refusal; heartburn; hematemesis; hyperextension of head; nighttime awakening; nighttime coughing; odynophagia; regurgitation; repetitive swallowing; reports "something stuck"; unexplained irritability surrounding mealtimes; volume limiting; vomiting; vomitus on pillow

Related Factors

Congenital Defects

Behavioral feeding problem; conditions with significant hypotonia; congenital heart disease; failure to thrive; history of enteral feeding; mechanical obstruction; neuromuscular impairment; protein-energy malnutrition; respiratory condition; self-injurious behavior; upper airway abnormality

Neurological Problems

Achalasia; acquired anatomic defects; brain injury (e.g., cerebrovascular impairment, neurological illness, trauma, tumor); cerebral palsy; cranial nerve involvement; developmental delay; esophageal reflux disease; laryngeal abnormality; laryngeal defect; nasal defect; nasopharyngeal cavity defect; neurological problems; oropharynx abnormality; prematurity; tracheal defect; trauma; upper airway anomaly

Client Outcomes

Client Will (Specify Time Frame)

- Demonstrate effective swallowing without signs of aspiration (see defining characteristics above)
- Remain free from aspiration (e.g., lungs clear, temperature within normal range)

Nursing Interventions

▲ Do not feed clients with impaired swallowing orally until an appropriate diagnostic workup is completed.

▲ Ensure proper nutrition by consulting with a health care provider regarding alternative nutrition and hydration when oral nutrition is not safe/adequate.

▲ Refer to a speech-language pathologist for evaluation and diagnostic evaluation of swallowing to determine swallowing problems and solutions as soon as oral and/or pharyngeal dysphagia is suspected.

▲ Observe the following feeding guidelines:
  ○ Before giving oral feedings, determine the client's readiness to eat (e.g., alert, able to hold head erect, follow instructions, move tongue in mouth, and manage oral secretions).

• = Independent   ▲ = Collaborative

○ Monitor client during oral feedings and provide cueing as needed to ensure client follows swallowing guidelines/aspiration precautions recommended by speech-language pathologist or dysphagia specialist. NOTE: General aspiration precautions include the following: sit at 90 degrees for all oral feedings; take small bites/sips, slow rate, no straws. However, client-specific strategies will be determined via bedside and/or instrumental swallowing evaluation performed by dysphagia specialist.

○ If the client is older or has gastroesophageal reflux disease, ensure the client is kept in an upright posture for an hour after eating.

• During meals and all oral intake, observe for signs associated with swallowing problems such as coughing, choking, spitting of food, drooling, difficulty handling oral secretions, double swallowing or delay in swallowing, watering eyes, nasal discharge, wet or gurgling voice, decreased ability to move the tongue and lips, decreased mastication of food, decreased ability to move food to the back of the pharynx, slow or scanning speech.

▲ Watch for uncoordinated chewing or swallowing; coughing immediately after eating or delayed coughing; pocketing of food; wet-sounding voice; sneezing when eating; delay of more than 1 second in swallowing; or a change in respiratory patterns. If any of these signs of dysphagia and/or aspiration are present, remove all food from the oral cavity, stop feedings, and consult with speech and language pathologist and dysphagia team.

▲ If signs of aspiration or pneumonia are present, auscultate lung sounds after feeding. Note new onset of crackles or wheezing, or elevated temperature.

▲ Watch for signs of malnutrition and dehydration and keep a record of food intake.

▲ Evaluate nutritional status daily. Weigh the client weekly to help evaluate nutritional status. If the client is not adequately nourished, work with the dysphagia team to determine whether the client needs therapeutic feeding only or needs enteral feedings until the client can swallow adequately.

▲ Assist client in following dysphagia specialist's recommendations and provide open, accurate, and effective communication with dysphagia team regarding client's diet tolerance.

S

• = Independent   ▲ = Collaborative

▲ Document and notify the health care provider and dysphagia team of changes in medical, nutritional, or swallowing status.

▲ Work with the client on swallowing exercises prescribed by the dysphagia team.

▲ If needed, provide meals in a quiet environment away from excessive stimuli, such as a community dining room, for some clients who are easily distracted.

▲ For many adult clients, avoid the use of straws if recommended by the speech pathologist.

▲ Recognize that the client can aspirate oral feedings, even if there are no symptoms of coughing or distress.

▲ Ensure oral hygiene is maintained.

▲ Check the oral cavity for proper emptying after the client swallows and after the client finishes the meal. Provide oral care at the end of the meal. It may be necessary to manually remove food from the client's mouth. If this is the case, use gloves and keep the client's teeth apart with a padded tongue blade.

▲ Praise the client for successfully following directions and swallowing appropriately.

▲ Keep the client in an upright position for 45 minutes to an hour after a meal.

▲ Recognize that impaired swallowing may be caused by the medications the client is taking. Side effects of medications include xerostomia (antidepressants, anticholinergics, antihistamines, bronchodilators, antineoplastic, anti-Parkinson), central nervous system depression (anticonvulsants, benzodiazepines, antispasmodics, antidepressants, antipsychotics), myopathy (corticosteroids, lipid-lowering agents, colchicines), and decreased esophageal sphincter tone (antihistamines, diuretics, opiates, antipsychotics, antihypertensives, anticholinergics).

▲ For clients receiving mechanical ventilation with a tracheostomy tube, request a referral to speech-language pathologist or dysphagia specialist for an instrumental swallowing evaluation before beginning oral diet.

Pediatric

▲ Refer a child who has difficulty swallowing and symptoms such as difficulty manipulating food, delayed swallow response, and pocketing of a bolus of food to speech-language pathologist (or dysphagia specialist) and a dietitian.

• = Independent   ▲ = Collaborative

▲ Consult with speech-language pathologist or dysphagia specialist regarding modifications to nipple; appropriate positioning and feeding strategies; and other therapeutic activities deemed most appropriate based on bedside and instrumental swallowing evaluation.

▲ The following are general feeding guidelines. Specific strategies to eliminate aspiration and maximize intake should be individualized and determined by swallowing specialist through bedside and instrumental swallowing evaluation.

• Attempt feedings when infant is in an optimal behavioral feeding state (e.g., awake, alert, and not agitated) and halt feedings if infant is not able to maintain or regain a proper feeding state.

• In preterm infant, provide opportunities for patterned nonnutritive sucking (NNS).

• In preterm infant, alter nipple flow rate to one that is easily managed by infant to facilitate intake while achieving physiologic stability.

• Watch for indicators of aspiration and physiologic instability during feeding: coughing, a change in vocal quality or wet vocal quality, perspiration and color changes, sneezing, apnea, and/or increased heart rate and breathing. Infants and children with silent aspiration may only have indicators of increased respiratory mucous, congestion and chronic wheeze or rhonchi, recurrent bronchitis, or recurrent pneumonia (Tutor & Gosa, 2012).

• Watch for warning signs of reflux: sour-smelling breath after eating, sneezing, lack of interest in feeding, crying and fussing extraordinarily when feeding, pained expressions when feeding, and excessive chewing and swallowing after eating.

• Observe infant's behavior and cues and adjust feeding to promote a safe, pleasurable feeding experience while eliminating aspiration and maximizing intake.

Geriatric

▲ Recognize that age-related changes can impact swallowing and these changes have a more pronounced effect when superimposed on disease such as neurological and other chronic medical problems.

▲ Evaluate medications the client is presently taking and consult with the pharmacist for assistance in monitoring for incorrect doses and drug interactions that could result in dysphagia.

• = Independent   ▲ = Collaborative

▲ Ensure all nursing home residents are screened for swallowing problems.

▲ Encourage and provide good oral hygiene when indicated.

▲ Consult with occupational therapist for adaptive equipment when appropriate.

▲ Recognize that the older client with dementia may need a longer time to eat and is often easily distracted. Help optimize hydration and nutrition using the following techniques:

○ Encourage six small meals and hydration breaks per day.

○ Offer foods that are sweet, spicy, or sour to increase sensory input.

○ Allow clients to touch food and self-feed, if necessary (Tanner, 2013).

○ Eliminate from the tray or table nonfoods such as salt and pepper, or anything that can be distracting.

○ Keep desserts out of sight until the end of the meal.

○ Offer finger foods to the client who has trouble holding still to eat.

○ Allow clients to eat immediately when they come for the meal.

○ Recognize that the client with advanced dementia, who is unable to swallow, may or may not benefit from enteral tube feedings.

S

Home Care

▲ Refer to speech therapy. Speech-language pathologists can work with clients to enhance swallowing ability and teach compensatory strategies.

Client/Family Teaching and Discharge Planning

▲ Teach the client and family exercises prescribed by the dysphagia team.

▲ Teach the client a systematic method of swallowing effectively as prescribed by the dysphagia team.

• Educate the client, family, and all caregivers about rationales for food consistency and choices.

• Teach the family how to monitor the client to prevent and detect aspiration during eating.

• = Independent   ▲ = Collaborative

Risk for imbalanced body Temperature

NANDA-I Definition

Vulnerable to failure to maintain body temperature within normal parameters, which may compromise health

Risk Factors

Acute brain injury; alteration in metabolic rate; condition affecting temperature regulation; decreased sweat response; dehydration; extremes of age; extremes of environmental temperature; extremes of weight; inactivity; inappropriate clothing for environmental temperature; increase in oxygen demand; increased body surface area to weight ratio; insufficient nonshivering thermogenesis; insufficient supply of subcutaneous fat; pharmaceutical agent; sedation; sepsis; vigorous activity

Client Outcomes, Nursing Interventions, and Client/Family Teaching and Discharge Planning

Refer to care plans for Ineffective **Thermoregulation** (fever), **Hyperthermia,** or **Hypothermia.**

Risk for Thermal injury

NANDA-I Definition

Vulnerable to extreme temperature damage to skin and mucous membranes, which may compromise health

Risk Factors

Alteration in cognitive functioning; extremes of age; extremes of environmental temperature; fatigue; inadequate protective clothing (e.g., flame-retardant sleepwear, gloves, ear covering); inadequate supervision; inattentiveness; insufficient knowledge of safety precautions (client, caregiver); intoxication (alcohol, drug); neuromuscular impairment; neuropathy; smoking; treatment regimen; unsafe environment

Client Outcomes

Client Will (Specify Time Frame)

- Be free of thermal injury to skin or tissue
- Explain actions he or she can take to protect self and family from thermal injury
- Explain actions he or she can take to protect self and others in the work environment

• = Independent   ▲ = Collaborative

Nursing Interventions

- Teach the following interventions to prevent fires in the home, to handle any possible fire, and to have a readily available exit from the home:
  - ○ Avoid plugging several appliance cords into the same electrical socket.
  - ○ Do not use open candles or allow smoking in the home.
  - ○ Keep a fire extinguisher within reach in case a fire should occur.
  - ○ Install smoke alarms on every level of the home and in every sleeping area.
  - ○ Keep furniture and other heavy objects out of the way of doors and windows.
  - ○ Develop a fire escape plan that includes two ways out of every room and an outside meeting place. Practice the escape plan at least twice a year.
- Teach the following activities to those living in homes with small children:
  - ○ Lock up matches and lighters out of sight and reach.
  - ○ Do not leave a hot stove unattended.
  - ○ Do not allow small children to use the microwave until they are at least 7 or 8 years of age.
  - ○ Keep all portable heaters out of children's reach and at least 3 feet away from anything that can burn.
  - ○ Install thermostatic mixer valves in hot water system to prevent extreme hot water that can cause scalding burns.
- Apply sunscreen as directed on the container when out in the sun. Use sun-blocking clothing, and stay in the shade if possible.
- Teach the following to prevent fires in the home where medical oxygen is in use:
  - ○ Never smoke in a home where medical oxygen is in use. "No smoking" signs should be posted inside and outside the home.
  - ○ All ignition sources (e.g., matches, lighters, candles, gas stoves, appliances, electric razors, and hair dryers) should be kept at least 10 feet away from the point where the oxygen comes out.
  - ○ Do not wear oxygen equipment while cooking. Oils, grease, and petroleum products can spontaneously ignite when exposed to high levels of oxygen. Also, do not use oil-based lotions, lip balm, or aerosol sprays.

• = Independent   ▲ = Collaborative

- ○ Homes with medical oxygen must have working smoke alarms that are tested monthly.
- ○ Keep a fire extinguisher within reach. If a fire occurs, turn off the oxygen and leave the home.
- ○ Develop a fire escape plan that includes two ways out of every room and an outside meeting place. Practice the escape plan at least twice a year.
- Be aware that thermal injury also includes injury from cold materials and environmental conditions, including freezing injury, nonfreezing injury, and hypothermia (Kiss, 2012).
- Provide adequate environmental temperatures. Older clients and others at risk for temperature dysregulation can easily become hypothermic in air-conditioned environments (e.g., a surgical suite) or with inadequate clothing (e.g., patient gowns).
  - ○ Monitor temperature in vulnerable clients. Core temperature is the best measure to assess for hypothermia. If a pulmonary artery catheter is not available, use a thermometer calibrated for lower body temperature (Moola & Lockwood, 2011).
  - ○ Use active warming measures to help clients maintain body temperature (e.g., warming blankets, warm intravenous fluids, forced warm-air warming devices, foil wraps, and radiant warmers) as indicated.
- Ensure that exposed skin is protected from cold with adequate clothing.
- Monitor for development of cold thermal injury by checking peripheral circulation, temperature, sensation, and fine motor coordination, which decreases as a very early sign of hypothermia.
- Check the temperature of all equipment and other materials before allowing them to contact client skin especially if client has increased risk factors for thermal injury.

Ineffective Thermoregulation
NANDA-I Definition

Temperature fluctuation between hypothermia and hyperthermia
Defining Characteristics

Cyanotic nail beds; fluctuations in body temperature above and below the normal range; flushed skin; hypertension; increase in body temperature above normal range; increase in respiratory rate; mild shivering; moderate

• = Independent   ▲ = Collaborative

pallor; piloerection; reduction in body temperature below normal range; seizures; skin cool to touch; skin warm to touch; slow capillary refill; tachycardia

Related Factors (r/t)

Extremes of age; fluctuating environmental temperature; illness; trauma

Client Outcomes

Client Will (Specify Time Frame)

• Maintain temperature within normal range
• Explain measures needed to maintain normal temperature
• Describe two to four symptoms of hypothermia or hyperthermia
• List two or three self-care measures to treat hypothermia or hyperthermia

Nursing Interventions

Temperature Measurement

• Measure and record the client's temperature using a consistent method of temperature measurement every 1 to 4 hours depending on severity of the situation or whenever a change in condition occurs (e.g., chills, change in mental status).
• Select core, near core, or peripheral temperature monitoring mode based on ability to obtain an accurate temperature from that site and clinical situation dictating the need for mode of temperature monitoring required for clinical treatment decisions.
• Caution should be taken in interpreting extreme values of temperature (less than 35°C or greater than 39°C) from a near core temperature site device.
• Evaluate the significance of a decreased or increased temperature.
▲ Notify the health care provider of temperature according to institutional standards or written orders, or when temperature reaches 100.5°F (38.3°C) and above (Saltzberg 2013; O'Grady et al, 2008). Also notify the health care provider of the presence of a change in mental status and temperature greater than 38.3°C or less than 36°C.

Fever (Pyrexia)

• Recognize that fever is characterized as a temporary elevation in internal body temperature 1°C to 2°C higher than the client's normal body temperature.
• Recognize that fever is a normal physiological response to a perceived threat by the body, frequently in response to an infection.

• = Independent   ▲ = Collaborative

▲ Review client history to include current medical diagnosis, medications, recent procedures/interventions, and review of laboratory analysis for cause of ineffective thermoregulation.

• Recognize that fever may be low grade (36°C to 38°C) in response to an inflammatory process such as infection, allergy, trauma, illness, or surgery. Moderate to high-grade fever (38°C to 40°C) indicates a more concerted inflammatory response from a systemic infection. Hyperpyrexia (40°C and higher) occurs as a result of damage of the hypothalamus, bacteremia, or an extremely overheated room (Scrase & Tranter, 2011; Kenny et al, 2014).

• Recognize that fever has a predictable physiological pattern.

• Monitor and intervene to provide comfort during a fever by:
  ○ Obtaining vital signs and accurate intake and output
  ○ Checking laboratory analysis trends of white blood cell counts and other markers of infection
  ○ Providing blankets when the client complains of being cold, but removing surplus of blankets when the client is too warm
  ○ Encouraging fluid and nutritional intake
  ○ Limiting activity to conserve energy
  ○ Providing frequent oral care (Scrase et al, 2011)

Hypothermia

• Take vital signs frequently, noting changes associated with hypothermia: increased blood pressure, pulse, and respirations that then advance to decreased values as hypothermia progresses.

• Monitor the client for signs of hypothermia (e.g., shivering, cool skin, piloerection, pallor, slow capillary refill, cyanotic nailbeds, decreased mentation, dysrhythmias) (Pitoni et al, 2011).

• See the care plan for **Hypothermia** as appropriate.

Hyperthermia

• Note changes in vital signs associated with hyperthermia: rapid, bounding pulse; increased respiratory rate; and decreased blood pressure, accompanied by orthostatic hypotension, and signs and symptoms of dehydration (Dinarello et al, 2011).

• Monitor the client for signs of hyperthermia (e.g., headache, nausea and vomiting, weakness, extreme fatigue, delirium, and coma). Adjust clothing to facilitate passive warming or cooling as appropriate.

• See the care plan for **Hyperthermia** as appropriate.

T

• = Independent   ▲ = Collaborative

Pediatric

- For routine measurement of temperature, use an electronic thermometer in the axilla in infants younger than 4 weeks; for a child up to 5 years of age, use an electronic thermometer in the axilla or an infrared temporal artery thermometer.
- Recognize that pediatric clients have a decreased ability to adapt to temperature extremes. Take the following actions to maintain body temperature in the infant/child:
  - ○ Keep the head covered.
  - ○ Use blankets to keep the client warm.
  - ○ Keep the client covered during procedures, transport, and diagnostic testing.
  - ○ Keep the room temperature at 72° F (22.2° C).
- Recognize that the infant and small child are both vulnerable to develop heat stroke in hot weather; ensure that they receive sufficient fluids and are protected from hot environments.
- Antipyretic treatments typically are not indicated unless the child's temperature is higher than 38.3° C and may be given to provide comfort.

Geriatric

- Do not allow an older client to become chilled. Keep the client covered when giving a bath and offer socks to wear in bed. Be aware of factors such as room temperature (heating/air conditioning), clothing (layered/loose), and fluid intake.
- Recognize that the older client may have an infection without a significant rise in body temperature.
- Fever does not put the older adult at risk for long-term complications; thus, fever should not be treated with antipyretic agents or other external methods of cooling, unless there is serious heart disease present.
- Ensure that older clients receive sufficient fluids during hot days and that they stay out of the sun.
- Assess the medication profile for the potential risk of drug-related altered body temperature.

Home Care

Treating Fever

- Instruct client/parents on the physiological benefits of fever and provide interventions to treat fever symptoms, avoiding antipyretic agents and external cooling interventions.

• = Independent   ▲ = Collaborative

- Ensure that client/parents know when to contact a health care provider for fever-related concerns.

Prevention of Hypothermia in Cold Weather

See the care plan for **Hypothermia.**

Prevention of Hyperthermia in Hot Weather

See the care plan for **Hyperthermia.**

Client/Family Teaching and Discharge Planning

- Teach the client and family the signs of fever, hypothermia, and hyperthermia and appropriate actions to take if either condition develops.
- Teach the client and family an age-appropriate method for taking the temperature.
- Teach the client to avoid alcohol and medications that depress cerebral function.

Impaired Tissue integrity

NANDA-I Definition

Damage to the mucous membrane, cornea, integumentary system, muscular fascia, muscle, tendon, bone, cartilage, joint capsule, and/or ligament

Defining Characteristics

Damaged tissue; destroyed tissue

Related Factors

Alteration in metabolism; alteration in sensation; chemical injury agent (e.g., burn, capsaicin, methylene chloride, mustard agent); excess fluid volume; extremes of age; extremes of environmental temperature; high-voltage power supply; humidity; imbalanced nutritional state (e.g., obesity, malnutrition); impaired circulation; impaired mobility; insufficient fluid volume; insufficient knowledge about maintaining tissue integrity; insufficient knowledge about protecting tissue integrity; mechanical factor; peripheral neuropathy; pharmaceutical agent; radiation; surgical procedure

Client Outcomes

Client Will (Specify Time Frame)

- Report any altered sensation or pain at site of tissue impairment
- Demonstrate understanding of plan to heal tissue and prevent reinjury
- Describe measures to protect and heal the tissue, including wound care
- Experience a wound that decreases in size and has increased granulation tissue

• = Independent ▲ = Collaborative

Nursing Interventions

- Assess the site of impaired tissue integrity and determine the cause and type of wound (e.g., acute or chronic wound, burn, dermatological lesion, pressure ulcer, leg ulcer, skin failure).
- Determine the size (length, width) and depth of the wound (e.g., full-thickness wound, deep tissue injury, stage III or IV pressure ulcer).
- ▲ Classify pressure ulcers using national guidelines and definitions (http://www.npuap.org/resources/educational-and-clinical-resources/npuap-pressure-ulcer-stagescategories)
  - ○ **Pressure Ulcer:** localized injury to the skin and/or underlying tissue usually over a bony prominence, as a result of pressure or pressure in combination with shear (NOTE: friction is not included in the definition) (National Pressure Ulcer Advisory Panel [NPUAP] and European Pressure Ulcer Advisory Panel [EPUAP], 2014).
  - ○ **Category/Stage III:** Full-thickness tissue loss. Subcutaneous fat may be visible, but bone, tendon, or muscle is not exposed. Slough may be present but does not obscure the depth of tissue loss. May include undermining and tunneling. The depth of a category/stage III pressure ulcer varies by anatomical location. The bridge of the nose, ear, occiput, and malleolus do not have (adipose) subcutaneous tissue and can be shallow. In contrast, areas of significant adiposity can develop extremely deep category/stage III pressure ulcers. Bone/tendon is not visible or directly palpable.
  - ○ **Category/Stage IV:** Full-thickness tissue loss with exposed bone, tendon, or muscle. Slough or eschar may be present on some parts of the wound bed. Often includes undermining and tunneling. The depth of a category/stage IV pressure ulcer varies by anatomical location. The bridge of the nose, ear, occiput, and malleolus do not have (adipose) subcutaneous tissue and can be shallow. Category IV ulcers can extend into muscle and/or supporting structures (e.g., fascia, tendon, or joint capsule), making osteomyelitis possible. Exposed bone/tendon is visible or directly palpable.
  - ○ **Suspected Deep Tissue Injury:** Purple or maroon localized area of discolored intact skin or blood-filled blister due to damage of underlying soft tissue from pressure and/or shear. The area may

be preceded by tissue that is painful, firm, mushy, boggy, warmer
or cooler as compared to adjacent tissue. Suspected deep tissue
injury may be difficult to detect in individuals with dark skin
tones. Evolution may include a thin blister over a dark wound
bed. The wound may further evolve and become covered by thin
eschar. Evolution may be rapid, exposing additional layers of
tissue even with optimal treatment.

○ **Unstageable (Depth Unknown):** Full-thickness tissue loss in
which the base of the ulcer is covered by slough (yellow, tan, gray,
green, or brown) and/or eschar (tan, brown, or black) in the
wound bed. Until enough slough and/or eschar are removed to
expose the base of the wound, the true depth and, therefore,
category/stage cannot be determined. Stable (dry, adherent, intact
without erythema or fluctuance) eschar on the heels serves as a
natural cover and should not be removed.

- Inspect and monitor the site of impaired tissue integrity at least once
daily for color changes, redness, swelling, warmth, pain, and other
signs of infection or per facility/agency policy. Determine whether
the client is experiencing changes in sensation or pain. Pay special
attention to all high-risk areas such as bony prominences, skin folds,
sacrum, and heels.

- Monitor the status of the skin around the wound. Monitor the
client's skin care practices, noting type of soap or other cleansing
agents used, temperature of water, and frequency of skin cleansing.

- Monitor the client's continence status and minimize exposure of the
skin impairment site and other areas to moisture from urine or stool,
perspiration, or wound drainage.

- Monitor for correct placement of tubes, catheters, and other devices.
Assess the skin and tissue affected by the pressure of the devices and
tape used to secures these devices. A medical device–related pressure
ulcer is defined as a localized injury to the skin or underlying tissue
as a result of sustained pressure from a medical device, and the skin/
tissue injury will often have the same configuration as the device
(NPUAP/EPUAP, 2014; Black et al, 2010).

- Assess frequently for correct placement of foot boards, restraints,
traction, casts, or other devices, and assess skin and tissue integrity.
Frequently assess for signs and symptoms of compartment syndrome
(refer to the care plan for Risk for **Peripheral Neurovascular**
dysfunction).

T

• = Independent   ▲ = Collaborative

- Implement and communicate a comprehensive treatment plan for the topical treatment of the skin impairment site.
▲ Identify a plan for debridement if necrotic tissue (eschar or slough) is present and if consistent with overall client management goals (i.e., curative vs. palliative care).
- Select a topical treatment that maintains a moist, wound-healing environment and also allows absorption of exudate and filling of dead space.
- Avoid positioning the client on the site of impaired tissue integrity. Evaluate for the use of support surfaces (specialty mattresses, beds) chair cushion, or devices as appropriate (Brienza et al, 2012; Lippoldt et al, 2014).
- If the goal of care is to keep the client comfortable (e.g., for a terminally ill client), repositioning may not be appropriate.
▲ Assess the client's nutritional status. Refer for a nutritional consult and/or institute dietary supplements as necessary.
▲ Develop a comprehensive plan of care that includes a thorough wound assessment, treatment interventions, support surfaces, nutritional products, adjunctive therapies, and evaluation of the outcome of care.

Home Care
- Some of the interventions previously described may be adapted for home care use.
▲ Assess the client's current phase of wound healing (inflammation, proliferation, maturation) and stage of injury; initiate appropriate wound management.
- Instruct and assist the client and caregivers in understanding how to change dressings and in the importance of maintaining a clean environment. Provide written instructions and observe them completing the dressing change.
▲ Initiate a consultation in a case assignment with a wound specialist or wound, ostomy, and continence nurse to establish a comprehensive plan as soon as possible. Plan case conferencing to promote optimal wound care.
▲ Consult with other health care disciplines to provide a thorough, comprehensive assessment.

Client/Family Teaching and Discharge Planning
- Teach skin and wound assessment and ways to monitor for signs and symptoms of infection, complications, and healing.

• = Independent   ▲ = Collaborative

- Teach the client why a topical treatment has been selected. Explain wound bed changes that the caregiver can expect to see. Instruct on when the dressing needs to be changed.
▲ Teach the use of pillows, foam wedges, and pressure-reducing devices to prevent pressure injury. The use of effective pressure-reducing seat cushions for older wheelchair users significantly prevented sitting-acquired pressure ulcers (Brienza et al, 2012).

Risk for Impaired Tissue integrity
NANDA-I Definition

Vulnerable to damage to the mucous membrane, cornea, integumentary system, muscular fascia, muscle, tendon, bone, cartilage, joint capsule, and/or ligament, which may compromise health

Risk Factors

Alteration in metabolism; alteration in sensation; chemical injury agent (e.g., burn, capsaicin, methylene chloride, mustard agent); excessive fluid volume; extremes of age; extremes of environmental temperature; high-voltage power supply; humidity; imbalanced nutritional state (e.g., obesity, malnutrition); impaired circulation; impaired mobility; insufficient fluid volume; insufficient knowledge about maintaining tissue integrity; insufficient knowledge about protecting tissue integrity; mechanical factor; peripheral neuropathy; pharmaceutical agent; radiation therapy; surgical procedure

Client Outcomes, Nursing Interventions, and Client/Family Teaching and Discharge Planning

Refer to care plan for Impaired **Tissue** integrity.

Ineffective peripheral Tissue Perfusion
NANDA-I Definition

Decrease in blood circulation to the periphery, which may compromise health

Defining Characteristics

Absence of peripheral pulses; alteration in motor function; altered skin characteristics (e.g., color, elasticity, hair, moisture, nails, sensation, temperature); ankle-brachial index (ABI) <0.90; capillary refill time >3 seconds; color does not return to lowered limb after 1 minute of leg

• = Independent   ▲ = Collaborative

elevation; decrease in blood pressure in extremities; decrease in pain-free distances achieved in the 6-minute walk test; decrease in peripheral pulses; delay in peripheral wound healing; distance in the 6-minute walk test below normal range (400 m to 700 m in adults); edema; extremity pain; femoral bruit; intermittent claudication; paresthesia; skin color pales with limb elevation

Related Factors

Diabetes mellitus; hypertension; insufficient knowledge of aggravating factors (e.g., smoking, sedentary lifestyle, trauma, obesity, salt intake, immobility); insufficient knowledge of disease process; sedentary lifestyle; smoking

Client Outcomes

Client Will (Specify Time Frame)

- Demonstrate adequate tissue perfusion as evidenced by palpable peripheral pulses, warm and dry skin, adequate urine output, and absence of respiratory distress
- Verbalize knowledge of treatment regimen, including appropriate exercise and medications and their actions and possible side effects
- Identify changes in lifestyle needed to increase tissue perfusion

Nursing Interventions

▲ Check the brachial, radial, dorsalis pedis, posterior tibial, and popliteal pulses bilaterally. If unable to find them, use a Doppler stethoscope and notify the health care provider immediately if new onset of absence of pulses along with a cold extremity.
- Note skin color and feel the temperature of the skin.
- Assess for pain in the extremities, noting severity, quality, timing, and exacerbating and alleviating factors. Differentiate venous from arterial disease.
- Check capillary refill.
- Note skin texture and the presence of hair, ulcers, or gangrenous areas on the legs or feet.
- Note the presence of edema in the extremities and rate severity on a four-point scale. Measure the circumference of the ankle and calf at the same time each day in the early morning (White, 2011).

Arterial Insufficiency

▲ Monitor peripheral pulses. If there is new onset of loss of pulses with bluish, purple, or black areas and extreme pain, notify the health care provider immediately.
▲ Measure ABI via Doppler imaging.

• = Independent   ▲ = Collaborative

- Avoid elevating the legs above the level of the heart. With arterial insufficiency, leg elevation decreases arterial blood supply to the legs.
▲ For early arterial insufficiency, encourage exercise such as walking or riding an exercise bicycle for 30 to 60 minutes per day as ordered by the health care provider.
- Keep the client warm and have the client wear socks and shoes or sheepskin-lined slippers when mobile. Do not apply heat. Clients with arterial insufficiency report being constantly cold; keep extremities warm to maintain vasodilation and blood supply. Heat application can easily damage ischemic tissues.
▲ Pay meticulous attention to foot care. Refer to a podiatrist if the client has a foot or nail abnormality. Ischemic feet are vulnerable to injury; meticulous foot care can prevent further injury.
- If the client has ischemic arterial ulcers, refer to the care plan for Impaired **Tissue** integrity.
▲ If the client smokes, aggressively counsel the client to stop smoking and refer to the health care provider for medications to support nicotine withdrawal and a smoking withdrawal program.

Venous Insufficiency

▲ Elevate edematous legs as ordered and ensure no pressure under the knees and heels to prevent pressure ulcers.
▲ Apply graduated compression stockings as ordered. Ensure proper fit by measuring accurately. Remove the stockings at least twice a day, in the morning with the bath and in the evening, to assess the condition of the extremity, then reapply. Knee length is preferred rather than thigh length.
- Encourage the client to walk with compression stockings on and perform toe-up and point-flex exercises.
- If the client is overweight, encourage weight loss to decrease venous disease.
- If the client has venous leg ulcers, encourage the client to avoid prolonged sitting, standing, and elevation of the involved leg. Encourage proper use of compression stockings. Pain may prevent compliance.
- Discuss lifestyle with the client to determine if the client's occupation requires prolonged standing or sitting, which can result in chronic venous disease (Longo et al, 2011).

• = Independent   ▲ = Collaborative

▲ If the client is mostly immobile, consult with the health care provider regarding use of a calf-high pneumatic compression device for prevention of DVT.

• Observe for signs of DVT, including pain, tenderness, swelling in the calf and thigh, and redness in the involved extremity. Take serial leg measurements of the thigh and calf circumferences. In some clients a tender venous cord can be felt in the popliteal fossa. Do not rely on Homan's sign.

▲ Note the results of a D-dimer test and ultrasounds.

• If DVT is present, observe for symptoms of a pulmonary embolism, including dyspnea, pleuritic chest pain, cough, and sometimes hemoptysis, especially with a history of trauma (Weitz, 2011).

▲ If the client develops DVT, after treatment and hospital discharge, recommend client wear below-the-knee elastic compression stockings during the day on the involved extremity.

Geriatric

• Complete a thorough lower extremity assessment. Document the smallest change from previous assessment, and implement a plan immediately.

• Change the client's position slowly when getting the client out of bed because of possible syncope.

• Recognize that older adults have an increased risk for development of pulmonary embolism; if pulmonary embolism is present, the symptoms are nonspecific and often mimic those of heart failure or pneumonia (Weitz, 2011).

Home Care

• The interventions previously described may be adapted for home care use.

• If arterial disease is present and the client smokes, aggressively encourage smoking cessation.

• Examine the feet carefully at frequent intervals for changes and new ulcerations.

▲ Assess the client's nutritional status, paying special attention to obesity, hyperlipidemia, and malnutrition. Refer to a dietitian if appropriate.

• Monitor for development of gangrene, venous ulceration, and symptoms of cellulitis (redness, pain, and increased swelling in an extremity).

• = Independent   ▲ = Collaborative

Client/Family Teaching and Discharge Planning

- Explain the importance of good foot care. Teach the client and family to wash and inspect the feet daily. Recommend that the diabetic client wear comfortable shoes and break them in slowly, watching for blisters.
- ▲ Teach the diabetic client that he or she should have a comprehensive foot examination at least annually (which includes an analysis for predicting foot ulceration risk), also including assessment of sensation using the Semmes-Weinstein monofilaments. If good sensation is not present, refer to a footwear professional for fitting of therapeutic shoes and inserts, the cost of which is covered by Medicare.
- For arterial disease, stress the importance of not smoking, following a weight loss program (if the client is obese), carefully controlling a diabetic condition, controlling hyperlipidemia and hypertension, maintaining intake of antiplatelet therapy, and reducing stress.
- Teach the client to avoid exposure to cold; limit exposure to brief periods if going out in cold weather and wear warm clothing.
- For venous disease, teach the importance of wearing compression stockings as ordered, elevating the legs at intervals, and watching for skin breakdown on the legs.
- Teach the client to recognize the signs and symptoms that should be reported to a health care provider (e.g., change in skin temperature, color, or sensation or the presence of a new lesion on the foot).
- Provide clear, simple instructions about plan of care.
- Instruct and provide emotional support for client undergoing hyperoxygenation treatment.

T

Risk for ineffective peripheral Tissue Perfusion

NANDA-I Definition

Vulnerable to a decrease in blood circulation to the periphery, which may compromise health

Risk Factors

Diabetes mellitus; endovascular procedure; excessive sodium intake; hypertension; insufficient knowledge of aggravating factors (e.g., smoking, sedentary lifestyle, trauma, obesity, salt intake, immobility); insufficient

• = Independent   ▲ = Collaborative

knowledge of disease process; insufficient knowledge of risk factors; sedentary lifestyle; smoking; trauma

Client Outcomes, Nursing Interventions, and Client/Family Teaching and Discharge Planning

Refer to care plan for Ineffective peripheral **Tissue Perfusion.**

Impaired Transfer ability

NANDA-I Definition

Limitation of independent movement between two nearby surfaces

Defining Characteristics

Impaired ability to transfer between bed and chair; impaired ability to transfer between bed and standing position; impaired ability to transfer between car and chair; impaired ability to transfer between chair and floor; impaired ability to transfer between chair and standing position; impaired ability to transfer between floor and standing position; impaired ability to transfer between uneven levels; impaired ability to transfer in or out of bath tub; impaired ability to transfer in or out of shower; impaired ability to transfer on or off a commode; impaired ability to transfer on or off a toilet

Related Factors (r/t)

Alteration in cognitive functioning; environmental barrier (e.g., bed height, inadequate space, wheelchair type, treatment equipment, restraints); impaired balance; impaired vision; insufficient knowledge of transfer techniques; insufficient muscle strength; musculoskeletal impairment; neuromuscular impairment; obesity; pain; physical deconditioning

NOTE: Specify level of independence using a standardized functional scale.

Client Outcomes

Client Will (Specify Time Frame)

- Transfer from bed to chair and back successfully
- Transfer from chair to chair successfully
- Transfer from wheelchair to toilet and back successfully
- Transfer from wheelchair to car and back successfully

Nursing Interventions

▲ Request consult for a physical and/or occupational therapist (PT and OT) to develop exercise and strengthening program early in the client's recovery.

• = Independent   ▲ = Collaborative

▲ Obtain a consult for a PT, OT, or orthotist to evaluate and fit clients with proper orthoses, braces, collars, and walking aids before helping them stand.

• Help client put on/take off collars, braces, prostheses in bed, as well as antiembolism stockings and abdominal binders. Applying antiembolism stockings while the client is in bed may reduce the risk of the client developing a deep vein thrombosis (DVT).

• Assess client's dependence, weight, strength, balance, tolerance to position change, cooperation, fatigue level, and cognition plus available equipment and staff ratio/experience to decide whether to do a manual or device-assisted transfer (Nelson et al, 2008; Cohen et al, 2010).

▲ Collaborate with PT and OT to use algorithms to identify technological aids to handle and transfer dependent and obese clients; do not use under-axilla method (Cohen et al, 2010).

• Implement and document type of transfer (e.g., slide board, pivot), weight-bearing status (non–weight-bearing, partial), equipment (walker, sling lift), and level of assistance (standby, moderate) on care plan, white board in room, and/or electronic medical record.

• Apply a gait belt with handles before transferring clients with partial weight-bearing abilities; keep the belt and client close to provider during the transfer.

• Help clients with wearing shoes with nonskid soles and socks/hose.

• Remove or swivel wheelchair armrests, leg rests, and footplates to the side, especially with squat or slide board transfers.

• Adjust transfer surfaces so they are similar in height. For example, lower a hospital bed to about an inch higher than commode height.

• Place wheelchair and commode at a slight angle toward the surface onto which client will transfer.

• Teach client to consistently lock brakes on wheelchair/commode/ shower chair before transferring.

• Give clear, simple instructions, allow client time to process information, and let him/her do as much of the transfer as possible.

▲ Remind clients to comply with weight-bearing restrictions ordered by their health care provider.

• Place client in set position before standing him or her—for example, sitting on edge of surface with bilateral weight bearing on buttocks and hips, with knees flexed, balls of feet aligned under knees, and head in midline.

• = Independent ▲ = Collaborative

- Support and stabilize client's weak knees by placing one or both of your knees next to or encircling client's knees, rather than blocking them.
  - Squat transfer: client leans well forward, slightly raises flexed hips off the surface, pivots, and sits down on new surface.
  - Standing pivot transfer: client leans forward with hips flexed and pushes up with hands from seat surface (or arms of chair), then stands erect, pivots, and sits down on new surface.
  - Slide board transfer: client should have on pants or have a pillowcase over the board. Remove arm and leg rest from wheelchair on one side, then slightly angle chair toward new surface. Help client lean sideways, thus shifting his/her weight so transfer board can be placed well under the upper thigh of the leg next to new surface. Make sure board is safely angled across both surfaces. Help client to sit upright and place one hand on board and the other hand on surface. Remind and help client perform a series of push-ups with arms while leaning slightly forward and lifting (not sliding) hips in small increments across board with each push-up.
- Position walking aids appropriately so a standing client can grasp and use them once he/she is upright.
- Reinforce to clients who use walkers to place one hand on walker and push with opposite hand against chair arm or surface from which they are arising to stand up.
- Use ceiling-mounted or bedside mechanical bariatric lifts to transfer dependent bariatric (extremely obese) clients.
- Use bariatric devices and use available safe client handling equipment for lifting, transferring, positioning, and sliding client (Cohen et al, 2010).
- Place a mechanical lift sling in the wheelchair preventively. Place two transfer sheets or a slide board under bariatric client. Reinforce so that head is leaning forward and knees are level with hips; help hold wheelchair in place as therapist directs/helps client with a scoot transfer.
- Perform initial and subsequent fall risk assessment.
▲ Collaborate with PT, OT, and pharmacist for individualized preventive/postfall plans, for example, scheduled toileting, balance and strength training, removal of hazards, chair alarms, call system/phone in reach, and review of medications.

• = Independent   ▲ = Collaborative

- Encourage an exercise component such as tai chi, physical therapy, or other exercise for balance, gait, and strength training in group programs or at home.
- Modify environment for safety; recommend vision assessment and consideration for cataract removal.
- Recommend polypharmacy assessment with special consideration to sedatives, antidepressants, and drugs affecting the central nervous system; recommend evaluation for orthostatic hypotension and irregular heartbeats; and recommend vitamin D supplementation of 800 IU per day (Barclay, 2011).

Home Care

▲ Obtain referral for OT and PT to teach home exercises and balance as well as fall prevention and recovery. They also evaluate for potential modifications such as an entry ramp, elevated toilet seat/toilevator (raised base under toilet), tub seat or shower chair, need for shower stall with built-in seat or wheel-in shower stall without a curb/threshold, handheld flexible shower head, lever-type facets, pull-out drawers with loop handles versus cupboards, standing lift, and so on.

- Assess for adequate lighting and hazards such as throw/area rugs, clutter, cords, and unfitted bedspreads. Suggest safe floor surfaces, such as use of adhesive nonslip strips in tubs/thresholds/areas where floor height changes; removal of wax from slippery floors; and installing low-pile carpet/nonglazed or nonglossy tiles/wood/linoleum coverings. Stress relocating commonly used items to shelves/drawers in reach, applying remote controls to appliances, and optimizing furniture placement for function, maneuverability, and stability.
- Nurses can provide further safety assessments by suggesting installation of hand rails in bathrooms and by stairs, ensuring client's slippers and clothes fit properly, and recommending repairing or discarding broken equipment in the home (Taylor et al, 2011).

▲ Involve social worker or case manager to educate clients about potential assistive technology, financial cost and benefits, regulations of payers, and local resources.

▲ Implement approaches for home care staff and family to safely handle and transfer clients.

- For further information, refer to care plans for Impaired physical **Mobility** and Impaired **Walking.**

• = Independent   ▲ = Collaborative

Client/Family Teaching and Discharge Planning

- Assess for readiness to learn and use teaching modalities conducive to personal learning styles, including written instructions for home use.
- Supervise practice sessions in which client and family apply items such as gait belts, braces, and orthoses. Check skin once aids are removed.
- Teach and monitor client/family for consistent use of safety precautions for transfers (e.g., nonskid shoes, correctly placed equipment/chairs, locked brakes, leg rests swiveled away) and for correct performance of transfer or use of lifts/slings.
- Teach client/family how to check brakes on chairs to ensure they engage and how to check tires for adequate air pressure; advise routine inspection and annual tune-up of devices.
- Offer information on safe use of shower and commode chairs to prevent discomfort, pressure, and falls during transfer, transport, care, and hygiene.
- For further information, refer to the care plans for Impaired physical **Mobility,** Impaired **Walking,** and Impaired wheelchair **Mobility.**

Risk for Trauma

T

NANDA-I Definition

Vulnerable to accidental tissue injury (e.g., wound, burn, fracture), which may compromise health

Risk Factors

External

Absence of call for aid device; absence of stairway gate; absence of window guard; access to weapon; bathing in very hot water; bed in high position; children riding in front seat of car; defective appliance; delay in ignition of gas appliance; dysfunctional call for aid device; electrical hazard (e.g., faulty plug, frayed wire, overloaded outlet/fuse box); exposure to corrosive product; exposure to dangerous machinery; exposure to radiation; exposure to toxic chemicals; extremes of environmental temperature; flammable object (e.g., clothing, toys); gas leak; grease on stove; high crime neighborhood; icicles hanging from roof; inadequate stair rails; inadequately stored combustible (e.g., matches, oily rags); inadequately stored corrosive (e.g., lye); insufficient lighting; insufficient protection from heat source; misuse of headgear (e.g., hard hat, motorcycle helmet); misuse of seat restraint;

• = Independent   ▲ = Collaborative

insufficient anti-slip material in bathroom; nonuse of seat restraints; obstructed passageway; playing with dangerous object; playing with explosive; pot handle facing front of stove; proximity to vehicle pathway (e.g., driveway, railroad track); slippery floor; smoking in bed; smoking near oxygen; struggling with restraints; unanchored electric wires; unsafe operation of heavy equipment (e.g., excessive speed, while intoxicated, without required eyewear); unsafe road; unsafe walkway; use of cracked dishware; use of throw rugs; use of unstable chair; use of unstable ladder; wearing loose clothing around open flame

Internal

Alteration in cognitive functioning; alteration in sensation (e.g., resulting from spinal cord injury, diabetes mellitus); decrease in eye-hand coordination; decrease in muscle coordination; economically disadvantaged; emotional disturbance; history of trauma (e.g., physical, psychological, sexual); impaired balance; insufficient knowledge of safety precautions; insufficient vision; weakness

Client Outcomes

Client Will (Specify Time Frame)

• Remain free from trauma
• Explain actions that can be taken to prevent trauma

Nursing Interventions

• Provide vision aids for visually impaired clients.
• Assist the client with ambulation. Encourage the client to use assistive devices in activities of daily living (ADLs) as needed.
• Evaluate client's risk for burn injury.
• Assess the client for causes of impaired cognition.
• Provide assistive devices in the home.
▲ Question the client concerning his/her sense of safety.
▲ Assess for a substance abuse problem and refer to appropriate resources for drug and alcohol education.
• Review drug profile for potential side effects that may inhibit performance of ADLs.
• See care plans for Risk for **Aspiration,** Risk for **Falls,** Impaired **Home** maintenance, Risk for **Injury,** Risk for **Poisoning,** and Risk for **Suffocation.**

Pediatric

• Assess the client's socioeconomic status.
• Never leave young children unsupervised.

T

• = Independent   ▲ = Collaborative

- Keep flammable and potentially flammable articles out of reach of young children.
- Lock up harmful objects such as guns.

Geriatric

- Assess the geriatric client's cognitive level of functioning.
- Assess for routine eye examinations.
- Perform a home safety assessment and recommend the following preventive measures: keep electrical cords out of the flow of traffic; remove small rugs or make sure they are slip resistant; increase lighting in hallways and other dark areas; place a light in the bathroom; keep towels, curtains, and other items that might catch fire away from the stove; store harmful products away from food products; provide at least one grab bar in tubs and showers; check prescribed medications for appropriate labels; store medications in original containers or in a dispenser of some type (e.g., egg carton, 7-day plastic dispenser). If the client cannot administer medications according to directions, secure someone to administer medications. Mark stove knobs with bright colors (yellow or red) and outline the borders of steps.
- Discourage driving at night.
- Encourage the client to participate in resistance and impact exercise programs as tolerated.

Client/Family Teaching and Discharge Planning

- Educate the family regarding age-appropriate child safety precautions, environmental safety precautions, and intervention in an emergency.
- Teach the family to assess the child care provider's knowledge regarding child safety.
- Educate the client and family regarding helmet use during recreation and sports activities.
- Encourage the proper use of car seats and safety belts.
- Teach parents to restrict driving for teens.
- Teach parents the importance of monitoring children after school.
- Teach firearm safety.
- For further information, refer to care plans for Risk for **Aspiration,** Risk for **Falls,** Impaired **Home** maintenance, Risk for **Injury,** Risk for **Poisoning,** and Risk for **Suffocation.**

• = Independent   ▲ = Collaborative

Unilateral Neglect
NANDA-I Definition

Impairment in sensory and motor response, mental representation, and spatial attention of the body and the corresponding environment characterized by inattention to one side and overattention to the opposite side; left-side neglect is more severe and persistent than right-side neglect

Defining Characteristics

Alteration in safety behavior on neglected side; disturbance of sound lateralization; failure to dress neglected side; failure to eat food from portion of plate on neglected side; failure to groom neglected side; failure to move eyes in the neglected hemisphere; failure to move head in the neglected hemisphere; failure to move limbs in the neglected hemisphere; failure to move trunk in the neglected hemisphere; failure to notice people approaching from the neglected side; hemianopia; impaired performance on line cancellation, line bisection, and target cancellation tests; left hemiplegia from cerebrovascular accident; marked deviation of the eyes to stimuli on the non-neglected side; marked deviation of the trunk to stimuli on the non-neglected side; omission of drawing on the neglected side; perseveration; representational neglect (e.g., distortion of drawing on the neglected side; substitution of letters to form alternative words when reading; transfer of pain sensation to the non-neglected side; unaware of positioning of neglected limb; unilateral visuospatial neglect; use of vertical half of page only when writing)

Related Factors (r/t)

Brain injury (e.g., cerebrovascular impairment, neurological illness, trauma, tumor)

Client Outcomes
Client Will (Specify Time Frame)

- Use techniques that can be used to minimize unilateral neglect
- Care for both sides of the body appropriately and keep affected side free from harm
- Return to the highest functioning level possible based on personal goals and abilities
- Remain free from injury

Nursing Interventions

- Assess the client for signs of unilateral neglect (UN; e.g., not washing, shaving, or dressing one side of the body; sitting or lying inappropriately on affected arm or leg; failing to respond to

• = Independent ▲ = Collaborative

environmental stimuli contralateral to the side of the lesion; eating food on only one side of plate; or failing to look to one side of the body).

▲ Collaborate with health care provider for referral to a rehabilitation team (including, but not limited to, rehabilitation clinical nurse specialist, physical medicine and rehabilitation health care provider, neuropsychologist, occupational therapist, physical therapist, and speech and language pathologist) for continued help in dealing with UN.

• Use the principles of rehabilitation to progressively increase the client's ability to compensate for UN by using assistive devices, feedback, and support.

• Set up the environment so that essential activity is on the unaffected side:
   ○ Place the client's personal items within view and on the unaffected side.
   ○ Position the bed so that client is approached from the unaffected side.
   ○ Monitor and assist the client to achieve adequate food and fluid intake.

• Implement fall prevention interventions. Clients with right hemisphere brain damage are twice as likely to fall as those with left hemisphere damage (Jepson et al, 2008).

• Position affected extremity in a safe and functional manner.

• Teach the client to be aware of the problem and modify behavior and environment.

Home Care

• Many of the previously listed interventions may be adapted for use in the home care setting.

• Position bed at home so that client gets out of bed on unaffected side.

Client/Family Teaching and Discharge Planning

• Engage discharge planning specialists for comprehensive assessment and planning early in the client's stay.

• Encourage family participation in care and exercise.

• Explain pathology and symptoms of unilateral neglect to both the client and family.

• Teach the client how to scan regularly to check the position of body parts and to regularly turn head from side to side for safety when ambulating, using a wheelchair, or doing self-care tasks.

• = Independent   ▲ = Collaborative

- Reinforce the client's use of adaptive devices such as prisms prescribed by rehabilitation professionals (Shiraishi et al, 2008).
- Teach caregivers to cue the client to the environment.

Impaired Urinary elimination

NANDA-I Definition

Dysfunction in urine elimination

Defining Characteristics

Dysuria; frequent voiding; hesitancy; nocturia; urinary incontinence; urinary retention; urinary urgency

Related Factors

Anatomic obstruction; multiple causality; sensory motor impairment; urinary tract infection (UTI)

Client Outcomes

Client Will (Specify Time Frame)

- State absence of pain or excessive urgency during urination
- Demonstrate voiding frequency no more than every 2 hours

Nursing Interventions

- Ask the client about urinary elimination patterns and concerns.
- Question the client regarding the following:
  o Presence of symptoms such as incontinence, dribbling, frequency, urgency, dysuria, and nocturia
  o Presence of pain in the area of the bladder
  o The pattern of urination and approximate amount
  o Possible aggravating and alleviating factors for urinary problems
- Ask the client to keep a bladder diary/bladder log.
- For interventions on urinary incontinence, refer to the following nursing diagnosis care plans as appropriate: Stress urinary **Incontinence,** Urge urinary **Incontinence,** Reflex urinary **Incontinence,** Overflow urinary **Incontinence,** or Functional urinary **Incontinence.**
- ▲ Perform a focused physical assessment including inspecting the perineal skin integrity, percussion, and palpation of the lower abdomen looking for obvious bladder distention or an enlarged kidney.
- ▲ Check for costovertebral tenderness.

U

• = Independent   ▲ = Collaborative

▲ Review results of urinalysis for the presence of urinary infection: white blood cells, red blood cells, bacteria, positive nitrites. If urinalysis results are not available, request a midstream specimen of urine (urine obtained during voiding, discarding the first and last portions) for a urinalysis (Norrby, 2011).

▲ If blood or protein is present in the urine, recognize that both hematuria and proteinuria are serious symptoms, and the client should be referred to a urologist to receive a workup to rule out pathology.

• Inquire about the client's history of smoking.

Urinary Tract Infection

▲ Consult the provider for a culture and sensitivity testing and antibiotic treatment in the individual with evidence of a symptomatic UTI.

▲ Teach the client to recognize symptoms of UTI: dysuria that crescendos as the bladder nears complete evacuation; urgency to urinate followed by micturition of only a few drops; suprapubic aching discomfort; malaise; voiding frequency; sudden exacerbation of urinary incontinence with or without fever, chills, and flank pain. Recognize that cloudy or malodorous urine, in the absence of other lower urinary tract symptoms, may not indicate the presence of a UTI and that asymptomatic bacteriuria in the older adult does not justify a course of antibiotics.

▲ Refer the individual with chronic lower urinary tract pain to a urologist or specialist in the management of pelvic pain.

Geriatric

▲ Perform urinalysis in all older adults who experience a sudden change in urine elimination patterns such as new-onset incontinence, lower abdominal discomfort, acute confusion, or a fever of unclear origin.

• Encourage older women to consume one to two servings of fresh blueberries and consider drinking at least 10 oz of cranberry juice daily or supplement the diet with cranberry concentrate capsules as ordered.

▲ Refer the older woman with recurrent UTIs to her health care provider for possible use of topical estrogen creams for treatment of atrophic vaginal mucosa from decreased hormonal stimulation, which can predispose to UTIs (Buhr et al, 2011; Norrby, 2011; Aydin et al, 2014).

• = Independent   ▲ = Collaborative

▲ Recognize that UTIs in older men are typically associated with prostatic hyperplasia or strictures of the urethra. Refer to a urologist (Norrby, 2011).

Client/Family Teaching and Discharge Planning

- Teach the client/family methods to keep the urinary tract healthy. Refer to Client/Family Teaching in the care plan for Readiness for enhanced **Urinary** elimination.
- Teach the following measures to women to decrease the incidence of UTIs:
  ○ Urinate at appropriate intervals. Do not ignore need to void, which can result in stasis of urine.
  ○ Drink plenty of liquids, especially water.
  ○ Wipe from front to back.
  ○ Wear underpants that have a cotton crotch.
  ○ Avoid potentially irritating feminine products.
- Teach the sexually active woman with recurrent UTIs prevention measures including:
  ○ Void after intercourse to flush bacteria out of the urethra and bladder.
  ○ Use a lubricating agent as needed during intercourse to protect the vagina from trauma and decrease the incidence of vaginitis.
  ○ Watch for signs of vaginitis and seek treatment as needed.
  ○ Avoid use of diaphragms with spermicide.
- Teach clients with spinal cord injury and neurogenic bladder dysfunction to consider adding cranberry extract tablets or cranberry juice, or fruits containing D-mannose (e.g., apples, oranges, peaches, blueberries) on a daily basis, monitor fluid intake. The client is encouraged to discuss the use of probiotics and antibiotic therapy with the provider for frequent recurrent symptomatic UTIs.
- Teach all persons to recognize hematuria and to promptly seek care if this symptom occurs.

U

Readiness for enhanced Urinary elimination

NANDA-I Definition

A pattern of urinary functions for meeting eliminatory needs, which can be strengthened

• = Independent   ▲ = Collaborative

Defining Characteristics

Expresses desire to enhance urinary elimination

Client Outcomes

Client Will (Specify Time Frame)

- Urinate every 3 to 4 hours while awake
- Remain free of undetected symptoms of a urinary tract infection (UTI) or cancer of the kidney or bladder
- Drink fluids at a sufficient level to have light yellow (e.g., straw-colored) urine

Nursing Interventions

- Ask the client questions regarding any bothersome or concerning urinary symptoms such as frequency, nocturia, urgency, dysuria, or retention of urine.
- Question the client regarding presence of incontinence. If incontinence is present, refer to the appropriate care plan: Stress urinary **Incontinence,** Urge urinary **Incontinence,** Functional urinary **Incontinence,** or Reflex urinary **Incontinence.**
- Question the client regarding history of UTIs. If the client has had UTIs in the past, provide teaching for prevention as outlined in the care plan for Impaired **Urinary** elimination.
- Ask the client to complete a bladder diary of diurnal and nocturnal urine elimination patterns and patterns of urinary leakage.

Pediatric

- Encourage children and adolescents to maintain normal weight because obesity has been related to cancers of the urinary tract.

Geriatric

- Encourage older women to consume one to two servings of fresh blueberries and consider drinking at least 10 oz of cranberry juice daily or supplement the diet with cranberry concentrate capsules as ordered.
- Older adults with toileting disability have increased care costs and dependency.

Client/Family Teaching and Discharge Planning

- Teach the client general guidelines for health of the urinary system.
- ▲ Ensure good hydration. Total daily fluid intake should be approximately 2.7 L per day for women and 3.7 L per day for men (Newman & Willson, 2011).

• = Independent   ▲ = Collaborative

▲ Recommend the client have a physical exam, a metabolic panel of laboratory tests, and a urinalysis done yearly.

▲ Recommend that the client not hold urine for long periods of time before emptying the bladder. It is normal to urinate every 3 to 4 hours.

▲ Recommend that the client with frequency, urgency in the morning, or possible incontinence consider reducing or eliminating caffeine intake.

• If the client has constipation at intervals, share measures to alleviate or prevent constipation, including adequate consumption of dietary fluids, dietary fiber, exercise, and regular bowel elimination patterns.

• Advise clients to stop smoking because of the association with damage to the kidney and bladder, including chronic kidney disease, bladder cancer, urinary incontinence, and bothersome lower urinary tract symptoms in men.

▲ Encourage the client to eat a healthy diet, avoiding processed meats with sodium nitrate as a preservative to decrease incidence of cancer of the bladder.

Urinary Retention
NANDA-I Definition

Incomplete emptying of the bladder

Defining Characteristics

Absent urinary output; bladder distention; dribbling of urine; dysuria; frequent voiding; overflow incontinence; residual urine; sensation of bladder fullness; small voiding

Related Factors

Blockage in urinary tract; high urethral pressure; reflex arc inhibition; strong sphincter

Client Outcomes

Client Will (Specify Time Frame)

• Demonstrate consistent ability to urinate when desire to void is perceived

• Have measured urinary residual volume of less than 200 to 250 mL

• Experience correction or relief from dysuria, nocturia, postvoid dribbling, and voiding frequently

• Be free of a urinary tract infection

• = Independent   ▲ = Collaborative

Nursing Interventions

- Obtain a focused urinary history including questioning the client about episodes of acute urinary retention (complete inability to void) or chronic retention (documented elevated postvoid residual volumes), as well as symptoms such as dysuria, nocturia, postvoid dribbling, and voiding frequently.
- Question the client concerning specific risk factors for urinary retention including:
  - Spinal cord injuries
  - Ischemic stroke
  - Metabolic disorders such as diabetes mellitus, chronic alcoholism, and related conditions associated with polyuria and peripheral polyneuropathies
  - Herpetic infection
  - Heavy-metal poisoning (lead, mercury) causing peripheral polyneuropathies
  - Advanced-stage human immunodeficiency virus (HIV) infection
  - Medications including antispasmodics/parasympatholytics, alpha-adrenergic agonists, antidepressants, sedatives, narcotics, psychotropic medications, illicit drugs
  - Recent surgery requiring general or spinal anesthesia
  - Vaginal delivery within the past 48 hours
  - Bowel elimination patterns, history of fecal impaction, encopresis
  - Recent surgical procedures
  - Recent prostatic biopsy
- Complete a pain assessment including pain intensity using a self-report pain tool, such as the 0 to 10 numerical pain rating scale. Also determine location, quality, onset/duration, intensity, aggravating/alleviating factors, and effects of pain on function and quality of life.
- Perform a focused physical assessment including perineal skin integrity and inspection, percussion, and palpation of the lower abdomen, looking for obvious bladder distention or an enlarged kidney.
- Recognize that unrelieved obstruction of urine can result in kidney damage and, if severe, kidney failure. Urinary retention can be a medical emergency and should be reported to the primary health care provider as soon as possible.

• = Independent   ▲ = Collaborative

- Review laboratory test results including serum electrolytes, blood urea nitrogen (BUN) and creatinine, along with calcium, phosphate, magnesium, uric acid, and albumin.
- Monitor for signs of dehydration, peripheral edema, elevated blood pressure, and heart failure.
- Ask the client to complete a bladder diary including patterns of urine elimination, urine loss (if present), nocturia, and volume and types of fluids consumed for a period of 3 to 7 days.
- Consult with the provider concerning eliminating or altering medications suspected of producing or exacerbating urinary retention.
- Advise the male client with urinary retention related to benign prostatic hyperplasia (BPH) to avoid risk factors associated with acute urinary retention:
  - Avoid over-the-counter cold remedies containing a decongestant (alpha-adrenergic agonist) or antihistamine such as diphenhydramine that has anticholinergic effects.
  - Avoid taking over-the-counter dietary medications (frequently contain alpha-adrenergic agonists).
  - Discuss voiding problems with a health care provider before beginning new prescription medications.
  - After prolonged exposure to cool weather, warm the body before attempting to urinate.
  - Avoid overfilling the bladder by regular urination patterns and refrain from excessive intake of alcohol.
- Provide the client who is unable to void with specific strategies to manage this potential medical emergency as follows:
  - Attempt urination in complete privacy.
  - Place the feet solidly on the floor.
  - If unable to void using these strategies, take a warm sitz bath or shower and void (if possible) while still in the tub or shower.
  - Drink a warm cup of caffeinated coffee or tea to stimulate the bladder, which may promote voiding.
- If unable to void within 6 hours or if bladder distention is producing significant pain, seek urgent or emergency care.
- Perform sterile (in acute care) or clean intermittent catheterization at home as ordered for clients with urinary retention. Refer to care plan for Reflex urinary **Incontinence** for more information about intermittent catheterization.

U

• = Independent   ▲ = Collaborative

- ▲ Insert an indwelling catheter only as ordered by a health care provider. Catheter-associated urinary tract infections (CAUTI) are among the most common health care–associated infections. Each CAUTI episode is estimated to cost $600, rising to $2800 per episode when a CAUTI leads to a bloodstream infection. While certain conditions among hospitalized clients may require the use of a urinary catheter, limiting their use and decreasing the length of use are the most effective methods of reducing clients' exposure to CAUTIs (Choosing wisely.org, 2014).
- Nurse-led and computer-based reminders are both successful in reducing how long urinary catheters remain in place (Bernard et al, 2012).
- Nurse-driven practice recommendations to reduce CAUTI risk include securing catheters; maintaining drainage bags lower than level of bladder; emptying drainage bags every 8 hours, when two-thirds full, and before any transfer; daily evaluation of catheter indication/need to promote removal; and use of bladder scanner to prevent reinsertion.
- Current practice recommendations support aseptic catheter insertions, while the use of hydrophilic-coated catheters for clean intermittent catheters can reduce the rate of CAUTIs. Suprapubic catheterization is not more effective than urethral catheterization in reducing the incidence of catheter-related bacteremia.
- For the individual with urinary retention who is not a suitable candidate for intermittent catheterization, recognize that the catheter can be a significant cause of harm to the client through development of a CAUTI or through genitourinary trauma when the catheter is pulled.
- Advise clients with indwelling catheters that bacteria in the urine is an almost universal finding after the catheter has remained in place for more than 1 week and that only symptomatic infections warrant treatment.
- Use the following strategies to reduce the risk for CAUTI whenever feasible:
  - ○ Insert the indwelling catheter with sterile technique, only when insertion is indicated.
  - ○ Remove the indwelling catheter as soon as possible; acute care facilities should institute a policy for regular review of the necessity of an indwelling catheter.

• = Independent   ▲ = Collaborative

- ○ Maintain a closed drainage system whenever feasible.
- ○ Maintain unobstructed urine flow, avoiding kinks in the tubing and keeping the collecting bag below the level of the bladder at all times.
- ○ Regularly cleanse the urethral meatus with a gentle cleanser to remove apparent soiling.
- ○ Change the long-term catheter every 4 weeks; more frequent catheter changes should be reserved for clients who experience catheter encrustation and blockage.
- Educate staff about the risks for CAUTI development and specific strategies to reduce these risks.

Postoperative Urinary Retention
- Urinary retention is a common complication of surgery, anesthesia, and advancing age. If conservative measures do not help the client pass urine, the bladder needs to be drained using either an intermittent catheter or indwelling urethral catheter, which places the client at risk for development of CAUTI (Steggall et al, 2013).
- Remove the indwelling urethral catheter at midnight in the hospitalized postoperative client to reduce the risk for acute urinary retention.
- Perform a bladder scan before considering inserting a catheter to determine postvoid residual volume following surgery.

Geriatric
- Aggressively assess older clients, particularly those with dribbling urinary incontinence, urinary tract infection, and related conditions for urinary retention.
- Assess older clients for impaction when urinary retention is documented or suspected.
- Monitor older male clients for retention related to BPH or prostate cancer.

Home Care
- Encourage the client to report any inability to void.
- Maintain an up-to-date medication list; evaluate side-effect profiles for risk of urinary retention.
- Refer the client for health care provider evaluation if urinary retention occurs.

U

• = Independent   ▲ = Collaborative

Client/Family Teaching and Discharge Planning

• Teach the client with mild to moderate obstructive symptoms to double void by urinating, resting in the bathroom for 3 to 5 minutes, and then trying again to urinate.

• Teach the client with urinary retention and infrequent voiding to urinate by the clock.

• Teach the client with an indwelling catheter to assess the tube for patency, maintain the drainage system below the level of the symphysis pubis, and routinely cleanse the bedside bag as directed.

• Teach the client with an indwelling catheter or undergoing intermittent catheterization the symptoms of a significant urinary infection, including hematuria, acute-onset incontinence, dysuria, flank pain, fever, and acute confusion.

Risk for Vascular Trauma

NANDA-I Definition

Vulnerable to damage to vein and its surrounding tissues related to the presence of a catheter and/or infusion solutions, which may compromise health

Risk Factors

Difficulty visualizing artery or vein; inadequate anchoring of catheter; inappropriate catheter type; inappropriate catheter width; insertion site; irritating solution (e.g., concentration, temperature, pH); length of time catheter is in place; rapid infusion rate

Client Outcomes

Client Will (Specify Time Frame)

• Remain free from vascular trauma
• Remain free from signs and symptoms that indicate vascular trauma
• Remain free from impaired tissue and/or skin
• Maintain skin integrity, tissue perfusion, and usual tissue temperature, color, and pigment
• Report any altered sensation or pain
• State site is comfortable

Nursing Interventions

Client Preparation

▲ Verify objective and estimate duration of treatment. Check health care provider's order.

• = Independent   ▲ = Collaborative

- Assess client's clinical situation when venous infusion is indicated.
- Assess if client is prepared for an intravenous (IV) procedure. Explain the procedure if necessary to decrease stress.
- Provide privacy and make the client comfortable during the intravenous insertion.
- Teach the client what symptoms of possible vascular trauma he should be alert to and to immediately inform staff if any of these symptoms are noticed.

Insertion

- Wash hands before and after touching the client, as well as when inserting, replacing, accessing, repairing, or dressing an intravascular catheter (O'Grady et al, 2011; Society for Health Care Epidemiology of America, 2014).
- Maintain aseptic technique for the insertion and care of intravascular catheters.
- Assess the condition of the client's veins, possible age-related influence, and previous intravenous site use.
- In cases of hard-to-access veins, consider strategies such as the use of ultrasound to assist in vein localization and safe venipuncture.
- Avoid areas of joint flexion and bony prominences.
- Choose an appropriate vascular access device (VAD) based on the types and characteristics of the devices and insertion site. Consider the following:
  - Peripheral cannulae: short devices that are placed into a peripheral vein; can be straight, winged, or ported and winged
  - Midline catheters or peripherally inserted central catheters (PICCs) with ranges from 7.5 to 20 cm
  - Central venous access devices (CVADs) are terminated in the central venous circulation and are available in a range of gauge sizes; they can be nontunneled catheters, skin-tunneled catheters, implantable injection ports, or PICCs.
  - Polyurethane venous devices and silicone rubber may cause less friction and consequently may reduce the risk of mechanical phlebitis (Phillips, 2014).
- ▲ Choose a device with consideration of the nature, volume, and flow of prescribed solution.
- If possible, choose the venous access site considering the client's preference. Engaging the client in choosing venous access site, when possible, may facilitate line patency.

V

• = Independent   ▲ = Collaborative

- Select the gauge of the venous device according to the duration of treatment, purpose of the procedure, and size of the vein.
- Verify whether client is allergic to fixation or device material.
- Disinfect the venipuncture site. Assess that skin is dry before puncturing to achieve maximal benefit of disinfection agent.
- Provide a comfortable, safe, hypoallergenic, easily removable stabilization dressing, allowing for visualization of the access site.
- Peripheral catheter intended dwell time is 72 to 96 hours and central catheters is 7 days (Helm et al, 2015).
- Use sterile, transparent, semipermeable dressing to cover catheter site.
- Document insertion date, site, type of VAD, number of punctures performed, other occurrences, and measures/arrangements.
- Always decontaminate the device before infusing medication or manipulating IV equipment (Xue, 2014; Helm et al, 2015).
- ▲ Verify the sequence of drugs to be administrated. Vesicants should always be administered first in a sequence of drugs (Loubani & Green, 2015).

Monitoring Infusion

- Monitor permeability and flow rate at regular intervals.
- Monitor catheter-skin junction and surrounding tissues at regular intervals, observing possible appearance of burning, pain, erythema, altered local temperature, infiltration, extravasation, edema, secretion, tenderness, or induration. Remove promptly.
- ▲ Replace device according to institution protocol.
- ▲ Flush vascular access according to organizational policies and procedures, and as recommended by the manufacturer.
- Remove catheter on suspected contamination; if the client develops signs of phlebitis, infection, or a malfunctioning catheter; or when no longer required.
- Encourage clients to report any discomfort such as pain, burning, swelling, or bleeding (Xue, 2014).

Pediatric

- The preceding interventions may be adapted for the pediatric client.
- Inform the client and family about the IV procedure; obtain permissions, maintain client's comfort, and perform appropriate assessment prior to venipuncture. Assess the client for any allergies or sensitivities to tape, antiseptics, or latex.

• = Independent   ▲ = Collaborative

- The use of an appropriate device to obtain blood samples reduces discomfort in the pediatric client.
- Avoid areas of joint flexion and bony prominences.
- ▲ Consider whether sedation or the use of local anesthetic is suitable for insertion of a catheter, taking into consideration the age of the pediatric client.
- ▲ Use diversion while carrying out the procedure.

Geriatric
- The preceding interventions may be adapted for the geriatric client.
- Consider the physical, emotional, and cognitive changes related to older adults.
- Use strict aseptic technique for venipuncture of older clients.

Home Care
- Some devices may remain after discharge. Provide device-specific education to the client and family members about care of the selected device.
- Help in the choice of actions that support self-care. The nurse can provide valuable information that can be used to guide decision-making to maximize the self-care abilities of clients receiving home infusion therapy.
- Select, with the client, the insertion site most compatible with the development of activities of daily living (Xue, 2014; McGowan, 2014).
- Minimize the use of continuous IV therapy whenever possible.

V

Impaired spontaneous Ventilation
NANDA-I Definition

Decreased energy reserves resulting in an inability to maintain independent breathing that is adequate to support life

Defining Characteristics

Alteration in metabolism; apprehensiveness; decrease in arterial oxygen saturation; decrease in cooperation; decrease in partial pressure of oxygen; decrease in tidal volume; dyspnea; increase in accessory muscle use; increase in heart rate; increase in partial pressure of carbon dioxide; restlessness

Related Factors

Alteration in metabolism; respiratory muscle fatigue

• = Independent   ▲ = Collaborative

Client Outcomes

Client Will (Specify Time Frame)

- Maintain arterial blood gases within safe parameters
- Remain free of dyspnea or restlessness
- Effectively maintain airway
- Effectively mobilize secretions

Nursing Interventions

▲ Collaborate with the client, family, and health care provider regarding possible intubation and ventilation. Ask whether the client has advanced directives and, if so, integrate them into the plan of care with clinical data regarding overall health and reversibility of the medical condition.

• Assess and respond to changes in the client's respiratory status. Monitor the client for dyspnea, increase in respiratory rate, use of accessory muscles, retraction of intercostal muscles, flaring of nostrils, decrease in O_2 saturation, cyanosis, and subjective complaints (Burns, 2011; Parshall et al, 2011).

• Have the client use a numerical scale (0-10) or visual analog scale to self-report dyspnea before and after interventions.

• Assess for history of chronic respiratory disorders when administering oxygen.

▲ Collaborate with the health care provider and respiratory therapists in determining the appropriateness of noninvasive positive pressure ventilation (NPPV/NIV) for the decompensated client with COPD. Ventilatory support in a COPD exacerbation can be provided by either noninvasive or invasive ventilation (Burns, 2011; GOLD, 2015). NIV improves respiratory acidosis and decreases respiratory rate, severity of breathlessness, incidence of ventilator-associated pneumonia (VAP), and hospital length of stay (GOLD, 2015; Mas & Masip, 2014).

▲ Assist with implementation, client support, and monitoring if NPPV is used.

• If the client has apnea, respiratory muscle fatigue, somnolence, hypoxemia, and/or acute respiratory acidosis, prepare the client for possible intubation and mechanical ventilation.

Ventilator Support

▲ Explain the endotracheal intubation and mechanical ventilation process to the client and family as appropriate, and during intubation

V

• = Independent   ▲ = Collaborative

administer sedation for client comfort according to the health care provider's orders.

- Secure the endotracheal tube in place using either tape or a commercially available device, auscultate bilateral breath sounds, use a CO_2 detector, and obtain a chest radiograph to confirm endotracheal tube placement.
- Review ventilator settings with the health care provider and respiratory therapist to ensure support is appropriate to meet the client's minute ventilation requirements (Grossbach et al, 2011; Stacy, 2013; Chacko et al, 2015).
▲ Suction as needed and hyperoxygenate according to facility policy. Refer to the care plan for Ineffective **Airway** clearance for further information on suctioning.
- Check that monitor alarms are set appropriately at the start of each shift.
- Respond to ventilator alarms promptly. If unable to immediately locate the source/cause of an alarm, use a manual self-inflating resuscitation bag to ventilate the client while waiting for assistance.
- Prevent unplanned extubation by maintaining stability of endotracheal tube.
- Drain collected fluid from condensation out of ventilator tubing as needed.
- Note ventilator settings of flow of inspired oxygen, peak inspiratory pressure, tidal volume, and alarm activation at intervals and when removing the client from the ventilator for any reason (Burns, 2011; Grossbach et al, 2011).
▲ Administer analgesics and sedatives as needed to facilitate client comfort and rest. Use behavioral and sedation scales for nonverbal clients to provide a consistent way of monitoring pain and sedation levels and ensuring that therapeutic outcomes are being met (Balas et al, 2012; Barr et al, 2013). Clients receiving mechanical ventilation frequently require sedation to help attenuate the anxiety, pain, and agitation associated with this intervention (Balas et al, 2012; Barr et al, 2013). The overall goal of sedation during mechanical ventilation is to provide physiological stability, ventilator synchrony, and comfort for clients.
- Tools such as the Riker Sedation-Agitation Scale, the Motor Activity Assessment Scale, the Ramsey Scale, or the Richmond

Agitation-Sedation Scale may be useful in monitoring levels of sedation.

• Alternatives to medications for decreasing anxiety should be attempted, such as music therapy with selections of the client's choice played on headphones at intervals.

• Analyze and respond to arterial blood gas results, end-tidal CO_2 levels, and pulse oximetry values.

• Use an effective means of verbal and nonverbal communication with the client. Barriers to communication include endotracheal tubes, sedation, and general weakness associated with a critical illness. Basic technologies should be readily available to the client, including eyeglasses and hearing aids (Grossbach et al, 2011; Khalaila et al, 2011). A variety of communication devices are available, including electronic voice output communication aids, alphabet boards, picture boards, computers, and writing slates. Ask the client for input into their care as appropriate (Grossbach et al, 2011; Khalaila et al, 2011).

• Move the endotracheal tube from side to side at least every 24 hours, and tape it or secure it with a commercially available device. Assess and document client's skin condition, and ensure correct tube placement at lip line (National Pressure Ulcer Advisory Panel, 2013).

• Implement steps to prevent ventilator-associated events (VAE), such as ventilator-associated pneumonia (VAP), including continuous removal of subglottic secretions, elevation of the head of bed to 30 to 45 degrees (Siela, 2010; Hospital Quality Institute, 2015) unless medically contraindicated, change of the ventilator circuit no more than every 48 hours, and wash hands before and after contact with each client.

• Use endotracheal tubes that allow for the continuous aspiration of subglottic secretions (Siela, 2010; Frost et al, 2013).

• Position the client in a semirecumbent position with the head of the bed at a 30 to 45 degree angle to decrease the aspiration of gastric, oral, and nasal secretions (Siela, 2010; Bell, 2011; Hospital Quality Institute, 2015). Consider use of kinetic therapy, using a kinetic bed that slowly moves the client with 40 degree turns.

• Perform handwashing using both soap and water and alcohol-based solution before and after all mechanically ventilated client contact to prevent spread of infections (Makic et al, 2013; Centers for Disease Control and Prevention, 2014).

• = Independent   ▲ = Collaborative

- Provide routine oral care using tooth brushing and oral rinsing with an antimicrobial agent if needed (Siela, 2010; Martin, 2010; Joanna Briggs Institute, 2014; Ames, 2011).
- Maintain proper cuff inflation for both endotracheal tubes and cuffed tracheostomy tubes with minimal leak volume or minimal occlusion volume to decrease risk of aspiration and reduce incidence of VAP (Siela, 2010; Bell, 2011; Skillings & Curtis, 2011; Stacy, 2013).
- Reposition the client as needed. Use rotational bed or kinetic bed therapy in clients for whom side-to-side turning is contraindicated or difficult.
- ▲ If the client is intubated and stable, consider getting the client up to sit at the edge of the bed, transfer to a chair, or walk as appropriate and an effective interdisciplinary team is developed to keep the client safe (Gosselink et al, 2008; Balas et al, 2012).
- Assess bilateral anterior and posterior breath sounds every 2 to 4 hours and as needed; respond to any relevant changes (Burns, 2011).
- Assess responsiveness to ventilator support; monitor for subjective complaints and sensation of dyspnea (Burns, 2011).
- ▲ Collaborate with the interdisciplinary team in treating clients with acute respiratory failure (Grap, 2009; Balas et al, 2012). Collaborate with the health care team to meet the client's ventilator care needs and avoid complications (Grossbach et al, 2011).

Geriatric

- Recognize that critically ill older adults have a high rate of morbidity when mechanically ventilated.
- ▲ NPPV may be used during acute treatment of older clients with impaired ventilation.

Home Care

- ▲ Some of the interventions listed previously may be adapted for home care use. Begin discharge planning as soon as possible with the case manager or social worker to assess the need for home support systems, assistive devices, and community or home health services.
- ▲ With help from a medical social worker, assist the client and family to determine the fiscal effect of care in the home versus an extended care facility.
- Assess the home setting during the discharge process to ensure the home can safely accommodate ventilator support (e.g., adequate space and electricity).

• = Independent   ▲ = Collaborative

- Have the family contact the electric company and place the client residence on a high-risk list in case of a power outage.
- Assess the caregivers for commitment to supporting a ventilator-dependent client in the home.
- Be sure that the client and family or caregivers are familiar with operation of all ventilation devices, know how to suction secretions if needed, are competent in doing tracheostomy care, and know schedules for cleaning equipment. Have the designated caregiver or caregivers demonstrate care before discharge.
- Assess client and caregiver knowledge of the disease, client needs, and medications to be administered via ventilation-assistive devices. Avoid analgesics. Assess knowledge of how to use equipment. Teach as necessary.
- Establish an emergency plan and criteria for use. Identify emergency procedures to be used until medical assistance arrives. Teach and role play emergency care.

Client/Family Teaching and Discharge Planning

- Explain to the client the potential sensations that will be experienced, including relief of dyspnea, the feeling of lung inflations, the noise of the ventilator, and the reality of alarms.
- Explain to the client and family about being unable to speak, and work out an alternative system of communication. See previously mentioned interventions.
- Demonstrate to the family how to perform simple procedures, such as suctioning secretions in the mouth with a tonsil-tip catheter, providing range-of-motion exercises, and reconnecting the ventilator immediately if it becomes disconnected.
- Offer both the client and family explanations of how the ventilator works and answer any questions.

Dysfunctional Ventilatory weaning response

NANDA-I Definition

Inability to adjust to lowered levels of mechanical ventilator support that interrupts and prolongs the weaning process

• = Independent ▲ = Collaborative

Defining Characteristics

Mild

Breathing discomfort; fatigue; fear of machine malfunction; increase in focus on breathing; mild increase of respiratory rate over baseline; perceived need for an increase in oxygen; restlessness; warmth

Moderate

Abnormal skin color (e.g., pale, dusky, cyanosis); apprehensiveness; decrease in air entry on auscultation; diaphoresis; facial expression of fear; hyperfocused on activities; impaired ability to cooperate; impaired ability to respond to coaching; increase in blood pressure from baseline (<20 mm Hg); increase in heart rate from baseline (<20 beats/min); minimal use of respiratory accessory muscles; moderate increase in respiratory rate over baseline

Severe

Abnormal skin color (e.g., pale, dusky, cyanosis); adventitious breath sounds; agitation; asynchronized breathing with the ventilator; decrease in level of consciousness; deterioration in arterial blood gases from baseline; gasping breaths; increase in blood pressure from baseline (≥20 mm Hg); increase in heart rate from baseline (≥20 beats/min); paradoxical abdominal breathing; profuse diaphoresis; shallow breathing; significant increase in respiratory rate above baseline; use of significant respiratory accessory muscles

Related Factors (r/t)

Physiological

Alteration in sleep pattern; ineffective airway clearance; inadequate nutrition; pain

Psychological

Anxiety; decrease in motivation; fear; hopelessness; insufficient knowledge of weaning process; insufficient trust in health care professional; low self-esteem; powerlessness; uncertainty about ability to wean

Situational

Environmental barrier (e.g., distractions, low nurse-to-client ratio, unfamiliar health care staff); history of unsuccessful weaning attempt; history of ventilator dependence longer than 4 days; inappropriate pace of weaning process; insufficient social support; uncontrolled episodic energy demands

V

Client Outcomes

Client Will (Specify Time Frame)

- Wean from ventilator with adequate arterial blood gases
- Remain free of unresolved dyspnea or restlessness
- Effectively clear secretions

Nursing Interventions

- Assess client's readiness for weaning as evidenced by the following:
  - ○ Physiological and psychological readiness. There has been little research devoted to the study of psychological readiness to wean.
  - ○ Resolution of initial medical problem that led to ventilator dependence
  - ○ Hemodynamic stability
  - ○ Normal hemoglobin levels
  - ○ Absence of fever
  - ○ Normal state of consciousness
  - ○ Metabolic, fluid, and electrolyte balance
  - ○ Adequate nutritional status with serum albumin levels >2.5 g/dL
  - ○ Adequate sleep
  - ○ Adequate pain management and minimal sedation
- For successful weaning, ensure that the client is in an optimal physiological and psychological state before introducing the stress of weaning (Burns, 2011a).
- Involve family as appropriate to help the client provide a maximal effort during weaning readiness measurements (Burns, 2011a).
- Provide adequate nutrition to ventilated clients, using enteral feeding when possible.

- Use evidence-based weaning and extubation protocols as appropriate.
- Identify reasons for previous unsuccessful weaning attempts, and include that information in development of the weaning plan.
- ▲ Collaborate with an interdisciplinary team (health care provider, nurse, respiratory therapist, physical therapist, and dietitian) to develop a weaning plan with a timeline and goals; revise this plan throughout the weaning period. Use a communication device, such as a weaning board or flow sheet (Burns, 2011b; Grossbach et al, 2011).
- In clients with chronic obstructive pulmonary disease who fail extubation, noninvasive ventilation (NIV) facilitates weaning, prevents reintubation, and reduces mortality. Early NIV after extubation reduces the risk for respiratory failure and lowers 90-day

• = Independent   ▲ = Collaborative

mortality in clients with hypercapnia during a spontaneous breathing trial (Epstein, 2009; Mas & Masip, 2014).

- Assist client to identify personal strategies that result in relaxation and comfort (e.g., music, visualization, relaxation techniques, reading, television, family visits). Support implementation of these strategies (Pattison & Watson, 2009). Music intervention can be used to allay anxiety and can be a powerful distractor from distressful sounds and thoughts in the intensive care unit (ICU) (Tracy & Chlan, 2011).
- Provide a safe and comfortable environment.
- If unable to stay, make the call light button readily available and assure the client that needs will be met responsively.
▲ Coordinate pain and sedation medications to minimize sedative effects.
- Administer analgesics and sedatives as needed to facilitate client comfort and rest. Use behavioral and sedation scales for nonverbal clients to provide a consistent way of monitoring pain and sedation levels and ensuring that therapeutic outcomes are being met (Barr et al, 2013).
- Tools such as the Riker Sedation-Agitation Scale, the Motor Activity Assessment Scale, the Ramsey Scale, or the Richmond Agitation-Sedation Scale may be useful in monitoring levels of sedation (Balas et al, 2012; Barr et al, 2013).
- Schedule weaning periods for the time of day when the client is most rested. Cluster care activities to promote successful weaning. Avoid other procedures during weaning; keep the environment quiet and promote restful activities between weaning periods.
- Promote a normal sleep-wake cycle, allowing uninterrupted periods of nighttime sleep.
- During weaning, monitor the client's physiological and psychological responses; acknowledge and respond to fears and subjective complaints. Validate the client's efforts during the weaning process.
- Monitor subjective and objective data (breath sounds, respiratory pattern, respiratory effort, heart rate, blood pressure, oxygen saturation per oximetry, amount and type of secretions, anxiety, and energy level) throughout weaning to determine client tolerance and responses (Burns, 2011c; Grap, 2009).
- Involve the client and family in the weaning plan. Inform them of the weaning plan and possible client responses to the weaning process (e.g., potential feelings of dyspnea). Foster a partnership

V

between clients and nurses in care planning for weaning (Pattison & Watson, 2009).

- Coach the client through episodes of increased anxiety. Remain with the client or place a supportive and calm significant other in this role. Give positive reinforcement; with permission, use touch to communicate support and concern.
- Terminate weaning when the client demonstrates predetermined criteria or when the following signs of weaning intolerance occur:
  - ○ Tachypnea, dyspnea, or chest and abdominal asynchrony
  - ○ Agitation or mental status changes
  - ○ Decreased oxygen saturation: Sao_2 <90%
  - ○ Increased $PaCO_2$ or $ETCO_2$
  - ○ Change in pulse rate or blood pressure or onset of new dysrhythmias
- ▲ If the dysfunctional weaning response is severe, consider slowing weaning to brief periods (e.g., 5 minutes). Continue to collaborate with the team to determine whether an untreated physiological cause for the dysfunctional weaning pattern remains. Consult with health care provider regarding use of noninvasive ventilation immediately after discontinuing ventilation. Consider an alternative care setting (subacute, rehabilitation facility, home) for clients with prolonged ventilator dependence as a strategy that can positively affect outcomes.

Geriatric
- Recognize that older clients may require longer periods to wean.

Home Care
- Weaning from a ventilator at home should be based on client stability and comfort of the client and caregivers under an intermittent care plan.

Risk for other-directed Violence
NANDA-I Definition

Vulnerable to behaviors in which an individual demonstrates that he or she can be physically, emotionally, and/or sexually harmful to others

Risk Factors

Access to weapon; alteration in cognitive functioning; cruelty to animals; fire setting; history of childhood abuse (e.g., physical, psychological, sexual); history of substance abuse; history of witnessing family violence;

V

impulsiveness; motor vehicle offense (e.g., traffic violations, use of a motor vehicle to release anger); negative body language (e.g., rigid posture, clenching of fists/jaw, hyperactivity, pacing, threatening stances); neurological impairment (e.g., positive electroencephalogram, head trauma, seizure disorders); pathological intoxication; pattern of indirect violence (e.g., tearing objects off walls, urinating/defecating on floor, stamping feet, temper tantrum, throwing objects, breaking a window, slamming doors, sexual advances); pattern of other directed violence (e.g., hitting/kicking/spitting/scratching others, throwing objects/biting someone, attempted rape, rape, sexual molestation, urinating/defecating on a person); pattern of threatening violence (e.g., verbal threats against property/people, social threats, cursing, threatening notes/gestures, sexual threats); pattern of violent anti-social behavior (e.g., stealing, insistent borrowing, insistent demands for privileges, insistent interrupting, refusal to eat/take medication, ignoring instructions); perinatal complications; prenatal complications; psychotic disorder; suicidal behavior

Client Outcomes

Client Will (Specify Time Frame)

- Stop all forms of abuse (physical, emotional, sexual; neglect; financial exploitation)
- Have cessation of abuse reported by victim
- Display no aggressive activity
- Refrain from verbal outbursts
- Refrain from violating others' personal space
- Refrain from antisocial behaviors
- Maintain relaxed body language and decreased motor activity
- Identify factors contributing to abusive/aggressive behavior
- Demonstrate impulse control or state feelings of control
- Identify impulsive behaviors
- Identify feelings/behaviors that lead to impulsive actions
- Identify consequences of impulsive actions to self or others
- Avoid high-risk environments and situations
- Identify and talk about feelings; express anger appropriately
- Express decreased anxiety and control of hallucinations as applicable
- Displace anger to meaningful activities
- Communicate needs appropriately
- Identify responsibility to maintain control
- Express empathy for victim
- Obtain no access or yield access to harmful objects
- Use alternative coping mechanisms for stress

• = Independent   ▲ = Collaborative

V

- Obtain and follow through with counseling
- Demonstrate knowledge of correct role behaviors

Victim (and Children if Applicable) Will (Specify Time Frame)

- Have safe plan for leaving situation or avoiding abuse
- Resolve depression or traumatic response

Parent Will (Specify Time Frame)

- Monitor social/play contacts
- Provide supervision and nurturing environment
- Intervene to prevent high-risk social behaviors

Nursing Interventions

Client Violence

▲ Monitor the environment, evaluate situations that could become violent, and intervene early to de-escalate the situation. Know and follow institutional policies and procedures concerning violence. Consider that family members or other staff may initiate violence in all settings. Enlist support from other staff rather than attempting to handle situations alone.

- Assess causes of aggression: social versus biological.
- Assess the client for risk factors of violence, including those in the following categories: personal history (e.g., past violent behavior, especially violent behavior in the community within 2 weeks of admission), psychiatric disorders (particularly psychoses, paranoid or bipolar disorders, substance abuse, post-traumatic stress disorder [PTSD], antisocial personality, or borderline personality disorder), neurological disorders (e.g., head injury, temporal lobe epilepsy, cardiovascular accident, dementia or senility), medical disorders (e.g., hypoxia, hypoglycemia, or hyperglycemia), psychological precursors (e.g., low tolerance for stress, impulsivity, hostility), coping difficulties (e.g., inability to plan solutions or see long-term consequences of behavior), younger age, risk of suicide, and childhood or adolescent disorders (e.g., conduct disorders, hyperactivity, autism, learning disability).
- Measures of violence may be useful in predicting or tracking behavior, and serving as outcome measures.
- Assess the client with a history of previous assaults, especially violent behavior in the community within 2 weeks of admission. Listen to

V

and acknowledge feelings of anger, observe for increased motor activity, and prepare to intervene if the client becomes aggressive.

- Assess the client for physiological signs and external signs of anger. Internal signs of anger include increased pulse rate, respiration rate, and blood pressure; chills; prickly sensations; numbness; choking sensation; nausea; and vertigo. External signs include increased muscle tone, changes in body posture (clenched fists, set jaw), eye changes (eyebrows lower and drawn together, eyelids tense, eyes assuming a "hard" appearance), lips pressed together, flushing or pallor, goose bumps, twitching, and sweating.
- Assess for the presence of hallucinations.
- Apply STAMPEDAR as an acronym for assessing the immediate potential for violence.
- Determine the presence and degree of homicidal or suicidal risk. A number of questions will elicit the necessary information: Have you been thinking about harming someone? If yes, who? How often do you have these thoughts, and how long do they last? Do you have a plan? What is it? Do you have access to the means to carry out that plan? What has kept you from hurting the person until now? Refer to the care plan for Risk for **Suicide.** Psychotherapists are required to report harm or threats of harm to another person, referred to as the "duty to warn." State laws and mental health codes should be checked to determine local mandates for threat reporting by specific health care professionals.
- Take action to minimize personal risk: use nonthreatening body language. Respect personal space and boundaries. Maintain at least an arm's length distance from the client; do not touch the client without permission (unless physical restraint is the goal). Do not allow the client to block access to an exit. If speaking with the client alone, keep the door to the room open. Be aware of where other staff is at all times. Notify other staff of where you are at all times. Take verbal threats seriously and notify other staff. Wear clothing and accessories that are not restricting and that will not be dangerous (e.g., sandals or shoes with heels can lead to twisted ankles; necklaces or dangling earrings could be grabbed). Ensure staff training to deal with violence.
- Remove potential weapons from the environment. Be prepared to remove obstructions to staff response from the environment. Search

V

the client and his or her belongings for weapons or potential weapons on admission to the hospital as appropriate.

- Inform the client of unit expectations for appropriate behavior and the consequences of not meeting these expectations. Emphasize that the client must comply with the rules of the unit. Give positive reinforcement for compliance. Increase surveillance of the hospitalized client at smoking, meal, and medication times.

- Assign a single room to the client with a potential for violence toward others. The client will be able to take time away from unit stimulation to calm self as needed. Another client will not be placed at risk as a roommate.

- Maintain a calm attitude in response to the client. Provide a low level of stimulation in the client's environment; place the client in a safe, quiet place, and speak slowly and quietly. Anxiety is contagious.

- Redirect possible violent behaviors into physical activities (e.g., walking, jogging) if the client is physically able. Using a punching bag or hitting a pillow is not indicated, because these are not calming activities and they continue patterning violent behavior. However, activities that distract while draining excess energy help build a repertoire of alternative behaviors for stress reduction.

- Provide sufficient staff if a show of force is necessary to demonstrate control to the client.

- De-escalation is the first and most important action in response to anger, hostility. Constant special observation may be implemented.

- Protect other clients in the environment from harm. Remove other individuals from the vicinity of a violent or potentially violent client. Follow safety protocols of the department. The risk of a violent client to others in the area (other clients, visitors) should be anticipated, even as efforts proceed to de-escalate the situation with the client.

- Maintain a secluded area for the client to be placed when violent. Ensure that staff are continuously present and available to client during seclusion.

▲ Recognize legal requirements that the least restrictive alternative of treatment should be used with aggressive clients. The hierarchy of intervention is as follows: promote a milieu that provides structure and calmness, with negotiation and collaboration taking precedence over control; maintain vigilance of the unit and respond to behavioral changes early; talk with client to calm and promote

• = Independent   ▲ = Collaborative

understanding of emotional state; use chemical restraints as ordered; increase to manual restraint if needed; increase to mechanical restraint and seclusion as a last resort.

▲ Use mechanical restraints if ordered and as necessary. Physical restraint can be therapeutic to keep the client and others safe.

▲ Follow the institutional protocol for releasing restraints. Observe the client closely, remain calm, and provide positive feedback as the client's behavior becomes controlled.

▲ After a violent event on a unit, debriefing and support of both staff and clients should be made available.

• Form a therapeutic alliance with the client, remaining calm, identifying the source of anger as external to both nurse and client, and using the therapeutic relationship to prevent the need for seclusion or restraint. The development of a therapeutic relationship before aggressive behavior occurs provides an alternative for working through anger and frustration. Assisting the client to identify a source of anger or frustration that is external to both the nurse and client prevents the need for defensiveness by both and directs energy at solving an external problem.

• Allow, encourage, and assist the client to verbalize feelings appropriately either one-on-one or in a group setting. Actively listen to the client; explore the source of the client's anger, and negotiate resolution when possible. Teach healthy ways to express feelings/anger, appropriate gender roles, and how to communicate needs appropriately.

• Identify with client the stimuli that initiate violence and the means of dealing with the stimuli. Have the client keep an anger diary and discuss alternative responses together. Teach cognitive behavioral techniques. Assisting the client to identify situations and people that upset him/her provides information needed for problem solving. The client may then identify alternative responses (e.g., leaving the stimulus; using relaxation techniques, such as deep breathing; initiating thought stopping; initiating a distracting activity; responding assertively rather than aggressively).

▲ Initiate and promote staff attendance at aggression management training programs.

Intimate Partner Violence (IPV)/Domestic Violence
NOTE: Before implementation of interventions in the face of domestic violence, nurses should examine their own emotional responses to abuse,

their knowledge base about abuse, and systemic elements within the emergency department (ED) to ensure that interventions will be compassionate and appropriate.

- Screen for possible abuse in women or children with a pattern of multiple injuries, particularly if any suspicion exists that the physical findings are inconsistent with the explanation of how the injuries were incurred.
▲ Report suspected child abuse to Child Protective Services. Refer women suspected of being in a spousal abuse situation to an area crisis center and provide phone number of area crisis hotline. Rapid screening tools are helpful to identify IPV. All nurses are required by law to report suspected child abuse.
- Assess for physical and mental concerns of women, including risk of HIV.
- Assist the client in negotiating the health care system and overcoming barriers.
- With women who repeatedly experience injuries from domestic violence, maintain a nonjudgmental approach and continue to offer resources/referrals. If the woman voices a willingness to leave her situation, assist with developing an emergency plan that will consider all contingencies possible (e.g., safe location, financial resources, care of children, when to leave safely). A woman in a domestic violence situation may change her mind several times before actually leaving. Proactive organization of an emergency plan helps increase the possibility that women will be able to leave safely. The most dangerous time of a domestic violence situation is when the spouse tries to leave.
- Maintain a nonjudgmental response when clients return to husbands or refuse to leave them. Women have many reasons for remaining in an abusive relationship, including economic concerns (especially with children), socialization about the woman's role, political or legal obstacles, powerlessness, and a realistic fear of retaliation or death. Refer to the care plan for **Powerlessness.** Experienced nurses working with abused women define success as client personal growth over time, rather than the woman leaving the relationship.
- Focus on providing support, ensuring safety, and promoting self-efficacy while encouraging disclosure about IPV events.

• = Independent   ▲ = Collaborative

- Screen pregnant women for the potential for domestic violence during pregnancy, especially in teenage pregnancies.
- Women with physical or mental disabilities require extended assessment, including a comprehensive functional assessment, with attention to cultural issues, the nature of the disability, and needed resources. Women with disabilities may experience abuse from multiple sources, and particular attention should be paid to the additional emotional stressors present. Difficulties leaving home, physical needs that shelter may not be able to accommodate, and the undesirability of nursing home placement are just a few stressors. Personal assistance providers may be abusive or take advantage financially.
▲ Referral for spiritual counseling may be considered, but be aware that clergy vary in their helpfulness.
- Identify risk factors such as ongoing mental illness of a parent, and monitor family closely.
- Be aware that IPV may arise or continue under circumstances of medical illness.
- Consider risk versus benefit when deciding if, when, and in how great a depth to explore client responses to abuse or violence.
▲ When spouse or child abuse accompanies substance abuse, refer the abusive client to a substance abuse treatment program. Refer the spouse receiving abuse to Al-Anon and the children to Alateen.
▲ When an adult reveals a history of unresolved/untreated sexual abuse as a child, referral to a local Adults Molested as Children (AMAC) group may be helpful. Refer to the care plans for Risk for **Suicide, Self-Mutilation,** and Risk for **Self-Mutilation.**
▲ Referral of women for psychiatric/psychological treatment or parenting classes should be considered as an appropriate intervention.
▲ Referral of children for psychiatric/psychological treatment should be considered as an appropriate intervention.
▲ Refer to batterer intervention programs that are often available and may be court mandated.

Social Violence

- Assess for acute stress disorder (ASD) and PTSD among victims of violence.

▲ Assess the support network of women who become victims of violent crime and refer for appropriate levels of assistance. Of particular concern would be women who do not have family or friends to provide support or who have difficulty accessing other types of assistance.

• Be aware that hate crime is increasing, particularly toward gay and transgendered individuals, and it requires support and advocacy for victims.

▲ Victims of violence seen in the ED should receive an assessment for needed services and assignment to case management.

Rape-Trauma Syndrome

• Assist client to cope with potential stalking activity.

• Approach client with sensitivity.

▲ Monitor for paradoxical drug reactions, and report any to the health care provider. Violent behavior can be stimulated by a medication intended to calm the client.

• Assess for brain insults, such as recent falls or injuries, strokes, or transient ischemic attacks. Clients with brain injuries may respond to stimulus control, problem solving, social skills training, relaxation training, and anger management to reduce aggressive behaviors. Brain injuries, lowered impulse control, and reduced coping can cause violent reactions to self or others. Brain injury symptoms may be mistaken for mental illness.

• Decrease environmental stimuli if violence is directed at others. Removal of the client to a quiet area can reduce violent impulses. Use a calm voice to "talk down" the client.

• Assess holistic needs of the client.

• Discuss with client her wishes regarding use of an emergency contraceptive.

Pediatric

• Assess for predictors of anger that can lead to violent behavior.

• Be alert for both shaken baby syndrome and exposure of children to violence.

• Pregnant teens should be assessed for abuse, particularly if they are with an older partner.

▲ In the case of child abuse or neglect, refer for early childhood home visitation.

• = Independent   ▲ = Collaborative

Geriatric

▲ If abuse or neglect of an older client is suspected, report the suspicion to an adult protective services agency with jurisdiction over the geographical area where the client lives.

- Be alert to the potential for elder abuse in clients, including the possibility of psychological abuse.
- Assess for presence or client history of mental illness or treatment.
- Assess and observe for aggressive behavior in older clients at long-term care facilities.
- Observe clients for dementia and delirium.
- Be aware of laws and regulations in the appropriate jurisdiction where client is located.
- Document and record suspected elder abuse according to mandatory regulations.
- Apart from mandated requirements, abide by the older client's wishes regarding action to be taken in response to abuse. Avoid interventions that increase the risk of abuse.
- Develop a safety plan and provide referrals to all relevant agencies or services.

Multicultural

- Exercise cultural competence when dealing with domestic violence.
- Identify and respond to unique needs of immigrant women who experience IPV.
- Assist with acculturation and activating social support.

Home Care

- Be alert to the potential for violent behavior in the home setting. Respond to verbal aggression with interventions to de-escalate negative emotional states. Violence is a process that can be recognized early. De-escalation involves reducing client stressors, responding to the client with respect, acknowledging the client's feeling state, and assisting the client to regain control. If de-escalation does not work, the nurse should leave the home.
- Assess family members or caregivers for their ability to protect the client and themselves. The safety of the client between home visits is a nursing priority. Caregivers often need assistance with recognizing or admitting fear of or danger from a loved one.
- Include an initial and ongoing assessment and evaluation of potential abuse and neglect. Photograph evidence of abuse or neglect when possible. Refer to the care plan for **Powerlessness.**

V

▲ If neglect or abuse is suspected, identify an emergency plan that addresses the problem immediately, ensures client safety, and includes a report to the appropriate authorities. Discuss when to use hotlines and 911. Role-play access to emergency resources with the client and caregivers.

• Encourage appropriate safety behaviors in abused women; call the client at intervals during a 6-month period to determine whether safety behaviors are being carried out.

• Assess the home environment for harmful objects. Have the family remove or lock objects as able.

▲ Refer for homemaker or psychiatric home health care services for respite, client reassurance, and implementation of a therapeutic regimen. Responsibility for a person who may become violent provides high caregiver stress. Respite decreases caregiver stress. The presence of caring individuals is reassuring to both the client and caregivers, especially during periods of client anxiety. Individuals exhibiting violent behaviors can respond to the interventions described previously, modified for the home setting.

▲ If the client is taking psychotropic medications, assess client and family knowledge of medication and its administration and side effects. Teach as necessary. Knowledge of the medical regimen supports compliance.

▲ Evaluate effectiveness and side effects of medications. Accurate clinical feedback improves the health care provider's ability to prescribe an effective medical regimen specific to a client's needs.

• If client displays mildly intensifying aggressive behavior, attempt to diffuse anger or violence (e.g., ask for a glass of water to distract client). Later in the visit, explain that aggressive behavior is not acceptable and present consequences of continued aggressive behavior (i.e., right of agency to discontinue services).

• Document all acts or verbalizations of aggression. Safety of the staff is a primary responsibility of home health agencies. Law enforcement intervention may be necessary.

▲ If client verbalizes or displays threatening behavior, notify your supervisor and plan to make joint visits with another staff person or a security escort.

• If the client's behavior is not overtly threatening but makes the nurse uncomfortable, a meeting may be held outside the home in sight of others (e.g., front porch).

• = Independent   ▲ = Collaborative

- Never enter a home or remain in a home if aggression threatens your well-being.
▲ Never challenge a show of force, such as a gun threat. Leave and notify your supervisor and the appropriate authorities. Document the incident.
▲ If client behaviors intensify, refer for immediate mental health intervention. The degree of disturbance and ability to manage care safely at home determines the level of services needed to protect the client.

Client/Family Teaching and Discharge Planning
- Instruct victims of IPV in the dynamics and prognosis of domestic violence behavior, as well as the effect on children who witness or are victims of domestic violence.
- Teach relaxation and exercise as ways to release anger and deal with stress.
- Teach cognitive behavioral activities, such as active problem solving, reframing (reappraising the situation from a different perspective), or thought stopping (in response to a negative thought, picture a large stop sign and replace the image with a prearranged positive alternative). Teach the client to confront his or her own negative thought patterns (or cognitive distortions), such as catastrophizing (expecting the very worst), dichotomous thinking (perceiving events in only one of two opposite categories), magnification (placing distorted emphasis on a single event), or unrealistic expectations (e.g., "should get what I want when I want it").
▲ Refer to individual or group therapy.
- Teach the adolescent client violence prevention, and encourage him/her to become involved in community service activities. School programs that couple community service with classroom health instruction can have a measurable effect on violent behaviors of young adolescents at high risk for being both the perpetrators and victims of peer violence. Community service programs may be a valuable part of multicomponent violence prevention programs.
- Teach the use of appropriate community resources in emergency situations (e.g., hotline, community mental health agency, ED, 911 in most places in the United States, the toll-free National Domestic Violence Hotline [1-800-799-SAFE]). Internet resources are increasing and should be made available to clients. It is necessary to get immediate help when violence occurs.

V

• = Independent   ▲ = Collaborative

- Encourage the use of self-help groups in nonemergency situations.
- Inform the client and family about any applicable medication actions, side effects, target symptoms, and toxic reactions.

Risk for self-directed Violence
NANDA-I Definition

Vulnerable to behaviors in which an individual demonstrates that he or she can be physically, emotionally, and/or sexually harmful to self

Risk Factors

Age ≥45 years; age 15 to 19 years; behavioral cues (e.g., writing forlorn love notes, directing angry messages at a significant other who has rejected the person, giving away personal items, taking out a large life insurance policy); conflict about sexual orientation; conflict in interpersonal relationships; employment concern (e.g., unemployed, recent job loss/failure); engagement in autoerotic sexual acts; history of multiple suicide attempts; insufficient personal resources (e.g., achievement, insight, affect unavailable and poorly controlled); marital status (e.g., single, widowed, divorced); mental health issue (e.g., depression, psychosis, personality disorder, substance abuse); occupation (e.g., executive, administrator/owner of business, professional, semi-skilled worker); pattern of difficulties in family background (e.g., chaotic or conflictual, history of suicide); physical health issue; psychological disorder; social isolation; suicidal ideation; suicidal plan; verbal cues (e.g., talking about death, "better off without me," asking about lethal dosage of medication)

Client Outcomes, Nursing Interventions, and Client/Family Teaching and Discharge Planning

Refer to care plans for Risk for **Suicide, Self-Mutilation,** and Risk for **Self-Mutilation.**

Impaired Walking
NANDA-I Definition

Limitation of independent movement within the environment on foot

Defining Characteristics

Impaired ability to climb stairs; impaired ability to navigate curbs; impaired ability to walk on decline; impaired ability to walk on incline; impaired ability to walk on uneven surface; impaired ability to walk required distance

• = Independent   ▲ = Collaborative

Related Factors

Alteration in cognitive functioning; alteration in mood; decrease in endurance; environmental barriers (e.g., stairs, inclines, uneven surfaces, obstacles, distances, lack of assistive device); fear of falling; impaired balance; impaired vision; insufficient knowledge of mobility strategies; insufficient muscle strength; musculoskeletal impairment; neuromuscular impairment; obesity; pain; physical deconditioning

Client Outcomes

Client Will (Specify Time Frame)

- Demonstrate optimal independence and safety in walking
- Demonstrate the ability to direct others on how to assist with walking
- Demonstrate the ability to properly and safely use and care for assistive walking devices

Nursing Interventions

- Progressively mobilize clients (e.g., gradual elevation of head of bed [HOB], sitting in reclined chair, standing).
- Assist clients to apply orthosis, immobilizers, splints, and braces as prescribed before walking.
- Apply thromboembolic deterrent stockings (TEDs) and/or elastic leg wraps; raise HOB slowly in small increments to sitting; have clients move feet/legs up and down then stand slowly; avoid prolonged standing.
- Carefully monitor blood pressure of older adults at least from 30 to 90 minutes after meals before walking. There are significant differences in systolic and diastolic pressure over time, with the biggest drop in systolic and diastolic blood pressure occurring at 45 minutes after a meal (Son & Lee, 2012; Lee, 2013).
- Maintain partial head elevation when resting in bed to help decrease orthostatic hypotension.
- Compare morning lying/sitting/standing blood pressures. If systolic pressure falls 20 mm Hg or diastolic pressure falls 10 mm Hg from lying to standing within 3 minutes, and/or if lightheadedness, dizziness, syncope, or unexplained falls occur, consult a health care provider (Lee, 2013).
- Detection of orthostatic hypotension is key to fall prevention.
- ▲ Implement thromboembolism prophylaxis/treatment as prescribed (e.g., anticoagulants, antiembolic stockings, elastic leg wraps, sequential compression devices, feet/ankle exercises, and hydration). Refer to care plan for Ineffective peripheral **Tissue Perfusion.**

• = Independent   ▲ = Collaborative

- Reinforce correct use of prescribed mobility devices and remind clients of weight-bearing restrictions. Canes provide stability in persons with hemiparesis; canes are prescribed to improve gait and balance and to alleviate joint pain and are usually used on the contralateral side of the affected limb.
  - ○ Teach clients with leg amputations to correctly don stump socks, liner, and immediate postoperative prostheses or traditional prosthesis before standing/walking.
  - ○ Teach client importance of avoiding prolonged hip and knee flexion. If contractures occur, the client may have difficulty with prosthesis fit and use.
- Emphasize the importance of wearing properly fitting, low-heeled shoes with nonskid soles, and socks/hose, and of seeking medical care for foot pain or problems with abnormal toenails, corns, calluses, or diabetes.
- Use a snug gait belt with handles and assistive devices while walking clients, as recommended by the physical therapist (PT).
- Walk clients frequently with an appropriate number of people; have one team member state short, simple motor instructions.
- Cue and manually guide clients with unilateral neglect to prevent clients from bumping into objects/people.
- Document the number of helpers, level of assistance (e.g., maximum, standby), type of assistance, and devices needed on the care plan and room white board (if used).
- Take pulse rate/rhythm and pulse oximetry before walking clients, and reassess within 5 minutes of walking, then ongoing as needed. If either is abnormal, have the client sit 5 minutes, then reassess. If still abnormal, walk clients more slowly and with more help or for a shorter time or notify the health care provider.
- If uncontrolled diabetes/angina/arrhythmias/tachycardia ($\geq$100 bpm) or resting systolic blood pressure $\geq$200 mm Hg or diastolic blood pressure $\geq$110 mm Hg occur, do not initiate walking exercise without consulting the health care prescriber.

Refer to the care plan for **Activity** intolerance.

- Perform initial/ongoing screening for risk of falling and perform postfall assessments including medications and lab results to prevent further falls.
- Individualize interventions to prevent falls, e.g., scheduled toileting, monitored rooms, bed alarms, wheelchair alarms, balance/strength

W

• = Independent   ▲ = Collaborative

training, sleep hygiene, education on risk of medication/alcohol use, removal of hazards, and attention to safe handling during any transfers, wound care, toileting, showering/bathing (Cohen et al, 2010).

Geriatric

▲ Assess for swaying, poor balance, weakness, and fear of falling while older adults stand/walk. If present, refer to PT.

▲ Review medications for polypharmacy and those that place older adults at risk for falls; consult with pharmacy as needed. More than five drugs indicates polypharmacy and puts the client at risk for adverse drug reactions, drug-drug interactions, and overall low adherence to drug therapy due to too many drugs to take (Hovstadius et al, 2010).

▲ Encourage an exercise component such as tai chi, physical therapy, or other exercise for balance, gait, and strength training in group programs or at home; modify environment for safety; recommend vision assessment for corrective lenses and consideration for cataract removal; conduct polypharmacy assessment with special consideration to sedatives, antidepressants, and drugs affecting the central nervous system; evaluate for orthostatic hypotension and dysrhythmia; recommend vitamin D supplementation of 800 IU per day (National Institutes of Health, 2014).

• Assess fall risk, then implement fall precautions, such as clearing obstacles, reviewing medications, and using a visual identifier on clients starting exercise/education programs.

Home Care

▲ Establish a support system for emergency and contingency care (e.g., remote monitoring, emergency call system, alert local EMS).

▲ Assess for and modify any barriers to walking in the home environment to promote safety.

▲ Obtain prescription for PT home visits for individualized strength, balance retraining, and an exercise plan.

▲ Make referrals for home health services for support and assistance with activities of daily living (ADLs). This is a key component of discharge planning. Listen to and support client/caregivers; refer to support groups that meet or are online. Refer to care plan for **Caregiver Role Strain.**

W

• = Independent ▲ = Collaborative

Client/Family Teaching and Discharge Planning

- Teach clients to check ambulation devices weekly for cracks, loose nuts, or worn tips; clean dust and dirt on tips; remove all items from stairways; be certain hand rails are strong and secure; position furniture to allow a 36-inch-wide unobstructed pathway when possible; and remove electrical cords or loose objects from walking paths (Boelens et al, 2013).
- Teach clients with diabetes that they are at risk for foot ulcers and train them in preventive interventions.
- Instruct anyone at risk for osteoporosis or hip fractures to bear weight, walk, engage in resistance exercise (with appropriate adjustments for conditions), take good nutrition, especially adequate intake of calcium and vitamin D, stop smoking, monitor alcohol intake, and consult a health care provider for antiresorptive therapy.
- For more information, refer to the care plans for Impaired **Transfer** ability and Impaired wheelchair **Mobility.**

Wandering

NANDA-I Definition

Meandering; aimless or repetitive locomotion that exposes the individual to harm; frequently incongruent with boundaries, limits, or obstacles

Defining Characteristics

Continuous movement from place to place; eloping behavior; frequent movement from place to place; fretful locomotion; haphazard locomotion; hyperactivity; impaired ability to locate landmarks in a familiar setting; locomotion into unauthorized spaces; locomotion resulting in getting lost; locomotion that cannot be easily dissuaded; long periods of locomotion without an apparent destination; pacing; periods of locomotion interspersed with periods of non-locomotion (e.g., sitting, standing, sleeping); persistent locomotion in search of something; scanning behavior; searching behavior; shadowing a caregiver's locomotion; trespassing

Related Factors (r/t)

Alteration in cognitive functioning; cortical atrophy; overstimulating environment; physiological state (e.g., hunger, thirst, pain, need to urinate); premorbid behavior (e.g., outgoing, sociable personality); psychological disorder; sedation; separation from familiar environment; time of day

Client Outcomes

Client Will (Specify Time Frame)

- Maintain psychological well-being and reduce any felt need to wander
- Decrease the amount of time getting lost
- Engage in meaningful activities daily
- Remain safe and free from falls and elopement
- Maintain physical activity and remain comfortable and free of pain
- Maintain appropriate body weight and be well nourished and well hydrated
- Be physically well rested and demonstrate absence of fatigue

Caregiver Will (Specify Time Frame)

- Be able to explain interventions he/she can use to provide a safe environment for a care receiver who displays wandering behavior
- Develop strategies to reduce caregiver stress levels

Nursing Interventions

Acute Care Hospital: Wandering

- Screen clients with cognitive impairment at the time of admission and when the client is transferred to another unit in the hospital. Assess for concerns that the client will wander from family members and health care professionals. In addition, assess for the client's ability to walk independently or with minimal assistance.
- If the client is at risk for wandering in the hospital setting, the following interventions may be implemented: dress the client in a brightly colored hospital gown that is easily identifiable, provide appropriate supervision and surveillance of the at-risk client, identify in the chart (electronic record) the client's risk for wandering, discuss with the client and family the risks of wandering, set up appropriate alarm systems, consult with geriatric or mental health advanced practice nurse regarding wandering risks and individualized interventions, and have a current client photograph on file to help with identification in case the client leaves unattended.

Nursing Care Facilities: Wandering

- Assess and document the amount (frequency and duration), percentage of hours with wandering, and 24-hour distribution of wandering behavior over 3 days.
- Assess and document the quantity and qualities of wandering behaviors (e.g., persistent walking, repetitive walking, eloping behaviors, spatial disorientation, goal directed, negative outcomes).

W

• = Independent   ▲ = Collaborative

- Obtain a history of personality characteristics and behavioral responses to stress.
- Evaluate for neurocognitive strengths and limitations, particularly language, attention, and visuospatial skills.
- Assess for level of cognitive and emotional status and age.
- Assess for changes in cognition and signs and symptoms of medical illness such as pneumonia or cardiovascular disease.
- Assess and monitor for drug-induced akathisia (motor restlessness).
- Discontinue use of medications and physical restraints that are used for the sole purpose of controlling wandering behavior.
- Assess for emotional or psychological distress, such as anxiety, fear, or feeling lost.
- Assess for physical distress or unmet needs (e.g., hunger, thirst, pain discomfort, elimination) with the Need-Driven Dementia-Compromised Behaviors (NDB) model.
- Observe wandering episodes for antecedents and consequences.
- Observe the location where and environmental conditions in which wandering is occurring and modify those that appear to induce wandering.
- Assess regularly for the presence of or potential for negative outcomes of wandering (e.g., elopement, declining social skills, onset of falls, becoming lost, and injuries).
- Weigh the client at defined intervals to detect onset of weight loss, and watch for symptoms associated with inadequate food intake, including constipation, dehydration, muscle wasting, and starvation.

- For the client who displays wandering behavior during mealtimes, use behavioral interventions to shape behavior, including verbal statements, nonverbal social behavior, and systematic extinguishing of undesirable client behavior.
- Provide for safe ambulation with comfortable and well-fitting clothes, shoes with nonskid soles and foot support, and any necessary walking aids (e.g., a cane or walker).
- Refer to physical therapy for core therapeutic exercise, balance, gait, and assistive device training.
- Provide safe and secure surroundings that deter accidental elopements, using perimeter control devices or electronic tracking systems.
- There are ethical concerns in the use of tracking technologies.

• = Independent   ▲ = Collaborative

- During periods of inactivity, position the wanderer so that desirable destinations (e.g., bathroom) are within the client's line of vision and undesirable destinations (e.g., exits or stairwells) are out of sight.
- Facilitate way-finding through therapeutic environmental design.
- Enhance the physical environment by increasing visual appeal and provide interesting views and opportunities to sit.
- Engage wanderers in social interaction and structured activity such as painting or coloring, especially when wanderers appear distressed or otherwise uncomfortable, or their wandering presents a challenge to others in the setting.
- Provide headphones and iPod with individualized preferred music while the person with dementia is wandering, or encourage the person to participate in a music group.
- If wandering has a pacing quality, attempt to identify and address any underlying problems or concerns. Offer stress-reducing approaches, such as music, massage, or rocking. Attempts to distract or redirect the pacing wanderer may worsen wandering.
- Provide a regularly scheduled and supervised exercise or walking program, particularly if wandering occurs excessively during the night or at times that are inconvenient in the setting.
- Use soft tactile hand massage before the times of day or events that induce wandering.

Multicultural

- Recognize that wandering occurs with little variation in expression among individuals with dementia regardless of culture or ethnicity.
- Assess for the influence of cultural beliefs, norms, and values on the family's understanding of wandering behavior.
- ▲ Refer the family to social services or other supportive services to assist with the impact of caregiving for the wandering client.
- Encourage the family to use support groups or other service programs.

Home Care

- Help the caregiver set up a plan to deal with wandering behavior using the interventions mentioned earlier.
- Assess the home environment for modifications that will protect the client and prevent elopement.
- Assist the family to set up a plan of exercise for the client, including safe walking.

W

• = Independent   ▲ = Collaborative

- Enroll wanderers in the Safe Return Program of the Alzheimer's Association, and help the caregiver develop a plan of action to use if the client elopes.
- Help the caregiver develop a plan of action to use if the client elopes.
- Refer for homemaker or psychiatric home health care services for respite, client reassurance, and implementation of a therapeutic regimen. Refer to the care plan for **Caregiver Role Strain.**

Client/Family Teaching and Discharge Planning

- Use a broad range of descriptions for the term "wandering" to enhance caregivers' understanding.
- Inform the client and family of the meaning of and reasons for wandering behavior. An understanding of wandering behavior will enable the client and family to provide the client with a safe environment.
- Teach the caregiver/family methods to deal with wandering behavior using the interventions mentioned in nursing interventions.

Nursing Care Plans for Hearing Loss and Vision Loss

Hearing Loss

Definition

A condition where there is the inability to detect some or all frequencies of sound and may involve complete or partial impairment of the ability to hear

NOTE: **Hearing Loss** is not a NANDA-I accepted diagnosis but is included here because of the frequency of occurrence of hearing loss, especially in the geriatric population.

Defining Characteristics

Inability to hear in noisy environments; difficulty following conversations with more than one person; change in speech; change in usual response to stimuli; disorientation; impaired communication; irritability; poor concentration; restlessness; sensory distortions

Related Factors (r/t)

Altered sensory integration; altered sensory reception; altered sensory transmission; biochemical imbalance; electrolyte imbalance; excessive noise exposure; psychological stress

Client Outcomes

Client Will (Specify Time Frame)

- Demonstrate understanding by a verbal, written, or signed response
- Demonstrate relaxed body movements and facial expressions
- Explain plan to modify lifestyle to accommodate hearing impairment
- Demonstrate familiarity with hearing assistive devices

Nursing Interventions

- Observe for signs of hearing loss, especially in people exposed to loud noise and people older than 60 years.
- Use the National Institutes of Health (NIH) Toolbox to test hearing as available.

- Recognize that certain populations are especially vulnerable to noise-induced hearing loss, including farmers, industrial workers, firefighters, construction workers, musicians, and music lovers using personal listening devices.
▲ Refer to otolaryngologist and/or audiologist.
- Keep background noise to a minimum. Turn off the television and radio when communicating with the client. If in a noisy environment, take the client to a private room and shut the door.
- Stand or sit directly in front of the client when communicating. Make sure adequate light is on the nurse's face, avoid chewing gum or covering mouth or face with hands while speaking, establish eye contact, and use nonverbal gestures.
- Speak clearly in lower voice tones if possible. Do not overenunciate or shout at the client.
- Verify that the client understands critical information by asking the client to repeat the information.
- If necessary, provide a communication board, personnel who know sign language, or any method helpful to increase understanding for the hearing impaired client.
- Prepare pictures or diagrams depicting tests or procedures; have books with relevant pictures available for more detailed discussions.
- Watch for signs of depression such as withdrawal, impaired sleep, or flat affect, and refer for treatment if needed.
- Encourage the client to wear a hearing aid if available.
- Recognize that clients with a hearing aid may choose to wear the hearing aid intermittently because hearing aids can create distortion of speech and extraneous noise that is bothersome (Shah & Lotke, 2013).

Critical Care

- Develop a communication cart to foster communication with hearing impaired clients. Contents can include spiral notebooks, felt tip markers, clipboards, communication boards (picture, word, whole phrases, alphabet), hearing aid batteries, and electronic speech generators.
- Develop good communication skills to interact with hearing impaired clients. It is unfair to expect critically ill older adults to understand what is being said to them only through auditory means.

• = Independent　　　　▲ = Collaborative

Pediatric

▲ Refer infants or children for hearing tests as indicated so that treatment/therapy begins early as needed.

- In the child, recommend parents watch for signs of hearing loss including worsening speech or school performance, withdrawal from social activities, playing alone, and playing the television and music increasingly louder (Shah & Lotke, 2013).

- Refer the child to the use of a language wizard player with Baldi, a computer-animated tutor for teaching vocabulary.

- Recognize that children who are deaf or hard of hearing are particularly vulnerable to abuse, both by parents/caregivers and by sexual predators (Shah & Lotke, 2013).

- Recommend that teenagers avoid use of personal listening devices, or try to keep the volume down. Use culturally appropriate teaching materials.

Geriatric

▲ Routinely screen geriatric clients for presence of hearing loss because up to two thirds of all people 70 or older have a hearing loss (Bainbridge & Wallhagen, 2014).

▲ Inspect the ear canal for wax buildup.

- Work with the client to ensure contact with others and maintenance of meaningful activities to strengthen the social network and maintain cognitive abilities.

Home Care

- The previously listed interventions are applicable in the home care setting.

- Recommend that the client change the home environment if needed for better acoustics. Avoid glossy walls, high and reflective ceilings, reflective glass counters, and tiled floors. Use acoustic paneling if needed.

- Suggest installation of devices such as strobe lights for the telephone; alarm clock, fire alarms, and doorbell; sensors that detect an infant's cry; alarm clocks that vibrate the bed; and closed caption decoders for television sets. Other helpful devices include telephone amplifiers, speakerphones, cell phones with text messaging or instant messaging, pocket talker personal listening systems, and FM and infrared amplification systems that connect directly to a TV or audio output jack. Also available is a telecommunication device, a typewriter keyboard with an alphanumeric display that allows the hearing

• = Independent   ▲ = Collaborative

impaired person to send typed messages over the telephone line. Use of hearing ear dogs (dogs specially trained to alert their owners to specific sounds) may also be helpful.

Client/Family Teaching and Discharge Planning

- Teach client to avoid excessive noise at work or at home and to wear hearing protection when necessary.
- Teach the client to avoid inserting objects such as cotton-tipped swabs or bobby pins into the ears.

Vision Loss

Definition

Decreased or absence of vision when it existed previously; vision loss can be either acute in onset or occur as a slow progressive chronic visual loss

NOTE: **Vision Loss** is not a NANDA-I nursing diagnosis. The authors have identified this health problem because vision loss is commonly seen in nursing practice.

Defining Characteristics

Change in behavior pattern; change in problem-solving abilities; disorientation; decreased visual acuity; loss of vision; visual hallucinations

Related Factors

Aging; diabetes mellitus; exposure to UV light; impaired visual function; impaired visual integration; impaired visual reception; impaired visual transmission; nutritional deficiency

(Adapted from the work of NANDA-I)

Client Outcomes

Client Will (Specify Time Frame)

- Demonstrate relaxed body movements and facial expressions
- Remain as independent as possible
- Explain plan to modify lifestyle to accommodate visual impairment
- Incorporate use of lighting to maximize visual abilities
- Demonstrate familiarity with vision assistive devices
- Remain free of physical harm resulting from loss of vision

Nursing Interventions

- Identify yourself immediately whenever you enter the client's area.
- Provide environmental predictability. Consistently remind staff, family members, and visitors to tell the client when something is added or removed from the environment.

• = Independent ▲ = Collaborative

- Assist with feeding at mealtimes if blindness is temporary.
- Keep side rails up using half rails; maintain bed in a low position.
- Converse with and touch the client frequently during care if frequent touch is within the client's cultural norm.
- Walk the client by having the client grasp nurse's elbow or shoulder and walk partially behind nurse.
- Walk a frightened or confused client by having the client place both hands on the nurse's shoulders or waist. Then have the nurse backs up in the desired direction while holding the client around the waist. This method helps the client feel secure and ensures safety.
- Keep the call light within the client's reach; check location of call light before leaving the room.
- Provide good lighting in rooms, task lights, and night lights.
- Make doorframes and light switches a contrasting color to the walls.
- Ensure access to eyeglasses or magnifying devices as needed. Vision aid devices include readers, microscopes, handheld magnifiers, and stand magnifiers (Ventocilla, 2013).
- Encourage expression of feelings and expect grieving behavior if onset of blindness is new. Blind people grieve the loss of vision and experience a loss of identity and control over their lives.
- Recommend client have vision evaluated by an optometrist or ophthalmologist as appropriate to determine whether an improvement in visual acuity is possible.
- Question the client regarding the presence of visual hallucinations. If present, reassure the client that the experience is common and does not mean he or she has a mental illness. It is helpful for the client to know that this is common and usually does not require treatment.
- Provide a CD player, radio, or books on tape as desired. These provide sensory stimulation and can help deal with the boredom of hospitalization.
- Take protective measures to prevent falls. Refer to the care plan for Risk for **Falls.**
- Explore and enhance available support systems to ensure a safe discharge. Caregivers and/or family members may not have the ability to assist the client after discharge. See care plan for Risk for **Injury** or Risk for **Falls.**
- Assess the client's visual and other sensory loss using valid and reliable tools.

- Encourage the client to implement lifestyle strategies that promote avoidance of cardiovascular disease and diabetes to prevent vision loss.

Multicultural

- Consider race/ethnicity as a possible related factor to vision loss.

Geriatric

- Keep environment quiet, soothing, and familiar. Use consistent caregivers. These measures are comforting to older adults with a sensory loss and help decrease confusion (Lawrence, 2011).
- Increase the amount of light in the environment for older eyes; ensure it is nonglare lighting.
- ▲ Determine origin of vision loss if possible.
- Cataract is a leading cause of reversible vision impairment and may increase the risk for falls in older adults.
- Hearing and vision rehabilitation services need to screen for dual sensory impairment.
- ▲ Refer to a comprehensive vision rehabilitation center early in the disease process of macular degeneration to prevent some of the negative consequences of vision loss (Maturi, 2011).
- Teach the client methods to preserve remaining vision as much as possible, including not smoking or breathing second-hand smoke, protecting the eyes from sunlight, and including fish and leafy green vegetables in the diet (Maturi, 2011).
- Vision impairment is independently associated with malnutrition.
- Monitor for signs of new onset of increased vision loss, such as not recognizing familiar people, difficulty seeing in bright light or low light, new problems with reading, the client complains of tired eyes and/or verbalizes vision problems with current glasses facilitating effective vision (Ventocilla, 2013).
- Age-related visual problems can also occur with stroke (Pollock et al, 2011). If vision loss is from a stroke, watch for hemianopia, an ability to see to one side only. Encourage clients to scan environment by turning head from side to side. Also assess for visual spatial misconception.
- ▲ Refer client to low-vision clinics or independent living programs, which are designed for individuals who are vision impaired or blind to help maintain independence.
- Work with the client to ensure contact with others, to maintain meaningful activities, and to strengthen the social network.

• = Independent   ▲ = Collaborative

- Watch for signs of depression: decreased appetite, withdrawal from usual life activities, flat affect, excessive time in bed, and somatization.
- For the client with both vision loss and dementia, provide nursing care including:
  - Recognize that vision loss can increase problems for the client with dementia, including decreased orientation, decreased recognition of others, less recall, impaired judgment, and possibly aggression (Barrand, 2011).
  - Use one-to-one conversations to maintain socialization.
  - Obtain and use visual aids to help maintain orientation and contact with the environment, including such things as talking clocks, speaking Freeview digital boxes to give an auditory version of what is on the television, and use of memory photo dial pads so that clients can use the telephone to maintain contact with others (Barrand, 2011).

Home Care

- Most of the listed interventions are applicable in the home care setting.
- Monitor home care clients for recent visual loss and resulting decrease in social activity.
- Enable the visually impaired client to do things for himself/herself to maintain independence as long as possible (Cattan, 2011).

Client/Family Teaching and Discharge Planning
Low Vision

- Use contrast to increase visibility of items; for example, place a dark background around the light switch so that it can be located more easily.
- Place red, yellow, or orange identifiers on important items that need to be seen, such as a red strip at the edge of steps, red behind a light switch, or a red dot on a stove or washing machine to indicate how far to turn knob, or use a dial marker that will offer a tactile cue to the client to turn on ovens, stoves, and washing machines.
- Use a watch or clock that verbally tells time, and a phone with large numerals and emergency numbers programmed into it (Ventocilla et al, 2013).
- Teach blind clients how to feed self; associate food on plate with hours on a clock so that the client can identify location of food.

- Use low-vision aids including magnifying devices for near vision and telescopes for seeing objects at a distance, a closed-circuit television that magnifies print, and guides for writing checks and envelopes.
- Teach the client with vision loss to do the following:
  - Use a magnifying mirror to shave or apply makeup. Use an electric razor only.
  - Put personal care products in brightly colored pump containers (red, yellow, or orange) for identification.
  - Use tactile clues such as safety pins or buttons placed in hems to help client match clothing. Or place matching outfits of clothing in separate plastic bags.
  - Use a prefilled medication organizer with large lettering or three-dimensional markers.
- Increase lighting in the home to help vision in the following ways:
  - Ensure adequate illumination of the entire home, add light fixtures and increase wattage of existing bulbs as needed.
  - Decrease glare; where light reflects on shiny surfaces, move or cover object.
  - Use nonglare wax on the floor.
  - Use motion lights that turn on automatically when a person enters the room for nighttime use.
  - Add indoor strip or "runway"-type lighting to baseboards.
- ▲ Refer the client to an occupational therapist for assistance in dealing with vision loss and learning how to meet personal needs to maintain maximum independence.
- Encourage the client to wear a hat and sunglasses when out in the sun.
- Work with the client to find rewarding recreational pursuits.

BIBLIOGRAPHY

Aderinto-Adike, A. O., & Quigley, E. M. (2014). Gastrointestinal motility problems in critical care: a clinical perspective. *J Dig Dis, 15*(7), 335–344.

Aitola, P., et al. (2010). Prevalence of fecal incontinence in adults aged 30 years or more in general population. *Colorect Dis, 12*(7), 687–691.

Allen, L. A., Stevenson, L. W., Grady, K. L., et al. (2012). Decision making in advanced heart failure: a scientific statement from the American Heart Association. *Circulation, 125*, 1928–1952.

Allison, J., & George, M. (2014). Using preoperative assessment and patient instruction to improve patient safety. *AORN, 99*(3), 364–375.

American Academy of Audiology. *How's your hearing?* From <http://www.howsyourhearing.org>, retrieved July 13, 2011.

American Academy of Nursing's Expert Panel on Acute and Critical Care. (2012). *Reducing functional decline in older adults during hospitalization: A best practice approach*, Issue Number 31. Retrieved from <http://consult gerirn.org/uploads/File/trythis/try_this_31.pdf>.

American Academy of Ophthalmology (AAO). (2013). Dry eye syndrome preferred practice patterns—2013. *The Ophthalmic News and Education Network*. Retrieved from <http://one.aao.org/preferred-practice-pattern/dry-eye-syndrome-ppp–2013>.

American Academy of Pediatrics (AAP). (2014a). *Preventing SIDS*. Retrieved from <http://www.healthychildren.org/English/ages-stages/baby/sleep/Pages/Preventing-SIDS.aspx>.

American Academy of Pediatrics (AAP). (2014b). *Winter safety tips*. Retrieved from <http://www.aap.org/en-us/about-the-aap/aap-press-room/news-features-and-safety-tips/Pages/Winter-Safety-Tips.aspx>.

American Association of Poison Control Centers. (2014). *Health Care Providers*. Retrieved from <http://www.aapcc.org/prevention/health-care-providers/>.

American College of Sports Medicine (ACSM). (2009). Progression models in resistance training for healthy adults. *Med Sci Sports Exerc, 41*(3), 687–708.

American College of Sports Medicine (ACSM). (2011). Quantity and quality of exercise for developing and maintaining cardiorespiratory, musculoskeletal, and neuromotor fitness in apparently healthy adults: guidance for prescribing exercise. *Med Sci Sports Exerc, 43*(7), 1334–1359.

American College of Sports Medicine (ACSM). (2011). *Selecting and effectively using a walking program*. From <http://www.acsm.org/docs/brochures/>, retrieved Sept. 20, 2012.

American College of Sports Medicine (ACSM). (2014). *American College of Sports Medicine's guidelines for exercise testing and prescription* (9th ed.). Philadelphia: Lippincott Williams & Wilkins.

American Dental Association (ADA). *MouthHealthy: ADA's Award-Winning Consumer Website*. From <http://www.ada.org/en/public-programs/mouthhealthy>, retrieved June 12, 2015.

American Dental Association (ADA). (2015a). *Oral Health*. From <http://www.mouthhealthy.org/en/az-topics/o/oral-health>, retrieved June 24, 2015.

American Dental Association (ADA). (2015b). *Mouth Healthy:* Halitosis. From <http://www.mouthhealthy.org/en/az-topics/h/Halitosis>, retrieved June 24, 2015.

American Dental Association (ADA). (2015c). *Dry mouth*. Retrieved June 25, 2015. From <http://www.mouthhealthy.org/en/az-topics/d/dry-mouth>.

American Diabetes Association (ADA). (2014b). *Checking your blood glucose*. Retrieved from <http://www.diabetes.org/living-with-diabetes/treatment-and-care/blood-glucose-control/checking-your-blood-glucose.html>.

American Diabetes Association (ADA). (2014a). Clinical practice recommendations. *Diabetes Care*, 37(Suppl. 1).

American Geriatrics Society 2012 Beers Criteria Update Panel. (2012). American Geriatrics Society updated Beers Criteria for potentially inappropriate medication use in older adults. *J Am Geriatr Soc*, 60(4), 616–631.

American Psychiatric Association (APA). (2015). *Practice guidelines for the treatment of psychiatric disorders: Compendium*. Retrieved from <http://psychiatryonline.org/guidelines>.

American Psychiatric Nurses Association. (2015). *Psychiatric-mental health nurse essential competencies for assessment and management of individuals at risk for suicide*. Retrieved from <http://www.apna.org/i4a/pages/index.cfm?pageid=5684>.

Amsterdam, E. A., Wenger, N. K., Brindis, R. G., et al. (2014). AHA/ACC guideline for the management of patients with non-ST elevation acute coronary syndromes: a report of the American College of Cardiology/American Heart Association Task Force on Practice Guidelines. *Circulation*, 23(30), e344–e426.

Anderson, K., Ewen, H., Miles, E., et al. (2010). The Grief Support in Healthcare Scale: Development and testing. *Nurs Res*, 59(6), 372–379.

Andrews, M., & Boyle, J. (2003). *Transcultural concepts in nursing* (4th ed.). Philadelphia: Lippincott Williams & Wilkins.

AORN. (2015a) *Clinical Practice Position Statements*. From <http://www.aorn.org/Clinical_Practice/Position_Statements/Position_Statements.aspx>, retrieved June 25, 2015.

AORN. (2015b). *Position statement on the care of the older adult in perioperative settings*. From <http://www.aorn.org/Clinical_Practice/Position_Statements/Position_Statements.aspx>, retrieved June 25, 2015.

Assaad, S., Popescu, W., & Perrino, A. (2013). Fluid management in thoracic surgery. *Curr Opin Anesthesiol*, 26, 31–39.

Attaluri, A., et al. (2011). Randomised clinical trial: dried plums (prunes) vs psyllium for constipation. *Aliment Pharmacol Ther*, 33, 822–828.

Avery, G. (2013). *Law and ethics in nursing and healthcare an introduction*. London: Sage Publications Inc.

Aydin, A., Ahmed, K., Zaman, I., et al. (2014). Recurrent urinary tract infections in women. *Int Urogyneocol J*, 26(6), 795–804.

Azmoon, S., et al. (2011). Neurological and cardiac benefits of therapeutic hypothermia. *Cardiol Rev*, 19(3), 108–114.

Badr, H., Acitelli, L. K., & Taylor, C. L. (2008). Does talking about their relationship affect couples' marital and psychological adjustment to lung cancer? *J Cancer Surviv*, 2(1), 53–64.

Baharestani, M. (2013). *Medical device related pressure ulcers: The hidden epidemic across the life span*. Presentation on Behalf of the National Pressure Ulcer Advisory Panel.

Bainbridge, K. E., & Wallhagen, M. I. (2014). Hearing loss in an aging American population: extent, impact and management. *Annu Rev Public Health*, *35*, 139–152.

Balas, M. C., Vasilevskis, E. E., Burke, W. J., et al. (2012). Critical care nurses' role in implementing the "ABCDE Bundle" into practice. *Crit Care Nurse*, *32*(2), 35–38, 40–48.

Balemans, C. E. A., et al. (2012). Epidemiology of contrast material-induced nephropathy in the era of hydration. *Radiology*, *263*(3), 706–713.

Baranoski, S., & Ayello, E. A. (Eds.), (2012). *Wound care essentials: practice principles* (3rd ed.). Ambler, PA: Lippincott Williams & Wilkins.

Barclay, L. (2011). *Updated guidelines to prevent falls in elderly*. Medscape Education Clinical Briefs. From <http://www.medscape.com/viewarticle/735 768>, retrieved July 16, 2015.

Barr, J., Fraser, G. L., Puntillo, K., et al. (2013). Clinical practice guidelines for the management of pain, agitation, and delirium in adult patients in the intensive care unit. *Crit Care Med*, *41*(1), 263–306.

Barrand, J. *Supporting sight loss and dementia*. (2013). Retrieved October 13, 2014 From <http://www.magonlinelibrary.com/doi/abs/10.12968/nrec.2011.13.9.448>, retrieved Oct. 13, 2014.

Basch, E., Prestrud, A. A., Hesketh, P. J., et al. (2011). Antiemetics: American Society of Clinical Oncology practice guideline update. *J Clin Oncol*, [Epub ahead of print 9/26/11].

Baumgartner, C. A., Bewyer, E., & Bruner, D. (2008). Management of communication and swallowing in intensive care: the role of the speech pathologist. *AACN Adv Crit Care*, *19*(4), 433–443.

Beaumont, T., & Leadbeater, M. (2011). Treatment and care of patients with metastatic breast cancer. *Nurs Stand*, *25*(40), 49–56.

Bell, L. (2011). AACN Practice Alert-Prevention of Aspiration. *American Association of Critical Care Nurses*. Retrieved from <http://www.aacn.org/wd/practice/docs/practicealerts/prevention-aspiration-practice-alert.pdf?menu=aboutus>.

Berger, A. M., Gerber, L. H., & Mayer, D. K. (2012). Cancer-related fatigue. *Cancer*, *118*(S8), 2261–2269.

Bhowmik, A., Chahal, K., & Austin, G. (2009). Improving mucociliary clearance in chronic obstructive pulmonary disease. *Respir Med*, *103*(4), 496–502.

Bickley, L. S., & Szilagyi, P. (2012). *Bate's guide to physical examination* (11th ed.). Philadelphia: Lippincott.

Black, J. M., Cuddigan, J. E., Walko, M. A., et al. (2010). Medical device related pressure ulcers in hospitalized patients. *Int Wound J*, *7*(5), 358–365.

Black, J. M., et al. (2011). MASD part 2: incontinence-associated dermatitis and intertriginous dermatitis. *J Wound Ostomy Continence Nurs*, *38*(4), 359–370.

Bliss, D. Z., et al. (2000). Fecal incontinence in hospitalized clients who are acutely ill. *Nurs Res*, *49*(2), 101–108.

Bliss, D. Z., et al. (2011). Incontinence-associated dermatitis in critically ill adults. *J Wound Ostomy Continence Nurs*, *38*(4), 433–445.

Boelens, C., Hekman, E. E. G., & Verkerke, G. J. (2013). Risk factors for falls of older citizens. *Technol Health Care*, *21*, 521–533.

Bonds, R. S., Asawa, A., & Ghazi, A. I. (2015). Misuse of medical devices: a persistent problem in self-management of asthma and allergic disease. *Ann Allergy Asthma Immunol*, *114*(1), 74–76, e2.

Borchert, K., et al. (2010). The incontinence-associated dermatitis and its severity instrument. *J Wound Ostomy Continence Nurs*, *37*(5), 527–535.

Bosnic, G. (2014). Nutritional requirements after bariatric surgery. *Crit Care Nurs Clin N Am*, *26*, 255–262.

Bouras, E. P., Vazquez, M. I., & Aranda-Michel, J. (2013). Gastroparesis: from concepts to management. *Nutr Clin Pract*, *28*(4), 437–447.

Bravo, P. E., & Kim, F. (2014). Enhancing approaches to therapeutic hypothermia in patients with sudden circulatory arrest. *Curr Atheroscler Rep*, *16*, 451–456.

Brege, D. J. (2009). Red flags: recognizing and treating heatstroke. *Nurs Made Incred Easy*, *7*(4), 13–18.

Brienza, D. M., et al. (2012). Pressure redistribution: seating, positioning, and support surfaces. In S. Baranoski & E. A. Ayello (Eds.), *Wound care essentials: practice principles* (3rd ed.). Ambler, PA: Lippincott, Williams & Wilkins.

Buck, H. G., & Zambroski, C. H. (2012). Upstreaming palliative care for patients with heart failure. *J Cardiovasc Nurs*, *27*(2), 147–153.

Buhr, G. T., Genao, L., & White, H. I. (2011). Urinary tract infections in long-term care residents. *Clin Geriatr Med*, *27*(2), 229–239.

Burns, S. M. (2008). Pressure modes of mechanical ventilation: the good, the bad, and the ugly. *AACN Adv Crit Care*, *19*(4), 399–411.

Burns, S. M. (2011). Indices of oxygenation. In D. J. Lynn-McHale (Ed.), *AACN procedure manual for critical care* (6th ed.). Philadelphia: Saunders Elsevier.

Burns, S. M. (2011). Invasive Mechanical Ventilation (through an artificial airway): volume and pressure modes. In D. J. Lynn-McHale (Ed.), *AACN procedure manual for critical care* (6th ed.). Philadelphia: Saunders Elsevier.

Burns, S. M. (2011). Noninvasive positive pressure ventilation: continuous positive airway pressure (CPAP) and bilevel positive airway pressure (BiPAP). In D. J. Lynn-McHale (Ed.), *AACN procedure manual for critical care* (6th ed.). Philadelphia: Elsevier Saunders.

Burns, S. M. (2011). Standard weaning criteria: negative inspiratory force or pressure, positive inspiratory pressure, spontaneous tidal volume, vital capacity, and rapid shallow breathing index. In D. J. Lynn-McHale (Ed.), *AACN procedure manual for critical care* (6th ed.). Philadelphia: Elsevier Saunders.

Burns, S. M. (2011). Weaning process. In D. J. Lynn-McHale (Ed.), *AACN procedure manual for critical care* (6th ed.). Philadelphia: Elsevier Saunders.

Burns, S. M., Fisher, C., Tribble, S. S., Lewis, R., Merrel, P., Conaway, M. R., & Bleck, T. P. (2010). Multifactor clinical score and outcome of mechanical ventilation weaning trials: Burns wean assessment program. *Am J Crit Care*, *19*(5), 431–440.

Cagir, B. (2013). *Ileus: Drugs and diseases*. Medscape. Retrieved from <http://emedicine.medscape.com/article/178948-overview>.

Cattan, M. (2011). How to assist residents with sight loss in your home. *Nursing Residential Care, 13*(2), 91–93.

Centers for Disease Control and Prevention (CDC). (2007). *Healthcare Infection Control Practices Advisory Committee: guideline for isolation precautions: preventing transmission of infectious agents in healthcare settings.* From <http://www.cdc.gov/ncidad/dh9p/pdf/guidelines/isolation2007.pdf>, retrieved July 28, 2014.

Centers for Disease Control and Prevention (CDC). (2009). Application of lower sodium intake recommendations to adults—United States, 1999–2006. *MMWR Morb Mortal Wkly Rep, 58*(11), 281–283.

Centers for Disease Control and Prevention (CDC). (2009). *Healthcare Infection Control Practices Advisory Committee: guideline for prevention of catheter-associated urinary tract infections.* From <http://www.cdc.gov/hicpac/pdf/CAUTI/CAUTIguideline2009final.pdf>, retrieved Aug. 1, 2014.

Centers for Disease Control and Prevention (CDC). (2011). Guideline for hand hygiene in health-care settings. Recommendations of the Healthcare Infection Control Practices Advisory Committee and the HICPAC/SHEA/APIC/IDSA Hand Hygiene Task Force. *MMWR Recomm Rep, 51*(RR-16), 1–45. From <http://www.cdc.gov/handhygiene/Guidelines.html>, retrieved July 21, 2014.

Centers for Disease Control and Prevention (CDC). (2011). *Guideline for the prevention of intravascular catheter related infections.* From <http://www.cdc.gov/hicpac>, retrieved May 8, 2014.

Centers for Disease Control and Prevention (CDC). (2011). *Healthy weight, it is not a diet, it is a lifestyle. BMI calculator.* From <http://www.cdc.gov/healthyweight/assessing/bmi/index.html>. <http://www.cdc.gov/hepatitis/hbv/perinatalxmtn.htm>, retrieved Sept. 20, 2014.

Centers for Disease Control and Prevention (CDC). (2011). Prevention and control of influenza: recommendations of the Advisory Committee on Immuniza tion Practices (ACIP). *MMWR Recomm Rep, 60*(33), 1128–1132.

Centers for Disease Control and Prevention (CDC). (2012). Vital signs: preventing *Clostridium difficile* infections. *MMWR Morb Mortal Wkly Rep, 61*(9), 157–162.

Centers for Disease Control and Prevention (CDC). (2013). Heat stress, *2013, NIOSH workplace safety and health tips.* From <http://www.cdc.gov/niosh/topics/heatstress>, retrieved June, 2015.

Centers for Disease Control and Prevention (CDC). (2013). *Immigrant and refugee health: Screening for lead during the domestic medical examination for newly arrived refugees.* Retrieved from <http://www.cdc.gov/immigrantrefugeehealth/guidelines/lead-guidelines.htl>.

Centers for Disease Control and Prevention (CDC). (2014). *Carbon monoxide (CO) poisoning prevention.* Retrieved from <http://www.cdc.gov/features/copoisoning/>.

Centers for Disease Control and Prevention (CDC). (2014). *Ebola (Ebola Virus Disease), Interim Guidance for Monitoring and Movement of Person with Ebola Virus Disease Exposure.* From <http://www.cdc.gov/vhf/ebola/hcp/monitoring-and-movement-of-persons-with-exposure.html>, retrieved Oct. 27, 2014.

Centers for Disease Control and Prevention (CDC). (2014). *Hand hygiene basics.* From <http://www.cdc.gov/handhygiene/Basics.html>, retrieved April 23, 2015.

Centers for Disease Control and Prevention. (CDC). (2014). *Preventing seasonal flu with vaccination.* From <www.CDC.gov/flu/protect/vaccine>, retrieved Dec. 8, 2014.

Centers for Disease Control and Prevention. (2014). Unintentional drowning; get the facts. *Home and Recreational Safety.* From <http://www.cdc.gov/homeandrecreationalsafety/water-safety/waterinjuries-factsheet.html>, retrieved Oct. 15, 2014.

Centers for Disease Control and Prevention (CDC). (2014). *Vaccine information Statement (VIS) Influenza,* July 2014.

Centers for Disease Control and Prevention (CDC). (Updated April 6, 2015). *Adult immunization schedules.* Retrieved from <http://www.cdc.gov/vaccines/schedules/hcp/adult.html>.

Centers for Disease Control and Prevention (CDC). (2015a). *Hepatitis A, Q & A for health professionals.* From <http://www.cdc.gov/hepatitis/hcv/cfaq.htm>, retrieved June 25, 2015.

Centers for Disease Control and Prevention (CDC). (2015b). *Viral Hepatitis, Perinatal Transmission.* Retrieved June 25, 2015.

Centers for Disease Control and Prevention (CDC). (2014c). *International adoption and prevention of lead poisoning.* Retrieved from <http://www.cdc.gov/nceh/lead.tips/adoption.htm>.

Cerantola, C., & Happ, M. B. (2012). Transitional care for communication impaired older adults: ICU to home. *Geriatr Nurs (Minneap), 33*(6), 489–492.

Chacko, B., et al. (2015). Pressure-controlled versus volume-controlled ventilation for acute respiratory failure due to acute lung injury (ALI) or acute respiratory distress syndrome (ARDS). *Cochrane Database Syst Rev* 2015, (1), Art. No.: CD008807.

Chang, C. C., & Roberts, B. (2011). Strategies for feeding patients with dementia. *Am J Nurs, 11*(4), 36–44.

Chang, J., et al. (2011). Diabetic gastroparesis—backwards and forwards. *J Gastroenterol Hepatol, 26,* 46–57.

Change, S. J., & Huang, H. H. (2013). Diarrhea in enterally fed patients: Blame the diet? *Curr Opin Clin Nutr Metab Care, 16,* 588–594.

Choosing Wisely and the American Academy of Nursing. (2014). *Ten things nurses and patients should question.* From <http://www.choosingwisely.org/wp-content/uploads/2015/02/AANursing-Choosing-Wisely-List.pdf>, retrieved April 24, 2015.

Chulay, M., & Seckel, M. (2011). Suctioning: Endotracheal tube or tracheostomy tube. In D. J. Lynn-McHale (Ed.), *AACN procedure manual for critical care* (6th ed.). Philadelphia: Saunders Elsevier.

Clarke, K., Tong, D., Pan, Y., et al. (2013). Reduction in catheter-associated urinary tract infections by bundling interventions. *Int J Qual Health Care, 25*(1), 43–49.

Coggrave, K., Norton, C., & Cody, J. D. (2014). Management of faecal incontinence and constipation in adults with central neurological diseases. *Cochrane Database Syst Rev,* (1), CD002115.

Coggrave, M. J., & Norton, C. (2010). The need for manual evacuation and oral laxatives in the management of neurogenic bowel dysfunction after spinal cord injury: a randomized controlled trial of a stepwise protocol. *Spinal Cord*, *48*, 504–510.

Cohen, M. H., et al. (2010). *Patient handling and movement assessments: a white paper*, The Facility Guideline Institute. From <http://www.fgiguidelines.org/pdfs/FGI_PHAMA_whitepaper_042810.pdf>, retrieved July 16, 2015.

Connolly, D., O'Toole, L., Redmond, P., & Smith, S. M. (2013). Managing fatigue in patients with chronic conditions in primary care. *Fam Pract*, *30*(2), 123–124.

Cragg, J., & Krassioukov, A. (2013). Autonomic dysreflexia: Five things to know about. *CMAJ*.

Croucher, B. (2014). The challenge of diagnosing dyspnea. *AACN Adv Crit Care*, *25*(3), 284–290.

Dang, C. V., & Su, M. (2014). *Acute Mesenteric Ischemia. Medscape Diseases*. Retrieved from <http://emedicine.medscape.com/article/189146-overview#aw2aab6b2b6>.

Danzl, D. F., et al. (2011). Hypothermia and frostbite. In A. S. Fauci (Ed.), *Harrison's principles of internal medicine* (18th ed.). New York: McGraw-Hill.

Davies, E. C., et al. (2008). The use of opioids and laxatives, and incidence of constipation, in patients requiring neck-of-femur (NOF) surgery: a pilot study. *J Clin Pharm Ther*, *33*, 561–566.

De Almeida, L. M., & Braga, C. G. (2006). Construction and validation of an instrument to assess powerlessness. *Int J Nurs Terminol Classif*, *17*, 67.

de Vugt, M. E., & Verhey, F. R. (2013). The impact of early dementia diagnosis and intervention on informal caregivers. *Prog Neurobiol*, *110*(11), 54–62.

Diamond, B. J., & Bailey, M. R. (2013). Ginkgo biloba: indications, mechanisms, and safety. *Psychiatr Clin North Am*, *36*(1), 73–83.

Dienstag, J., et al. (2012). Toxic and drug-induced hepatitis. In D. L. Longo (Ed.), *Harrison's principles of internal medicine* (18th ed.). New York: McGraw-Hill.

Dinarello, C., et al. (2012). Fever and hyperthermia. In A. S. Fauci (Ed.), *Harrison's principles of internal medicine* (18th ed.). New York: McGraw-Hill.

Donaldson, J., Haddad, B., & Khan, W. S. (2014). The pathophysiology, diagnosis and current management of acute compartment syndrome. *Open Orthop*, *8*(Suppl. 1), 185–193. Published online June 27, 2014.

Downing, L. J., Caprio, T. V., & Lyness, J. M. (2013). Geriatric psychiatry review: Differential diagnosis and treatment of the 3 D's—delirium, dementia, and depression. *Curr Psychiatry Rep*, *15*(6), 365.

Drennan, V. M., Greenwood, N., & Cole, L. (2014). *Continence care for people with dementia at home*. Nurs Times, February 21.

Eilers, J., Harris, D., Henry, K., et al. (2014). Evidence-based interventions for cancer treatment-related mucositis: Putting evidence into practice. *Clin J Oncol Nurs*, *18*(6), 80–96.

Environmental Protection Agency (EPA). (2014). *Protect your family*. Retrieved from <http://www2.epa.gov/lead>.

Epstein, S. K. (2009). Weaning from ventilatory support. *Curr Opin Crit Care*, *15*(1), 36–43.

Federal Emergency Management Agency (FEMA). (2014). *Individuals with disabilities or access and functional needs.* Retrieved from <http://www.cdc.ready.gov/individuals-access-functional-needs>.

Fielding, F., & Long, C. O. (2014). The death rattle dilemma. *J of Hospice & Palliative Nursing, 16*(8). Retrieved from <http://www.medscape.com/viewarticle/834898>.

Flaherman, V. J., Gay, B., Scott, C., Avins, A., Lee, K. A., & Newman, T. B. (2012). Randomised trial comparing hand expression with breast pumping for mothers of term newborns feeding poorly. *Arch Dis Child Fetal Neonatal Ed, 97*(1), F18–F23.

Fortinsky, R. H., Baker, D., Gottschalk, M., et al. (2008). Extent of implementation of evidence-based fall prevention practices for older patients in home health care. *J Am Geriatr Soc, 56*(4), 737–743.

Fortinsky, R. H., Delaney, C., Harel, O., Pasquale, K., Schjavland, E., Lynch, J., Kleppinger, A., & Crumb, S. (2014). Results and lessons learned from a nurse practitioner-guided dementia care intervention for primary care patients and their family caregivers. *Res Gerontol Nurs, 7*(3), 126–137.

Frost, S. A., et al. (2013). Subglottic secretion drainage for preventing ventilator associated pneumonia: a meta-analysis. *Aust Crit Care, 26*(4), 180–188.

Gillibrand, W. (2012). Faecal incontinence in the elderly: Issues and interventions in the home. *Br J Community Nurs, 17*(8), 364–368.

Gillman, P. K. (2010). Neuroleptic malignant syndrome: mechanisms, interactions and causality, a review. *Move Disord, 25*(12), 1780–1790.

GOLD. Global strategy for the diagnosis, management, and prevention of COPD (revised 2015). *Global Initiative for Chronic Obstructive Lung Disease.* From <http://www.goldcopd.org/uploads/users/files/GOLD_Report_2015_Apr2.pdf>, retrieved April 23, 2015.

Goodwin, V. A., Abbott, R. A., Whear, R., et al. (2014). Multiple component interventions for preventing falls and fall related injuries among older people: Systematic review and meta-analysis. *BMC Geriatr, 14*, 15–21.

Gooneratne, N. S., & Vitiello, M. V. (2014). *Sleep in older adults: normative changes, sleep disorders, and treatment options.*

Gosselink, R., Bott, J., Johnson, M., et al. (2008). Physiotherapy for adult patients with critical illness: recommendations of the European Respiratory Society and European Society of Critical Care Medicine Task Force on Physiotherapy for Critically Ill Patients. *Intensive Care Med, 34*(7), 1188–1199.

Grabiner, M. D. (2013). Exercise-based fall prevention programmes decrease fall-related injuries. *Evid Based Nurs, 17*(4), 125.

Grap, M. (2009). Not-so-trivial pursuit: Mechanical ventilation risk reduction. *Am J Crit Care, 18*(4), 299–309.

Gray, M. (2010). Reducing catheter-associated urinary tract infection in the critical care unit. *AACN Adv Crit Care, 21*(2), 247–257.

Gray-Miceli, D. (2008). Delirium: preventing falls in acute care. In E. Capezuti, D. Zwicker, M. Mezey, et al. (Eds.), *Geriatric nursing protocols* (3rd ed.). New York: Springer.

Greenberg, S. A. (2011). *Try this: best practices in nursing care to older adults.* In: The John A. Hartford Institute for Geriatric Nursing, *Falls Efficacy Scale-International (FES-I).* From <http://consultgerirn.org/uploads/File/trythis/try_this_29.pdf>, retrieved Sep. 9, 2011.

Grossbach, I., Chlan, L., & Tracy, M. F. (2011). Overview of mechanical ventilator support and management of patient- and ventilator-related responses. *Crit Care Nurse, 31*(3), 30–45.

Grossbach, I., Stanberg, S., & Chlan, L. (2011). Promoting effective communication for patients receiving mechanical ventilation. *Crit Care Nurse, 31*(3), 46–61.

Guandalini, S., Frye, R. E., Tamer, M. A., Liacouras, C. A., Windle, M. A., Schwartz, S. M., et al. (2014). *Diarrhea*. Medscape Reference. Retrieved December, 6, 2014. Retrieved from <http://emedicine.medscape.com/article/928598-overview>.

Guenter, P. (2010). Safe practices for enteral nutrition in critically ill patients. *Crit Care Nurs Clin North Am, 22*(2), 197–208.

Guess, K. F. (2006). Posttraumatic stress disorder: early detection is key. *Nurse Pract, 31*(3), 26–35.

Guly, H. (2011). History of accidental hypothermia. *Resuscitation, 82*(2), 122–125.

Gutierrez, J., Negron, J., & Garcia-Fragoso, L. (2011). Parental practices for prevention of home poisoning in children 1-6 years of age. *J Community Health, 36*, 845–848.

Hansson, L., & Bjorkman, T. (2005). Empowerment in people with a mental illness: reliability and validity of the Swedish version of an empowerment scale. *Scand J Caring Sci, 19*, 32.

Harvard Health Letter: Keep a lookout for sodium, 37(4):1, 2012.

Hauser, S. C. (2011). Vascular diseases of the gastrointestinal tract. In R. L. Cecil, et al. (Eds.), *Goldman-Cecil medicine* (24th ed.). Philadelphia: Elsevier Saunders.

Headley, J., & Giuliano, K. (2011). Continuous venous oxygen saturation monitoring. In D. J. Lynn-McHale (Ed.), *AACN procedure manual for critical care* (6th ed.). Philadelphia: Saunders Elsevier.

Health Protection Agency. (2013). *Ayliffe Hand Washing Technique*. Retrieved from <www.hpa.org.uk/Topics/InfectiousDiseases/infectionsAZ/Handwashing>.

Healthy People 2020. *Hearing and other sensory or communication disorders*. From <www.healthypeople.gov/2020/topicsobjectives2020/overviewaspx?topicid=20>, retrieved Sept. 12, 2014.

Helm, R. E., Klausner, J. D., Klemperer, J. D., et al. (2015). Accepted but unacceptable: Peripheral IV catheter failure. *J Infusion Nurs, 38*(3), 189–201.

Herter, R., & Kazer, M. W. (2010). Best practices in urinary catheter care. *Home Healthc Nurse*, (2896), 342–349.

Hill, E., & Fauerbach, L. A. (2014). Falls and fall prevention in older adults. *Journal of Legal Nurse Consulting, 25*(2), 24–29.

Hipp, B., & Letizia, M. J. (2009). Understanding and responding to the death rattle in dying patients. *Medsurg Nurs, 18*(1), 17–21.

Hogan, N. S., Worden, J. W., & Schmidt, L. A. (2004). An empirical study of the proposed complicated grief disorder criteria. *Omega (Westport), 48*(3), 263–277.

Hooper, L., Bunn, D., Jimoh, F. O., & Fairweather-Tait, S. J. (2014). Water loss dehydration and aging. *Mech Ageing Dev, 136-137*, 50–58.

Hooten, T. M., Bradley, S. F., Cardenas, D. D., et al. (2010). Diagnosis, prevention, and treatment of catheter-associated urinary tract infection in adults: 2009 International Clinical Practice Guidelines from the Infectious Diseases Society of America. *Clin Infect Dis, 50*, 625–663.

Hopkins, P. M. (2011). Malignant hyperthermia: pharmacology of triggering. *Br J Anaesth, 107*(1), 48–56.

Hospital Quality Institute. (2015). *Eliminating VAP/VAE. HQI Toolkit.* From http://www.hqinstitute.org/hqi-toolkit/eliminating-vapvae>, retrieved April 23, 2015.

Hovstadius, B., et al. (2010). Increasing polypharmacy—an individual based study of the Swedish population 2005–2008. *BMC Clin Pharmacol, 10*(16), 1–8.

Howatson-Jones, L., Standing, M., & Roberts, S. (Eds.), (2012). *Patient assessment and care planning in nursing.* London: Sage Publications Inc.

Hunt, R. (2005). *Introduction to community-based nursing* (3rd ed.). Philadelphia: Lippincott.

Institute of Medicine. (2002). *Speaking of health.* Washington, DC: National Academies Press.

International Foundation for Functional Gastrointestinal Disorders. (March, 2014). *Nutritional strategies for managing diarrhea.* From <http://www.iffgd.org/site/gi-disorders/functional-gi-disorders/diarrhea/nutrition>, retrieved April 13, 2015.

Irwin, M., & Johnson, L. A. (2014). *Putting evidence into practice: a pocket guide to cancer symptom management.* Pittsburgh, PA: Oncology Nursing Society.

Islam, N., et al. (2013). Impact of blood glucose levels on contrast induced nephropathy after percutaneous coronary intervention in patients not known to be diabetic with acute coronary syndrome. *Cardiovascular Journal, 6*(1), 23–30.

Jepson, R., Despain, K., & Keller, D. C. (2008). Unilateral neglect: assessment in nursing practice. *J Neurosci Nurs, 40*(3), 142–149.

Joanna Briggs Institute. (2013). *Endotracheal tube (ventilated patient) care.*

Joanna Briggs Institute. (2014). *Ventilator-associated pneumonia prevention.*

Johnson, D. M., Worell, J., & Chandler, R. K. (2005). Assessing psychological health and empowerment in women: The Personal Progress Scale Revised. *Women Health, 41*(1), 109.

Jootun, D., & McGhee, G. (2011). Effective communication with people who have dementia. *Nurs Stand, 25*(25), 40–46.

Jordan, A. H., & Litz, B. T. (2014). Prolonged grief disorder: Diagnostic, assessment, and treatment considerations. *Prof Psychol Res Pr, 45*(3), 180–187.

Kahn, S., et al. (2012). *Antithrombotic therapy and prevention of thrombosis* (9th ed.). American College of Chest Physician Evidence-Based Clinical Practice Guidelines Online Only Articles. *Chest, 141*(Suppl. 2), e195S–e226S.

Kaiser, A., Orangio, G. R., Zutshi, M., et al. (2014). Current status: New technologies for the treatment of patients with fecal incontinence. *Surg Endosc, 28*, 2277–2301.

Kelleher, A. D., Moorer, A., & Makic, M. B. F. (2012). Peer to peer nursing rounds and hospital-acquired pressure ulcer prevalence in a surgical intensive care unit: A quality improvement project. *JWOCN, 3992*, 152–157.

Kenney, W. L., et al. (2014). Blood pressure regulation III: What happens when one system must serve two masters: Temperature and pressure regulation? *Eur J Appl Physiol, 114,* 467–479.

Kerr, Z. Y., Marshall, S. W., Cornstock, D., et al. (2014). Exertional heat stroke management strategies in United States high school football. *Am J Sports Med, 42*(1), 70–81.

Khaalaila, R., Zbidat, W., Anwar, K., Bayya, A., Linton, D. M., & Sviri, S. (2011). Communication difficulties and psychoemotional distress in patients receiving mechanical ventilation. *Am J Crit Care, 20*(6), 470–479.

Kim, F., Bravo, P. E., & Nichol, G. (2015). What is the use of hypothermia for neuroprotection after out-of-hospital cardiac arrest? *Stroke, 46,* 592–597.

Kiss, T. K. (2012). Critical care for frostbite. *Crit Care Nurs Clin N Am, 24,* 581–591.

Koenig, S., Teixeira, J., & Yetzer, E. (2012). Promoting mobility and function. In K. L. Mauk (Ed.), *Rehabilitation nursing, a contemporary approach to practice.* Sudbury, MA: Jones & Bartlett Learning.

Kolcaba, K. (2003). *Comfort theory and practice.* New York: Springer.

Kolcaba, K. (2013). *Comfort theory and practice: a vision for holistic health care and research.* New York: Springer Publishing Company, Inc.

Kolcaba, K., et al. (2004). Efficacy of hand massage for enhancing the comfort of hospice patients. *Int J Palliat Nurs, 6*(2), 91–102.

Kolcaba, K., & DeMarco, M. (2005). Comfort theory and application to pediatric nursing. *Pediatr Nurs, 31*(3), 187–194.

Koornstra, R. H., Peters, M., Donofrio, S., van den Borne, B., & de Jong, F. A. (2014). Management of fatigue in patients with cancer—a practical overview. *Cancer Treat Rev, 40*(6), 791–799.

Kwekkeboom, K. L., Cherwin, C. H., Lee, J. W., & Wanta, B. (2010). Mind-body treatments for the pain-fatigue-sleep disturbance symptom cluster in persons with cancer. *J Pain Symptom Manage, 39*(1), 126–138.

Langemo, D., et al. (2011). Incontinence and incontinence-associated dermatitis. *Adv Skin Wound Care, 24*(3), 126–140.

Larson, J., et al. (2005). Spouse's life situation after partner's stroke: psychometric testing of a questionnaire. *J Adv Nurs, 52,* 300.

Lawrence, V. (2011). Caring for older people with dementia and sight loss. *Nursing Residential Care, 13*(4), 186–188.

Lee, Y. (2013). Orthostatic hypertension in older people. *J Am Assoc Nurse Pract, 25,* 451–458.

Leon, L. R., & Helwig, B. G. (2010). Heat stroke: role of the systemic inflammatory response. *J Appl Physiol, 109,* 1980–1988.

Lin, Y. B., & Gardiner, M. F. (2014). Fingernail-induced corneal abrasions: case series from an ophthalmology emergency department. I. *Cornea, 33*(7), 691–695.

Lippoldt, J., & Staudinger, T. (2014). Interface pressure at different degrees of backrest elevation with various types of pressure redistribution surfaces. *Am J Crit Care, 23*(2), 119–126.

Lo, E., Nicolle, L. E., Coffin, S. E., et al. (2014). Strategies to prevent catheter-associated urinary tract infections in acute care hospitals: 2014 update. *Infect Control Hosp Epidemiol, 35*(Suppl. 2), S32–S47.

Longo, D., et al. (2011). *Harrison's principles of internal medicine* (18th ed.). New York: McGraw-Hill.

Loscalzo, J. (2013). Hypoxia and cyanosis. In J. Loscalzo (Ed.), *Harrison's pulmonary and critical care medicine* (2nd ed., pp. 21–25). New York: McGraw Hill Education Medical.

Loubani, O. M., & Green, R. S. (2015). A systematic review of extravasation and local tissue injury from administration of vasopressors through peripheral intravenous catheters and central venous catheters. *J Cri Car, 30*(3), 653–659.

Luijten, M., Machielsen, M. W., Veltman, D. J., Hester, R., de Haan, L., & Franken, I. H. (2014). Systematic review of ERP and fMRI studies investigating inhibitory control and error processing in people with substance dependence and behavioural addictions. *J Psychiatry Neurosci, 39*(3), 149–169.

Mabvuure, N. T., et al. (2012). Acute compartment syndrome of the limbs: current concepts and management. *Open Ortho J, 6*, 535–543.

Magnil, M., Gunnarsson, R., & Björkelund, C. (2011). Using patient-centred consultation when screening for depression in elderly patients: a comparative pilot study. *Scand J Prim Health Care, 29*(1), 51–56.

Makic, M. B. F., et al. (2011). Evidence-based practice habits: putting more sacred cows out to pasture. *Crit Care Nurse, 31*, 38–62.

Makic, M. B. F., Martin, S. A., Burns, S., et al. (2013). Putting evidence into nursing practice: Four traditional practices not supported by the evidence. *Crit Care Nurse, 33*(2), 28–42.

Makris, M., Van Veen, J. J., Tait, C. R., et al. (2013). Guideline on the management of bleeding in patients on antithrombotic agents. *Br J Haematol, 160*, 35–46.

Mancini, A., Prati, G., & Black, S. (2011). Self worth mediates the effects of violent loss on PTSD symptoms. *J Trauma Stress, 24*, 116–120. Epub 2011 Jan 6].

Martin, B. (2010). AACN Practice Alert—Oral care for patients at risk for ventilator-associated pneumonia. *American Association of Critical Care Nurses.* From <http://www.aacn.org/wd/practice/docs/practicealerts/oral-care-patients-at-risk-vap.pdf?menu=aboutus>, retrieved April 15, 2015.

Martin-Plank, L. (2014). Chest disorders. In L. Kennedy-Malone, K. R. Fletcher, & L. Martin-Plank (Eds.), *Advanced practice nursing in the care of older adults.* Philadelphia: F.A. Davis Company.

Marzuillo, P., del Guidice, E. M., & Santoro, N. (2014). Pediatric fatty liver disease: Role of ethnicity and genetics. *World J Gastroenterol, 20*(23), 7347–7355.

Mas, A., & Masip, J. (2014). Noninvasive ventilation in acute respiratory failure. *Int J COPD, 9*, 837–852.

Matthews, E. (2011). *Nursing care planning.* London: Lippincott Williams & Wilkins.

Matthews, E. (2011). Sleep disturbances and fatigue in critically ill patients. *AACN Adv Crit Care, 22*(3), 204–224.

Mayo Clinic Health Letter: Risks of vitamin supplements, March 4, 2012.

McCarter-Bayer, A., Bayer, F., & Hall, K. (2005). Preventing falls in acute care: an innovative approach. *J Gerontol Nurs, 31*(3), 25.

McGowan, D. (2014). Peripheral intravenous cannulation: What is considered best practice? *Br J Nurs, 23*(14), S26–S28.

Meade, M. O., Cook, D. J., Guyatt, G. H., et al. (2008). Ventilation strategy using low tidal volumes, recruitment maneuvers, and high positive end-expiratory pressure for acute lung injury and acute respiratory distress syndrome: A randomized controlled trial. *JAMA, 299*(6), 637–645.

Meiner, S. E. (2010). *Gerontologic nursing.* St Louis: Mosby/Elsevier.

Melancon, M. O., Lorrain, D., & Dionne, I. J. (2014). Exercise and sleep in aging: Emphasis on serotonin. *Pathol Biol, 62*, 276–283.

Memorial Sloan Kettering Cancer Center. (2015). *Caring for your urinary catheter.* From <https://www.mskcc.org/cancer-care/patient-education/caring-your -urinary-foley-catheter>, retrieved June 26, 2015.

Merriman, J. D., Von Ah, D., Miaskowski, C., & Aouizerat, B. E. (2013). Proposed mechanisms for cancer- and treatment-related cognitive changes. *Semin Oncol Nurs, 29*(4), 260–269.

Morse, J. M., Tylko, S. J., & Dixon, H. A. (1987). Characteristics of the fall-prone patient. *Gerontologist, 27*(4), 516–522.

Naeim, A., Aapro, M., Subbarao, R., & Balducci, L. (2014). Supportive care considerations for older adults with cancer. *J Clin Oncol, 32*(24), 2627–2634.

Narayanasomy, A., et al. (2004). Responses to the spiritual needs of older people. *J Adv Nurs, 48*(1), 6–16.

National Cancer Institute. *Posttraumatic stress disorder*, 2013. From <http:// www.cancer.gov/cancertopics/pdq/supportivecare/post-traumatic-stress/ Patient/page4>, retrieved Oct. 23, 2014.

National Comprehensive Cancer Network. (2014). *NCCN clinical practice guidelines in oncology cancer–related fatigue version I.2014.* Retrieved from <http://www.nccn.org/professionals/physician_gls/pdf/fatigue.pdf>.

National Interagency Fire Center. (2014). *CISM Information Sheets.* From <http:// gacc.nifc.gov/wgbc/cism/effectsoftrauma.pdf>, retrieved Oct. 23, 2014.

National Kidney Foundation. (2013a). *Contrast dyes and the kidney.* Retrieved from <http://www.kidney.org/atoz/content/Contrast-Dye-and-Kidneys.cfm>.

National Kidney Foundation. (2013b). *Smoking and your kidneys.* Retrieved from <http://www.kidney.org/news/ekidney/May12/Smoking.cfm>.

National Pressure Ulcer Advisory Panel. (2011). Pressure ulcers: Avoidable or unavoidable? Results of the National Pressure Ulcer Advisory Panel Consensus Conference. *Ostomy Wound Mgmt, 57*(2), 24–37.

National Pressure Ulcer Advisory Panel (NPUAP) and European Pressure Ulcer Advisory Panel (EPUAP). (2014). E. Haesler (Ed.), *Prevention and treatment of pressure ulcers.* Perth, Australia: Cambridge Media.

Neifert, M., & Bunik, M. (2013). Overcoming clinical barriers to exclusive breastfeeding. *Pediatr Clin N Am, 60*(1), 115–145.

Nelson, A., et al. (2008). Myths and facts about safe patient handling in rehabilitation. *Rehabil Nurs, 33*(1), 10–17.

Neumer, R. W., et al. (2011). Implementation strategies for improving survival after out-of-hospital cardiac arrest in the United States. *Circulation, 123*, 2898–2911.

Newman, D., & Willson, M. (2011). Review of intermittent catheterization and current best practices. *Urol Nurs, 31*(1), 12–48.

Nielsen, S., et al. (2011). Adequacy of milk intake during exclusive breastfeeding: a longitudinal study. *Pediatrics, 128*(4), 907–914.

Norrby, S. R. (2011). Approach to the patient with urinary tract infection. In L. Goldman & A. Schafer (Eds.), *Goldman-Cecil Medicine* (24th ed.). St Louis: Saunders/Elsevier.

Nurko, S., & Scott, S. M. (2011). Coexistence of constipation and incontinence in children and adults. *Best Pract Res Clin Gastroenterol, 25*(1), 29–41.

Nutescu, E. A., Wittkowsky, A. K., Burnett, A., Merli, G. J., Ansell, J. E., & Garcia, D. A. (2013). Delivery of optimized inpatient anticoagulation therapy: Consensus statement from the Anticoagulation Forum. *Ann Pharmacother, 47*(5), 714–724.

Nutrition Action HealthLetter. *Eat smart: which foods are good for what*, December, 2011.

Odom-Forren, J., Hooper, V., Moser, D. K., et al. (2014). Postdischarge nausea and vomiting: Management strategies and outcomes over 7 days. *J Perianesth Nurs, 29*(4), 275–284.

Oerther, S. E. (2011). Plant poisonings: common plants that contain cardiac glycosides. *J Emerg Nurs, 37*(1), 102–103.

O'Grady, N. P., et al. (2011). *Guidelines for the prevention of intravascular catheter-related infections*. From <http://www.cdc.gov/hicpac/pdf/guidelines/bsi-guidelines-2011.pdf>, retrieved June 19, 2015.

Ortega, A., Sanchez-Manzanares, M., Gil, F., & Rico, R. (2013). Enhancing team learning in nursing teams through beliefs about interpersonal contexts. *J Adv Nurs, 69*(1), 102–111.

O'Shea, R. S., et al. (2010). Alcoholic liver disease. *Hepatology, 51*(1), 307–327.

Paden, M. S., Franjic, L., & Halcomb, E. (2013). Hyperthermia caused by drug interactions and adverse reaction. *Emerg Med Clin N Am, 31*, 1035–1044.

Pan American Health Organization. (2012). *Mental health and psychosocial support in disaster situations in the Caribbean*. Washington, DC: PAHO.

Parshall, M. B., Schwartzstein, R. M., Adams, L., et al. (2012). An official American Thoracic Society statement: Update on the mechanisms, assessment, and management of dyspnea. *Am J Respir Crit Care Med, 185*(4), 435–452.

Pasero, C., & McCaffrey, M. (2004). Comfort-function goals. *Am J Nurs, 104*(9), 77–81.

Pattison, N., & Watson, J. (2009). Ventilatory weaning: a case study of protracted weaning. *Nurs Crit Care, 14*(2), 75–85.

Paulus, R. A., Davis, K., & Steele, G. D. (2008). Continuous innovation in health care: implication of the Geisinger experience. *Health Aff, 27*(5), 1235–1245.

Pender, N. J., Murdaugh, C. L., & Parsons, M. A. (2015). *Health promotion in nursing practice* (7th ed.). Upper Saddle River, NJ: Prentice Hall.

Perme, C., & Chandrashekar, R. (2009). Early mobility and walking program for patients in intensive care units: creating a standard of care. *Am J Crit Care, 18*(3), 212–220.

Petrone, P. (2014). Management of accidental hypothermia and cold injury. *Curr Probl Surg, 51*(10), 417–431.

Peyrani, P. (2014). Pneumonia, In *APIC test of Infection Control and Epidemiology* (4th ed.). Washington, DC, Association for Professionals in Infection Control and Epidemiology, last revised 6/6/14, Accessed 01.08.14.

Phillips, L. D. (2014). *Manual of IV therapeutics: evidence-based practice for infusion therapy* (6th ed.). Philadelphia: FA Davis.

Pinto, S., Schub, T., & Pravikoff, D. (2013). *Hydration: Maintaining oral hydration in older adults*. Cinahl Information Systems, Evidence-based care sheet.

Pitoni, S., Sinclair, H. L., & Andrews, P. J. D. (2011). Aspects of thermoregulation physiology. *Curr Opin Crit Care, 17*(2), 115–121.

Pollock, A., et al. (2011). Interventions for visual field defects in patients with stroke. *Cochrane Database Syst Rev*, (10), CD008388.

Pryor, R. R., Casa, D. J., Holschen, J. C., et al. (2013). Exertional heat stroke: Strategies for prevention and treatment from the sports field to the emergency department. *Clin Ped Emerg Med, 14*(4), 267–278.

Pye, J. (2011). Travel-related health and safety considerations for children. *Nurs Stand, 25*(39), 50–56.

Quinlan, N., Marcantonio, E. R., Inouye, S. K., et al. (2011). Vulnerability: The crossroads of frailty and delirium. *J Am Geriatr Soc, 59*(Suppl. 2), S262–S268.

Radvansky, L. J., Pace, M. B., & Siddiqui, A. (2013). Prevention and management of radiation-induced dermatitis, mucositis, and xerostomia. *Am J Health Syst Pharm, 70*, 1025–1032.

Raholm, M.-B. (2012). The ethics of presence when bathing patients in a nursing home. *International Journal For Human Caring, 16*(4), 30–35.

Rees, H. C. (2013). Care of patients requiring oxygen therapy or tracheostomy. In D. Ignatavicius & M. L. Workman (Eds.), *Medical-surgical nursing: patient-centered collaborative care* (7th ed., pp. 562–580). St. Louis, MO: W.B. Saunders Company.

Rehman, T., & deBoisblanc, B. P. (2013). Persistent fever in the ICU. *Chest, 145*(1), 158–165.

Remke, S., & Chrastek, J. (2007). Improving care in the home for children with palliative care needs. *Home Healthc Nurse, 25*(1), 45–51.

Requejo, P. S., Furumasu, J., & Mulroy, S. J. (2015). Evidence-based strategies for preserving mobility for elders and aging manual wheelchair users. *Top Geriatr Rehab, 31*(1), 26–41.

Resnick, B. (2009). Promoting exercise for older adults. *J Am Acad Nurse Pract, 21*(2), 77–78.

Resnick, B., et al. (2008). A proposal for a new screening paradigm and toll called Exercise Assessment and Screening for You (EASY). *J Aging Phys Act, 16*(2), 215–233.

Resnick, B., et al. (2009). Nursing home resident outcomes from the Res-Care Intervention. *J Am Geriatr Soc, 57*(7), 1156–1165.

Resnick, B., et al. (2010). Perceptions and performance of function and physical activity in assisted living communities. *J Am Med Dir Assoc, 11*(6), 406–414.

Resnick, B., et al. (2011). Testing the effect of function-focused card in assisted living. *J Am Geriatr Soc, 59*, 2233–2240.

Resnick, B., & D'Adamo, C. (2011). Factors associated with exercise among older adults in a continuing care retirement community. *Rehabil Nurs, 36*(2), 47–53.

Resnick, B., & Galik, E. (2013). Using Function-Focused Care to increase physical activity among older adults. *Annu Rev Nurs Res*, *31*, 175–208.

Resnick, B., Hammersla, M., Michael, K., et al. (2014). Changing behavior in senior housing residents: Testing of phase I of the PRAISEDD-2 intervention. *Appl Nurs Res*, *27*(3), 162–169.

Resnick, B., & Jenkins, L. S. (2000). Testing the reliability and validity of the self-efficacy for exercise scale. *Nurs Res*, *49*(3), 154–159.

Resnick, B., Zimmerman, S., & Orwig, D. (2001). Model testing for reliability and validity of the outcome expectations for exercise scale. *Nurs Res*, *50*, 5.

Rhoads, J., & Murphy-Jensen, M. (2014). *Differential diagnoses for the advanced practice nurse*. New York: Springer Publishing Company.

Rich, M. W., & Nienaber, W. J. (2014). Polypharmacy and adverse drug reactions in the aging population with heart failure. In B. I. Jugdutt (Ed.), *Aging and heart failure* (pp. 107–116). New York: Springer.

Rodgers, G. B., Franklin, R. L., & Midgett, J. D. (2012). Unintentional paediatric ingestion poisonings and the role of imitative behavior. *Inj Prev*, *18*(2), 103–108.

Rodhe, N., et al. (2008). Bacteriuria is associated with urge urinary incontinence in older women. *Scand J Prim Health Care*, *26*(1), 35–39.

Rosenberg, M., Wood, L., Leeds, M., & Wicks, S. (2011). "But they can't reach that high …": Parental perceptions and knowledge relating to childhood poisoning. *Health Promot J Austr*, *22*(3), 217–222.

Rubin, F. H., Neal, K., Fenlon, K., et al. (2011). Sustainability and scalability of the hospital elder life program at a community hospital. *J Am Geriatr Soc*, *59*(2), 359–365.

Sadaka, F., & Veremakis, C. (2012). Therapeutic hypothermia for the management of intracranial hypertension in severe traumatic brain injury: A systematic review. *Brain Inj*, *26*(7-8), 899–908.

Sadler, C. (2011). When the heat is on. *Nurs Standard*, *25*(40), 18–20.

Safekids.org. (2014). *Medication safety policy brief, by the numbers*. Retrieved from <http://www.safekids.org/search?search_api_views_fulltext=poisoning+statistics&=Apply>.

Saint, S., Greene, T., Kowalski, C. P., et al. (2013). Preventing catheter-associated urinary tract infection in the United States. *JAMA Intern Med*, *173*(10), 874–879.

Saliakellis, E., & Fotoulaki, M. (2013). Gastroparesis in children. *Ann Gastroenterol*, *26*(3), 204–2011.

Sande, R., Noothroon, E., Wiersdma, A., Hellendoorn, E., Staak, C., Mulder, C., et al. (2013). Association between short-term structured risk assessment outcomes and seclusion. *Int J Ment Health Nurs*, *22*(6), 475–484.

Schallom, M., Dykeman, B., Kirby, J., & Pierce, J. (2015). Head-of-bed elevation and early outcomes of gastric reflux, aspiration, and pressure ulcers: A feasibility study. *Am J Crit Care*, *24*(1), 57–66.

Schnur, J., & John, R. M. (2014). Childhood lead poisoning and the new Centers for Disease Control and Prevention guidelines for lead exposure. *J Am Assoc Nurse Pract*, *26*(5), 238–247.

Schub, E., Schub, T., & Pravikoff, D. (2010b). Stomatitis (oral mucositis) therapy. *Nursing Reference Center: CINAHL Nursing Guide*, Oct. 29.

Schub, T., Grose, S., & Pravikoff, D. (2010a). Xerostomia. *Nursing Reference Center: CINAHL Nursing Guide*, Sept. 3.

Scirica, B. M. (2013). Therapeutic hypothermia after cardiac arrest. *Circulation*, *127*, 244–250.

Scott, R. A., Oman, K. S., Makic, M. B. F., et al. (2014). Reducing indwelling urinary catheter use in the emergency department: A successful quality-improvement initiative. *J Emerg Nurs*, *40*(3), 237–240.

Scrase, W., & Tranter, S. (2011). Improving evidence-based care for patients with pyrexia. *Nurs Stand*, *25*(29), 37–41.

Segal, K. L., Fleischut, P. M., Kim, C., et al. (2014). Evaluation and treatment of perioperative corneal abrasions. *J Ophthalmol*, 320–326.

Seifert, P. C., Wahr, J. A., Pace, M., et al. (2014). Crisis management of malignant hyperthermia in the OR. *AORN*, *100*(2), 189–202.

Seymour, C., Cross, B., & Cooke, C. (2009). Physiologic impact of closed-system endotracheal suctioning in spontaneously breathing patients receiving mechanical ventilation. *Respir Care*, *54*(3), 367–374.

Shah, R., & Lotke, M. (2013). *Hearing impairment*. Medscape. Retrieved from <http://emedicine.medscape.com/article/994159-overview#a0199>.

Shiraishi, H., et al. (2008). Long-term effects of prism adaptation on chronic neglect after stroke. *Neurorehabilitation*, *23*(2), 137–151.

Shukla, P., & Rishi, P. (2014). A correlational study of psychosocial & spiritual well being and death anxiety among advanced stage cancer patients. *American Journal of Applied Psychology*, *2*(3), 59–65.

Siela, D. (2010). Evaluation standards for management of artificial airways. *Crit Care Nurse*, *30*(4), 76–78.

Simons, S. R., & Abdallah, L. M. (2012). Bedside assessment of enteral tube placement aligning practice with evidence. *Am J Nurs*, *112*(2), 40–48.

Siniscalchi, A., Gallelli, L., Russo, E., & De Sarro, G. (2013). A review on antiepileptic drugs-dependent fatigue: Pathophysiological mechanisms and incidence. *Eur J Pharmacol*, *718*(1), 10–16.

Skillings, K., & Curtis, B. (2011). Tracheal tube cuff care. In D. J. Lynn-McHale (Ed.), *AACN procedure manual for critical care* (6th ed.). Philadelphia: Elsevier Saunders.

Society for Health Care Epidemiology of America (SHEA). (2014). *Expert CLABSI guidance adds real world implementation strategies*. From <http://www.shea-online.org/View/ArticleId/286/Expert-CLABSI-Guidance-Adds-Real-World-Implementation-Strategies.aspx>, retrieved June 19, 2015.

Sofka, K. (2011). *Technology Corner: It's All Downhill- Ramps*, Part 1, JNLCP XI.3:438 ff and Part 2, JNLCP XI.4: 476 ff.

Son, J. T., & Lee, E. (2012). Postprandial hypotension among older residents of a nursing home in Korea. *J Clin Nurs*, *21*(23-24), 3565–3573.

Soreide, K. (2014). Clinical and translational aspects of hypothermia in major trauma patients: from pathophysiology to prevention, prognosis and potential preservation. *Injury*, *45*(4), 647–654.

Spiller, H. A., Beuhler, M. C., Ryan, M. L., et al. (2013). Evaluation of changes in poisoning in young children 2000-2010. *Pediatr Emerg Care*, *29*(5), 635–640.

Spinzi, G., et al. (2009). Constipation in the elderly. *Drugs Aging*, *26*(6), 469–474.

Sprigle, S., & Sonenblum, S. (2011). Assessing evidence supporting redistribution of pressure for pressure ulcer prevention: A review. *J Rehabil Res Dev*, *48*(3), 203–214.

Stacy, K. M. (2013). Pulmonary therapeutic management. (2013). In L. D. Urden, K. M. Stacy, & M. E. Lough (Eds.), *Critical care nursing: diagnosis and management* (7th ed.). St. Louis: Elsevier.

Stanhope, M., & Lancaster, J. (2006). *Foundation of nursing in the community* (2nd ed.). St. Louis: Mosby.

Steggall, M., Treacy, C., & Jones, M. (2013). Post-operative urinary retention. *Nurs Stand Oct*, *28*(5), 43–48.

Steinke, E. E. (2013). Sexuality and chronic illness. *J Gerontol Nurs*, *39*(11), 18–27.

Steinke, E. E., & Jaarsma, T. (2014). Sexual counseling and cardiovascular disease: practical approaches. *Asian J Androl*, *16*, 1–8.

Steinke, E. E., Jaarsma, T., Barnason, S. A., et al. (2013a). Sexual counseling for individuals with cardiovascular disease and their partners: a consensus document from the American Heart Association and the ESC Council on Cardiovascular Nursing and Allied Health Professionals (CCNAP). *Circulation*, *128*, 2075–2076.

Steinke, E. E., Mosack, V., Barnason, S., & Wright, D. W. (2011). Progress in sexual counseling by cardiac nurses, 1994 to 2009. *Heart Lung*, *40*(3), e15–e24.

Steinke, E. E., Mosack, V. M., & Hill, T. J. (2013). Sexual self-perception and adjustment in cardiac patients: a psychometric analysis. *Journal of Research in Nursing*, *18*(3), 191–201.

Stevens, R. D., et al. (2009). A framework for diagnosing and classifying intensive care unit-acquired weakness. *Crit Care Med*, *37*(10), S299–S308.

Stewart, M. W. (2014). Anesthetic drugs and malignant hyperthermia. *JoPAN*, *29*(3), 253–255.

Suzumura, E. A., Figueiro, M., Normilio-Silva, K., et al. (2014). Effects of alveolar recruitment maneuvers on clinical outcomes in patients with acute respiratory distress syndrome: A systematic review and meta-analysis. *Intensive Care Med*, *40*, 1227–1240.

Swann, J. I. (2013). Dementia and reminiscence: not just a focus on the past. *Nursing & Residential Care*, *15*(12), 790–795.

Sykes, N. P. (2006). The pathogenesis of constipation. *J Support Oncol*, *4*(5), 213–218.

Tack, J., Muller-Lissner, S., Stanghellini, V., et al. (2011). Diagnosis and treatment of chronic constipation—a European perspective. *Neurogastroenterol Motil*, *23*(8), 697–710.

Tanner, D. (2013). CNA observations could save a resident: an interview. *Nursing Assistant*, Cengage Learning, *18*(8).

Tanner, D. C., & Culbertson, W. R. (2014). Avoiding negative dysphagia outcomes. *OJIN: The Online Journal of Issues in Nursing*, *19*(2).

Taylor, C. R., et al. (2011). Safety, security and emergency preparedness. In C. R. Taylor, et al. (Eds.), *Fundamentals of nursing, the art and science of nursing care* (7th ed.). Philadelphia: Lippincott Williams & Wilkins.

The Joint Commission. (2009). *National patient safety goals*. From <www.jointcommission.org/NR/rdonlyres/DB3D6A66-DA79-412B-97E5-6FC400663127/0/OME_NPSG_Outline.pdf2009>, retrieved March 31, 2009.

The Joint Commission on Accreditation of Healthcare Organizations. (2010). *Accreditation program: home care.* 2010 national patient safety goals. Goal 9. Reduce the risk of patient harm resulting from falls, 2009. From <www.jointcommission.org/NR/rdonlyres/E07E8A63–5867–4090 –A5AC-210D9565BCDB/0/RevisedChapter_OME_NPSG_20090924 .pdf>, retrieved Aug. 10, 2009.

Tinetti, M. E. (2003). Preventing falls in elderly persons. *N Engl J Med, 348*(1), 42–49.

Tracy, M. F., & Chlan, L. (2011). Nonpharmacological interventions to manage common symptoms in patients receiving mechanical ventilation. *Crit Care Nurse, 31*(3), 19–29.

Trollor, J. N., Chen, X., & Sachdev, P. S. (2009). Neuroleptic malignant syndrome associated with atypical antipsychotic drugs. *CNS Drugs, 23*(6), 477–492.

Turk, E. E. (2010). Hypothermia. *Forensic Sci Med Pathol, 6*, 106–115.

Tutor, J. D., & Gosa, M. M. (2012). Dysphagia and aspiration in children. *Pediatr Pulmonol, 47*(4), 321–337.

U.S. Department of Agriculture. (2014). *Weight Management, USDA Choose-MyPlate.gov. retrieved from WWW 6/21/15.*

U.S. Department of Health and Human Services. (2008). *Physical activity guidelines for Americans, 2008.* Washington, DC: Author.

U.S. Department of Health and Human Services. (2012). *Physical Activity Guidelines for Americans Midcourse Report Subcommittee of the President's Council on Fitness, Sports & Nutrition.* Strategies to Increase Physical Activity Among Youth. Washington, DC: U.S. Department of Health and Human Services.

U.S. Food and Drug Administration. (2014). *Consumer updates: Have a baby or young child with a cold? Most don't need medicines.* Retrieved from <http://www.fda.gov/ForConsumers/ConsumerUpdates/ucm422465.htm>.

Veenema, T. G. (2013). *Disaster nursing and emergency preparedness for chemical, biological and radiological terrorism and other hazards* (3rd ed.). New York: Springer.

Vollman, K., & Powers, J. (2011). Pronation therapy. In D. J. Lynn-McHale (Ed.), *AACN procedure manual for critical care* (6th ed.). Philadelphia: Saunders Elsevier.

Vollman, K., & Sole, M. (2011). Endotracheal tube and oral care. In D. J. Lynn-McHale (Ed.), *AACN procedure manual for critical care* (6th ed.). Philadelphia: Saunders Elsevier.

Vrtis, M. C. (2013). The economic impact of complex wound care on home health agencies. JWOCN, *40*(4), 360–363.

Wachholtz, A., & Pargament, K. (2008). Migraines and meditation: does spirituality matter? *J Behav Med, 31*(4), 351–366.

Wagner, K. D., & Hardin-Pierce, M. G. (2014). *High acuity nursing* (6th ed.). Boston, MA: Prentice Hall, Inc.

Watts, R., Adams, J., Yearwood, M., et al. (2011). Strategies to promote intermittent self-cauterization in adults with neurogenic bladders. JoAnna Briggs Institute. *Best Practice, 15*(7), 1–4.

Weitz, J. (2011). *Pulmonary embolism.* St. Louis: Saunders.

Weitzel, T., Robinson, S., Barnes, M. R., et al. (2011). The special needs of the hospitalized patient with dementia. *Medsurg Nurs, 20*(1), 13–18.

White, C. (2011). *Atherosclerotic peripheral arterial disease.* St. Louis: Saunders.

White, J., Guenter, P., & Gordon, J. (2012). Consensus statement of the Academy of Nutrition and Dietetics/American Society for Parenteral and Enteral Nutrition: characteristics recommended for the identification and documentation of adult malnutrition. *J Acad Nutr Diet, 112*, 730–738.

Whitehead, W. E., et al.. (2009) Conservative and behavioral management of constipation. *Neurogastroenterol Motil, 21*(Suppl. 2), 55–61.

Willson, M. M., Angyus, M., Beals, D., et al. (2014). Executive summary: A quick reference guide for managing fecal incontinence. *JWOCN, 41*(1), 61–69.

Wilson, B. (2011). Contrast media-induced compartment syndrome. *Radiol Technol, 83*(1), 63–77.

Wound, Ostomy, and Continence Nurses Society (WOCN). (2010). *Guideline for prevention and management of pressure ulcers. WOCN clinical practice guideline series no. 2.* WOCN: Mount Laurel, NJ.

Xue, Y. (2014). *Peripheral intravenous line: Insertion.* JoAnn Briggs Institute EBP Database. JB11841.

Yancy, C. W., Jessup, M., Bozkurt, B., et al. (2013). ACCF/AHA guideline for the management of heart failure: a report of the American College of Cardiology Foundation/American Heart Association Task Force on Practice Guidelines. *Circulation, 128*, e240–e327.

Yardley, L., Beyer, N., Hauer, K., et al. (2005). Development and initial validation of the Falls Efficacy Scale-International (FES-I). *Age Ageing, 34*(6), 614–619.

Yeom, H. A., Keller, C., & Fleury, J. (2009). Interventions for promoting mobility in community-dwelling older adults. *J Am Acad Nurse Pract, 21*(2), 95–100.

Zamor, P. J., & Russo, M. W. (2011). Liver function tests and statins. *Curr Opin Cardiol, 26*(4), 338–341.

INDEX